D1155861

Atlas of

Pediatric Orthopaedic Surgery

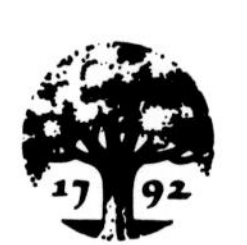

J. B. Lippincott Company
Philadelphia

Atlas of
Pediatric Orthopaedic Surgery

Raymond T. Morrissy, M.D.

Medical Director and Chief of Orthopaedics
Scottish Rite Children's Medical Center
Clinical Professor of Orthopaedics
Emory University School of Medicine
Atlanta, Georgia

Illustrated by Bernie Kida

Developmental Editor: Delois Patterson
Project Editor: Dina Kamilatos
Indexer: Helene Taylor
Design Coordinator: Doug Smock
Interior Designer: Arlene Putterman
Cover Designer: Arlene Putterman
Production Manager: Caren Erlichman
Production Coordinator: Kevin Johnson
Compositor: Bi-Comp, Incorporated
Printer/Binder: Arcata Graphics/Halliday

Printed in the United States of America. For information write J. B. Lippincott Company, 227 East Washington Square, Philadelphia, Pennsylvania 19106.

6 5 4 3 2 1

Library of Congress Cataloging-in-Publication Data

Morrissy, Raymond T.
Atlas of pediatric orthopaedic surgery / Raymond T. Morrissy ; illustrated by Bernie Kida.
p. cm.
Includes bibliographical references and index.
ISBN 0-397-50969-3
1. Pediatric orthopedics—Atlases. I. Title.
[DNLM: 1. Orthopedics—in infancy & childhood—atlases. WS 17 M883a]
RD732.3.C48M67 1992
617.3—dc20
DNLM/DLC
for Library of Congress 91-45983
CIP

The author and publisher have exerted every effort to ensure that drug selection and dosage set forth in this text are in accord with current recommendations and practice at the time of publication. However, in view of ongoing research, changes in government regulations, and the constant flow of information relating to drug therapy and drug reactions, the reader is urged to check the package insert for each drug for any change in indications and dosage and for added warnings and precautions. This is particularly important when the recommended agent is a new or infrequently employed drug.

To three role models who have had a significant and lasting effect on my career as an orthopaedic physician and surgeon:

Philip O. Lichtblau, M.D.

whose example, kindness, and interest led me, as a high school senior, into a career of medicine and orthopaedics;

William H. Harris, M.D.

whose tireless pursuit of important questions for better patient care indelibly stamped my approach to patient care when I was a research fellow; and

John E. Hall, M.D.

whose intellectual honesty, mastery of surgery, and practice of the art of medicine was a shining example to me as an orthopaedic resident, and has remained a beacon to me as an orthopaedic surgeon.

Preface

The *Atlas of Pediatric Orthopaedic Surgery* was conceived with the notion that learning surgery is primarily visual and that narrative descriptions of a surgical procedure are complementary to the visual input. Thus, the illustrations attempt to give a level of detail that will require little labeling and a sense of realism that will simulate the actual operative field. To this end, the vast majority of the procedures illustrated in this atlas were first drawn in the operating room during the actual procedure.

The purpose of *Lovell and Winter's Pediatric Orthopaedics* was not to deal with surgical procedures; the purpose of this atlas is not to discuss the indications for the various procedures but rather their technical performance. The tremendous responsibility that surgeons take with them into the operating room requires knowledge of both. As residents and fellows in training we learn many new procedures. As surgeons in a rapidly advancing field we are faced with the necessity of performing surgical procedures that we were not taught in our residency or fellowship training. Searching the literature usually yields only a terse description and a few sketchy line drawings that do not always accurately and unambiguously convey all of the details that the surgeon would like to have.

It is hoped that this atlas will help the resident, fellow, and practicing orthopaedic surgeon to better understand the technical aspects of some of the surgical procedures required in the orthopaedic care of infants, children, and adolescents.

Raymond T. Morrissy, M.D.

Acknowledgments

The contents of *Atlas of Pediatric Orthopaedic Surgery* are not uniquely mine as I did not invent surgery and have not been an originator of new tools, prostheses, and procedures. I first learned to operate during my residency and the credit for that must go to those who took the time and interest to teach me. However, I have learned much more since then, and for that the credit must go to my colleagues in orthopaedics, including many of the residents and fellows with whom I have been associated over the years.

The unique aspect of this atlas, the detailed illustrations, are the work of a very talented illustrator, Mr Bernie Kida. Without him this atlas would have been something very different—I suspect something less. In addition, his patience and perseverance in working with me for two years on the details of each of the drawings is another of his talents that has contributed significantly to this atlas.

In view of the cost of artwork today, there is a question as to whether or not an atlas such as this is economically feasible. To that end I would like to thank J. B. Lippincott for their support in undertaking this project. I offer a special thanks to Darlene Cooke for both her encouragement and badgering. Both were necessary to get me through a project that became much more than I had expected.

Finally I would like to express my gratitude to those colleagues who lent me direct support in reviewing and commenting on the art work and text of a particular procedure. Special thanks go to Deborah Bell, Charles Price, and Gary Lourie for their time and effort, as well as Louis G. Bayne, M.D., Atlanta, Georgia; Deborah F. Bell, M.D., FRCSC, Toronto, Canada; H. M. Bell, M.D., FRCSC, Vancouver, Canada; Michael T. Busch, M.D., Atlanta, Georgia; Norris C. Carroll, M.D., FRCSC, Chicago, Illinois; Sherman S. Coleman, M.D., Salt Lake City, Utah; John E. Hall, M.D., FRCSC, Boston, Massachusetts; J. Anthony Herring, M.D., Dallas, Texas; Douglas K. Kehl, M.D., Atlanta, Georgia; Gary M. Lourie, M.D., Atlanta, Georgia; Richard E. McCarthy, M.D., Little Rock, Arkansas; Scott J. Mubarak, M.D., San Diego, California; Charles T. Price, M.D., Orlando, Florida; George T. Rab, M.D., Sacramento, California; Lynn T. Staheli, M.D., Seattle, Washington; Dennis S. Weiner, M.D., Akron, Ohio; Stuart L. Weinstein, M.D., Iowa City, Iowa; Robert A. Winquist, M.D., Seattle, Washington; and Robert B. Winter, M.D., Minneapolis, Minnesota.

Contents

Atlas of

Pediatric Orthopaedic Surgery

CHAPTER ONE
THE SPINE

1.1
Posterior Spinal Arthrodesis With Harrington Rod Instrumentation for Scoliosis

The Harrington rod was the first successful instrumentation for correction of scoliosis deformity. Although its use is giving way to newer methods of instrumentation, it still remains in use today. It has the longest follow-up of any technique and therefore is the standard of comparison for new techniques.

The main advantage of the Harrington instrumentation is the simplicity of its use: the insertion of two hooks and a rod. In light of newer methods of instrumentation, its disadvantages have become more apparent. The pure distraction force does nothing to affect rotation or sagittal contour directly. Various adaptations have been used to overcome these two deficiencies. First, the use of a square end that fits into a square hole in the distal hook and second, the addition of sublaminar wires. These adaptations allow the rod to be contoured and at the same time not to rotate into the scoliosis. The degree of correction in the sagittal plane, however, does not match what can be achieved with newer methods (*eg*, the Cotrel-Dubousset instrumentation). In addition, the fixation is precarious enough to require postoperative immobilization.

The technique of Harrington rod placement is useful in learning the fundamentals of other related techniques, especially regarding hook placement and arthrodesis. In the technique initially used by Harrington, a compression rod was placed on the convex side of the curve. This offered increased stability and at the same time shortened the spine or at least resisted the stretching of the spine produced by the distraction rod. It is this distraction that is thought in some instances to be responsible for the rare spinal cord injury seen after Harrington rod instrumentation. The compression increased the lordosis, however, which was usually present. Although not critically noted in the 1960s and early 1970s, this degree of thoracic hypokyphosis would not be acceptable by today's standards. Most surgeons never used the compression rod, finding it too difficult.

For Harrington instrumentation, the levels of fusion are selected according to the criteria proposed by King et al.[1]

Figure 1–1. The patient is placed in the prone position in such a way as to leave the abdomen free and thus reduce blood loss[2] (***Figure 1–1A***). The entire back as well as the posterior pelvis is in the operative field so that bone from the posterior iliac crest can be obtained for arthrodesis.

Except for the severest and rigid curves, the incision is straight. It should extend from just above the topmost vertebrae to be fused to just below the lower vertebrae to be fused. If the fusion is to end in the region of L1 or L2, a separate incision can be used to obtain the iliac graft (see later discussion on iliac graft). If the L3 or lower vertebrae is to be fused, however, it is easier to extend the incision to the sacrum remaining in the midline.

The incision is made partially through the dermis to mark the path. To aid in hemostasis a dilute solution of epinephrine and saline (1:500,000) is injected into the dermis, producing a *peau d'orange* effect and into the subcutaneous tissue (***Figure 1–1B***). Injection may also be used deeply along the spinous process down to the laminae (***Figure 1–1C***). Care should be taken to follow the direction of the spinous process, which angles cephalad from its tip in the thoracic spine, and to stay slightly wide of the midline to be in the area where the laminae overlap.

The incision is then made down to the tips of the spinous processes and the midline raphe identified. This is thinner in the thoracic region, and in cases with severe rotation may actually be hidden by the elevated and rotated paravertebral muscles on the convex side of the curve. This midline raphe including the cartilage caps of the spinous processes is incised. Subperiosteal dissection of the desired levels is performed from the tips of the spinous processes to the tips of the transverse processes. Care should be taken at this point to expose the entire facet, which is indicated by a line extending from the caudal edge of the transverse process to the caudal end of the spinous process (***Figure 1–1D***).

Until this point of the procedure bleeding should be minimal, and the wound should be dry. A frequent and obscure source of bleeding is from veins that can be seen to course along the exposed surface of the muscle. When the muscle is retracted the bleeding stops, and when it is released the bleeding resumes. At this point the most difficult part of the operation is complete, for if the surgeon can visualize the posterior spinal elements free of soft tissue and bleeding, the insertion of the hooks and rod, and the decortication is easy (***Figure 1–1E***). The superior facets have been removed from the convex side of the curve.

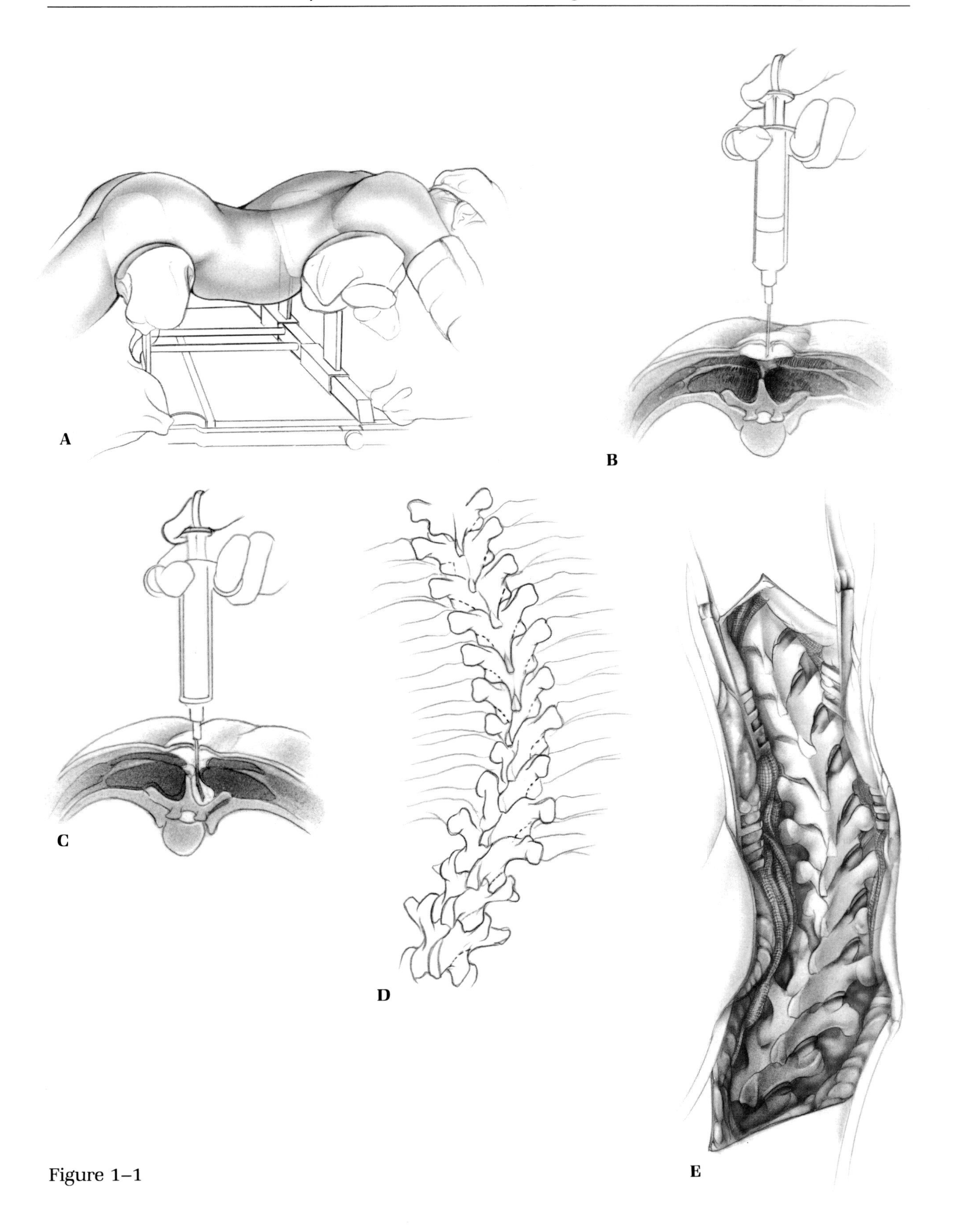

Figure 1–1

Figure 1–2. Hook placement on the concave side of the curve in the thoracic region is begun by removing a small portion of the caudal edge of the selected vertebrae (***Figure 1–2A***). This is done to allow the hook to move cephalad enough to be medial to the pedicle and within the confines of the spinal canal. This prevents its twisting out laterally. The notch in the lamina is made with a $\frac{1}{4}$-in osteotome. Care should be taken to rest the hand holding the osteotome and as much as possible aim the osteotome away from the spinal cord. Provided not too much bone is removed, the inferior facet will block the osteotome from penetrating into the canal.

Hook placement begins with a #1251 hook on a hook holder and with a pusher. This hook has a sharp edge that will aid in penetrating the remaining ligmentum flavum. The hook should be introduced so that it is medial to the pedicle (***Figure 1–2B***). After placement it should be removed to be certain that it is under both cortices of the lamina and has not split the lamina (***Figure 1–2C***). To accomplish this, the introduction of the hook should begin with it tilted downward (***Figure 1–2D***). It is useful to think of inserting it in such a way as to scrape the cartilage off of the inferior facet. Once in place it should be tested to be sure that it is medial to the pedicle. This can be done by pulling it lateral in an attempt to slide it out of the facet. This hook (or a #1253) may be left in place because there is no danger that it will be pushed into the canal, and its presence will serve as a reminder not to decorticate that lamina.

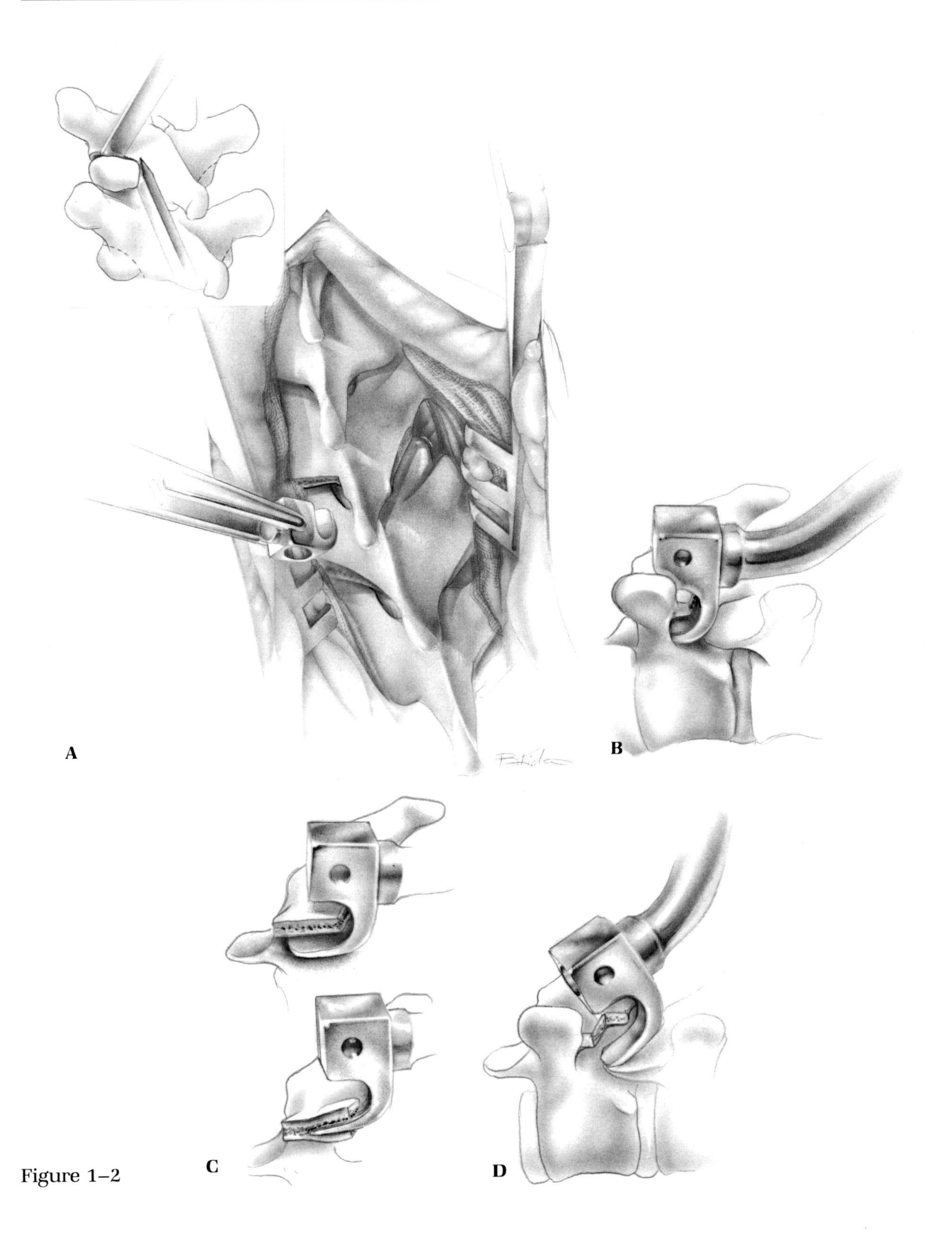

Figure 1–2

Figure 1–3. Placement of the distal hook in the lumbar region begins with gaining access to the spinal canal. This can most safely be done by nibbling away the ligment flavum in the midline cephalad to the selected vertebra. The caudal portion of the spinous process and the adjacent portion of the superior facet can also be removed to improve access (***Figure 1–3A***).

Next the superior edge of the selected vertebra is squared off with a Kerrison rongeur. Only enough bone to provide seating for the hook should be removed (***Figure 1–3B***). Additional bone may have to be removed to allow the actual placement of the hook, and this should be taken from the facet and lamina of the vertebra above.

A #1254 hook that is designed to fit on the collar end of the Harrington rod is now tried for fit. Like the thoracic hook it should lie medial to the pedicle within the spinal canal (***Figure 1–3C***). This hook should be removed because it could easily be pushed into the canal (***Figure 1–3D***).

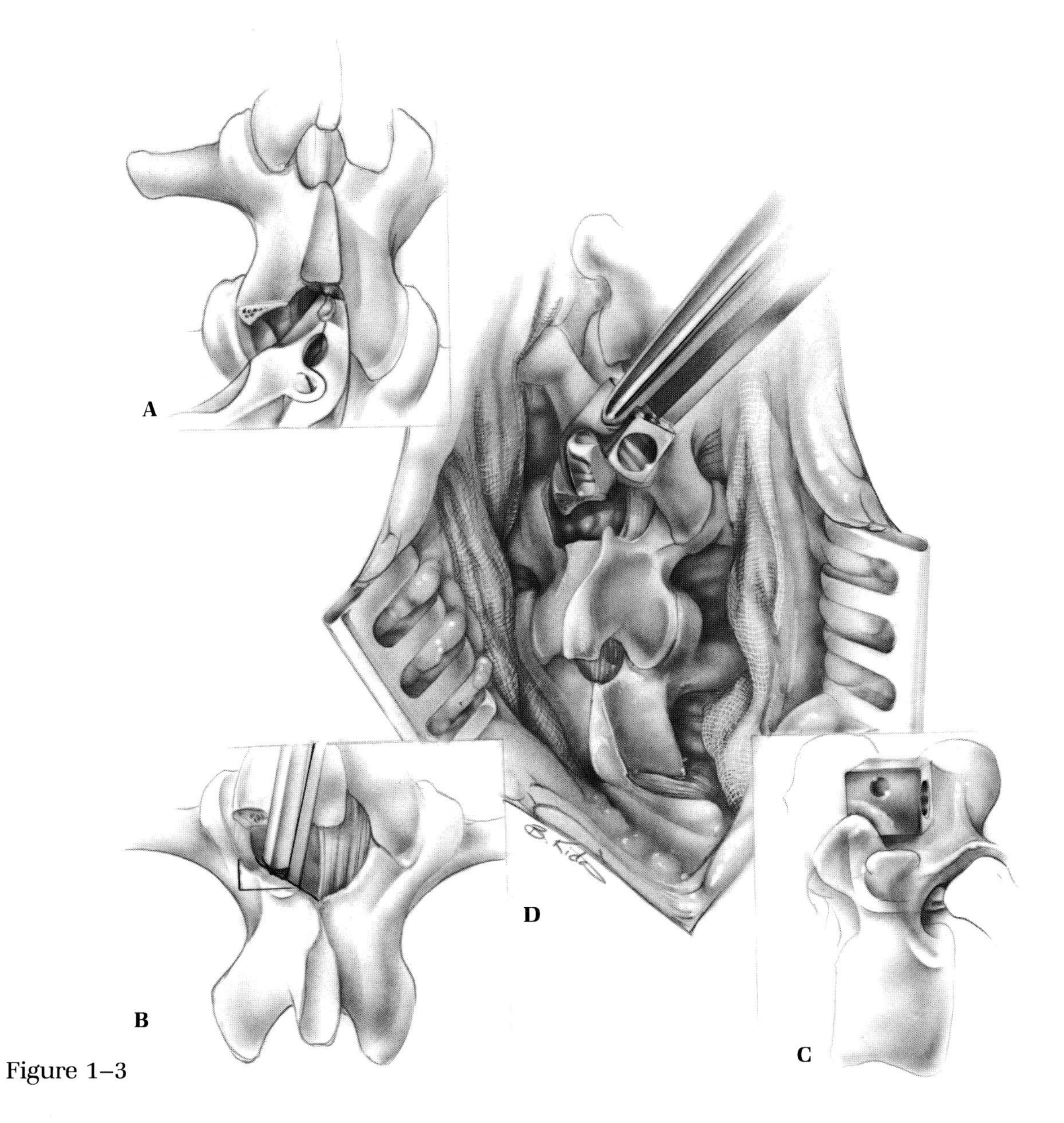

Figure 1–3

Figure 1–4. Before placement of the rod, all of the facets in the fusion area on both the concave and convex sides of the curve are excised. This is followed by a complete decortication of the spinous processes, laminae, and transverse processes in the area that will lie under the rod. Those laminae that support hooks should not be decorticated, however. Pieces of cancellous bone from the iliac crest should be packed into each facet.

Both hooks are then placed and held firmly with a hook holder. The rachet end of the rod is passed through the cephalad hook to the point where the distal collar end can be engaged in the caudal hook. The rod is now ready to be distracted by use of the spreader. The spine is pushed straight by an assistant while the distractor is used to force the superior hook along the rachets of the rod.

At the completion of distraction it is desirable to have as few rachets as possible below the cephalad hook because this is the weakest part of the rod. This means that at the beginning of distraction no rachets may be visible below the hook, and therefore the Harrington spreader cannot be used for distraction. Although there is a special tool available to accomplish distraction in this situation, a small vise grips can be locked onto the rod far enough below the hook for the Harrington spreader to push against. After distraction is complete the locking C ring is placed on the rachet adjacent to the hook to prevent the rod from slipping.

Figure 1–5. At the completion of distraction the remainder of the spine is decorticated and the bone graft which has been obtained from the iliac crest is carefully placed.

Prior to wound closure any bleeding from the muscle should be controlled. Any devitalized tissue resulting from the retractors or dissection should be debrided. Closure of the wound in three layers of runing suture can be accomplished rapidly. The use of drains is at the surgeon's discretion.

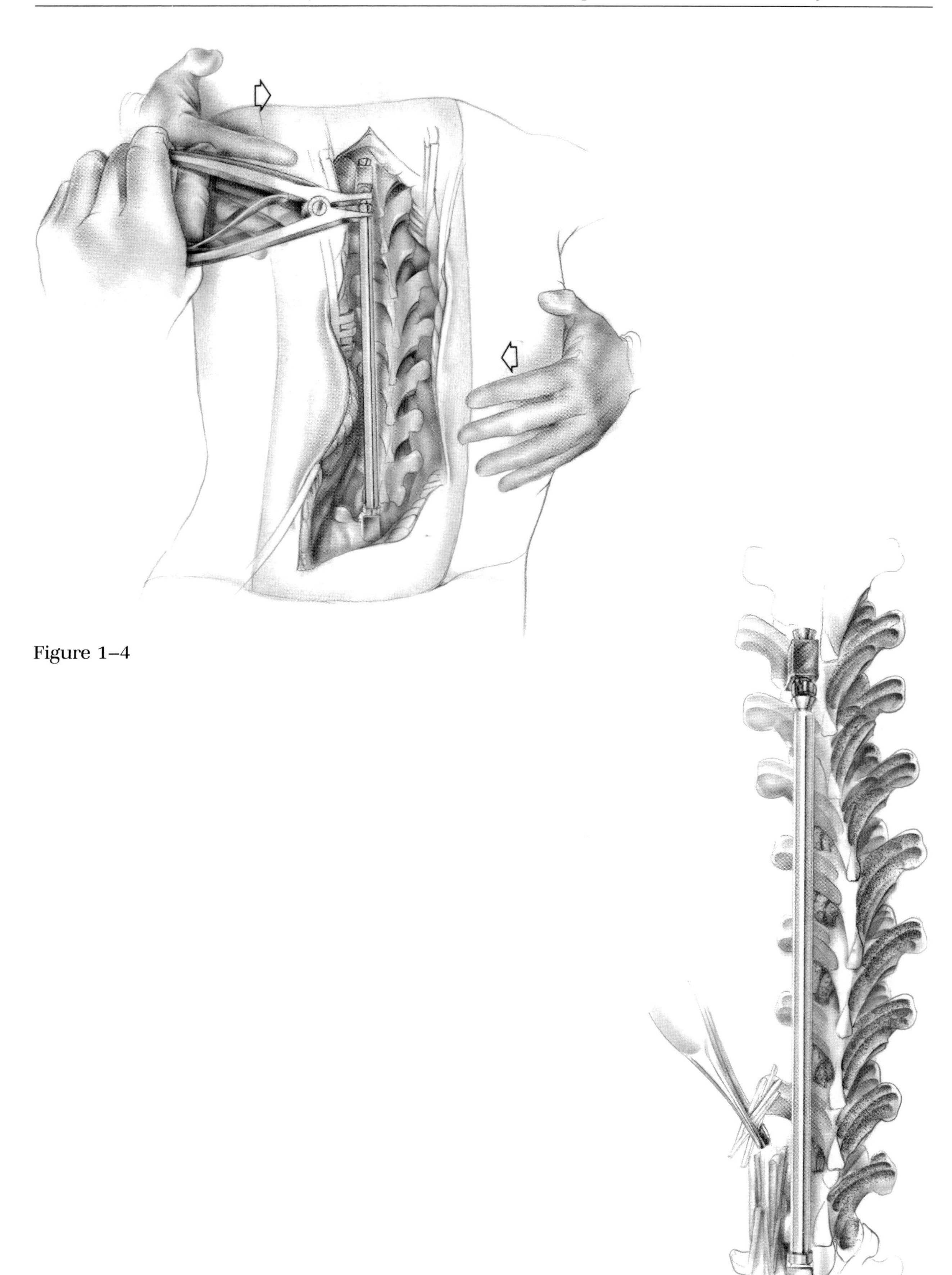

Figure 1–4

Figure 1–5

Figure 1–6. A comparison of the preoperative and postoperative radiographs in this 13-year-old girl demonstrates the correction of the scoliosis. The lack of correction of the hypokyphosis is particularly noticeable on the lateral radiograph. (Courtesy of Douglas K. Kehl, MD.)

POSTOPERATIVE CARE

It is likely that a properly placed Harrington rod is securer than is generally believed. The tension on the rod and thus the force on the hooks will decrease during the first hours and days. Thus, the likelihood that one of the laminae will break decreases. As the force of distraction lessens, however, there is greater likelihood that a hook may be dislodged. In addition, there is no fixation of the vertebrae between the two hooks, and considerable motion may occur between these vertebrae. This can be demonstrated at the time of surgery. For these reasons postoperative immobilization is considered necessary.

Initially the patient is managed by "log rolling." Full mobilization is delayed until a suitable spinal orthosis is available, or the patient has been placed in a cast. Pain is managed with morphine administered by a patient controlled analgesia (PCA) pump for the first 24 to 48 hours. Oral pain medication supplemented by intramuscular medication is then used. If a Foley catheter was used during surgery, it is best left in place until the morphine has been discontinued. Patients are followed at 3-month intervals with radiographs for the first year. The cast or orthosis can usually be discontinued at 6 months, and by 1 year the arthrodesis should be solid and the patient allowed to return to full activities.

REFERENCES

1. King HA, Moe JH, Bradford DS, Winter RB. The selection of fusion levels in thoracic idiopathic scoliosis. J Bone Joint Surg 1983;65A:1302.
2. Relton JES, Hall JE. An operation frame for spinal fusion: A new apparatus designed to reduce haemorrhage during operation. J Bone Joint Surg 1967;49B:327.

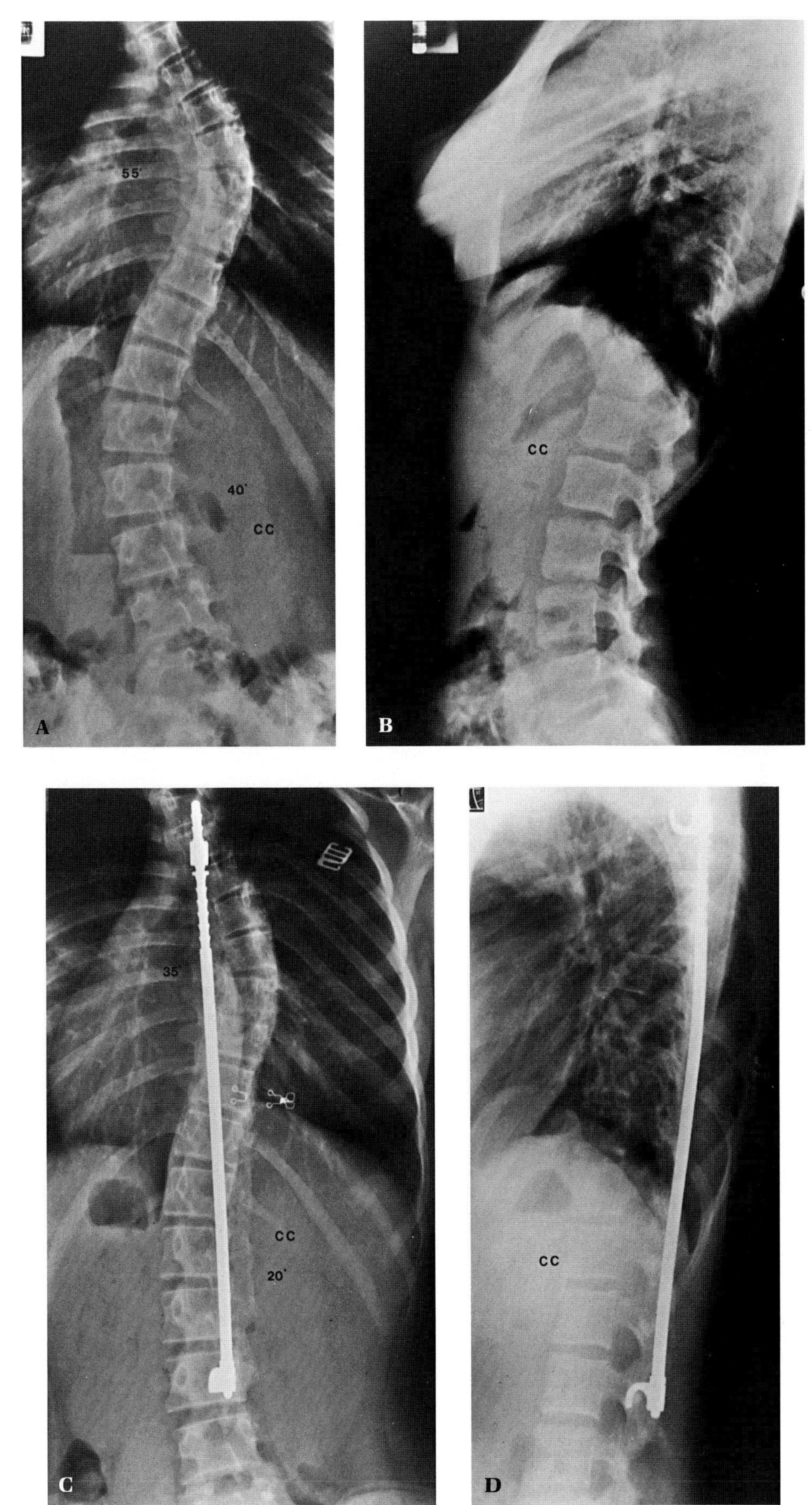

Figure 1–6

1.2 Harrington Rod Instrumentation With Sublaminar Wires for Scoliosis

As the techniques of spinal fixation evolved in an effort to gain better correction of both the coronal and sagittal deformities, it was inevitable that the technique of sublaminar wires with a Harrington distraction rod would be combined. This technique provides better correction of the sagittal contour and increased rigidity of fixation than the Harrington rod alone, but does not offer a substantial increase in correction of the coronal deformity. Because this technique requires contouring of the rod, it is essential that a square-ended rod be used so that the rod will not rotate into the deformity but rather will pull the deformity to the rod, thus gaining correction. This technique remains in wide use today by surgeons who have chosen not to embrace the concept of the Cotrel-Dubousset instrumentation.

The selection of the vertebrae to be fused is by the criteria of King et al.[1]

Figure 1–7. It is important that the rod be contoured so that it will have the desired configuration when the distal square end is inserted in the square-ended hook. Usually the distal square hook will sit with a 20-degree lateral tilt when inserted under the lamina (***Figure 1–7A***). An easy method to contour the rod is to hold it in a hook, which is held by a hook holder. The hook can then be inclined to the same degree of tilt that is observed when it is inserted and the rod contoured in this position (***Figure 1–7B***).

Figure 1–8. The technique for inserting the hooks is the same as for the Harrington rod, and the technique of passing the wires is described in the Luque technique. Wires should be passed around the laminae of all the vertebrae to be fused including the most superior and inferior vertebrae into which the hooks are inserted. This will provide additional stability for the hooks that are under different stresses from the Harrington technique.

The wires that pass around the rod will tend to pull the rod toward the midline. This force, applied to the most dorsal aspect of the hook, will tend to rotate the hook that is under the lamina in a lateral direction. Although this force should be resisted by the pedicle, additional stability will be obtained by passing the wire around the hook.

Figure 1–9. This technique can be accomplished fast enough to permit thorough facetectomy and decortication of the area that will lie under the rod without undue blood loss. The distraction is obtained before tightening the wires. The tightening starts at the ends and progresses toward the middle. In addition to an assistant pushing the spine straight, the rod is stabilized with a rod pusher.

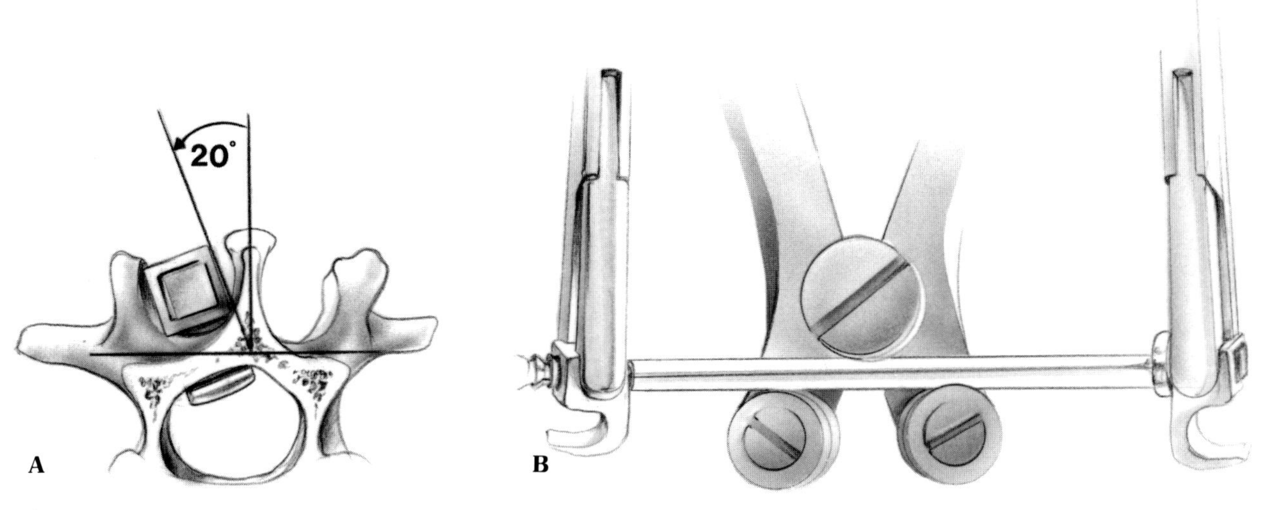

Figure 1–7

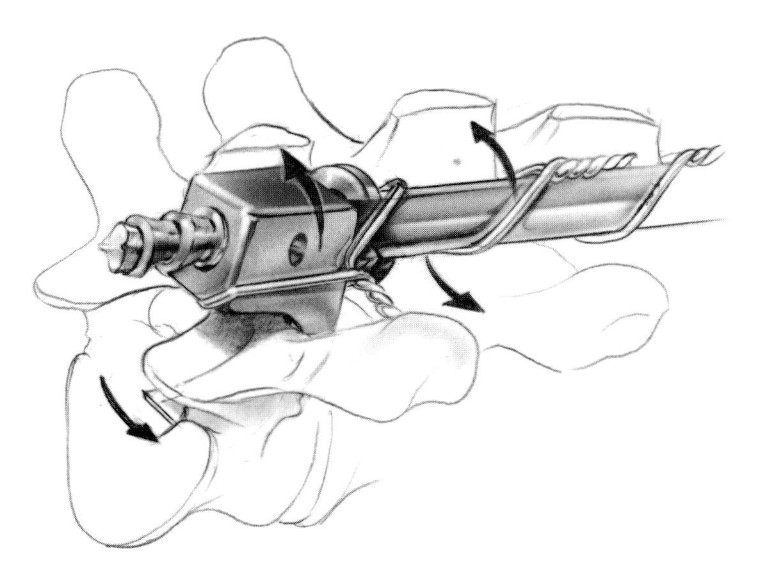

Figure 1–8

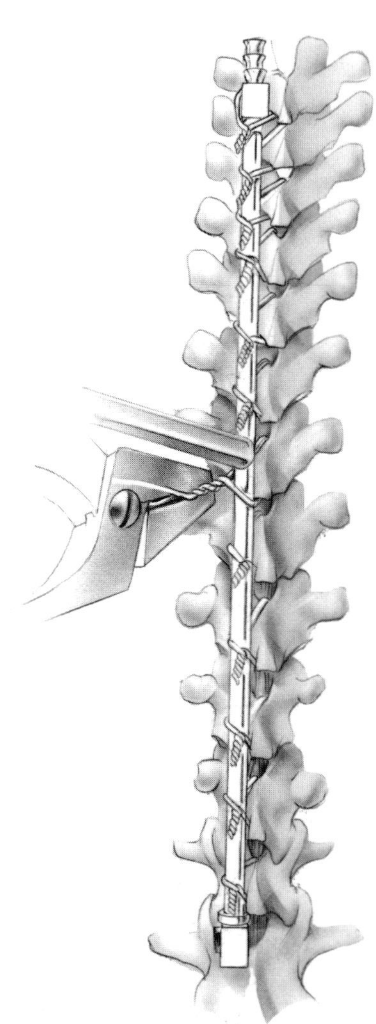

Figure 1–9

Figure 1–10. Preoperative (***Figure 1–10A***) and postoperative (***Figures 1–10B, C***) radiographs of a 14-year-old-girl with a single curve illustrate the correction of the scoliosis and the preservation of the normal lumbar lordosis. Although moderately effective in correcting the thoracic hypokyphosis, it offers little if any additional correction of the rotational deformity compared with the Harrington rod by itself.

POSTOPERATIVE CARE

These patients are cared for like those with a Harrington rod. The need for immobilization in the postoperative period is not so great, however. The author's treatment consists of an orthoplast jacket that is worn full-time for the first 3 months and for the next 3 months when ambulatory.

REFERENCE

1. King HA, Moe JH, Bradford DS, Winter RB. The selection of fusion levels in thoracic idiopathic scoliosis. J Bone Joint Surg 1983;65A:1302.

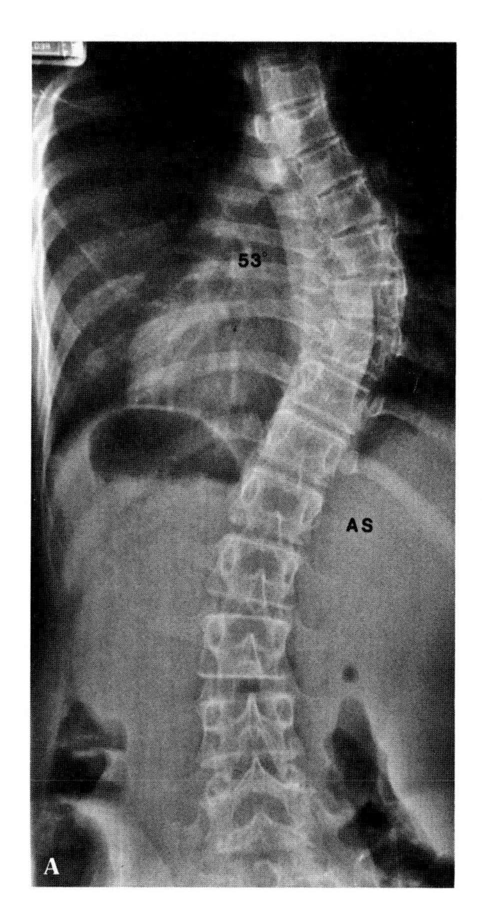

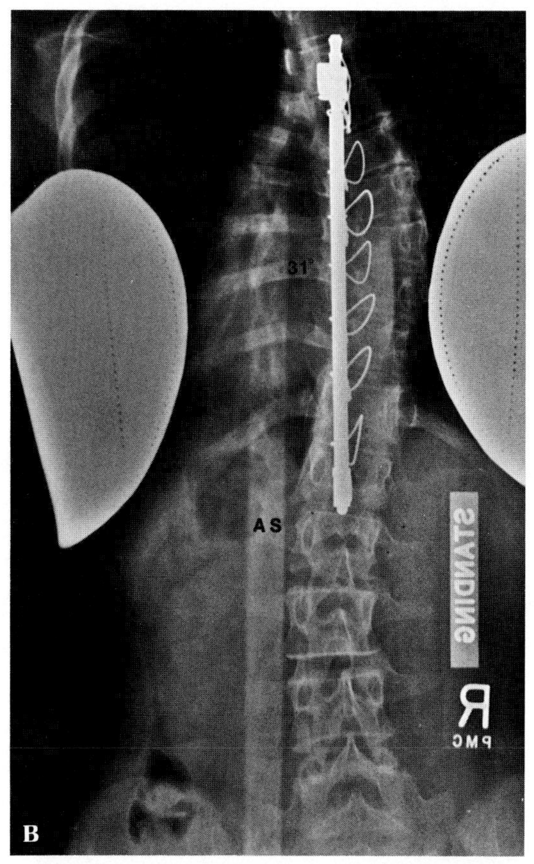

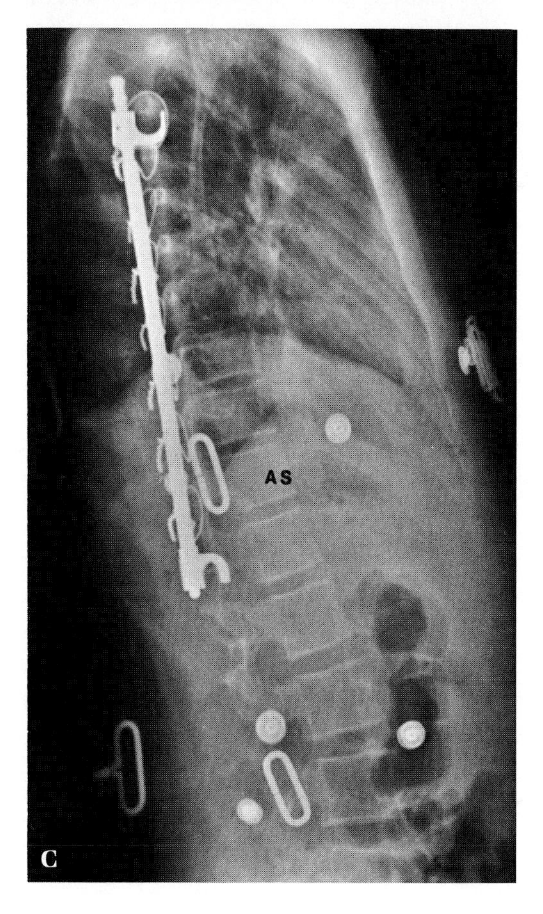

Figure 1–10

1.3
Interspinous Process Segmental Instrumentation (Wisconsin Instrumentation) for Scoliosis

Initial concepts of segmental spinal fixation used the spinous process for the segmental fixation.[1,2] This technique, also known as the Wisconsin technique, was developed to provide a means of segmental spinal fixation that was as secure as the Luque method but did not entail the risk of passing wires in the spinal canal. The technique has the additional theoretic advantage of combining distraction with a lateral corrective force.

Among the disadvantages of this technique is the limited ability to correct sagittal plane deformity unless a contoured, square-ended rod is used and the theoretic problem that tightening the wires around the Harrington distraction rod tends to worsen the rotational deformity.

Figure 1–11. The spine is exposed as in the Harrington rod procedure. The levels for fusion are selected based on the needs of the particular case and the two hook sites for the Harrington rod are prepared. The next step is to prepare the holes in the base of the spinous processes through which will pass the button-wire implants. These holes can be prepared by the use of special curved awls that were designed for this purpose. The author has found it easier to begin the holes on each side of the spinous process with a small air-driven burr, however. This provides excellent control. The two holes are then easily connected by passing a small curved hemostat or right-angled clamp through each side. These blunt-tip instruments are less likely to penetrate the cortical wall of the canal than a sharp awl.

It is important to be at the base of the spinous process and to direct the holes as deeply as possible without entering the spinal canal. If the holes are placed too close to the tip of the spinous processes, there will not be sufficient strength in the bone. This technique is not suitable for a kyphotic spine because in this particular deformity the spinous processes will thin and flatten out, providing little bone between the spinal canal and the tip of the spinous process.

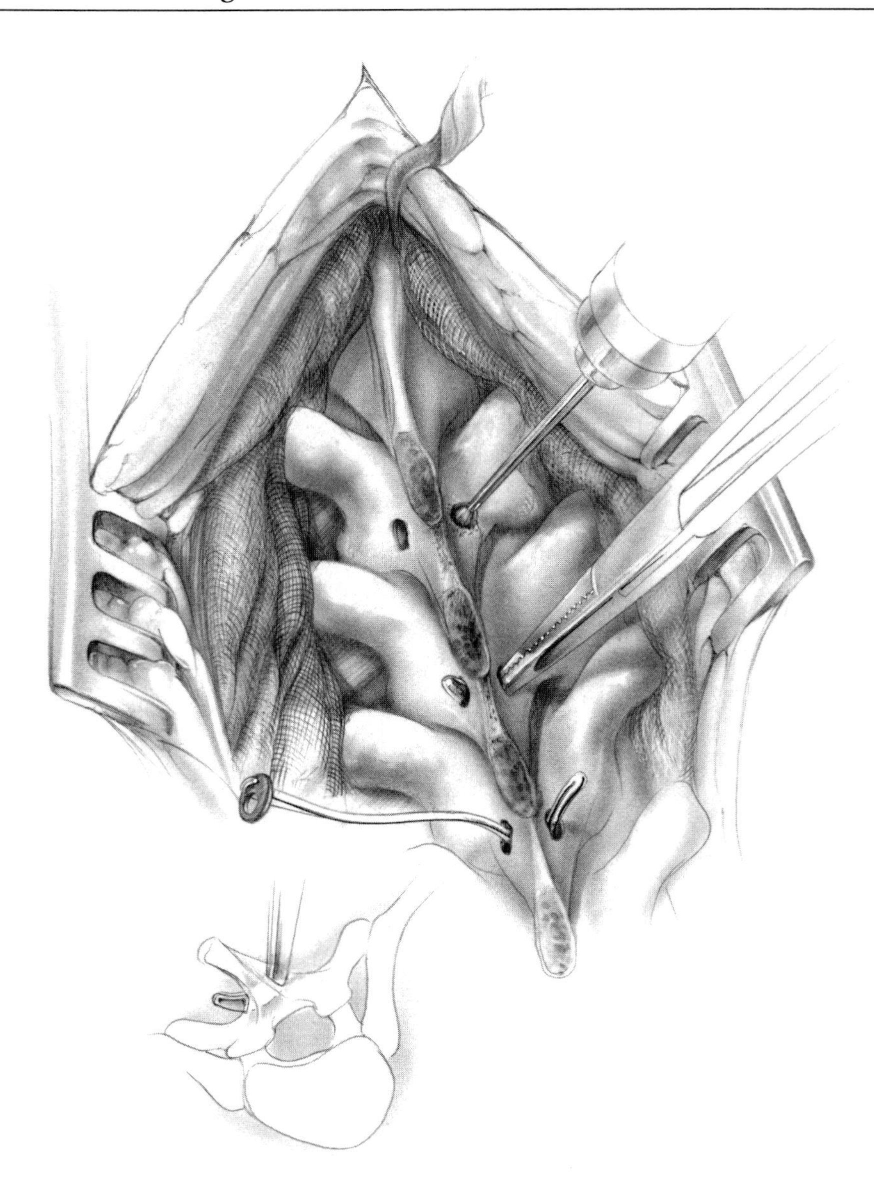

Figure 1–11

Figure 1–12. After the holes are made the button-wire implants are placed. Two of these are passed through each hole, one from each side. Each button has a hole in addition to the one through which the wire is attached. The wire from the opposite side is passed through this extra hole. When these wires are pulled through and the buttons are firmly seated against the base of the spinous process, there will be a wire loop projecting on each side of each spinous process to be instrumented. At this point all of the facets are excised, and the area of the spine that will lie under the Harrington rod is decorticated.

Figure 1–13. The hooks for the Harrington rod are put into their previously created holes, and the rod is placed into the hooks after being passed through the wire loops. The rod is then distracted and the wires are tightened around the rod, starting in those areas where the rod closely approximates the spine and working toward the apex of the curve.

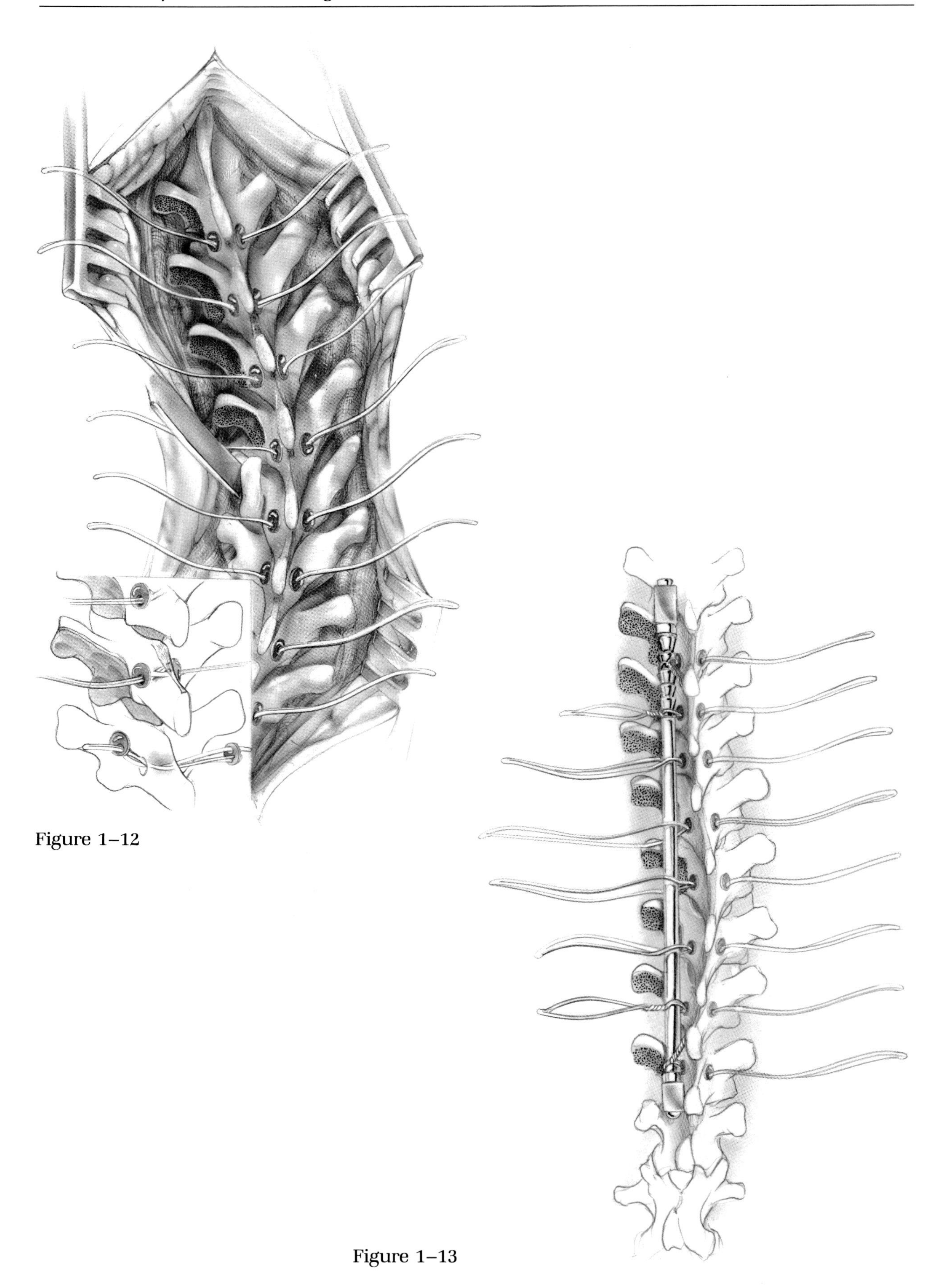

Figure 1–12

Figure 1–13

Figure 1–14. The Luque rod can now be placed on the convex side after it is decorticated. It is contoured to give the estimated amount of correction that can be obtained. Kyphosis and lordosis can also be contoured in this rod, but this will be more of a bother than help unless a contoured, square-ended Harrington rod has been used on the concave side. An "L" configuration should be placed at one or both ends of the rod to keep it from sliding because it will not be locked in place by rigid cross-links. This rod can then be tightened by the convex technique.[3]

Figure 1–15. ***Figure 1–15A*** is the radiograph of a 15-year-old girl with a severe rigid scoliosis. An anterior disectomy and fusion was performed to obtain better correction. At the same operative session, posterior arthrodesis with interspinous process segmental spinal instrumentation was performed. This method is rapid, combines distraction with lateral corrective force, and is rigid, making it a reasonable choice for this situation. ***Figure 1–15B*** shows the results 2 years later.

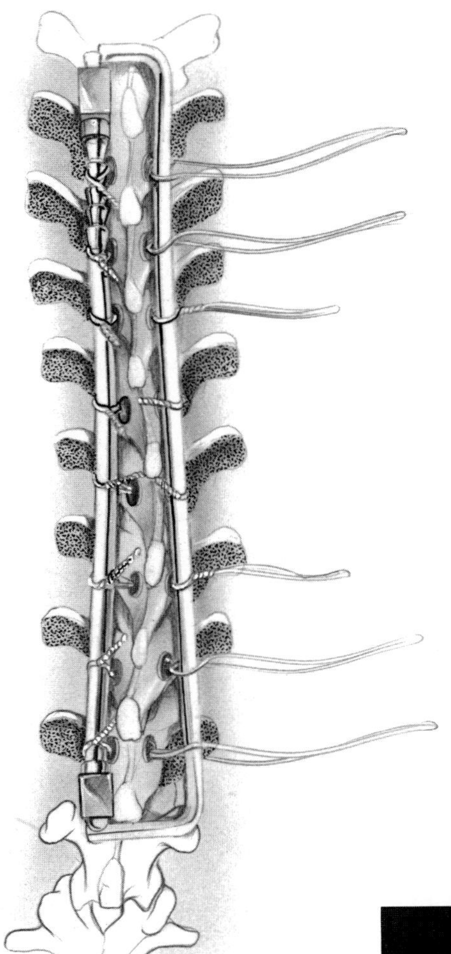

Figure 1–14

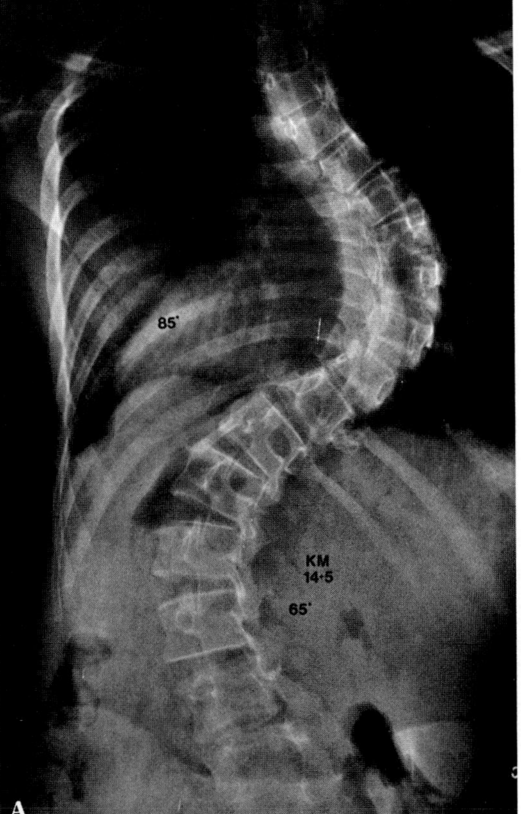

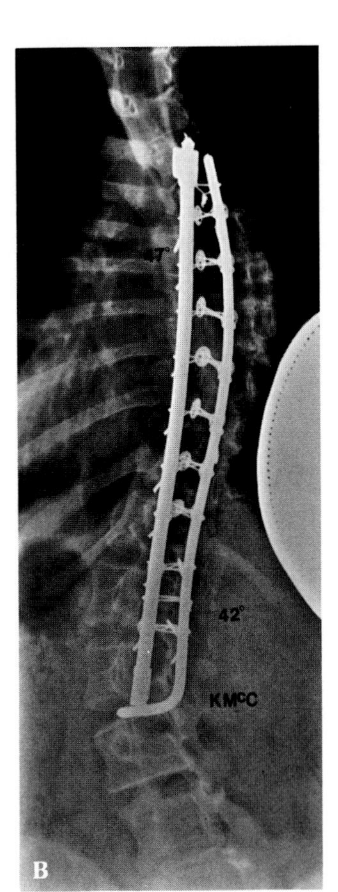

Figure 1–15

POSTOPERATIVE CARE

Postoperatively patients are treated in the same manner as any stable spinal instrumentation would allow. Little thought needs to be given to positioning or rolling the patient except for comfort. Early ambulation with or without an orthosis is possible depending on the surgeon's choice.

REFERENCES

1. Perry JO, Nickel VL, Bonnett C. Halo-button-traction wire technique of spine fusion in the non-ambulatory respiratory patient with spine instability. J Bone Joint Surg 1968;50A:1059.
2. Resina J, Ferreira-Alves A. A technique of correction and internal fixation for scoliosis. J Bone Joint Surg 1977;59B:159.
3. Allen BL, Ferguson RL. The Galveston technique for L rod instrumentation of the scoliotic spine. Spine 1982;7:276.

1.4 Bilateral Sublaminar Segmental Instrumentation (Luque Instrumentation) for Scoliosis

The double L-rod method of segmental spinal instrumentation, popularized by Luque, introduced the first practical application of segmental fixation to the spine. The final evolution of the technique has resulted in a method of fixation in which two stainless steel rods are secured to both laminae of each vertebrae in the fusion area.

These rods must be contoured to conform to the spine in its corrected position as the spine is moved to the rods and held there by wires to achieve correction. In addition, the rods can be contoured in the sagittal plane. Although this can be quite effective in maintaining or producing lumbar lordosis, it is less effective in correcting the hypokyphosis in thoracic scoliosis. Theoretically, better correction should be possible with this instrumentation because the geometric limitation of curve correction by distraction does not apply to lateral forces.[1] Because the force of correction is shared by each lamina in the fusion area, this technique is ideal for those cases in which the bone is not of normal strength (*eg*, neuromuscular scoliosis). The secure fixation produced by this technique lessens or obviates the need for postoperative immobilization.

This technique is far more difficult to master than the Harrington rod technique and probably remains the most difficult technique of spinal instrumentation today. The potential for neurologic injury with all of the wires in the spinal canal is great,[2] although many surgeons with wide experience in the technique report no complications from the wires. Reliance on the instrumentation rather than facetectomy, decortication, and bone grafting is a seductive trap that will probably result in an increased incidence of late pseudarthroses.

As with most other methods of instrumentation, the levels of fusion are determined by the upright (sitting) and bend films. Today this technique finds its widest use in neuromuscular scoliosis; therefore, the usual criteria for fusion of neuromuscular curves apply. In these cases the commonest error is to fuse too short cephalad. Fusion to the pelvis is an entirely different tissue that is undergoing reconsideration at the present time.

The rods come in two diameters: $\frac{3}{16}$ in (4.8 mm) and $\frac{1}{4}$ in (6.4 mm). The smaller $\frac{3}{16}$-in rods are somewhat flexible, and for that reason are more forgiving and easier to contour. This same flexibility may prove a disadvantage in gaining and maintaining correction, however, and in the author's opinion is rarely indicated.

The rods are secured to the spine with stainless steel wire, usually 16 gauge. The wire should be malleable and workable so that it does not break with bending and twisting. It can be obtained in precut lengths with a small bead on the ends.

Figure 1–16. Some surgeons prefer to prebend the rods based on the preoperative traction or bend film. The author finds it much easier to bend the rod after the spine is exposed, and with an assistant pushing the spine straight. In this way the rods can be bent, applied against the spine to check the fit, and adjusted in both the coronal and sagittal plane. Because correction will improve after all of the facets are excised, the rods are usually bent to gain slightly more correction than is apparent with an assistant pushing the spine straight. It should be possible to achieve correction equal to that seen on a forced bend film. At the completion of the surgery, the rods should lie in close contact with the laminae.

Figure 1–17. If the spine is not instrumented to the pelvis, an "L" is bent at one end of each rod. Initially one reason for this bend was to keep the rod from slipping through the wire. This potential problem is obviated by the use of the Texas Scottish Rite cross-links. The bend makes it easier to control the rotation of the rod as the wires are being tightened, however. One of these bent ends is placed cephalad and one on the opposite side caudad. At the caudal end the "L" may be passed through a hole in the base of the lumbar spinous process.

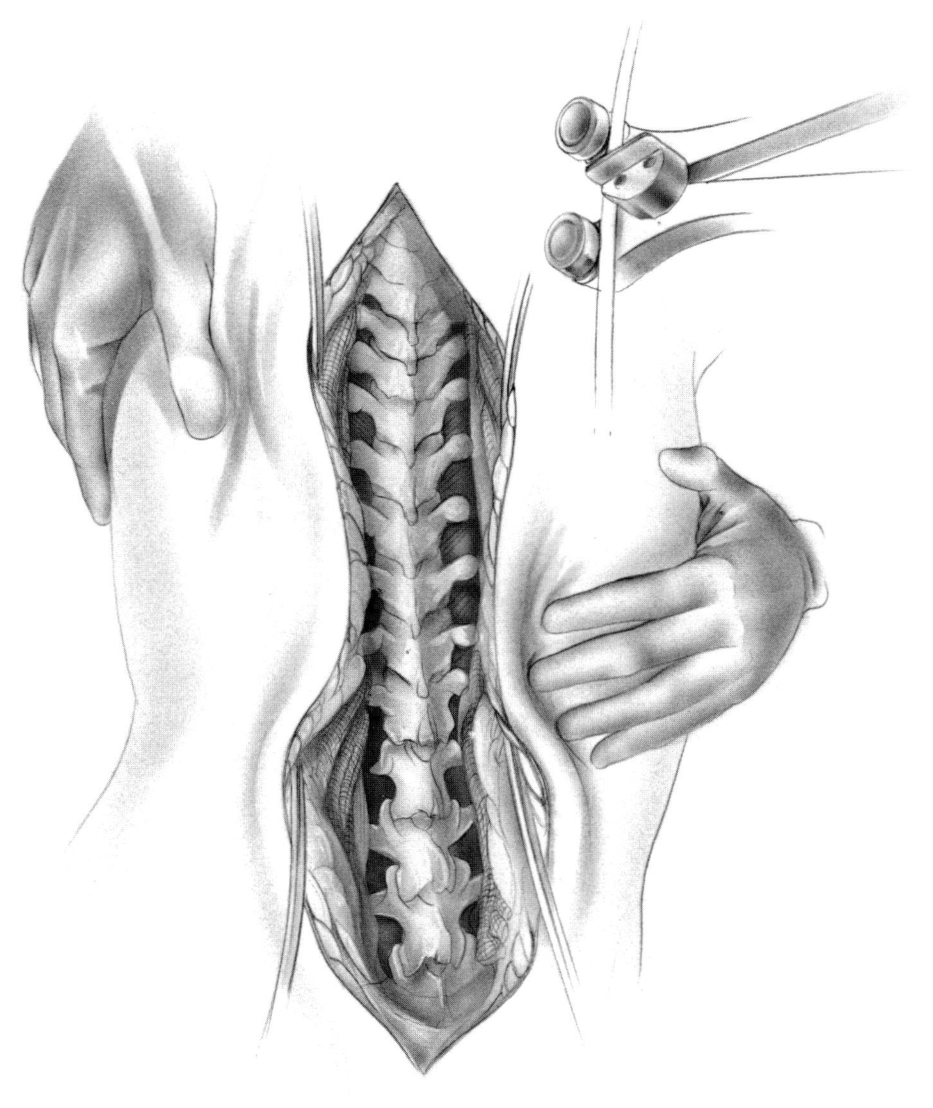

Figure 1–16

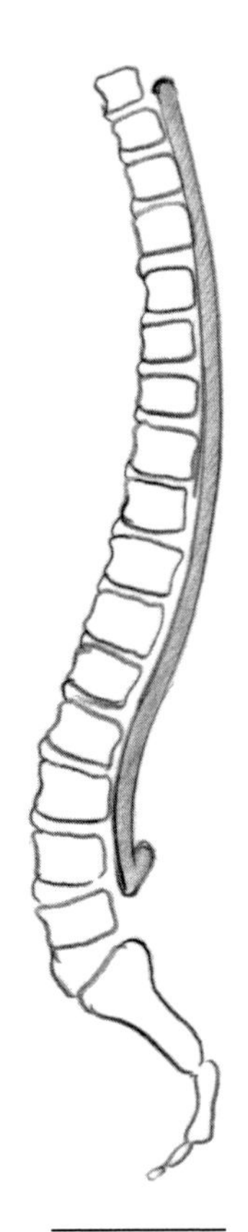

Figure 1–17

Figure 1–18. After the rods are contoured and before the next step, excision of the ligamentum flavum and all of the facets in the fusion area is performed. In the lumbar spine there is sufficient room between the spinous processes to excise a portion of the ligamentum flavum without removal of bone. In the thoracic spine the spinous processes overlap, however, obscuring the ligament. This overlapping portion of the spinous process can be removed with the same large rongeur or a bone biter. This is followed by excision of a small portion of the ligamentum flavum.

Figure 1–19. A large double-action rongeur is used to bite the ligament in the midline. It is usually possible with experience to bite through the ligamentum flavum with the large rongeur in a small area exposing the epidural fat. This hole can then be enlarged with a smaller and sharply angulated rongeur. A more cautious and time-consuming method is to take a small bite from the ligamentum flavum, thinning it out until the midline separation is found. This can then be separated with a small dissector and a Kerrison rongeur used to remove a portion of the ligament.

The removal of the ligamentum flavum should be just sufficient to permit passage of the wire. Extensive removal of the ligament does little to make passage of the wire easier and only creates more bleeding and opportunity for bone graft to fall into the spinal canal. As passage of the wire will be easier and safer on the convex side of a curve, enlargement of the opening in the ligament in this direction is best.

Figure 1–20. The bending of the wires is a matter that is critical if their passage is to be easy and may have some importance for safety. Pulling the wire through the canal is easier if no sharp bends are placed in the wire that is to be pulled under the lamina. The bend in the wire should be slightly longer than the width of the lamina so that the tip will emerge on the other side. Care is needed to avoid creating a curve with too large a radius, however, as this may impinge on the cord during passage.

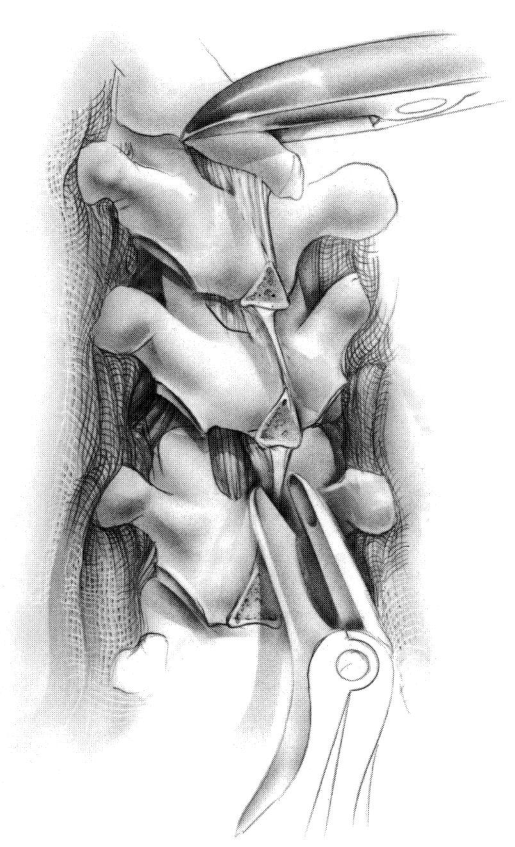

Figure 1–18

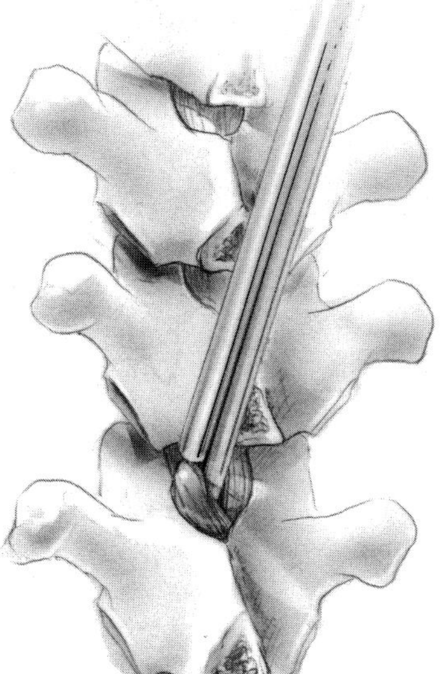

Figure 1–19

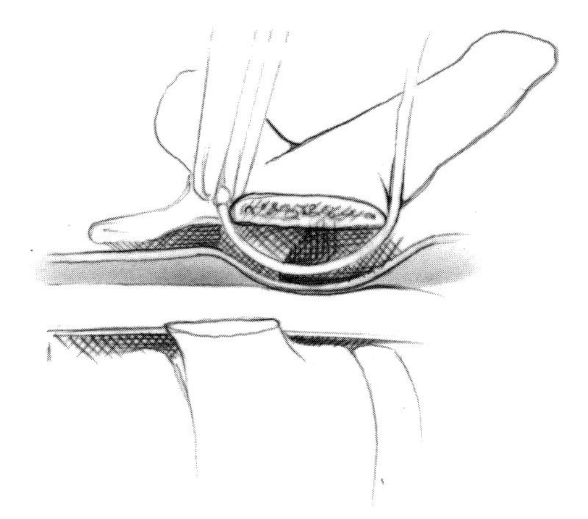

Figure 1–20

Figure 1–21. In situations in which the lamina is broad, it is better to bend only the tip, leaving the portion that is to be passed under the lamina flat. The wire can then easily be slid under the lamina without striking the spinal cord.

Figure 1–22. The wires are most easily passed from the caudad to cephalad direction. The wire must be controlled at all times and no force should be necessary to pass it. When the tip of the wire becomes visible at the cephalad end of the lamina, it is grasped with a large sturdy needle holder. As it is pulled through, a gentle upward force is maintained on the caudal end of the wire to help straighten the bend and be sure it does not impinge on the cord.

If both sides of the spine are to be secured with a rod as is usual in paralytic curves, a double segment of wire may be passed, the bent end cut off after passage, and the two resulting pieces secured on opposite laminae. (In these illustrations passage of a single wire is shown for clarity.) Double wires are often used on each side at the top and bottom of the rods where the stress may be greater.

Figure 1–23. After the wire is drawn under the lamina, it must be secured in such a way that if it is accidentally hit it will not be forced into the spinal canal. No matter how careful the operating team, it is difficult to avoid hitting the wires during the course of the surgery. The amount of force necessary to push a wire in against the spinal cord is so slight that it can occur without the surgeon being aware.

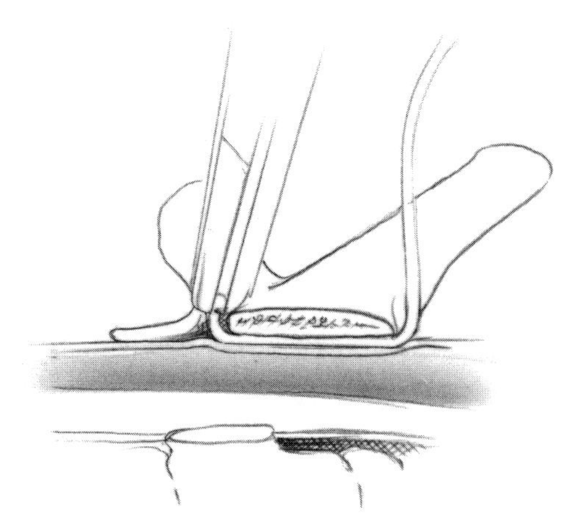

Figure 1–21

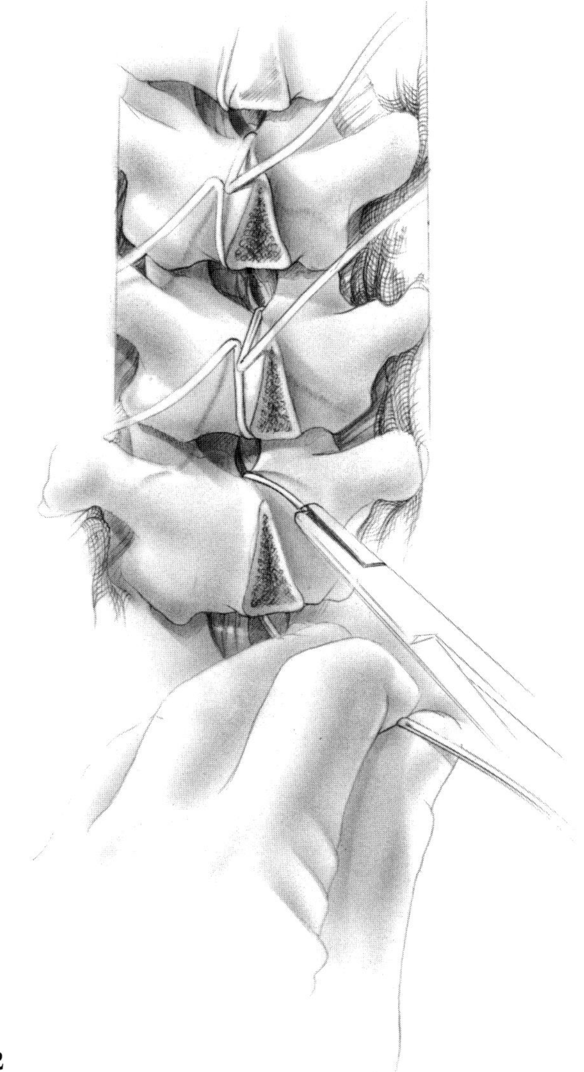

Figure 1–22

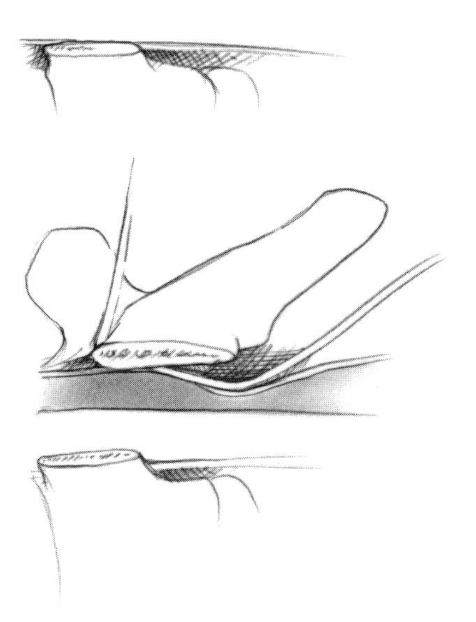

Figure 1–23

Figure 1–24. The best way to secure the wires is by bending each end of the wire securely over the lamina and then over the edge of the wound.

If complete decortication of the spine is to be done, it must be done now before the rods are wired in place. Desirable as it is, there are two major problems with doing a complete decortication of a paralytic spine at this stage: The bleeding may be excessive, and there is increased risk of neurologic injury in moving all of the wires from side to side. Therefore, in most cases the rods will be wired in place at this point, and decortication of the accessible bony surface will be done as the final step before closure—thus, the importance of previous complete excision of all facets. In addition, the more closely the rods lie against the lamina, the more bone that will be available for decortication lateral to them.

Figure 1–25. The technique of tightening the wires is important. The wires should not be used to pull the spine to the rod. Rather an assistant pushes the spine straight while the rod is stabilized with a rod holder or pusher. The wires are then tightened sequentially, holding the correction that is gained.

Figure 1–26. It can be difficult to determine when the wires are tight enough. As the wires are tightened with the wire twister, the twists will be at an angle of approximately 45 degrees to the axis of the wire.

Figure 1–27. When the newest twist, the one closest to the rod, changes direction to lie at 90 degrees to the axis of the wire, it is as tight as it can be made without risking breakage. During the tightening careful inspection of the L segment is necessary to be sure that it is not rotating. This segment can be held with a rod holder.

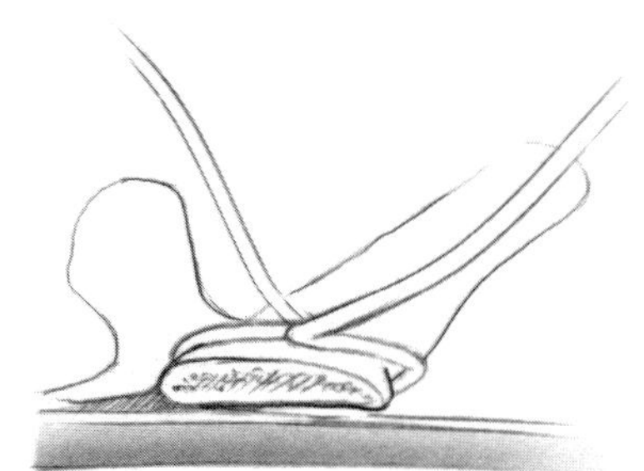

Figure 1–24

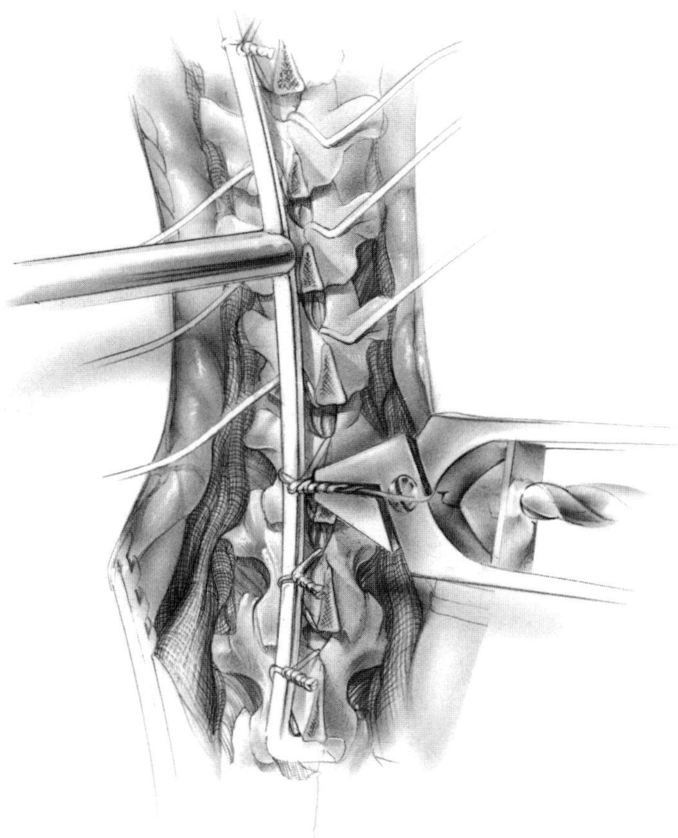

Figure 1–25

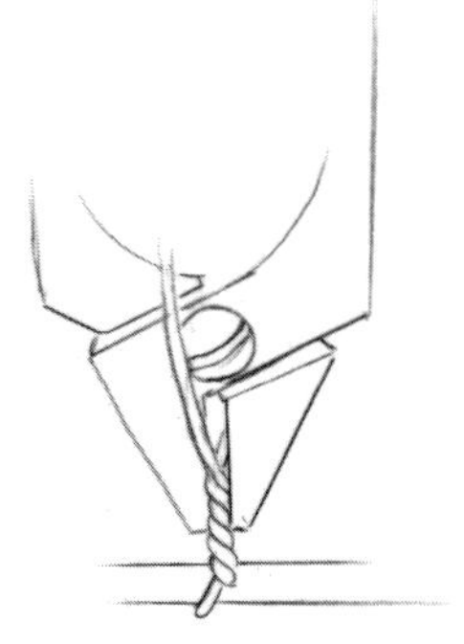

Figure 1–26

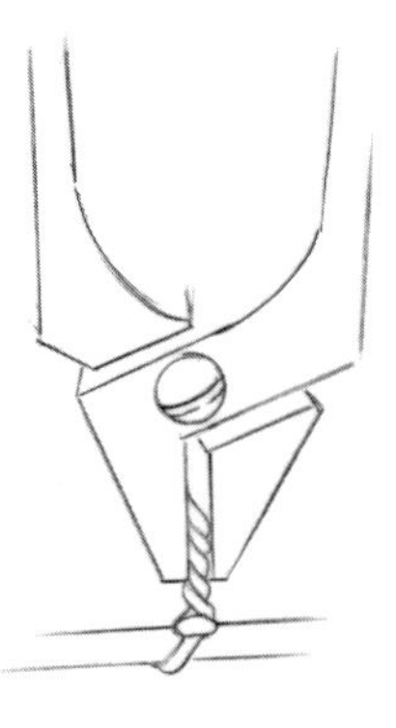

Figure 1–27

Figure 1–28. Two techniques for rod insertion are recommended: convex rod technique and concave rod technique.[3] In the usual paralytic C curve the author uses a simpler technique, first wiring in the concave rod completely and then wiring in the convex rod. The principle is to insert the rods and tighten the wires in the manner that most gradually applies force to the spine and thereby corrects the curve. Therefore, the wires tightened first are those where the rod is already closely in contact with the lamina. On the concave side these are the end wires progressing toward the apex of the curve. On the convex side the wires at the apex of the curve are tightened first, alternately progressing toward each end.

Figure 1–29. After all of the wires are tightened and retightened once, they are cut and bent over the rod. As they are bent they are twisted in the direction of the twist so as not to loosen them. The Texas Scottish Rite cross-link plates are then secured, and all of the exposed cortical surface is decorticated. Bone graft is added, and the wound is closed.

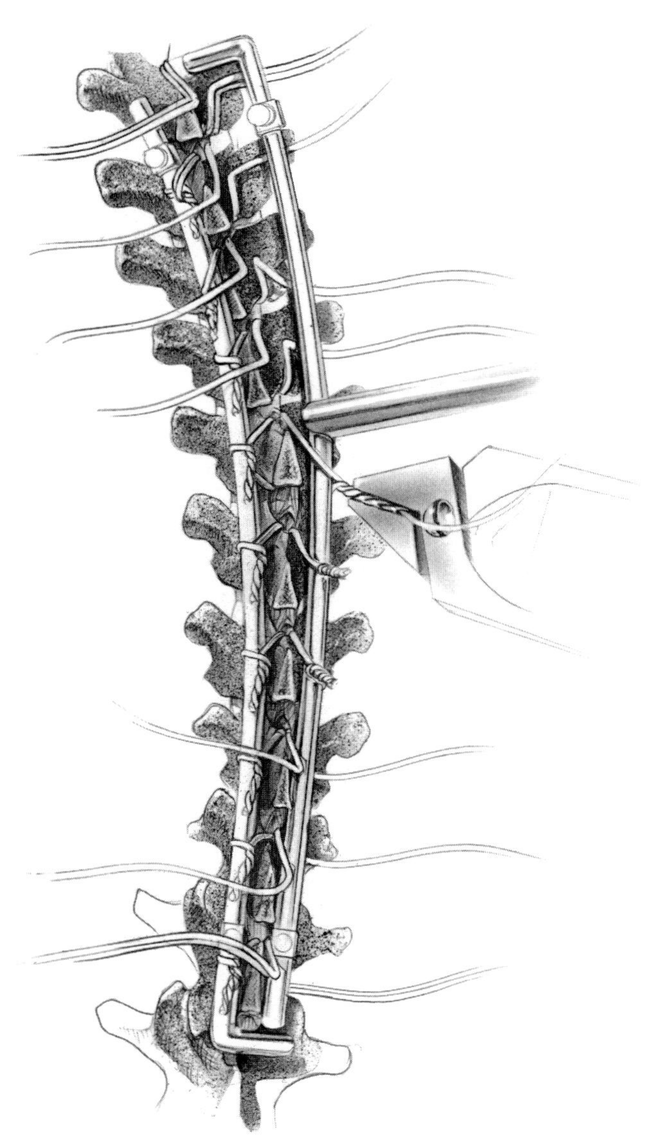

Figure 1–28

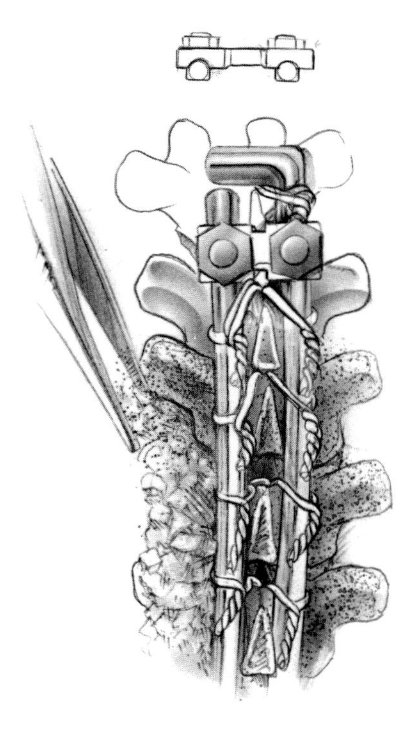

Figure 1–29

Figure 1–30. The postoperative radiographs of a 12-year-old girl with spastic quadriparesis demonstrate the use of Luque rods with Texas Scottish Rite cross-links and fixation to the pelvis by the Galveston technique. Note the failure of the instrumentation to derotate the lumbar spine, although the lumbar lordosis is well preserved.

POSTOPERATIVE CARE

Except in cases of unusually soft bone, no postoperative immobilization is required. Most of the patients in whom this technique is used tolerate casts and orthoses poorly. Early mobilization is possible with most patients, beginning with sitting on the third or fourth postoperative day. Although parents are often concerned about how they may lift and handle their children after surgery, they can be reassured that no changes in their usual routine are necessary.

REFERENCES

1. Schultz AB, Hirsch C. Mechanical analysis of techniques for improved correction of idiopathic scoliosis. Clin Orthop 1974;100:66.
2. Wilber G et al. Postoperative neurological deficits in segmental spinal instrumentation. J Bone Joint Surg 1984;66A:1178.
3. Allen BL, Ferguson RL. The Galveston technique for L rod instrumentation of the scoliotic spine. Spine 1982;7:276.

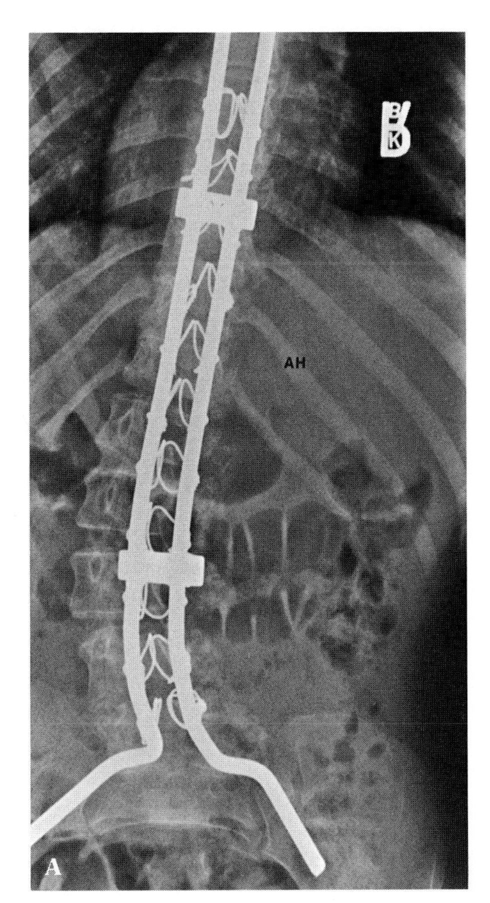

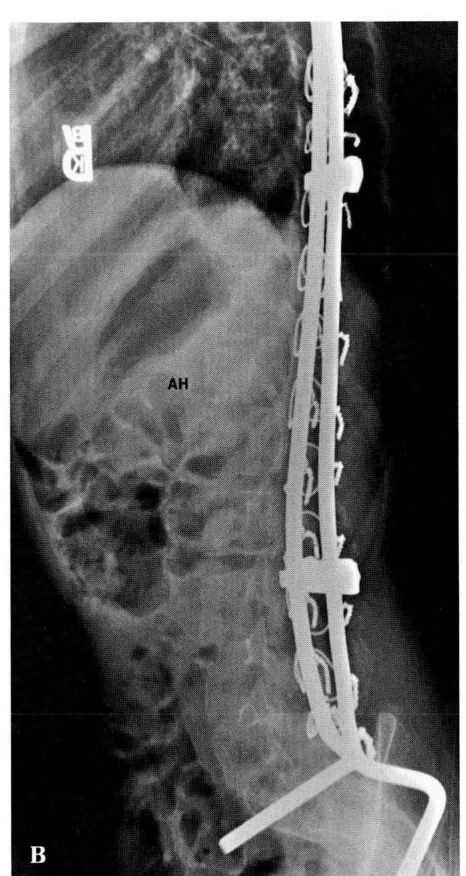

Figure 1–30

1.5 Galveston Pelvic Instrumentation

Figure 1–31. The Galveston technique of pelvic fixation has largely replaced the original technique described by Luque in which the bent segment of the rod was passed transversely through both tables of the ilium. In the Galveston technique the segment of the rod that is in the pelvis passes between the two tables of cortical bone in the thickest portion of the ilium—the transverse portion just cephalad to the sciatic notch.[1]

The foremost advantage of this method is the secure fixation it provides in all planes. The rods can be contoured at the operating table and do not require prebending with special instruments or techniques. The main disadvantage is the difficulty in bending the rods to fit properly. This can largely be overcome by understanding the proper technique as well as experience. Both are necessary. A theoretic disadvantage is that the instrumentation extends to an area outside of the fusion area. The motion that results is reflected in the loosening evidenced by the "windshield wiper" effect seen with the original Luque method. This has not proved to be of any clinical consequence.

Figure 1–32. From the midline incision both iliac crests are exposed. Unlike the exposure for obtaining a bone graft from a midline incision, this entire dissection is best carried out deep to the paravertebral muscles so that the rod can lie in contact with the bone and be covered with the muscle. Elevating the muscle is aided by a transverse cut at the caudal extent of the muscle. The periosteum over the posterior crest is incised, and the posterior crest as well as the outer table of the ilium is exposed. The sciatic notch should be visible as it serves as a guide to the pelvic segment of the rod. Bone graft can be obtained from the more cephalad portion of the ilium where it will not interfere with the purchase of the rod. In most cases in which this technique is used, however (*eg*, paralytic scoliosis), the ilium is very thin and what little bone is harvested does not make this worthwhile.

Figure 1–33. It will take two bends and one twist to produce the finished rod that will consist of three segments. The first segment is that which will lie between the two cortical tables of the ilium and is called the iliac segment (*A*). The second part of the rod will run from the ilium transversely to the area adjacent to the sacral spinous process and is called the sacral segment (*B*). The last segment is the one that will be fixed to the spinal vertebrae and is called the spinal segment (*C*).

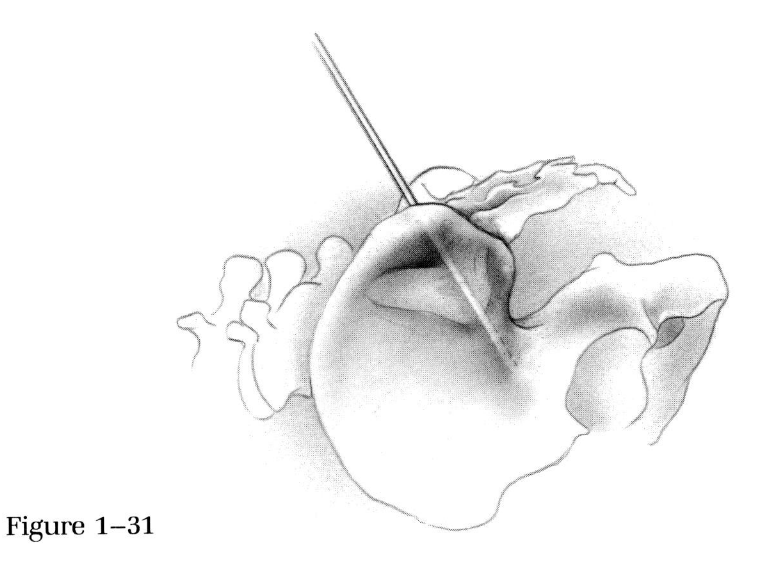

Figure 1–31

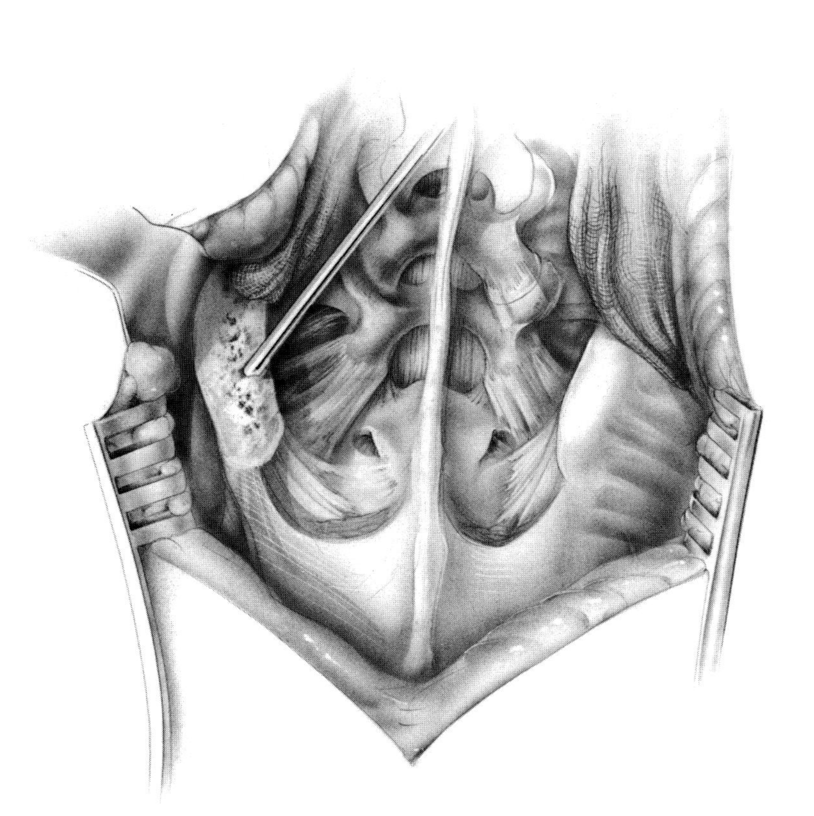

Figure 1–32

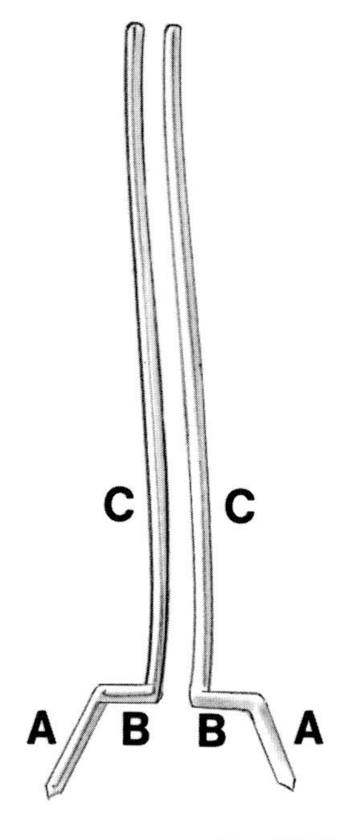

Figure 1–33

Figure 1–34. The hole for the iliac segment is made with a drill. If desired a guide pin can be inserted in this hole to be used with a special jigg to aid in bending the correct contours into the rod (see ***Figure 1–39***). After a little experience, however, it is easier simply to bend the rods and make minor adjustments with the rod in place. The hole is started slightly cephalad to the posterior inferior iliac spine and the drill directed between the two tables of the ilium to pass just cephalad to the sciatic notch. The depth of the hole will vary between 6 and 9 cm, depending on the size of the child.

Figure 1–35. The depth of the hole should be noted. It will usually be around 7 to 8 cm. This is the length of the iliac segment of the rod (*A*). In addition, the distance from the hole to a point adjacent to the sacral spinous process should be noted. This is usually 2 to 2.5 cm and represents the sacral segment of the rod (*B*). The rod is now bent with two tube rod benders to place a 60- to 80-degree bend in the rod at a distance from the end of the rod that is equal to the length of both the iliac and sacral segment of the rod (*A, B*). On the concave side of the curve, the rod will fit better if the bend is less (*ie,* about 60 degrees). On the convex side, 80 degrees is usually correct.

Figure 1–36. The next step is to place the bend that will separate the iliac segment from the sacral segment. With a tube bender on the iliac section and a rod clamp on the sacral segment, a bend is placed that will allow the rod to reach the sacral lamina when the iliac segment is inserted. In calculating the measurement with the bend, it should be remembered that the bend in the rod itself will account for at least 0.5 cm. It is also important to remember that although the technique for bending the opposite rods is identical, they will be mirror images of each other.

Figure 1–37. The three sections of the rod are now formed. At this point the rod cannot be placed.

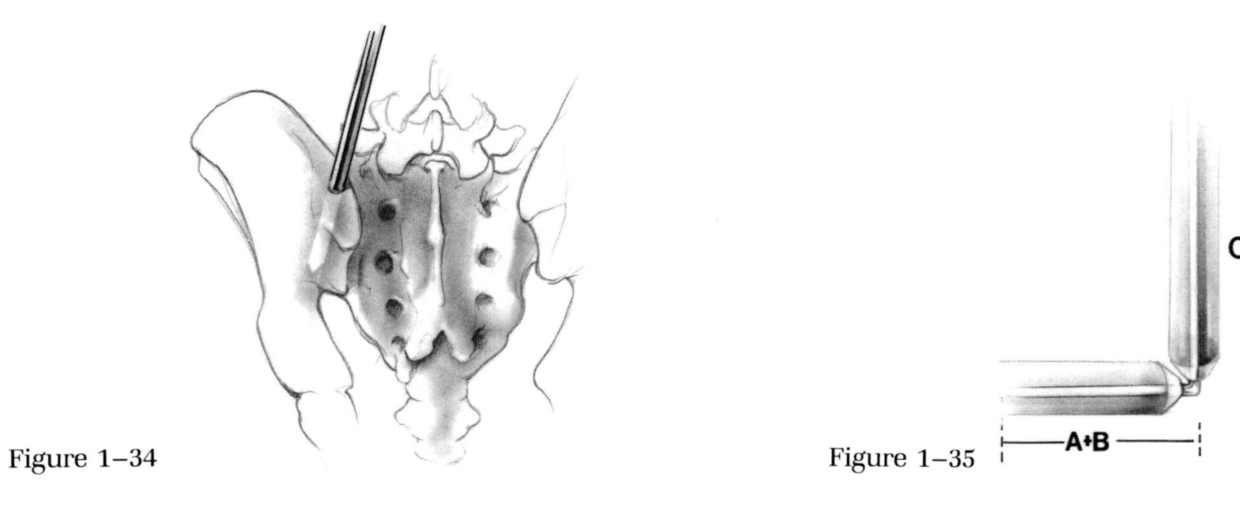

Figure 1–34

Figure 1–35

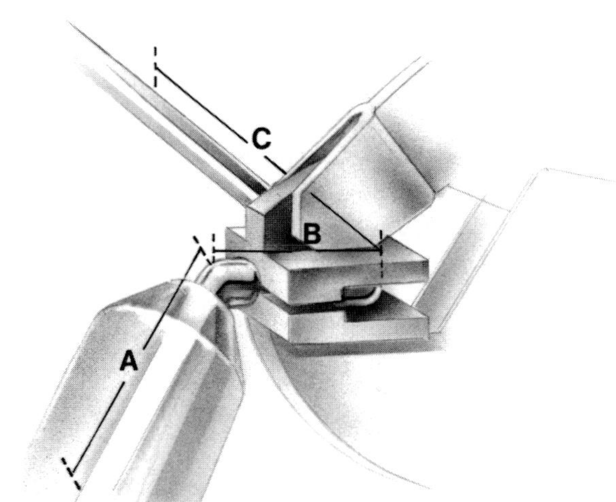

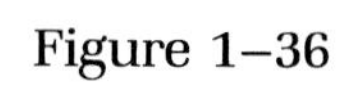
Figure 1–36

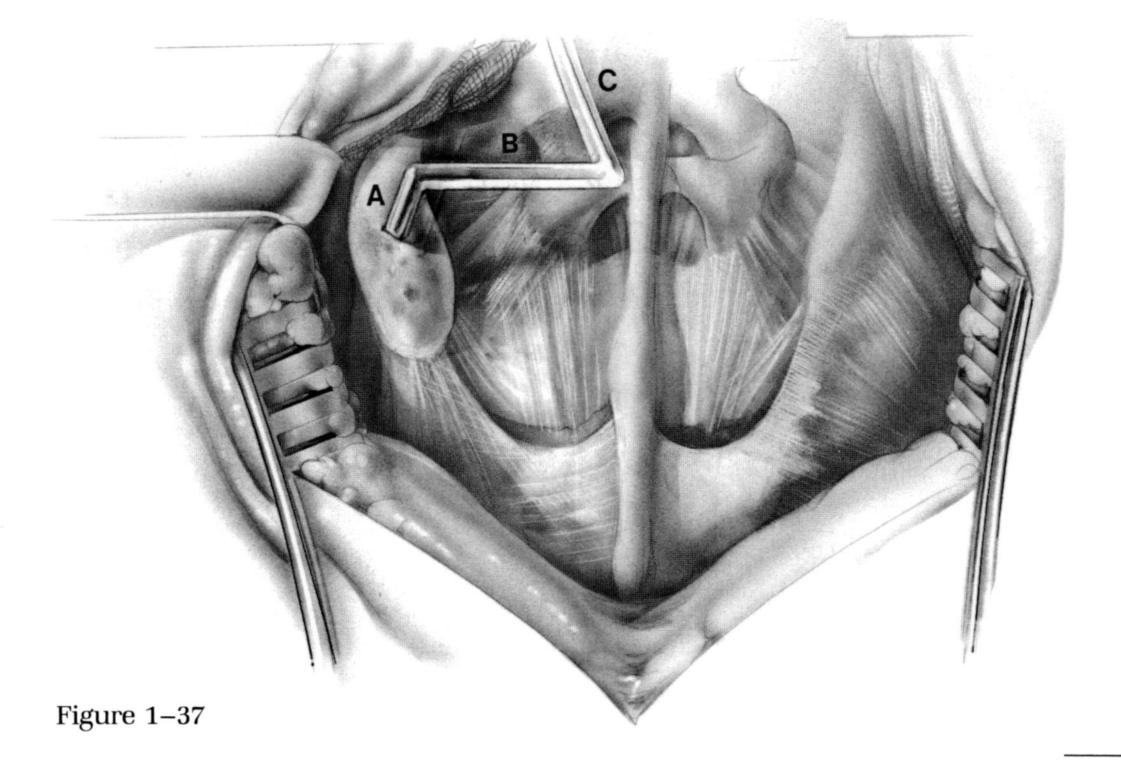

Figure 1–37

Figure 1–38. The last step is to place a twist in the rod in the sacral segment (***Figure 1–38B***). The purpose of this is to allow the rod to conform to the sacral inclination. Although this can be done to some extent by bending lordosis into the rod, it is usually difficult to bend in sufficient lordosis close enough to the junction of the sacral and spinal sections to have the rod lie on the sacral lamina. This twist is created by placing a tube rod bender on the spinal (*C*) and iliac segment (*A*). The benders are brought toward each other. This will produce a more ventrally directed spinal section, which will conform better to the sacrum. The amount of twist to be placed must be estimated because the rod cannot be placed at this point.

Figure 1–39. Finally the desired spinal contours are bent into the rod. It is best to start with lordosis because it will not be possible to place the rod in the iliac hole and next to the spine until this is done. Although a rod guide can be used with a pelvic guide pin in the iliac hole and the double-rod guide, this technique will usually result in less than a perfect fit and after a short learning curve is easily omitted.

Figure 1–40. After the rod is contoured and the proper fit of both rods is assured, the facet excision, any desired decortication, and passage of the sublaminar wires is completed. The rod can now be inserted and wired into place.

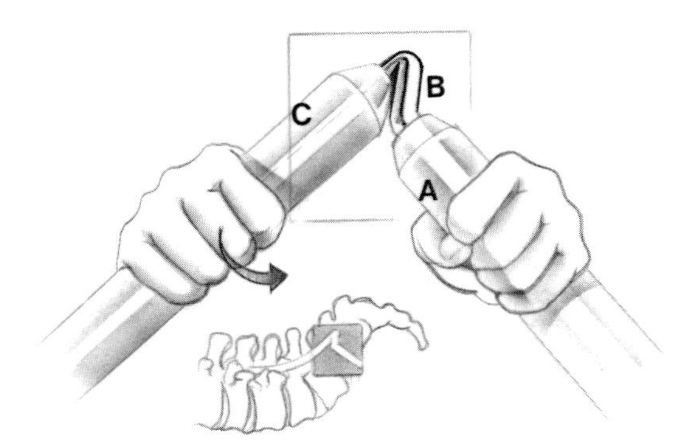

Figure 1–38

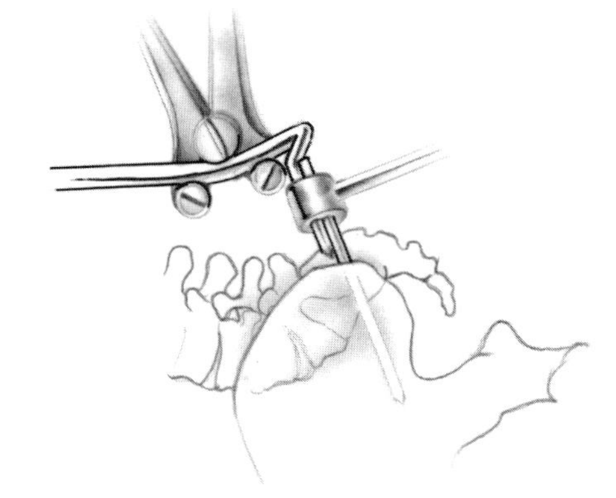

Figure 1–39

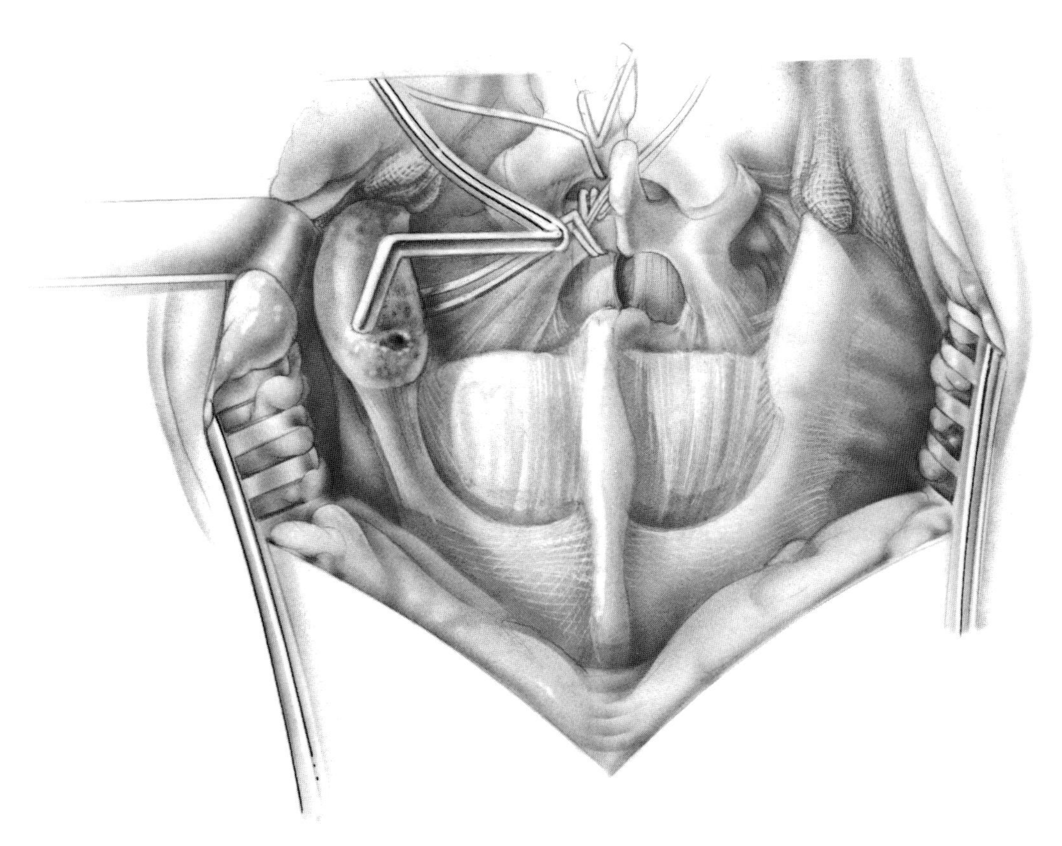

Figure 1–40

Figure 1–41. After the rods are in place, and even after some of the wires have been tightened, it is possible to make adjustments in the spinal segment with a pair of rod benders. The rod benders supplied with the Cotrel-Dubousset instrumentation are ideal because of their slim contours. After the first rod is in place, consideration should be given to placing the second rod. It is very likely that after tightening some of the wires on the spinal segment of the first rod, the contour of the spine will have changed. The contour of the spinal segment of the second rod may need to be adjusted.

POSTOPERATIVE CARE

In general postoperative immobilization is not used. Most of the patients in whom this pelvic fixation will be used have spinal deformity because of neuromuscular disease and therefore are not good candidates for immobilization. The fixation is extremely rigid, but the iliac segment will become loose with time because of the motion between the ilium and the sacrum. It is doubtful that cast immobilization will prevent this motion. There are no good long-term reports of many patients in which the fusion rate between L5 and the sacrum can be determined.

REFERENCE

1. Allen BL, Ferguson RL. The Galveston technique for L rod instrumentation of the scoliotic spine. Spine 1982;7:276.

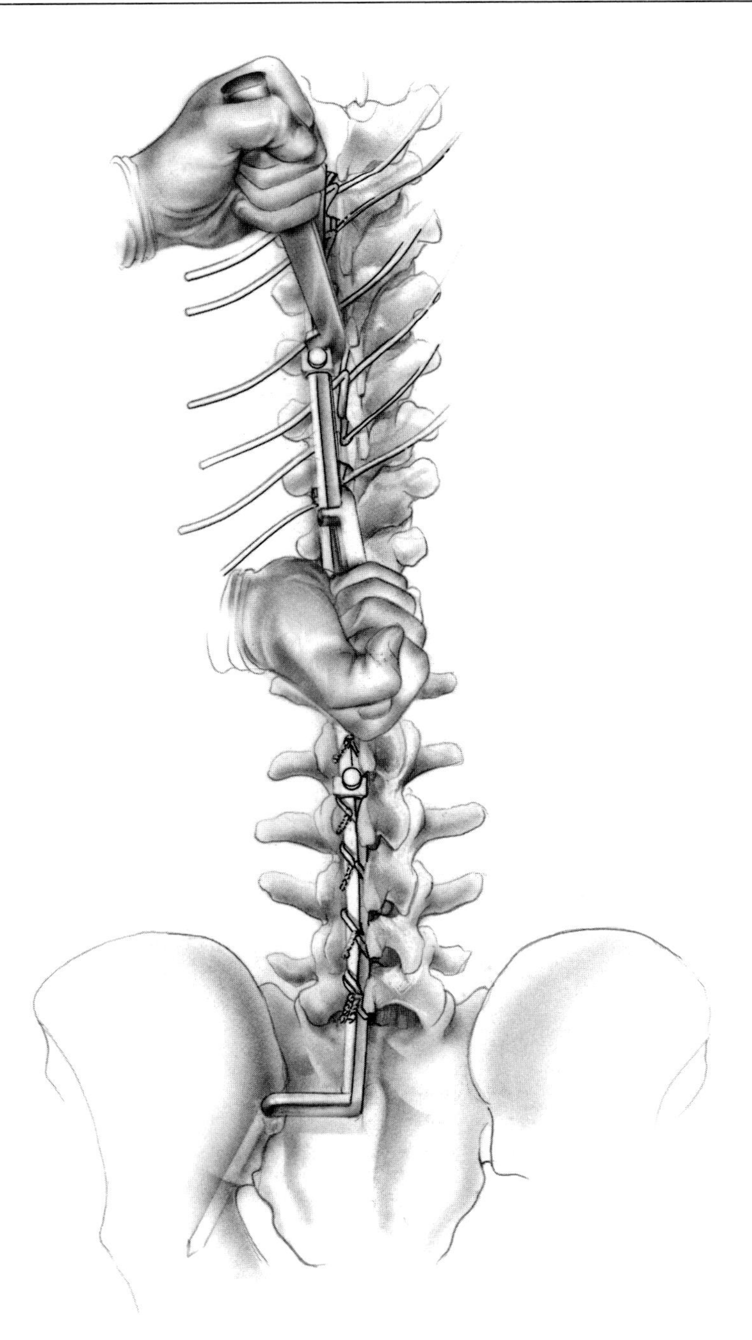

Figure 1–41

1.6 Dunn-McCarthy Pelvic Fixation

An alternative to the Galveston type of pelvic fixation is that described by McCarthy, Dunn, and McCullough.[1] In this technique the ends of the Luque rods are prebent to fit over the sacral ala in the manner of large alar hooks. This technique may be particularly indicated when the pelvis is very thin or small and is mechanically at its best in the correction of kyphosis, and contradicted in lordosis.

The end of the rod that is to fit over the sacral ala must be bent before the operation. The tight bends necessitate that the rods be flame heated to soften the metal before bending. Bends of two different dimensions can be made, one at each end of a long Luque rod. The one of these that fits the least well can be cut off at surgery and discarded. It is necessary that the rods be bent so that they are mirror images of each other.

Figure 1–42. Measurement from the preoperative radiographs will aid in achieving the correct dimensions of the bends. The first consideration is that the midportion of the sacral ala is lateral to the midportion of the lamina. This amount of lateral offset in the rod can be estimated by measuring the distance from the midportion of the L5 lamina to the midportion of the sacral ala (***Figure 1–42A***). This will usually be about 1 to 1.5 cm in the typical patient. The width of the segment that is to go over the sacral ala is measured from the lateral radiograph of the pelvis (***Figure 1–42B***). This width will usually be between 1 to 1.5 cm also. If this is to be used in the bifid myelodysplastic spine, careful preoperative planning is necessary to be sure that the rod lies in the desired position.

At surgery the sacral ala is cleaned as it would be for lumbosacral arthrodesis. It is important that the hook portion of the rod pass anterior to the alae, thus necessitating that the dissection be carried slightly more anterior than usual. Before seating the rod it should be possible to pass a finger around the front of the alae.

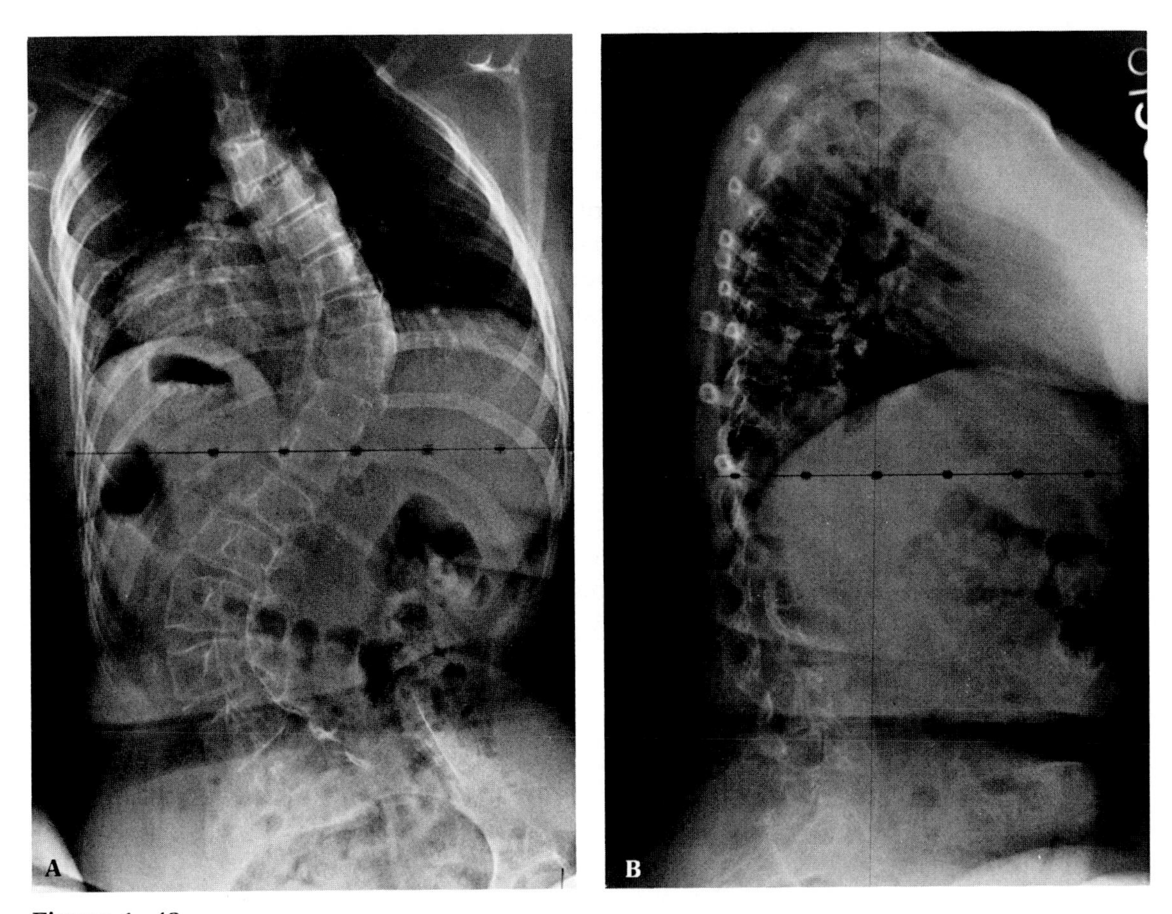

Figure 1–42

Figure 1–43. The prebent (***Figures 1–43A–C***) portion of the rod is hooked on the ala like a giant sacral hook. It does not penetrate the cortex. It is possible to make minor adjustments to the rods during surgery, but it is not possible to bend all of the necessary curves into the rod in the operating room. Contouring lordosis into the sacral segment of the rod will position it more firmly against the sacral alae. Use of the Texas Scottish Rite cross-links on the spinal segment of the rods will prevent movement of one rod in relation to one another and provide a rigid construct. The rod is held in place over the sacral alae by the sublaminar wires.

Figure 1–44. Anterior (***Figure 1–44A***) and posterior (***Figure 1–44B***) radiographs of the patient illustrated following posterior arthrodesis and instrumentation with the Dunn-McCarthy technique. (Courtesy of Richard McCarthy, MD.)

POSTOPERATIVE CARE

This fixation is as rigid as the Galveston fixation, and, therefore, may or may not require immobilization depending on the surgeon's choice and the circumstances.

REFERENCE

1. McCarthy RE, Dunn H, McCullough FL. Luque fixation to the sacral ala using the Dunn-McCarthy modification. Spine 1989;14:281.

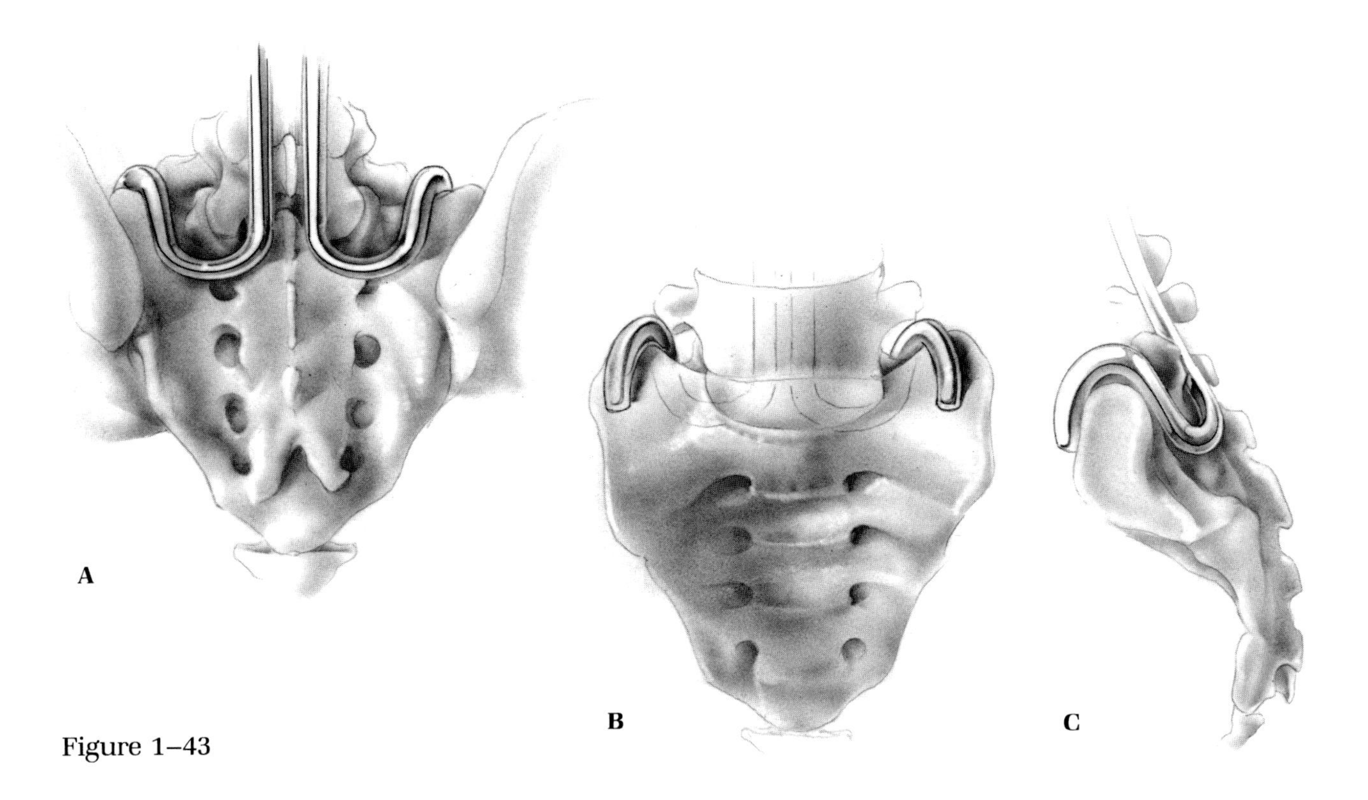

Figure 1–43

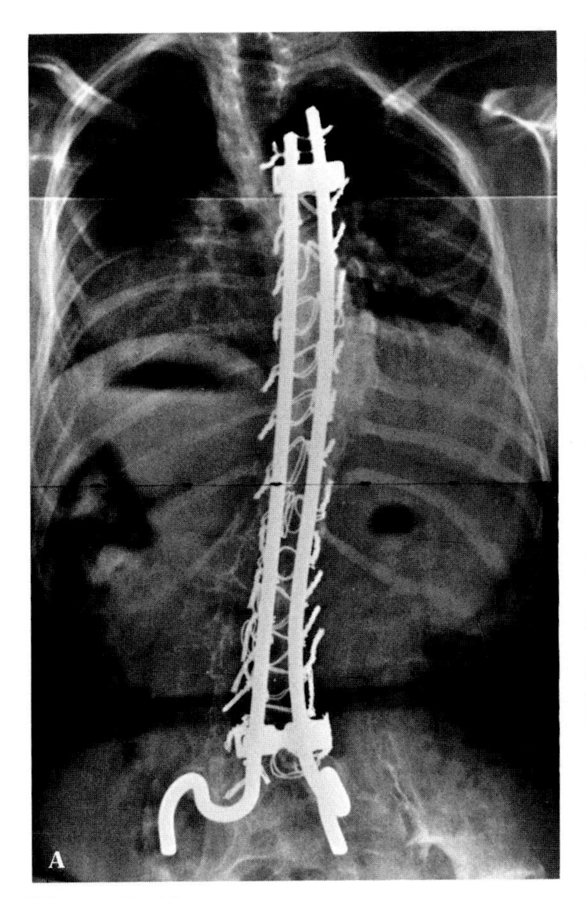

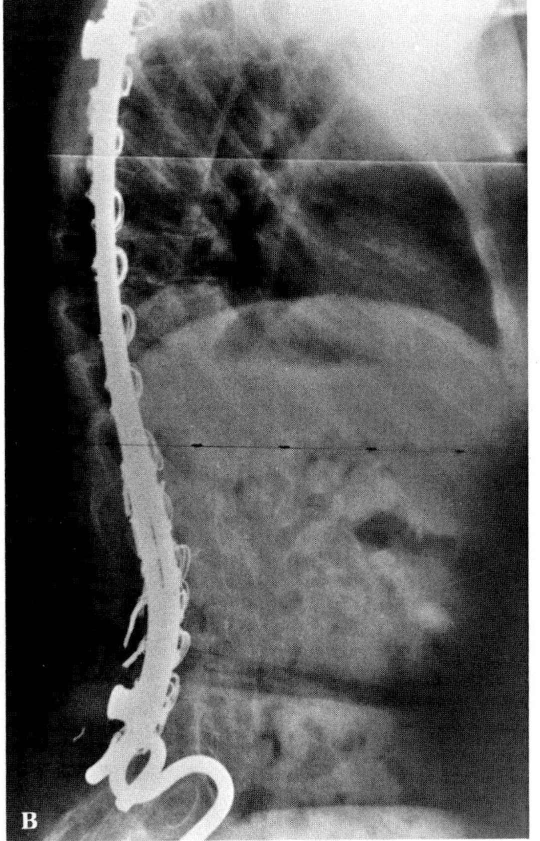

Figure 1–44

1.7 Cotrel-Dubousset Instrumentation for Scoliosis

The Cotrel-Dubousset instrumentation represents more than just different instrumentation for scoliosis deformity. It introduces several new concepts in instrumentation. It is designed and constructed in such a way that multiple hooks are placed on the same rod that allows for simultaneous compression and distraction forces on the same rod. The hooks can be rotated on the rod with correction being achieved mainly through rotation and not distraction. Two rods are used and linked together to produce a rigid, rectangular frame, obviating the need for postoperative immobilization.[1]

One of the main claims for the Cotrel-Dubousset instrumentation is that it derotates the spine. It has been observed that there is no definite relationship between the amount of rib deformity and the amount of vertebral rotation,[2] and that Harrington rod distraction can improve the rib deformity without affecting vertebral rotation.[3] Complete evaluation of the Cotrel-Dubousset instrumentation is not yet available; however, clinical experience to date supports the claim that Cotrel-Dubousset instrumentation reduces the rib deformity to a greater degree than any previous posterior instrumentation. Its effect on actually derotating the thoracic vertebrae is still debated, although there is general agreement that it does not produce much derotation of the lumbar vertebrae nor does it reduce the lumbar rotational deformity to the extent that it does in the thoracic spine. The ability to rotate, distract, and compress the hooks on the same rod results in correction and maintenance of the sagittal contour better than any other method. The rigidity and strength of the fixation allows freedom from postoperative immobilization.

Early evaluation has also demonstrated several potential disadvantages. The instrumentation is more complex than previous methods and has a steeper learning curve as witnessed by a slightly higher incidence of neurologic complications with this method.[4] The increased complexity of the instrumentation coupled with the increased surface occupied by the hooks (often on both lamina of a vertebra) both encourage and permit less thorough decortication. This is a potential problem in an operation that is primarily designed to achieve an arthrodesis. Finally, the instrumentation is very expensive.

Figure 1–45. The unique design principles of this instrumentation are two: a rod with a knurled surface on which each hook can be secured individually in any position and hooks that in some locations can grasp the pedicle for better rotational control. A variety of special instruments and knowledge of their use are also required.

There are two types of hooks: pedicle hooks that are bifid and are designed to straddle the pedicle (***Figures 1–45A, B***) and lamina hooks that are similar to the Harrington hooks (***Figures 1–45C–F***). There are two types of lamina hooks, thoracic (***Figures 1–45C, E***) and lumbar (***Figures 1–45D, F***), which vary in the depth and size of the blade portion. The part of the hook that attaches to the rod is either open or closed. The open hooks are secured to the rod by a blocker (***Figure 1–45G***), which slides onto the rod and then slides into the opening of the hook. Blockers and closed hooks are locked to the rod by set screws. The last component of the system is the C ring (***Figure 1–45H***), which is also furnished with a set screw. Tightening the set screw of the C ring adjacent to a hook in which the set screw is not tightened allows the hook to be firmly held in place in distraction and at the same time allows the rod to rotate on the hook.

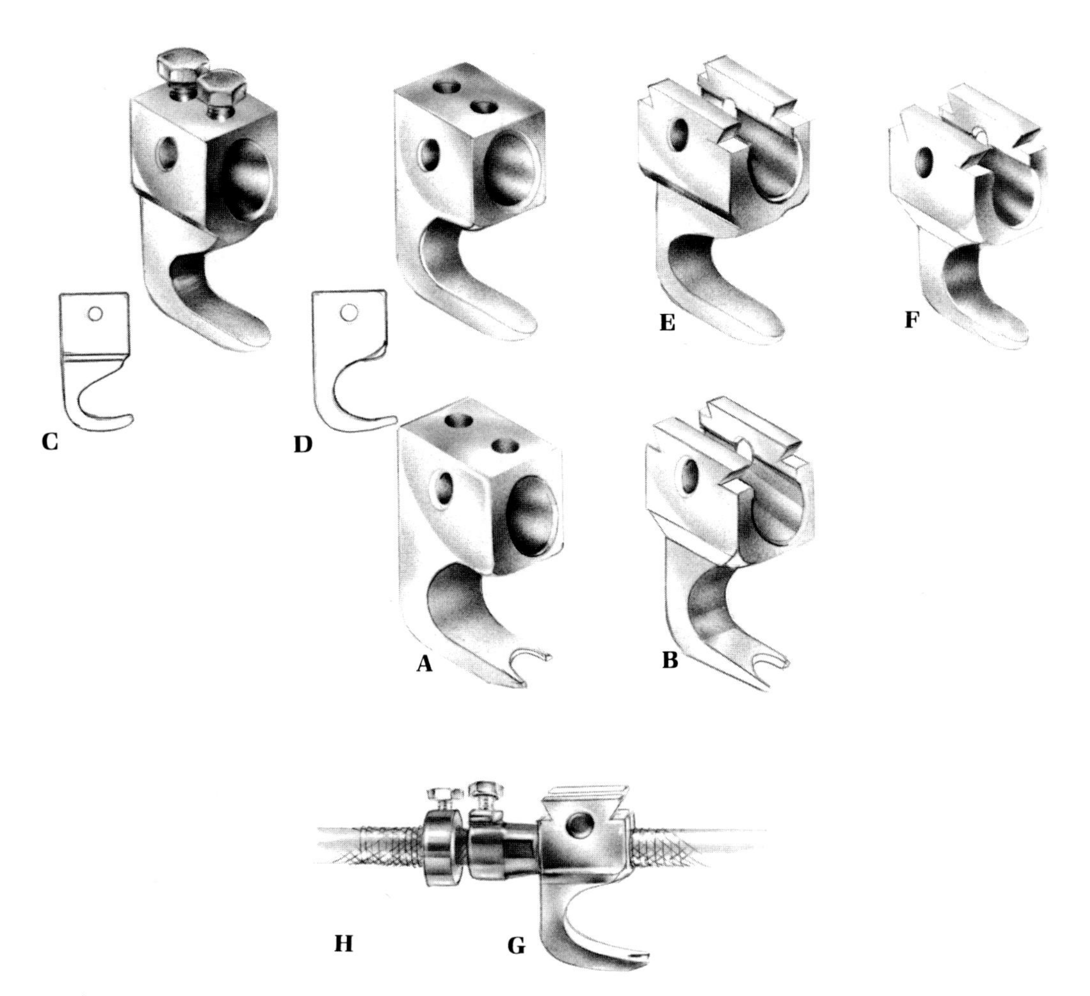

Figure 1–45

Figure 1–46. Preparation of the patient and exposure of the spine are the same as for Harrington instrumentation. Preplanning of hook placement is essential, however. This can be clearly marked on the preoperative radiograph to guide both the surgeon and the nurse (***Figure 1–46A***).

Selection of levels for fusion follows many of the principles outlined by King et al.[5] Experience has demonstrated one important exception related to selective fusion in the type II curve, however. The guidelines proposed by King et al[5] have frequently been noted to produce decompensation of the spine to the left when only the right thoracic curve is corrected in a type II curve. There is as yet no universal agreement on the proper selection of the most inferior vertebra to be instrumented when treating a type II curve with Cotrel-Dubousset instrumentation.

The use of the instrumentation is demonstrated on a single thoracic curve. The upper and lower vertebra on the concave side are selected on the criteria of King et al.[5] The cephalad vertebra should extend beyond the hypokyphosis seen on the lateral radiograph (***Figure 1–46B***). The stiffest segment of the spine as determined on the bending radiograph is noted (***Figure 1–46C***) and two hooks are placed on either side of this segment. On the convex side of the curve, the top and bottom vertebra are instrumented as is the apical vertebra. The lower hook on the convex side of the curve is the most frequent to dislodge. To help secure this a "claw" configuration can be used to securely lock it in place. Although the "claw" configuration using the transverse process of the most cephalad vertebra and the pedicle of the vertebra below is recommended for the top vertebra on the convex side, this seems unnecessarily difficult. A simple laminar hook in compression on the top vertebra is sufficient.

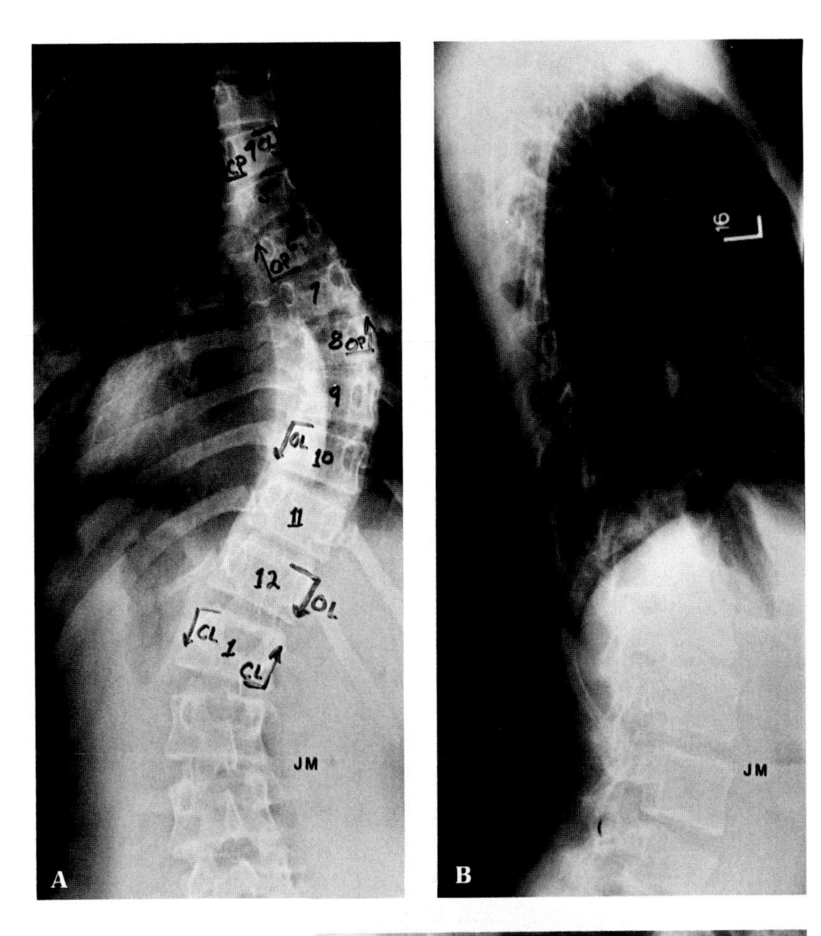

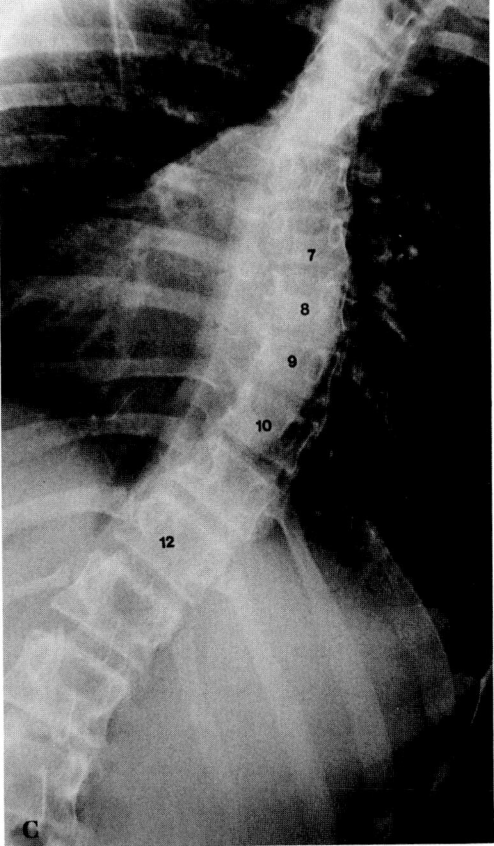

Figure 1–46

Figure 1–47. The thoracic hooks at or above T10 that are facing cephalad are pedicle hooks. The lamina is prepared for these hooks in much the same way as it is in the Harrington technique (***Figure 1–47A***). Sufficient lamina should be removed to permit the bifid portion of the pedicle hook to engage the pedicle (***Figures 1–47C, D***). After removing the caudal edge of the lamina, the pedicle finder is used to locate the pedicle (***Figures 1–47A, B***). Great care should be used with this tool, for as supplied there is no block on the tool to prevent it from sliding deep into the spinal canal. To ascertain that the pedicle has been engaged and thus identified, an attempt is made to move the pedicle finder medial and lateral. If the pedicle has not been engaged, the pedicle finder may strike the cord when it is moved medially, especially if it is also being pushed cephalad. After the pedicle is identified, the appropriate hook is inserted. Closed hooks are used at the ends and open hooks for the remainder. Hooks placed in the lumbar region and hooks facing caudal cannot engage the pedicle, and therefore laminar hooks are used in these areas in the same manner as Harrington distraction hooks. Lumbar hooks may be used in the thoracic spine and vice versa. Their use is dictated by which fits best. In this regard attention should be paid to the fact that a lumbar hook with its deeper blade placed on a small thoracic lamina may be pushed into the canal when the rod is rotated.

Figure 1–48. The hooks have been placed on the concave side. Notice that the facets have been excised on both sides, and the convex hook sites at T4, T8, T12, and L1 have been prepared. Excision of all of the facets is best done before any correction because it will increase the mobility of the spine. Decortication of the spine is done on each side before rod insertion on that side. Bone graft should be placed beneath the rod and in each facet.

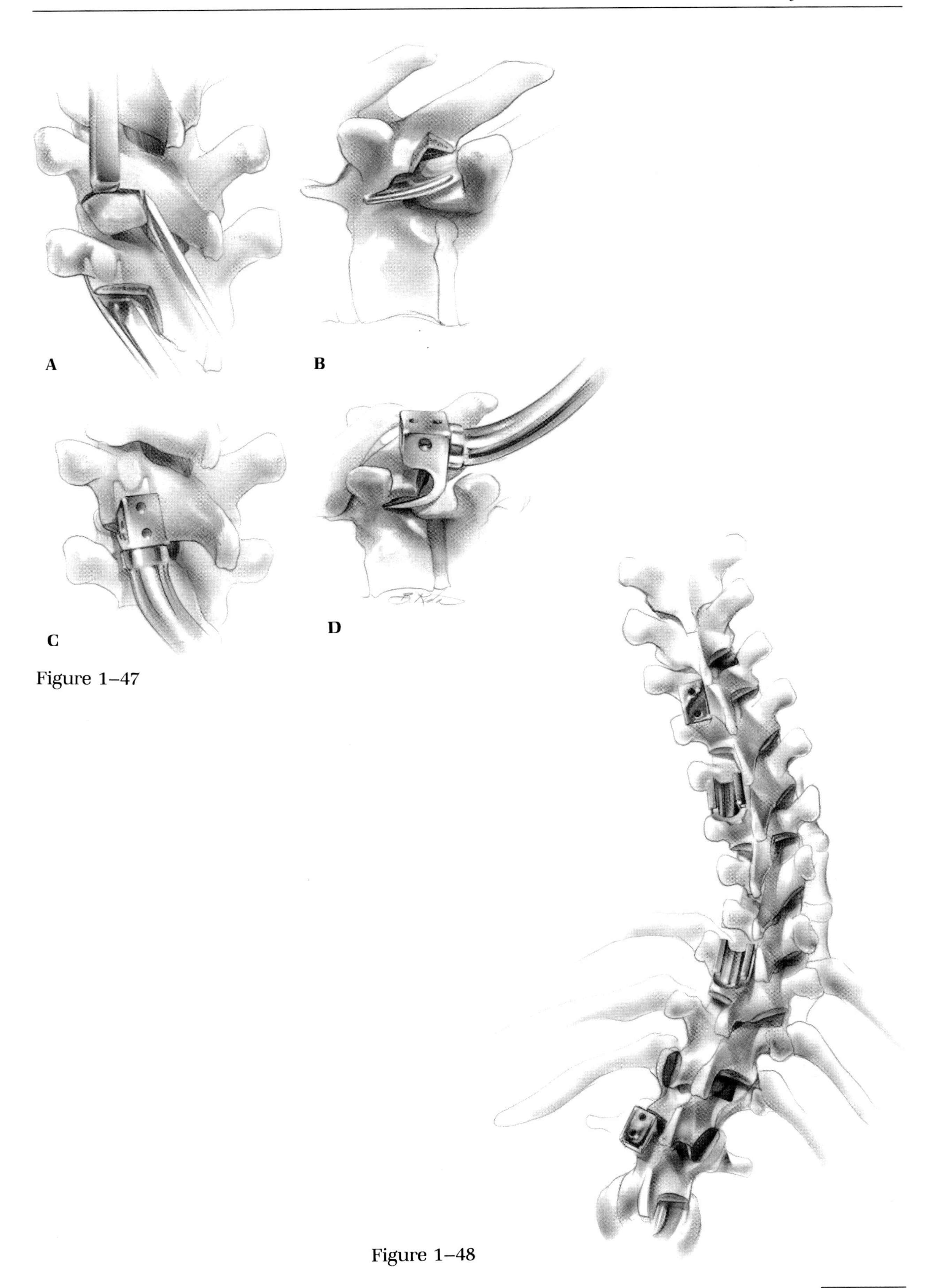

Figure 1–47

Figure 1–48

Figure 1–49. The rod is contoured to conform to the normal sagittal contour of the segment to be fused. In most areas this will nearly conform to the scoliosis when the rod is rotated 90 degrees. In other areas such as the open distraction hook at T11, however, the rod will usually not be close to the hook. The rod should not be contoured to make it easier for the rod to fit into the hook. Before placing the rod, care must be taken to put all of the blockers and attachments for the cross-links on the rod in their correct position. Note the two blockers facing in opposite directions for the two open hooks, and the two attachments for the Texas Scottish Rite cross-links (bolts for cross-links (*A*); blocker for cephalad-facing pedicle hook at T6 (*B*); and blocker for caudal-facing lamina hook at T9 (*C*)).

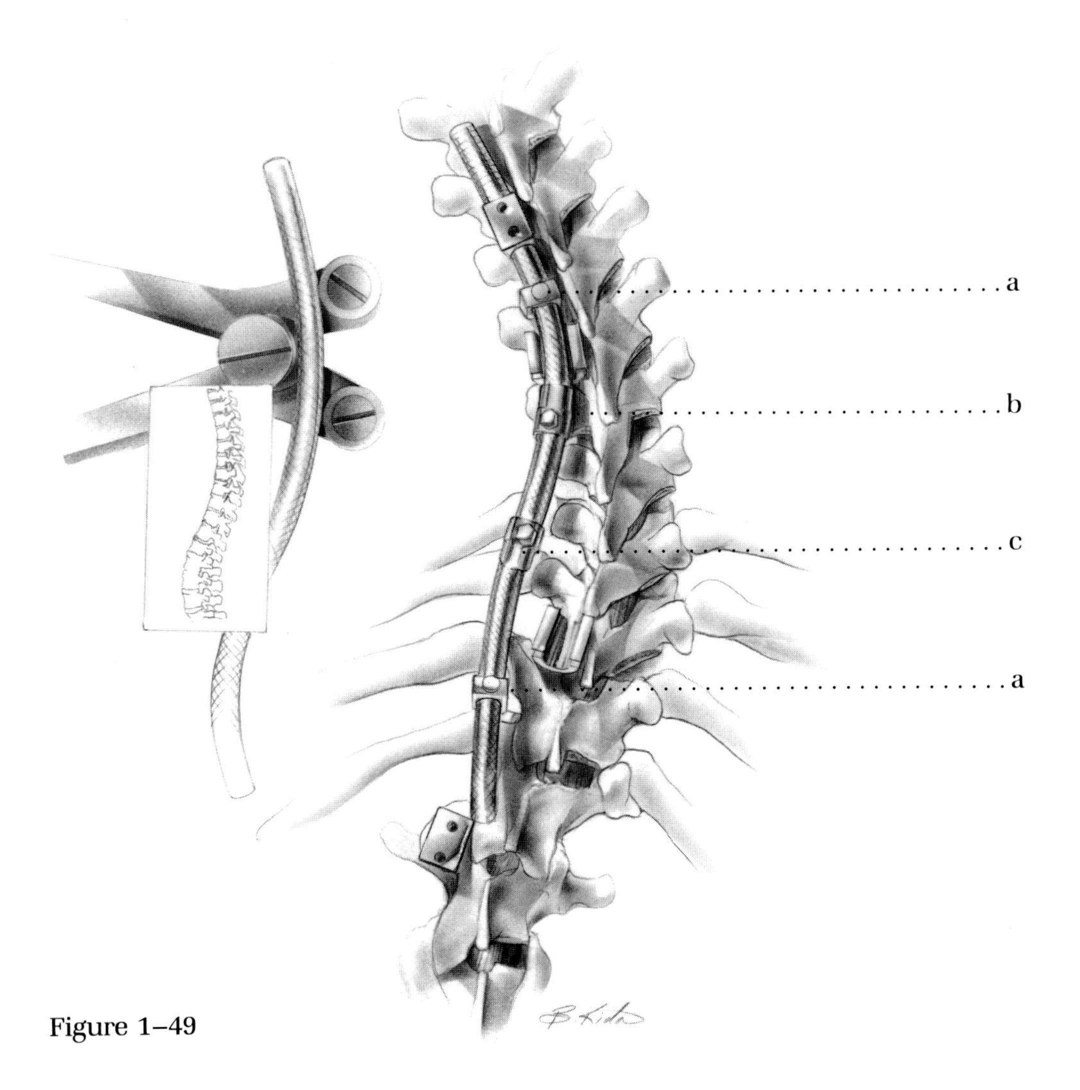

Figure 1–49

Figure 1–50. The rod is passed through the top closed hook and then pulled caudal and passed through the distal closed hook while these hooks are firmly held in place with a hook holder by an assistant. The bulb hook holder will be required to engage the rod with the hook at T10. This device is a hook holder that grasps the hook linked to a rod pusher that is screwed down on the rod, bringing the hook toward the rod (***Figure 1–50A***). As the bulb hook holder is tightened there is a tendency for the hook to pull out from under the lamina so it should be held firmly in place. After the rod is seated in the hook, the blocker is pushed into the hook securing it to the rod (***Figure 1–50B***). The set screw is partially tightened to secure the blocker.

After the rod has engaged all of the hooks, the C rings are applied. They are usually necessary only at the two intermediate hooks. These are necessary to hold the hook securely in place while at the same time allowing the rod to rotate on the hook. All of the set screws on the hooks and blockers should be loose to allow rotation of the rod. Before rotating the rod, it is important to set the hooks firmly so that they do not pull out. To do this a rod clamp is applied to the rod 2 to 3 cm from the hook, and the spreader is used to push against the C ring seating the hook firmly under the lamina (***Figures 1–50C, D***). The set screw of the C ring is then tightened but not broken off because this will later be removed. The set screw of the C ring should be placed toward the midline so that after rotation it will still be accessible for removal. Avoid the temptation to distract the spine at this point as excessive distraction may actually block rotation. Only enough force should be used to engage the hooks firmly so they do not disengage during rotation of the rod.

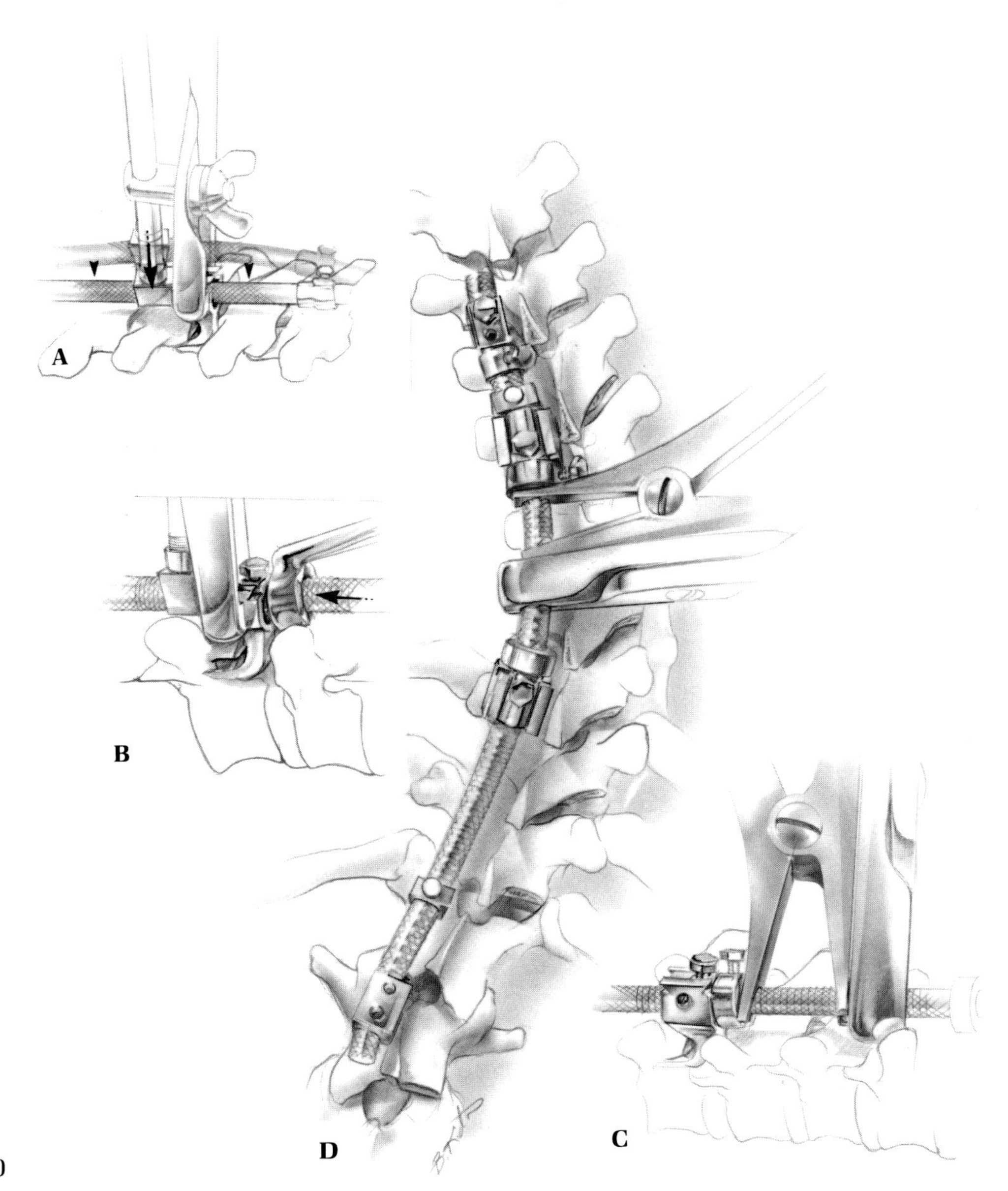

Figure 1–50

Figure 1–51. The rod is now grasped with two rod holders or vise grips, and rotation is begun. Rotation should be accomplished slowly with attention to the hooks to be sure they remain in place and show no signs of breaking a lamina. In particular, the top hook on the concave side has been reported to strike the spinal cord if this lamina breaks. As the rod is rotated the spine will be observed to straighten. This is accomplished by the curved portion of the rod moving dorsally and laterally. The degree of straightening is dependent on the flexibility of the spine, the correct contour of the rod, and the correct placement of the hooks. When rotation is completed the set screws on the hooks and blockers are tightened but not to the point of breaking them off. The C rings can then be removed.

In the typical curve illustrated here rotation of the rod will produce virtually all of the correction of the scoliosis that is obtained. After rotation is completed further distraction of each of the hooks can be obtained. This may produce some additional correction and will ensure that each of the hooks is firmly seated. To do this the spreader is opened between a rod clamp on the rod and the hook after the set screw is loosened.

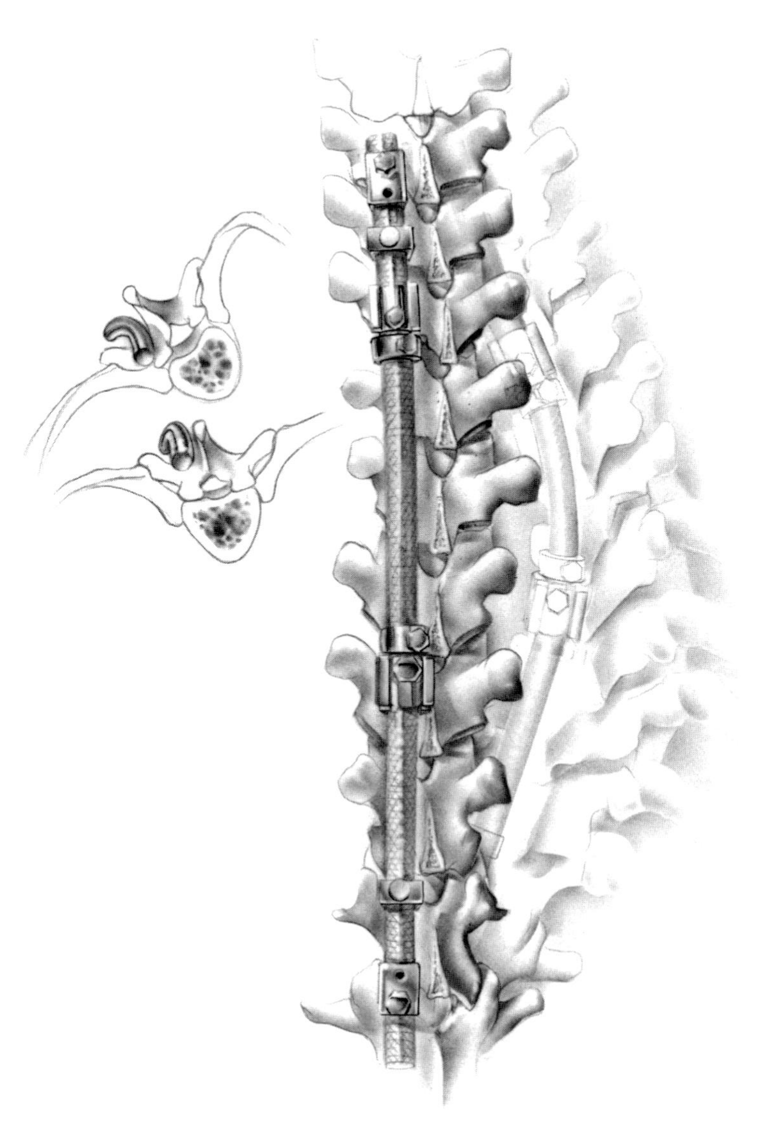

Figure 1–51

Figure 1–52. The convex rod is then inserted in a similar manner to the concave rod. It is recommended that the central portion of this rod be contoured flat so that when it is rotated the flat portion will tend to push down on the rotated vertebrae, producing further correction. It has been the author's observation that very little if any additional correction is gained with this rod in the usual curve. It does, however, provide additional rigidity by adding compression and allowing a rigid frame to be constructed (***Figure 1–52A***). The most cephalad hook is tightened first. The apical hook is then compressed against it and tightened. The most caudal hook is then compressed and tightened. Often there will be an insufficient amount of the rod protruding beyond the inferior hook for a rod clamp and spreader to be used. In this case a rod holder or C ring cephalad to the hook and the hook compression device can be used (***Figure 1–52B***). Finally, the hook on T12 is compressed against the hook on T1 and tightened, producing the "claw" configuration. Care should be taken to secure the most inferior hook, which has a tendency to dislodge. This can be done by deeply notching the lamina so the hook is well seated, compressing it securely, and, as illustrated in this case, using a "claw" configuration with an additional hook on T12.

The final stage is to secure the cross-links. The Texas Scottish Rite system is superior to other cross-link systems in that it provides torsional stiffness to the system.[6] The correct size must be selected so that the rod fits in the groove on the underside of the crossing plate. The rods may be pushed apart with a spreader or drawn closer together with a compression clamp if they do not fit exactly. Regardless of the length of the rods, two cross-links provide sufficient rigidity. Finally, all of the set screws (except on the C rings) are tightened until they break off. The C rings are then removed. This completes the instrumentation. Any remaining bone graft is added, and the wound is closed.

Figure 1–53. Postoperative radiographs demonstrate the correction of the scoliosis (*A*) and restoration of the sagittal contour (*B*).

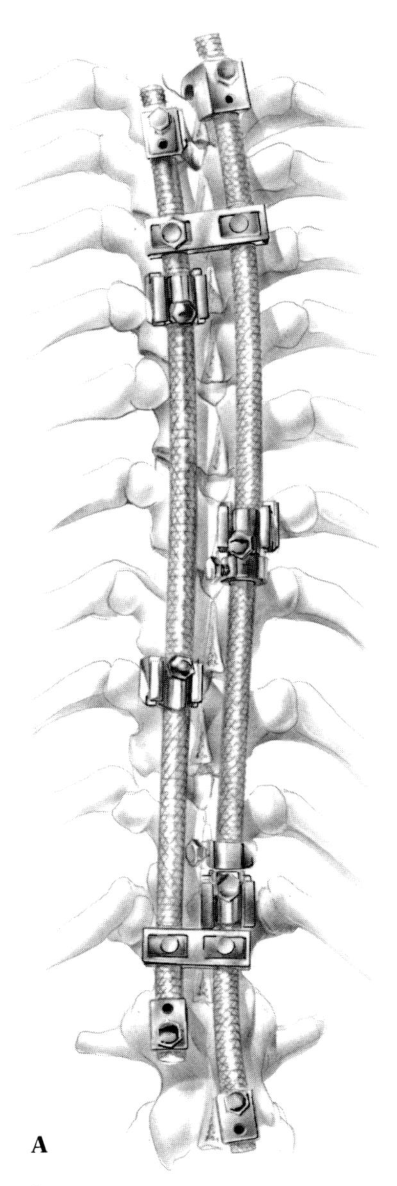

B

A

Figure 1–52

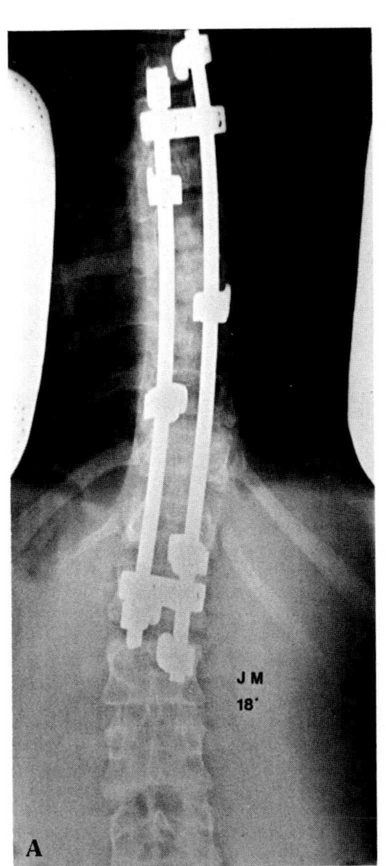

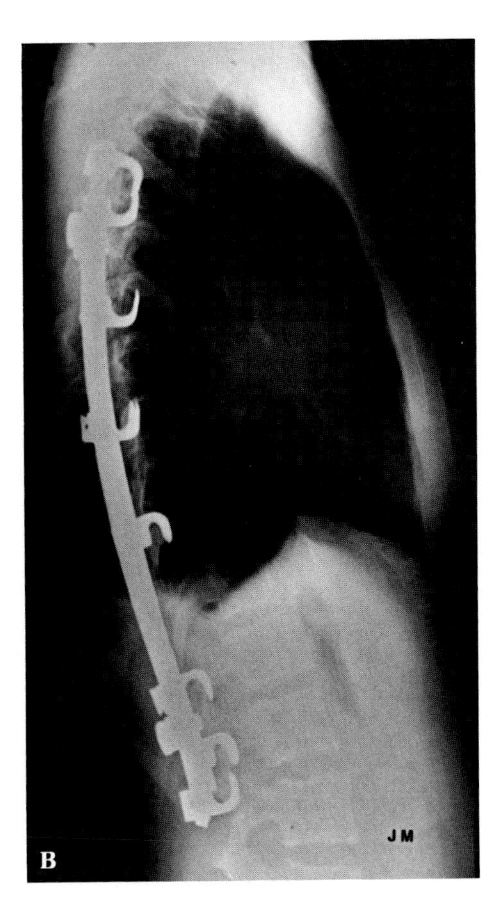

Figure 1–53

Figure 1–54. The use of the Cotrel-Dubousset instrumentation in a double curve is ideal from the viewpoint of preserving the normal lumbar lordosis while at the same time restoring the proper kyphosis to the thoracic spine (***Figure 1–54B, D***). It does not achieve the same degree of rotational correction in the lumbar spine as it does in the thoracic spine, however (***Figure 1–54A, C***).

POSTOPERATIVE CARE

The rigidity of the fixation is such that no special considerations need to be given in the immediate postoperative period to the movement or positioning of the patient. Patients are managed in the first 24 to 48 hours with pain medication delivered by a PCA pump, and "log rolling" in bed. On the second postoperative day the head of the bed is elevated, and by the third day the patient is assisted in sitting over the edge of the bed and standing. The patient is ambulatory by the fourth postoperative day, and is usually discharged on the sixth or seventh postoperative day. No postoperative immobilization is used. Patients are usually ready to attend school 3 weeks after the surgery. Patients are restricted from all strenuous and sporting activities for 6 to 9 months. Patients are seen at 1, 3, 6, and 9 months after surgery with radiographic assessment. After this period, follow-up is continued on a yearly basis.

REFERENCES

1. Cotrel Y, Dubousset J, Guillaumat M. New universal instrumentation in spinal surgery. Clin Orthop 1988;227:10.
2. Thulbourne T, Gillespie R. The rib hump in idiopathic scoliosis. J Bone Joint Surg 1976;58B:64.
3. Weatherley CR et al. The rib deformity in adolescent idiopathic scoliosis. J Bone Joint Surg 1987;69B:179.
4. Report on the Mortality and Morbidity Committee of the Scoliosis Research Society, 1987. (Unpublished)
5. King HA, Moe JH, Bradford DS, Winter RB. The selection of fusion levels in thoracic idiopathic scoliosis. J Bone Joint Surg 1983;65A:1302.
6. Ashman RB et al. Mechanical testing of spinal instrumentation. Clin Orthop 1988;227:113.

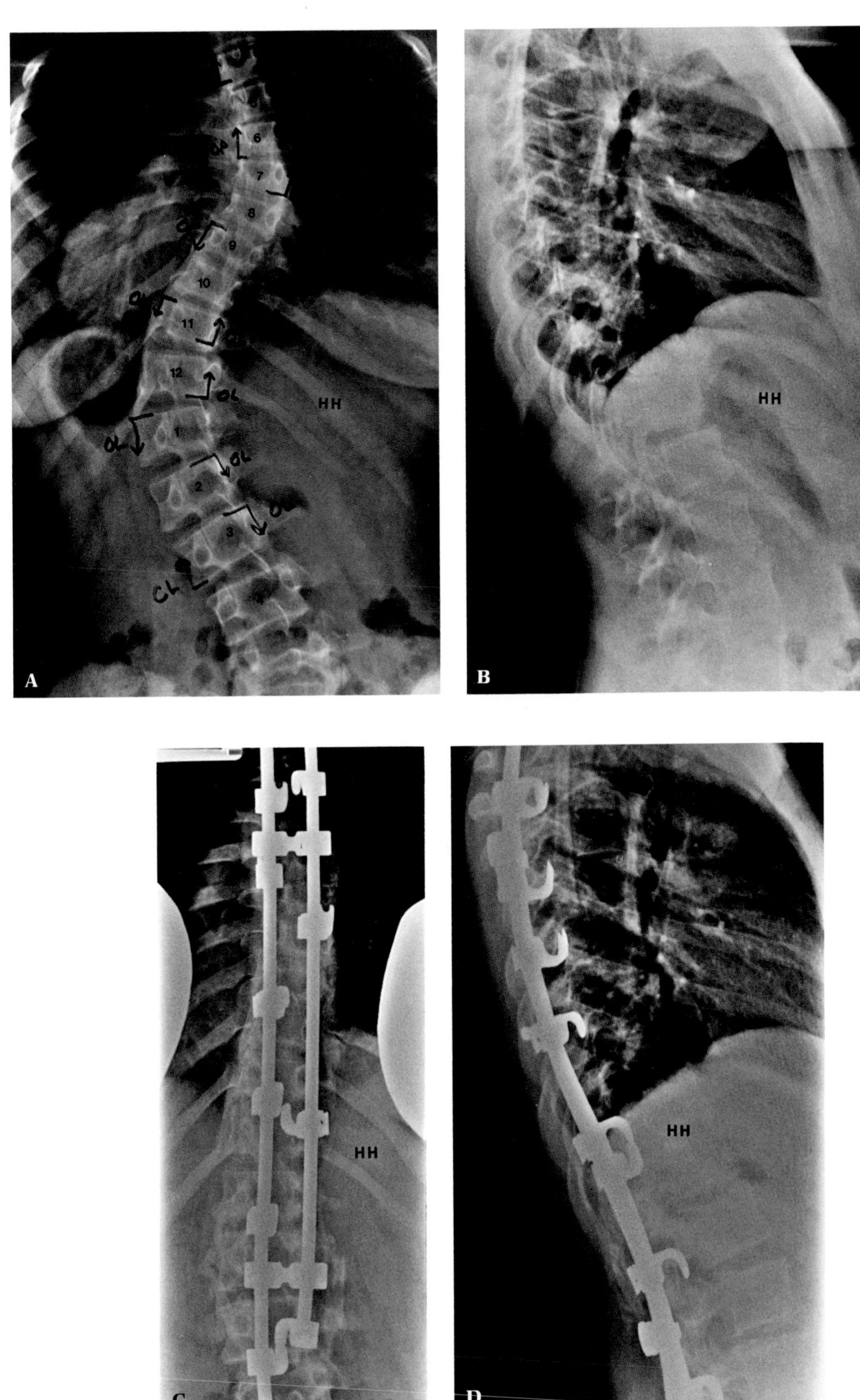

Figure 1–54

1.8 Anterior Thoracolumbar Arthrodesis With Zielke Instrumentation for Scoliosis

The Zielke instrumentation is the procedure of choice for many surgeons in the treatment of idiopathic thoracolumbar and lumbar curves,[1,2] and it is the instrumentation of choice for anterior instrumentation of scoliosis in general. It offers several improvements over the Dwyer instrumentation. The derotation possible with the Zielke system helps to minimize the creation of an iatrogenic kyphosis, while the adjustment of the correction is gradual and easily controlled. It is generally agreed that it is possible to fuse one less level caudal in the lumbar spine using the Zielke instrumentation compared with posterior techniques. This may be of considerable importance in the later incidence of low-back pain.[3] The Zielke, like the Dwyer, instrumentation is not indicated in thoracic curves because little correction can be gained through the narrow thoracic discs.

The instrumentation consists of screws with slotted heads into which a flexible, threaded rod fits. Nuts placed on the rod at the level of each screw secure the rod to the screw and move the screw on the rod. An outrigger can be used to derotate the spine.

Figure 1–55. In most curves it is safe to select the level based on the disc space that remains wedged on the bending film. Vertebrae that do not come to neutral or bend in the opposite direction on a bending film should be included in the instrumentation. This general rule assumes complete correction of the curve or slight overcorrection. In the thoracolumbar curve illustrated, the disc space between L3 and L4 definitely opens on the bending film, whereas the disc between L2 and L3 comes to neutral. Because of the rapid progression of this curve and the remaining growth, it was thought safest to include the L3 vertebra in the fusion. A bend film in the opposite direction is advisable to be sure that there is not a fixed lumbosacral curve in the opposite direction. There is no disadvantage to fusing one more level at the cephalad end of the curve. Because this is the screw most likely to fail, it is often wise to add an extra vertebra at this level and spread the force between the two most cephalad screws.

Figure 1–56. A thoracoabdominal approach is used to gain access to the vertebral bodies and discs that are to be included in the fusion area. The typical thoracolumbar curve illustrated would use an incision over the tenth rib extending across the costal margin into the abdominal wall. The incision in the abdominal wall stays lateral to the rectus sheath and is extended as far as necessary depending on the vertebra to be fused.

Figure 1–57. After the rib is removed and the pleural cavity opened, the costal cartilage is split. Teasing apart the muscle beneath will demonstrate the peritoneum.

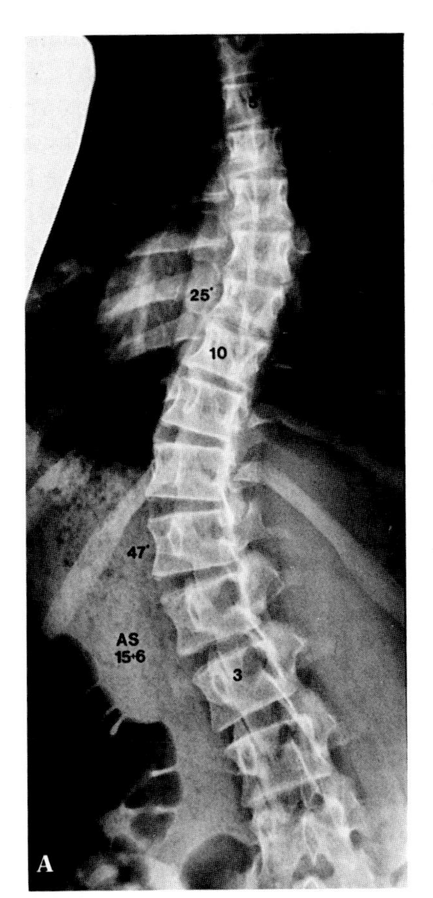

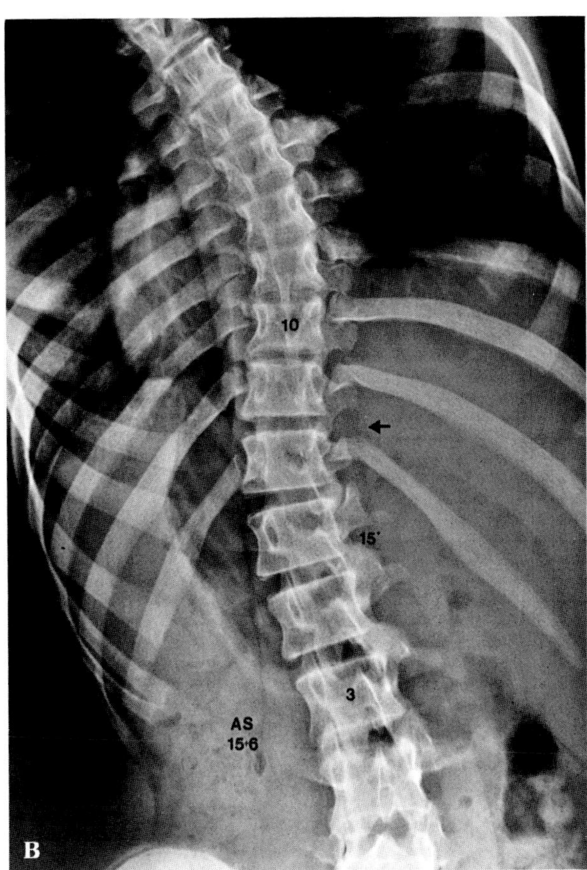

Figure 1–55

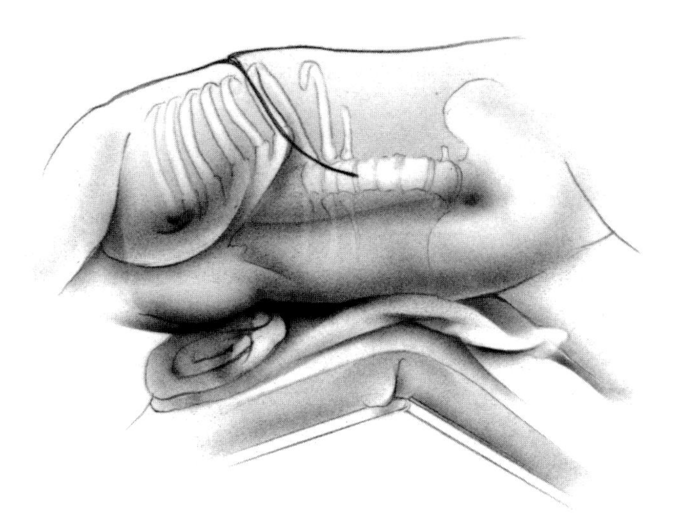

Figure 1–56

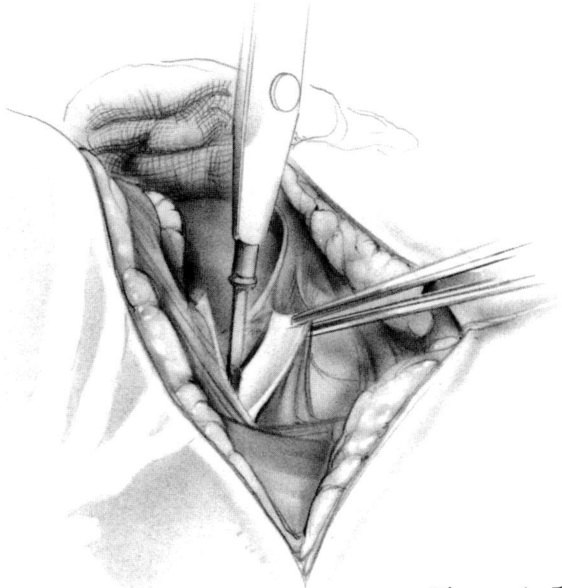

Figure 1–57

Figure 1–58. Because the peritoneum is adherent to both the underside of the diaphragm and the abdominal wall, it must be peeled off to avoid entering the peritoneal cavity and to gain access to the retroperitoneum. A small sponge wrapped over the finger aids in this dissection.

Figure 1–59. After the peritoneum is peeled from the underside of the diaphragm, the diaphragm is detached from its costal margin, leaving just enough on the chest wall to reattach it. Following this attachment in its posterior curving course will lead to the spine. After removing the peritoneum from the undersurface of the abdominal wall, it is also opened by cutting through the muscle layers lateral to the rectus sheath. The spine is now exposed by sweeping the peritoneum and the retroperitoneal fat forward off of the spine. The spleen, kidney, and aorta can all be palpated. The vena cava is best not seen. Care must be used with retractors and other instruments not to damage these structures.

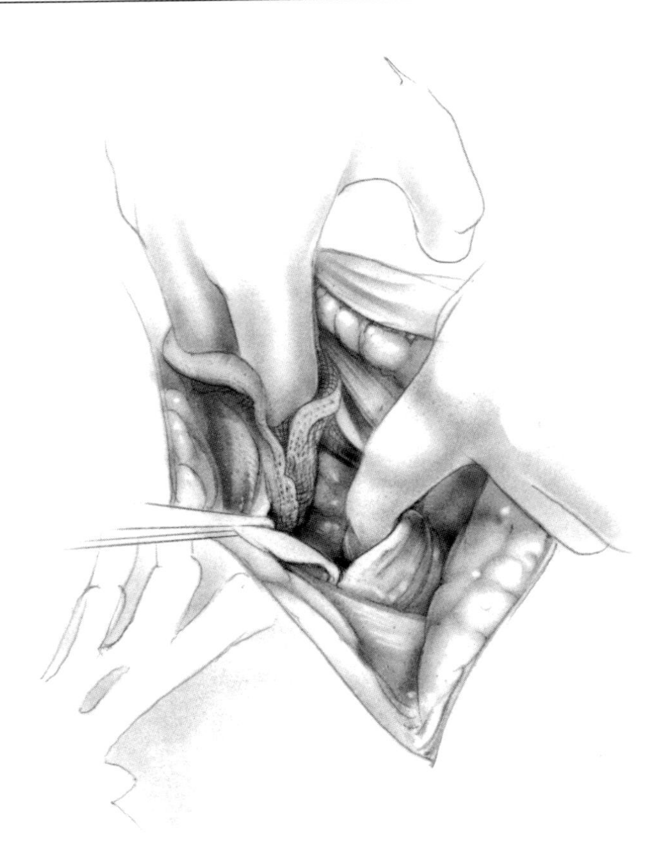

Figure 1–58

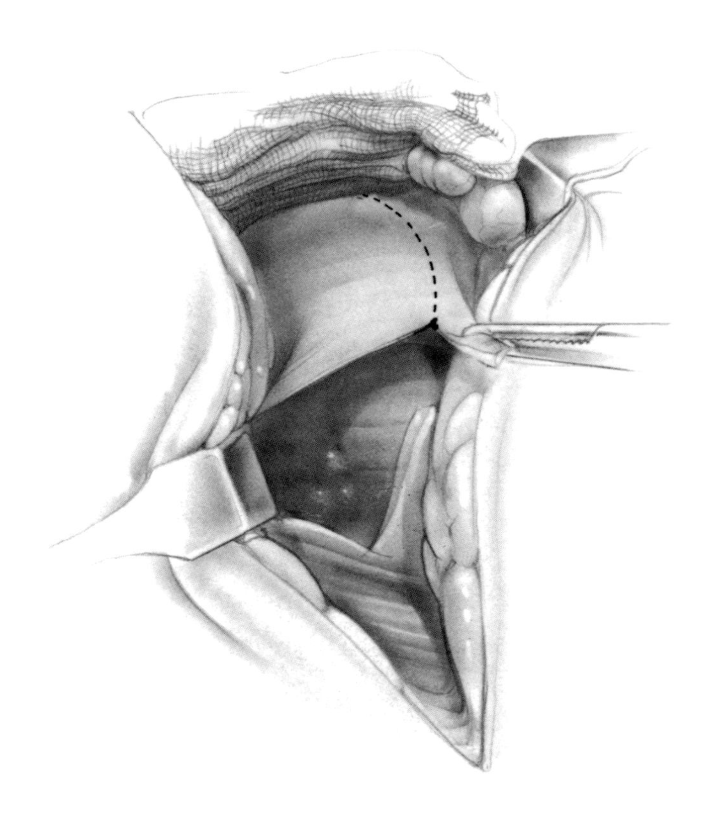

Figure 1–59

Figure 1–60. The parietal pleura covering the thoracic spine is opened. The discs and the segmental vessels crossing the vertebral bodies are easily seen. The lumbar spine will be covered with a fibrofatty layer and the psoas muscle. This fibrofatty investing layer is best opened by sharp dissection in the midline. This will expose the bulging discs, which is the safe avascular area in which to begin the circumferential dissection of the spine. Between the discs and crossing the concave center of the vertebral bodies are the segmental vessels. These are dissected free of the loose fascia and areolar tissue and ligated near the midline.

Figure 1–61. Exposure of the vertebrae and discs can be done either extraperiosteally by pushing the loose areolar tissue off of the periosteum, or by cutting the periosteum over the vertebrae and discs and elevating it as a continuous layer as illustrated here. The subperiosteal approach gives excellent exposure of the discs and end-plates and perhaps better healng at the expense of 20 minutes. The spine should be exposed to the base of the transverse processes on the convex side and as far past the midline as possible on the concave side. Regardless of the method used, it is advisable to bluntly dissect with a finger around each vertebral body to palpate the concave surface either directly or through the psoas. This will permit more accurate aiming of the screw, which is placed through the vertebral body and at the same time allows the surgeon to palpate the screw tip. This latter is important because it is necessary to be certain that the screw has penetrated the cortex on the concave side of the vertebral body (see **Figure 1–64**).

Figure 1–62. If the end-plates remain open, a broad chisel can be inserted between the end-plate and the bone of the vertebra. The chisel is advanced by gentle tapping with a mallet to avoid the plunges that can occur when pushing. Twisting and prying the chisel will loosen the end-plate and the disc for easy excision with a rongeur. Any remaining vertebral end-plate is removed with the Zielke ring curettes. Arthrodesis can be further enhanced by using a $\frac{1}{4}$-in curved osteotome to remove the compact bone beneath the vertebral end-plate exposing its cancellous bone. Because this will increase the bleeding, it is best left to the time when the graft is inserted. The excision of the disc should be thorough. The entire annulus should be removed from the transverse process of the convex side to a point past the midline, leaving the annulus on the concave side as a hinge. It is easy to be misled in the amount of disc and annulus that has been removed. The annulus on the concave side and the posterior longitudinal ligament posteriorly should be exposed. Care must be taken to note the rotation of the vertebral bodies and thus the changing location of the spinal canal.

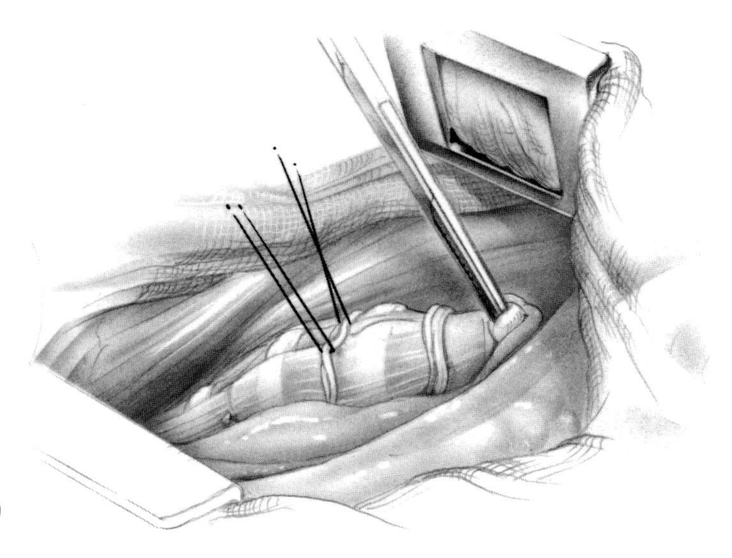

Figure 1–60

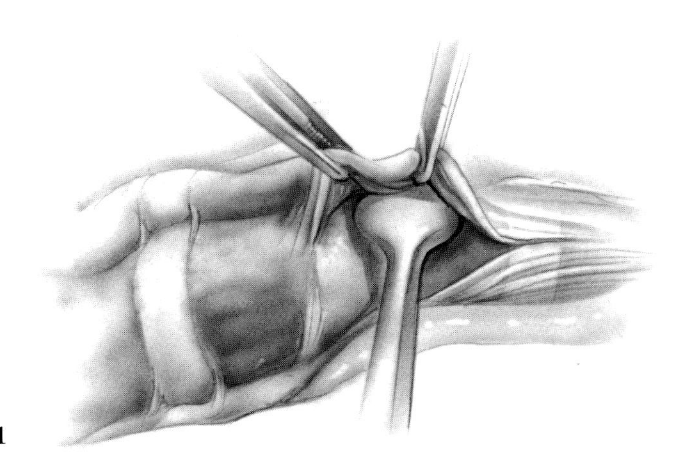

Figure 1–61

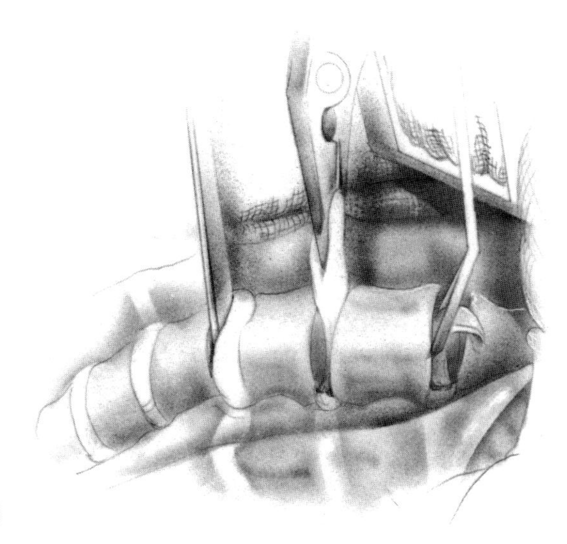

Figure 1–62

Figure 1–63. The placement of the screws is critical to the derotation effect. In principle each screw should parallel the posterior surface of the vertebral body. Because of the rotation of the vertebrae in the curve, the cephalad and caudad screws will be more ventral, whereas the screws at the apex will be more dorsal. Correction can be enhanced by placing the most caudal and cephalad screws approximately 1 cm more ventral than the screw at the apex. Fixation of the screws can be enhanced by angling them in a slightly posterior to anterior direction. When all of the screws are correctly placed, they will form a concave line ventrally. Later, the derotator will pull the apex of the rod (which conforms to this arch) forward, derotating the spine.

Figure 1–64. At the top and bottom vertebrae a staple is placed in the desired location with its blade best directed between the bone and the vertebral end-plate. On all other vertebrae a washer is used. If used in the manner that it was designed, concave surface facing up, it will fit the shape of the vertebral body better. In some instances, however, it will block the tightening of the nut. This can be avoided by placing the washer convex side up.

The depth of the screw can be measured by a caliper placed around the vertebral body if the dissection is sufficient. If not, a depth gauge can be inserted into the disc space along the exposed surface of the vertebral body. At least 5 mm will have to be added to this to account for the thickness of the annulus and the height of the washer. The hole is started in the vertebral body with an awl. A finger is placed on the concave side of the vertebra touching the transverse process, and the screw is directed toward the distal joint of the palpating finger. If the disc has been thoroughly removed, the proper direction of the screw can be confirmed by direct visualization of the posterior longitudinal ligament. The screw must penetrate the cortex on the far side of the vertebra to gain sufficient grip. Palpation is the best way to determine this. If soft porotic bone is encountered or if the screw tends to pull out, methylmethacrylate is injected into the screw hole, the screw is reinserted, and the cement allowed to set. It is recommended that the end screws be side opening, whereas the other screws be top opening. This uses the elasticity of the rod to lock it in place. It is often easier, especially in severe curves, to use all top-opening screws.

The rod is prepared by placing the nuts on it at the appropriate intervals. Double nuts may be used at each level or only at the top and bottom screws. Should the rod break, double nuts will prevent loss of correction at the other levels.

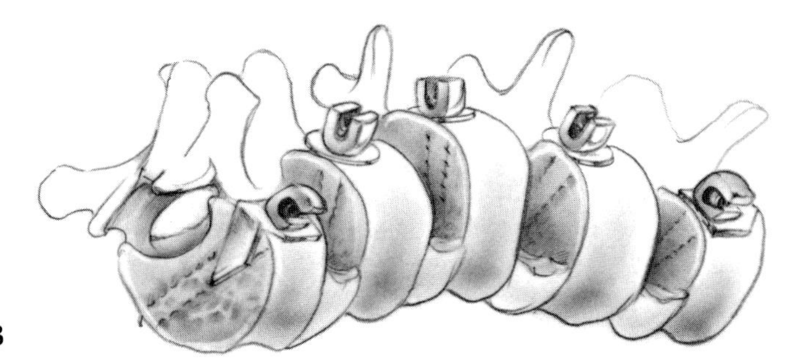

Figure 1–63

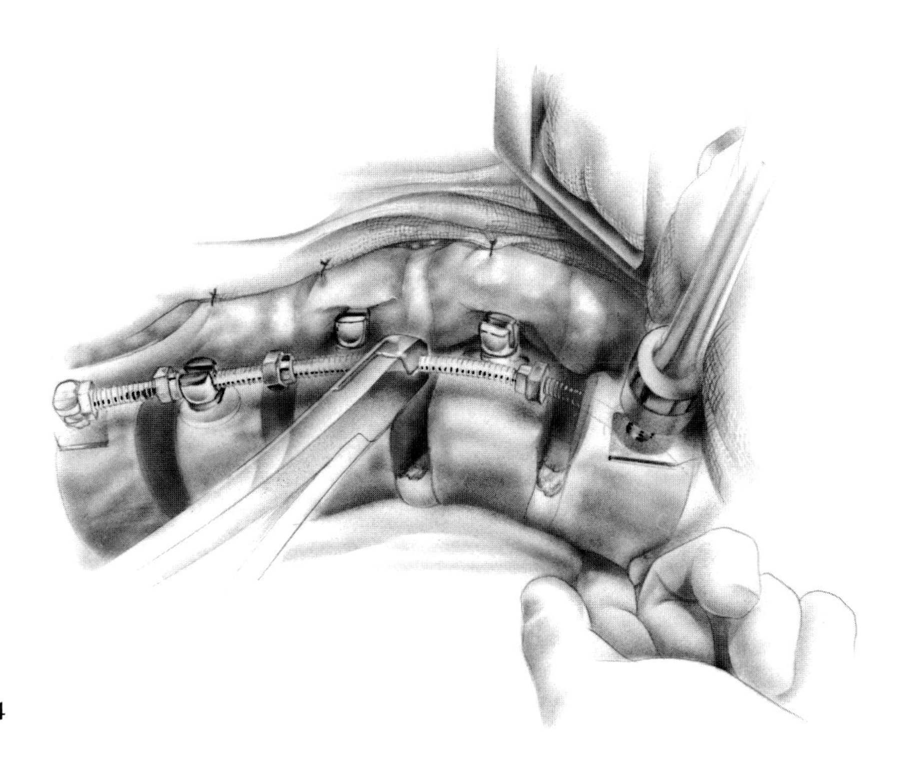

Figure 1–64

Figure 1–65. The rod is then inserted into the open slots of the screws and the nuts tightened enough to engage the head of the screw and thus hold the rod in the screw head. To do this it is often necessary to place a rod clamp on the side of the screw head opposite the nut being tightened to force the projection of the nut into the screw head. Compression of the opposing vertebral bodies should be avoided at this point.

Figure 1–66. Derotation of the spine is accomplished by first placing the articulated derotation bar on the rod. The wing screw on the derotator bar is tightened to secure the bar on the rod. The lever is placed on the bar and slowly and gently pulled ventral to derotate the apical vertebrae. Care must be taken with the derotation lever as an enormous amount of force can be applied. Actually the derotation can usually be accomplished by hand, but the lever is more out of the way to allow easier tightening of the nuts. As the apical vertebra is derotated, the disc spaces will be noted to open ventrally as lordosis is created.

To maintain the lordosis as the nuts are tightened, however, it is necessary to insert pieces of rib between adjacent vertebral bodies anteriorly in the midline (see **Figure 1–67**). These pieces of whole rib should span the cortical bone of the body so they do not sink into the cancellous bone. Excision of the annulus past the midline allows this graft to be placed anterior, creating lordosis and not blocking correction of the scoliosis.

Figure 1–67. After the bone graft is placed, the nuts are tightened beginning at the apex and moving cephalad and caudad. This will correct the remaining curve. If there is any question that the desired amount of correction has been obtained or fear that overcorrection has occurred, a radiograph can easily be obtained. As the tightening progresses, the apposition of the vertebral bodies should be observed as well as the screws. It is possible to tighten the nuts to the point that the top screw in the thoracic vertebra pulls out. After the desired correction is obtained, the threads of the rod are destroyed adjacent to each nut to prevent them from loosening. This can be done by twisting an old osteotome in the treads.

The parietal pleura is closed to cover the rod and screws in the thoracic spine, and the psoas muscle is allowed to cover the lumbar portion of the rod. It is critically important that no metal be left exposed in a position where it will come in contact with a major vessel as eventual erosion of the vessel will occur. This is particularly a problem when instrumentation is carried to the lower levels of the lumbar spine. The diaphragm is repaired and the wound closed with a chest tube in place.

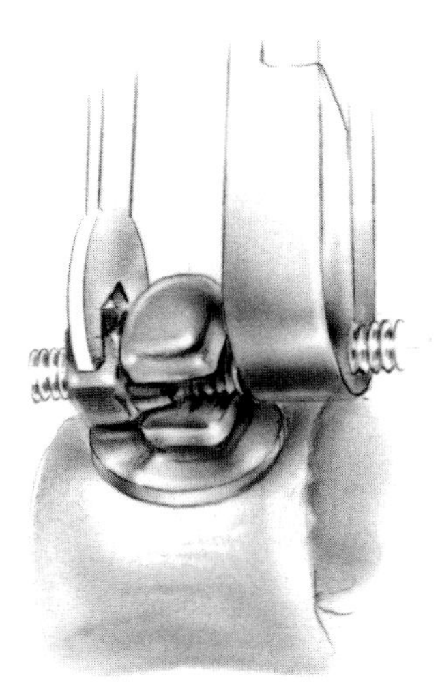

Figure 1–65

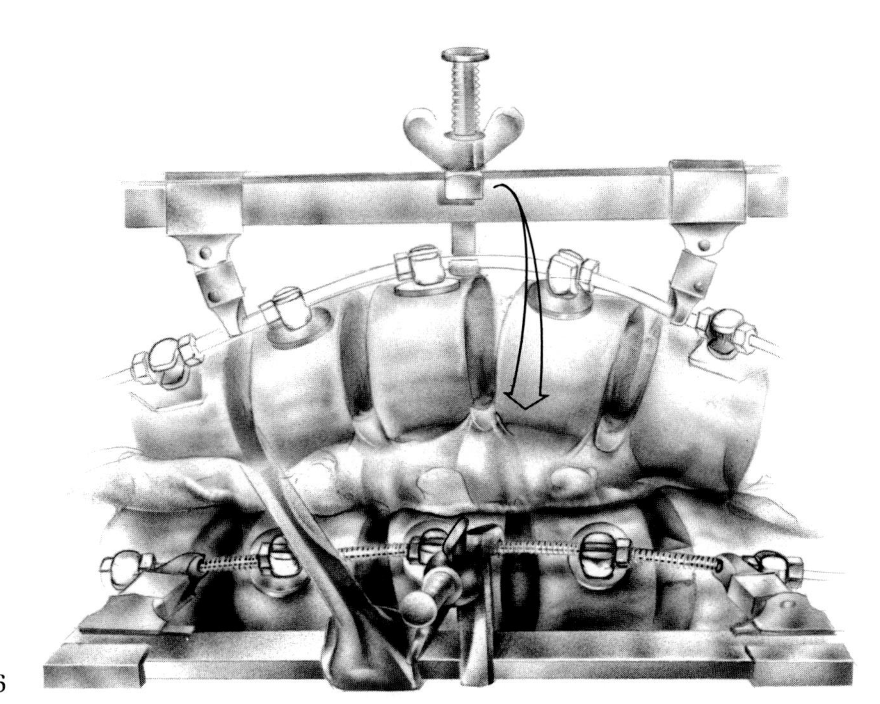

Figure 1–66

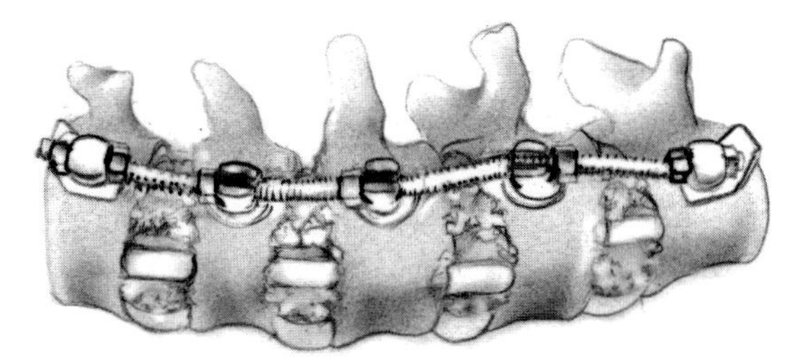

Figure 1–67

Figure 1–68. The postoperative radiographs demonstrate the excellent correction of both the scoliosis and the rotation. Although the anterior cortical rib grafts did not maintain the anterior disc space height, significant kyphosis was avoided.

POSTOPERATIVE CARE

When drainage from the chest tube is approximately 50 mL or less in 8 hours, it is removed. The bed is raised on the second postoperative day, the patient dangles his or her feet and stands at the bedside on the third postoperative day, and begins walking on the fourth. A small orthoplast jacket or similar device is made to immobilize the fusion area and is ready for the patient by the time of discharge on the sixth or seventh postoperative day. Ambulation does not have to await fitting of the jacket. The jacket is worn until arthrodesis of the vertebra is observed on the radiographs. This usually takes between 3 and 6 months.

REFERENCES

1. Winter RB. Adolescent idiopathic scoliosis (editorial). N Engl J Med 1986;314:1379.
2. Kaneda K, Fujiya N, Satoh S. Results with Zielke instrumentation for idiopathic thoracolumbar and lumbar scoliosis. Clin Orthop 1986;205:195.
3. Cochran T, Irstam L, Nachemson A. Long-term anatomic and functional changes in patients with adolescent idiopathic scoliosis treated by Harrington rod fusion. Spine 1983;8:576.

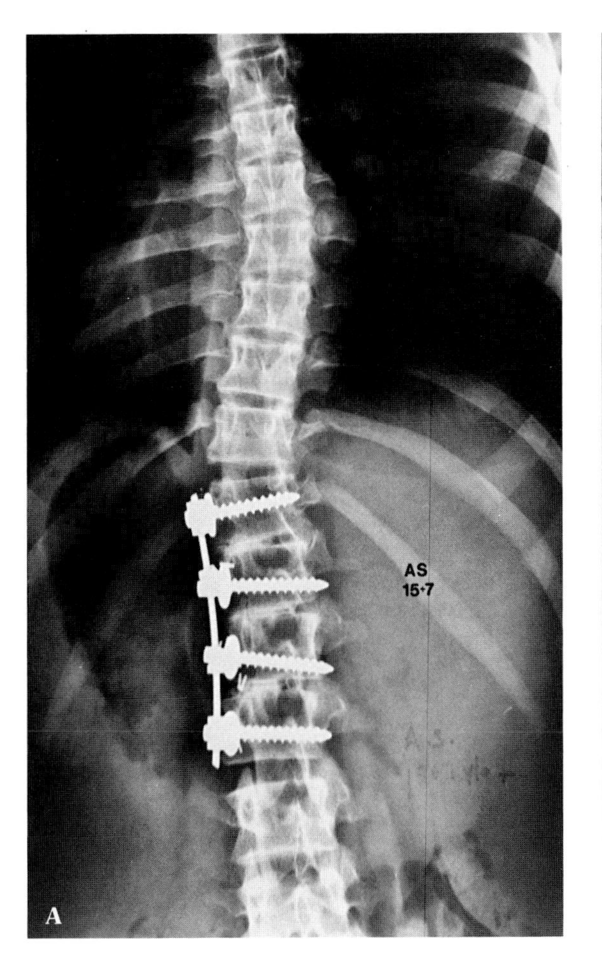

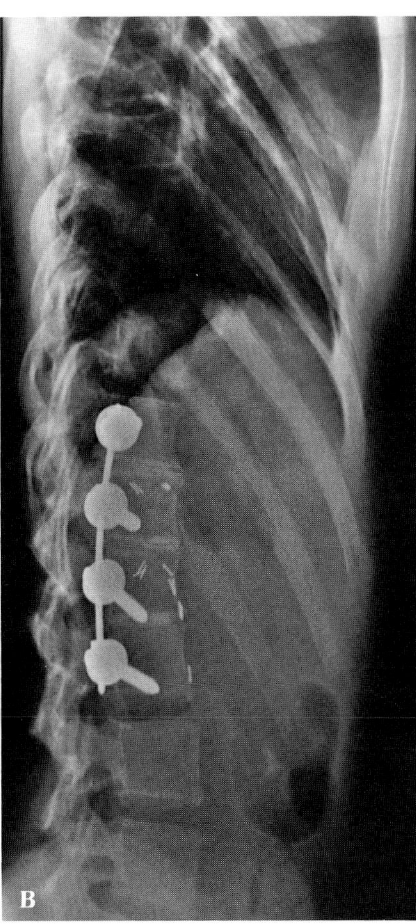

Figure 1–68

1.9 Posterior Harrington Compression Instrumentation for Kyphosis

The use of the heavy $\frac{1}{4}$-in Harrington compression rod (the small $\frac{3}{16}$-in rods are not strong enough and should not be used) and the #1256 hooks was the standard method of posterior instrumentation for kyphosis until the Cotrel-Dubousset instrumentation. The Harrington system still has many advantages to offset the disadvantages that the Cotrel-Dubousset instrumentation has alleviated. The main advantage of the Harrington system, which becomes a significant issue in severe kyphotic deformity, is that it is easier to insert, and the correction can be gained gradually at multiple levels. Although the hooks themselves are more difficult to insert than the Cotrel-Dubousset hooks because they must be on the rod, it is not so difficult as trying to get the Cotrel-Dubousset rod into the hooks. Probably the only true disadvantage of the Harrington compression system is that cast or orthotic support is required until arthrodesis is achieved.

The selection of the levels to be fused and the exposure of the spine is the same as for the Cotrel-Dubousset instrumentation. Again, it is important to extend the fusion into the normal lordotic segment of the spine below the kyphosis, usually L2.

There should be at least three and preferably four hooks on each side of the spine both above and below the kyphotic area. In the thoracic area the purchase sites can be a combination of lamina and transverse processes. The most cephalad purchase site must always be under the lamina. This is necessary to anchor the rod and prevent the hooks from sliding off of the transverse processes. In adolescent boys with strong bone and flexibility restored to the deformity by anterior disectomy, the most cephalad hook on each side can be under the lamina while the next three can be on the transverse processes. If the bone is porotic, the transverse processes are small, or the curve has remained stiff after the anterior release, more or all of the hooks should be under the lamina.

Figure 1–69. To prepare hook sites in the thoracic spine for compression it is first necessary to remove the overhanging portion of the spinous process and gain access to the spinal canal by removing a portion of the ligamentum flavum. A Kerrison rongeur is then used to remove portions of both the superior and inferior facet as illustrated at the top of the incision. The inferior hook site and the facetectomy and laminotomy are the same as when the procedure is done with the Cotrel-Dubousset instrumentation.

Figure 1–70. Although it is possible and often easier to seat the most cephalad hook and then pass the rod through it, this cannot be done with the remainder of the hooks. The $\frac{1}{4}$-in rod is too inflexible, and the threads will be destroyed in attempting to pull it through the hooks. Therefore, the hooks and the nuts that are used to tighten them are all placed on the rod before its insertion.

Because the hooks are on the rod, it is not possible to tilt the hook and slide it under the lamina. Therefore, to make seating of the hooks possible, the laminotomy that is prepared will have to be larger than in most other circumstances. It should be large enough to "drop" the hook into the spinal canal and then slide it forward under the lamina.

Figure 1–71. After the first rod is placed the surgeon will be tempted to tighten it to gain some correction that will make insertion of the second rod easier. This will create some compression of the opposite side, however, closing the holes that had been prepared for the hooks and making their insertion more difficult.

The hooks are tightened starting at the apex and moving from one side of the spine to the other to avoid creation of scoliosis. At the beginning, they can be tightened by the technique of spreading between a hook holder and a rod clamp. Following this the hooks are tightened with a wrench. As the nuts are tightened the interface between the hook and the bone should be observed so as not to overtighten the hooks and fracture the bone. If the surgeon is having difficulty judging the amount of correction, a cross-table lateral radiograph can be obtained. When tightening is completed, the threads behind each of the nuts are destroyed to keep them from loosening. This can be done with an old osteotome, twisting it in the threads.

Decortication of all bone that remains exposed is accomplished, and the graft is added before the wound is closed.

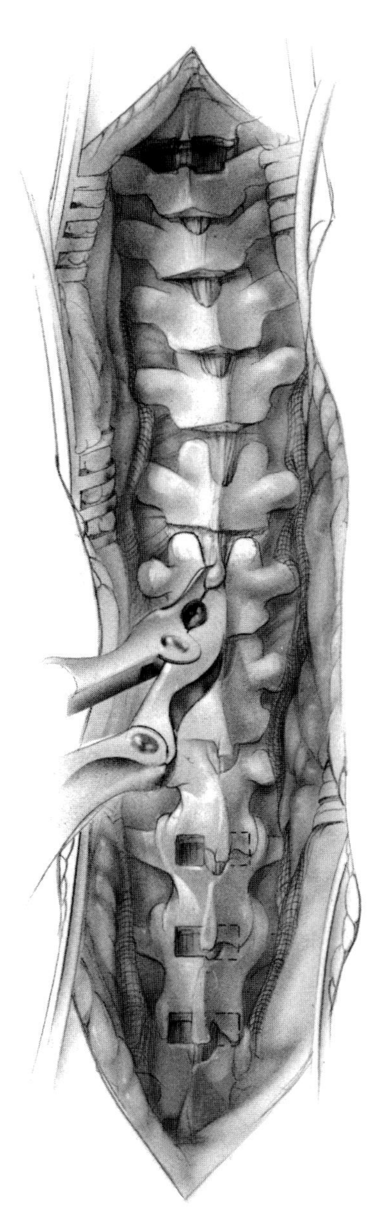

Figure 1–69

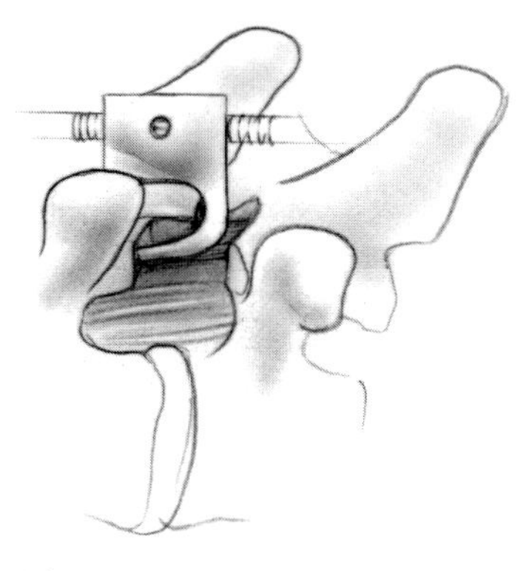

Figure 1–70

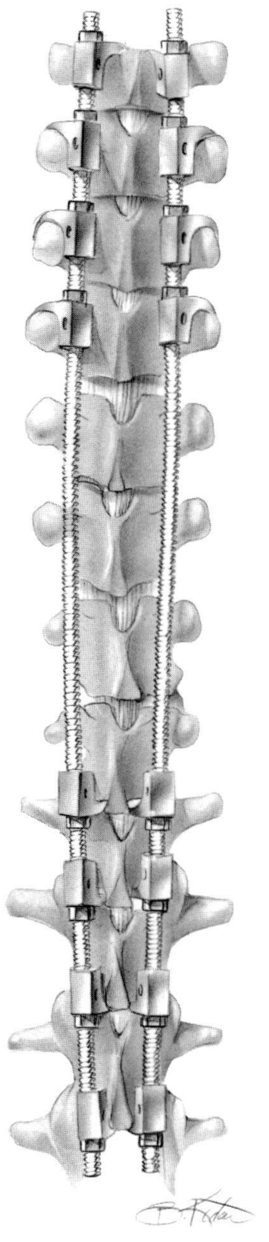

Figure 1–71

Figure 1–72. ***Figures 1–72A and B*** illustrate the radiographs of a 17-year-old boy with a history of deformity for the past 6 to 7 years, which his parents attributed to "poor posture." During the past 2 to 3 years he has had increasing aching in the region of the apex of the kyphosis. In addition, he was extremely displeased with his appearance. The correction achieved after anterior transthoracic disectomy and fusion along with posterior fusion and instrumentation with Harrington compression rods is illustrated in ***Figures 1–72C and D.***

POSTOPERATIVE CARE

The fixation is strong enough that no special concern is given to the initial management of the patient. The patient can be positioned as desired for comfort, and ambulation is usually started on the third or fourth postoperative day without any external support. At the time of discharge the patient is casted or fitted with an orthosis that is worn for 4 to 6 months.

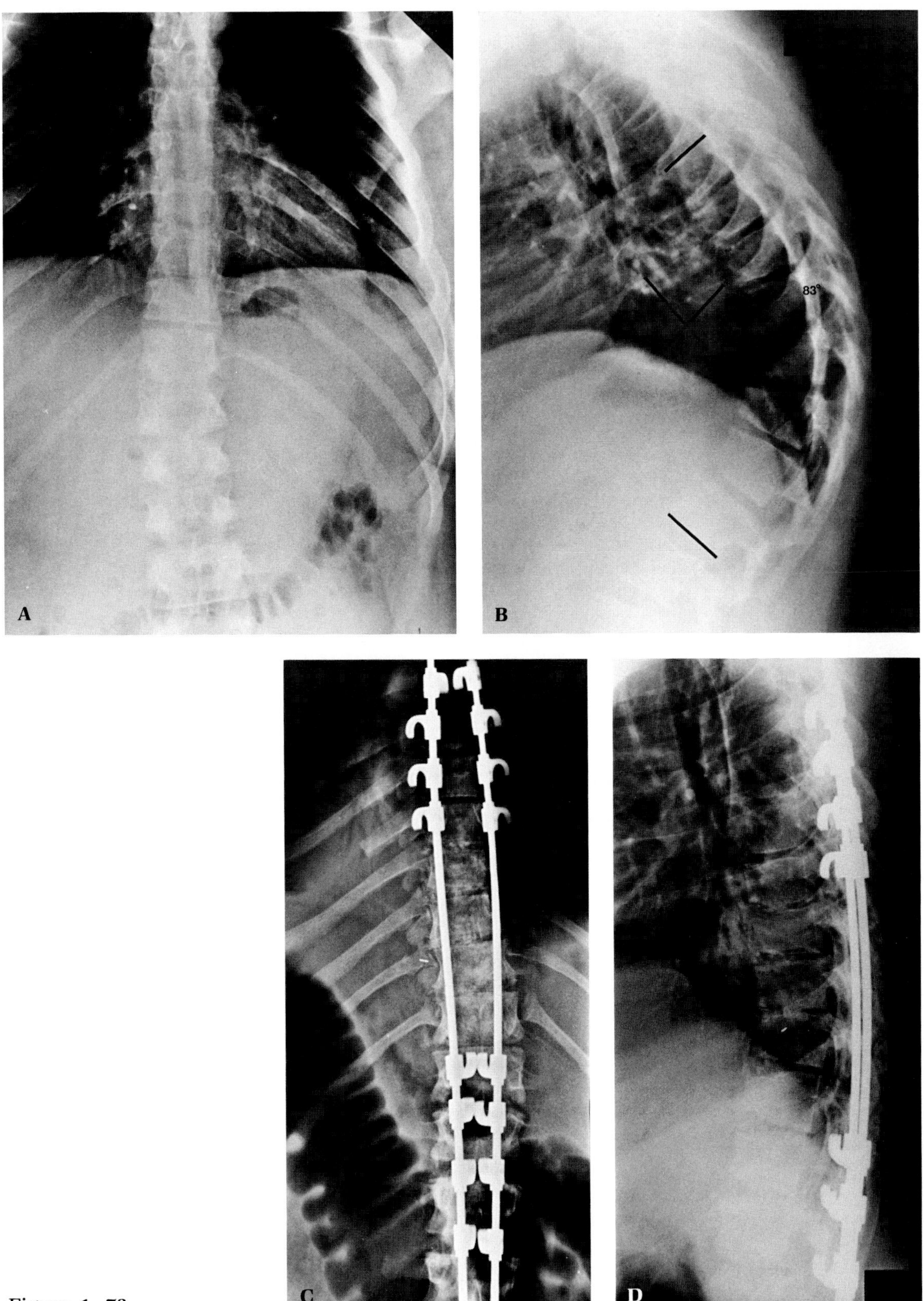

Figure 1–72

1.10 Posterior Cotrel-Dubousset Instrumentation for Kyphosis

The use of the Cotrel-Dubousset instrumentation for kyphosis has several attractive features. It is very rigid and probably requires no postoperative immobilization. In cases that also have significant scoliosis it has the ability to correct both the kyphosis and the scoliosis. The hooks can be placed without being on the rod (unlike the Harrington compression rod), which means that smaller holes need to be cut for their seating; it is not a problem to insert the hooks on the other side of the spine after the first hooks have been placed and tightened.

There are also disadvantages. The rods must be contoured to the desired correction, which means that most of the correction is obtained at once. This makes it difficult to get the rod into the inferior hooks after they have been placed in the superior hooks. In addition, it is often difficult to add compression on the hooks as they seem to bind on the rod and do not slide easily.

The area of the spine that is to be fused is exposed, and the hook sites are prepared. There are two methods of hook purchase that can be used in the instrumentation of kyphosis. They differ in the method used to place the hooks on the thoracic vertebrae.

Figure 1–73. The method of hook purchase illustrated here uses the "claw" configuration on the thoracic vertebrae. On the cephalad side of the kyphosis there should be at least three purchase sites on each side of the spine. The inferior edge of the lamina is cut to allow a pedicle hook to be placed as described in the use of the Cotrel-Dubousset instrumentation for scoliosis. On the same vertebra a transverse process hook is placed over the cephalad edge of the transverse process. This produces a rigid "claw" that is locked on the posterior element of the vertebra (***Figure 1–73A, B***). In the case to be illustrated here, only two "claw" configurations were used. The third hook was a simple transverse process hook. Side-opening hooks often facilitate seating the rod in this situation and can be interchanged with top-opening hooks as the situation demands.

An alternative method on the cephalad portion of the kyphos is to use lamina hooks inserted into every other lamina. These can be staggered on each side of the spine. For example, a lamina hook may be inserted on the lamina of T3, T5, and T7 on one side of the spine, and on the lamina of T4, T6, and T8 on the other side of the spine. These hooks are inserted on the cephalad aspect of the lamina so as to provide compression.

Inferior to the kyphosis three hook sites should be prepared on each side of the spine. It is important in selecting levels to extend the instrumentation into the normal lordosis. These hook sites are easily prepared by removing the inferior edge of the lamina and then the ligament flavum to allow the lamina hook to be seated within the spinal canal. The hook sites should be prepared on both sides of the spine before any hooks or rods are placed. If this is not done, the closing of the interlaminar spaces as a result of placing the first rod will make it more difficult to prepare the sites on the opposite side.

After this is completed, a radical facetectomy with removal of a significant portion of the inferior portion of the lamina is done in the area of the kyphosis to permit correction. This can be accomplished by entering the spinal canal in the midline and using a Kerrison ronguer to remove the bone. The bone that is removed will include the inferior portion of the lamina and the superior facet as well as a portion of the inferior facet.

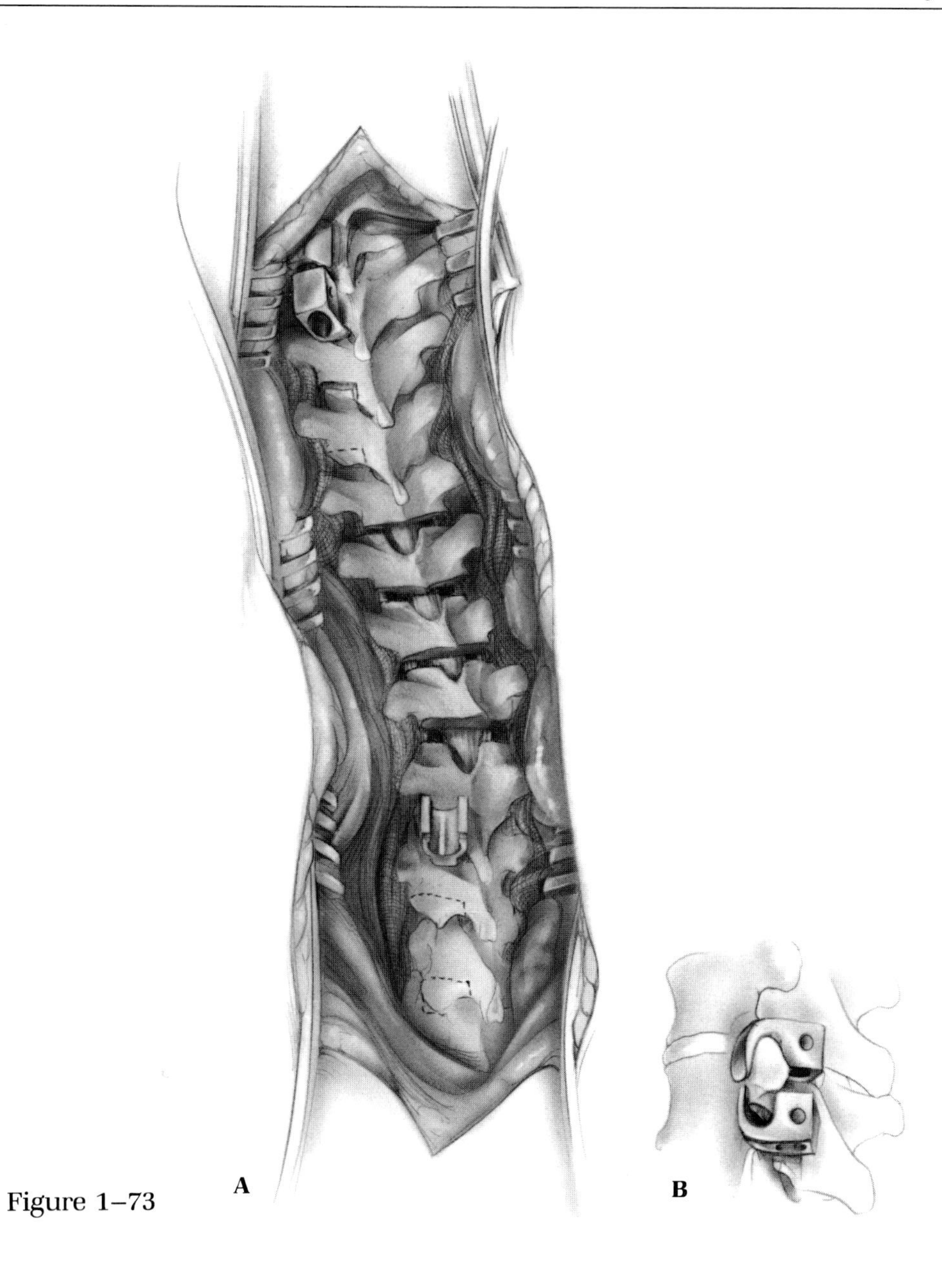

Figure 1–73

Figure 1–74. Now comes the most difficult part of this technique: placing the rods and hooks. It is difficult because the rods must first be contoured to the desired final degree of correction; therefore, when they are inserted, most of the correction is gained at one time. If all of the hooks and the rods are placed cephalad to the kyphosis it is not easy to push them down into the caudal hooks. In a severe kyphosis the surgeon has the distinct impression that something will break if he or she keeps pushing. Several tricks have been suggested to deal with this problem such as having an assistant push on the apex of the kyphos, trying to lift the pelvis, or placing one rod in the cephalad hooks and one rod in the caudal hooks and pushing both down toward their corresponding empty hooks at the same time as in a double-lever system. These tricks may work in flexible curves.

The most reliable method, however, is to apply a small Harrington compression rod to one side, tighten it to gain correction, and then place the Cotrel-Dubousset rod on the opposite side. The Harrington compression rod will then be removed and replaced with the second Cotrel-Dubousset rod (***Figure 1–74A***).

In the thoracic region the Harrington compression rod can be placed on the transverse processes (***Figure 1–74B***). These are usually strong enough for this temporary correction, and the hooks can be inserted rapidly.

Below the kyphosis the Harrington hooks can be placed in the holes that have been prepared for the Cotrel-Dubousset hooks.

Figure 1–75. Compression of this threaded rod is started in the middle on either side of the kyphosis and works toward the ends. Compression is accomplished by spreading the Harrington spreader between a hook holder on the hook and a rod clamp secured to the rod then advancing the nut by spinning it with a small periosteal elevator. It is not necessary to gain the correction by laboriously turning the nuts with a wrench.

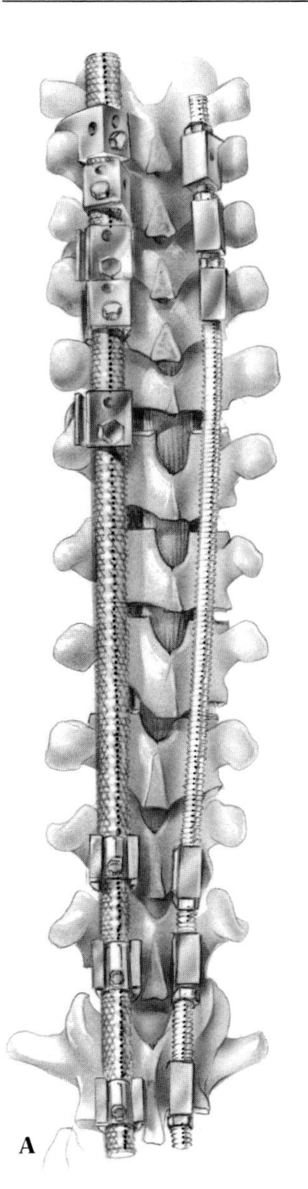

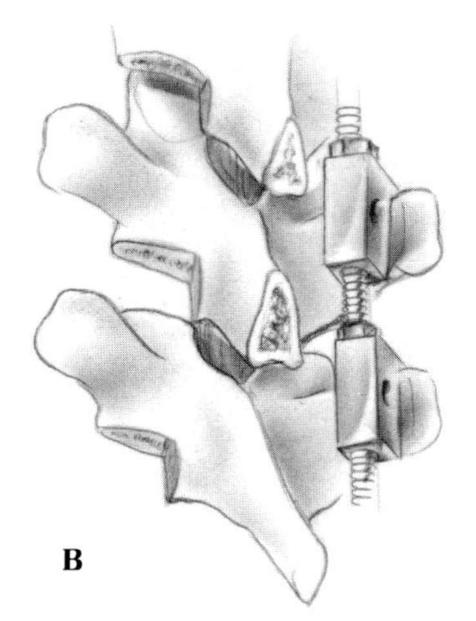

Figure 1–74

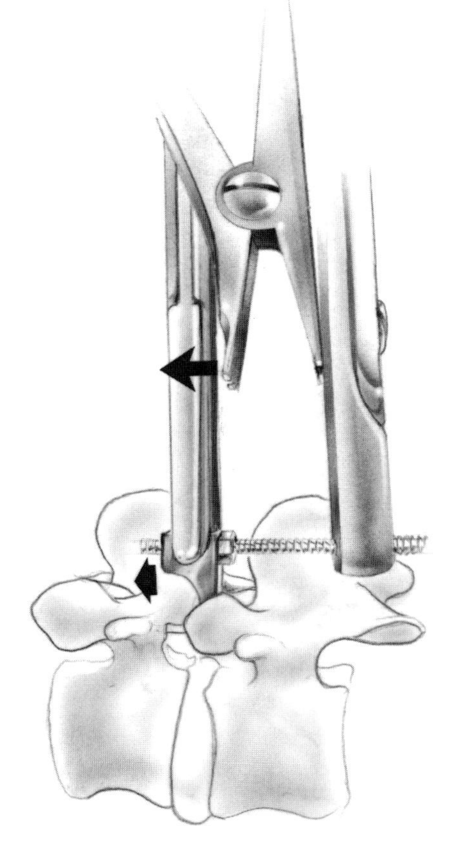

Figure 1–75

Figure 1–76. After the first Cotrel-Dubousset rod is placed, the Harrington compression rod is removed and replaced with the second Cotrel-Dubousset rod. At this point most of the correction will have been obtained. Some additional correction may be obtained by tightening the hooks in compression much as was done with the Harrington compression rod: spreading between the hook and a rod holder clamped onto the rod. This has the additional advantage of tightening the hook against the bone and should be done for each hook. To complete the operation, all possible decortication is accomplished, and a large amount of bone graft is added.

Figure 1–77. The anteroposterior and lateral radiographs of a 17-year-old boy with severe and persisting pain secondary to Scheurmann's kyphosis are shown in ***Figures 1–77A and B.*** The posterior radiographs with the Cotrel-Dubousset instrumentation in place are shown in ***Figures 1–77C and D.*** The upper hooks skipped a level to permit easier insertion, and the lower hooks were staggered to facilitate better decortication.

POSTOPERATIVE CARE

The advantage of the Cotrel-Dubousset instrumentation is that no external immobilization is needed. Therefore, immediate postoperative care is the same as for other spinal operations. The patient is mobilized as quickly as possible and followed the same as a patient with scoliosis treated with the Cotrel-Dubousset instrumentation.

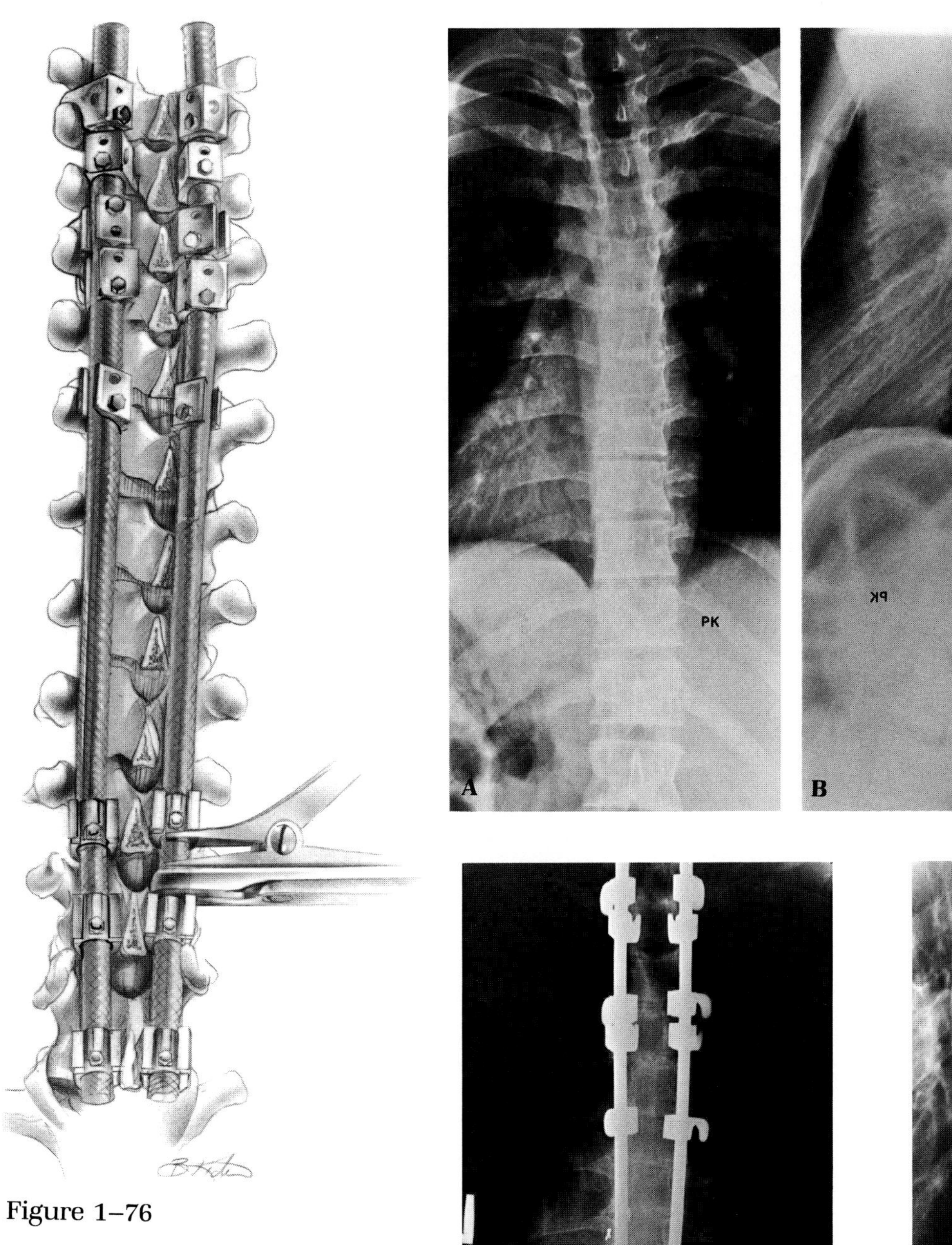

Figure 1–76

Figure 1–77

1.11 Posterior Arthrodesis C1–2, Gallie Technique

The commonest arthrodesis of the cervical spine is between the axis and the atlas because of the numerous congenital and developmental problems that affect this region. Although several techniques have been advocated to achieve arthrodesis of these vertebrae, the technique attributed to Gallie[1] is the most reliable and easiest to apply to the pediatric age group. In this technique the wire not only helps to pull C1 back into position and hold it there, but it also holds the bone graft firmly in place.[2,3] Occasionally the posterior arch of C1 will not be completely formed, making this technique impossible.

In cases in which there is a great deal of instability with chance for neurologic injury, the author prefers to place the patient in a halo vest or cast first. This can be done with local or general anesthesia as the circumstance demands. Reduction is achieved and confirmed by radiographs. If awake, the patient is now anesthetized and turned prone for the posterior fusion. No head rest is necessary, and there is little danger of neurologic injury while intubating and moving the patient.

Figure 1–78. The occipital region of the skull is shaved, and the posterior cervical area and the posterior iliac crest are prepared and draped. The incision extends in the midline from the base of the skull to the spinous process of C4. Dissection is carried down to the tips of the spinous processes. At this point a metal hub needle is placed in the spinous process of C2, and a lateral radiograph is taken. This is done to identify positively the correct vertebrae to be exposed. In the young child exposure of the base of the skull or any additional vertebrae may result in "creeping fusion."

Figure 1–79. When correctly identified, the posterior arch of C1 and the lamina of C2 are exposed subperiosteally by a combination of sharp and blunt dissection. It is important to remember that the vertebral arteries are unprotected by the bony foramen at the C1 level just lateral to the facets. In small children this is about 1 cm from the midline and in larger children about 1.5 cm from the midline.

To prepare the arch of C1 for passage of the wire beneath it, the periostium must be separated from its anterior surface. This can be accomplished with a small, angulated, neural elevator. The spinal canal does not need to be opened. After this a dental burr can be used to decorticate the exposed lamina of C1 and C2. This does not have to be as deep a decortication as is done in scoliosis.

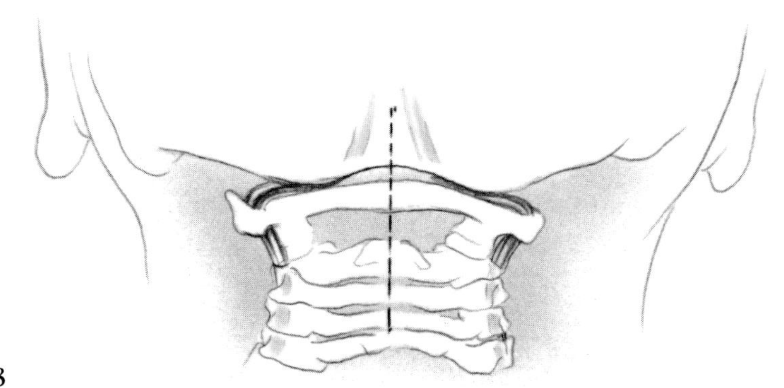

Figure 1–78

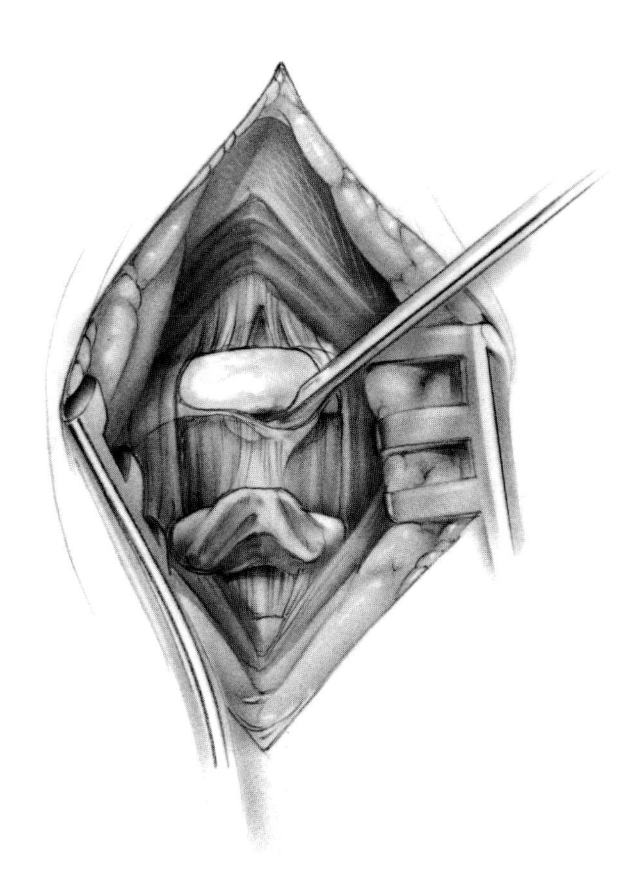

Figure 1–79

Figure 1–80. A loop of wire is passed under the arch of C1 from inferior to superior. The wire is bent back on itself, forming a smooth loop. Care should be taken not to introduce any sharp bends in the wire. The size of the wire will depend on both the size of the child and the desire of the surgeon. Anything from 18 gauge to 22 gauge can be used. Good quality, fully anealed flexible wire will allow a relatively larger size to be used because it will pull through easily without kinking.

Figure 1–81. The corticocancellous graft, which has previously been obtained and fashioned to fit over the lamina of C1 and C2, is now put in place. Small pieces of cancellous bone can be added beneath the corticocancellous graft. The loop of wire is pulled from under the arch of C1, over the graft, and placed around the spinous process of C2. A small notch cut in the base of the C2 spinous process helps to keep this in place.

Figure 1–82. The two ends of the wire that come out from under the arch of C1 inferiorly are pulled tight and brought around the sides and over the top of the graft. It is at this point, when the surgeon is pulling the wire tight, that the importance of a flexible wire that is not too large is realized. In working with the wire, it is best to keep it taut. This will minimize any chance of it impinging on the spinal cord and will make tightening easier. After the wire is pulled tight, it can be secured with a wire twister.

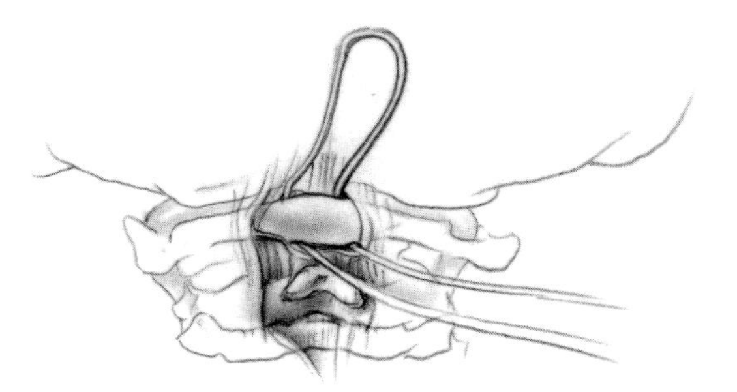

Figure 1–80

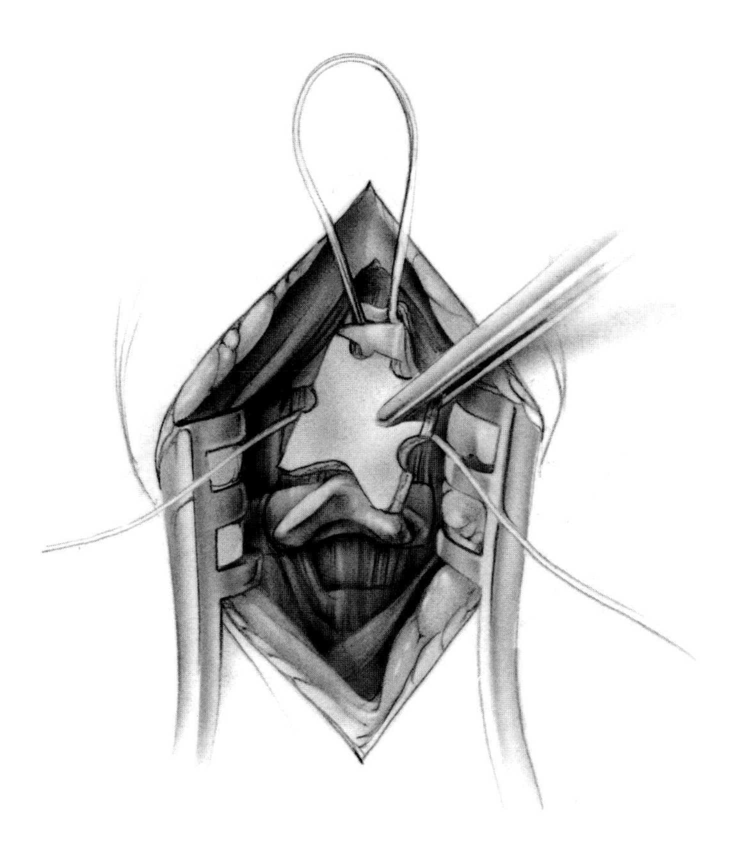

Figure 1–81

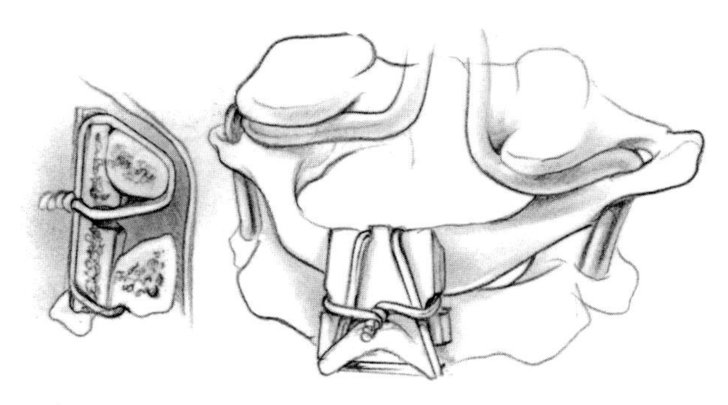

Figure 1–82

Figure 1–83. In children the spinous process of C2 is often small and does not provide much strength for fixation of the wire. A technique for circumventing this problem has recently been suggested.[4] In this technique a threaded K wire of appropriate size is passed through a small stab wound in the side of the neck, through the paravertebral muscles, and drilled through the spinous process of C2. It is cut so that approximately 1 cm is protruding on each side.

Figure 1–84. The corticocancellous graft is then put in place. It should fit under the K wire. The loop of wire that comes from under the arch of C1 is then drawn over the graft and looped around the spinous process of C2. The wire loop will be under the transverse Kirschner wire, however, which will keep it from slipping off of the spinous process.

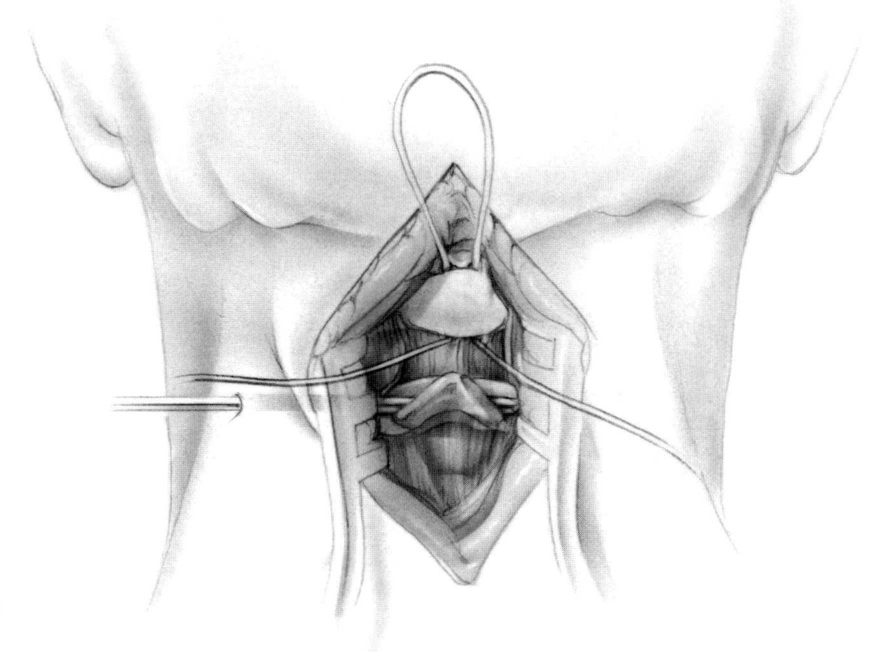

Figure 1–83

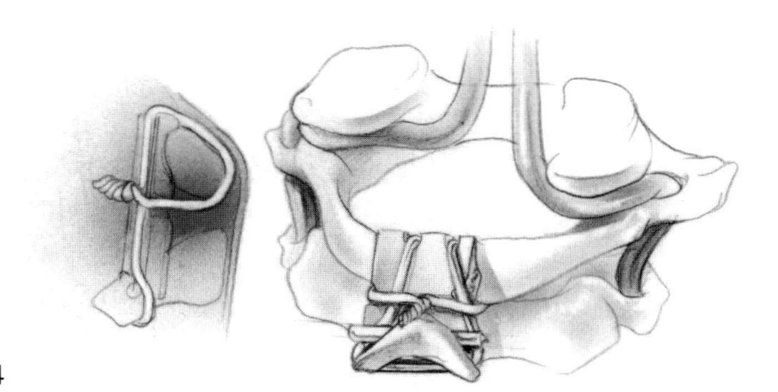

Figure 1–84

Figure 1–85. An 8-year-old child with a history of occipital headaches was noted by her orthodontist to have an absent odointoid. The extension lateral view of the cervical spine demonstrates the os odointoideum (***Figure 1–85A***). The flexion lateral radiograph demonstrates the instability (***Figure 1–85B***). One year following a posterior arthrodesis of C1 and C2 with fixation by the Gallie technique, the spine is stable (***Figure 1–85C***). Note the creeping fusion between the spinous processes of C2 and C3 where the interspinous ligament was cut.

POSTOPERATIVE CARE

There should be radiographic evidence of solid arthrodesis in 10 to 12 weeks. The postoperative care concerns what type of immobilization should be used until that time. The author's preference has been to leave the halo on for about 6 to 8 weeks in young and unreliable children, followed by some type of collar for an additional 4 weeks. In reliable adolescents in which the bone is stronger, a Philadelphia collar or similar device is usually adequate.

REFERENCES

1. Gallie WE. Fractures and dislocation of the cervical spine. Am J Surg 1939;46:495.
2. McGraw RW, Rusch RM. Atlanto-axial arthrodesis. J Bone Joint Surg 1973;55B:482.
3. Fielding JW, Hawkins RJ, Ratzan SA. Spine fusion for atlantoaxial instability. J Bone Joint Surg 1976;58A:400.
4. Mah JY et al. Threaded K-wire spinous process fixation of the axis for modified Gallie fusion in children and adolescents. J Pediatr Orthop 1989;9:675.

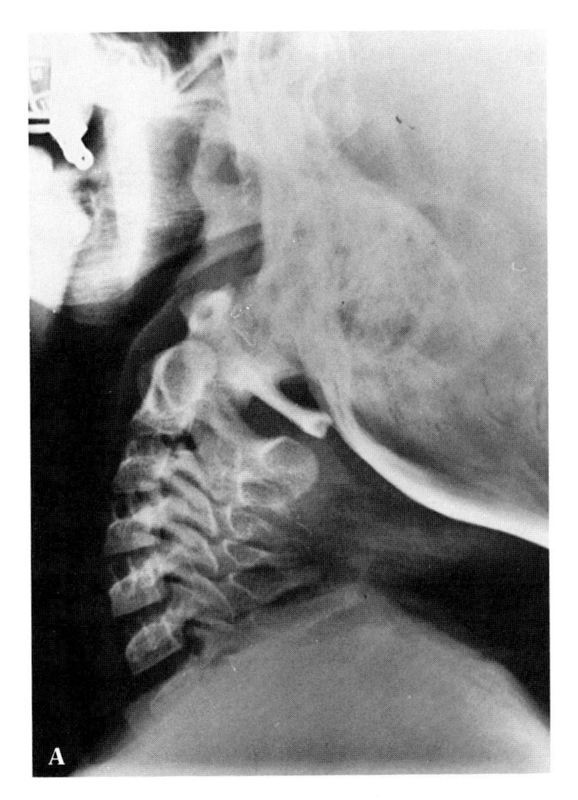

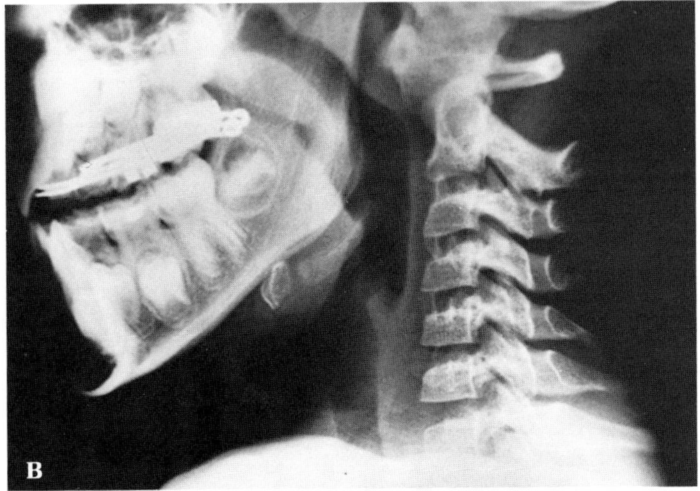

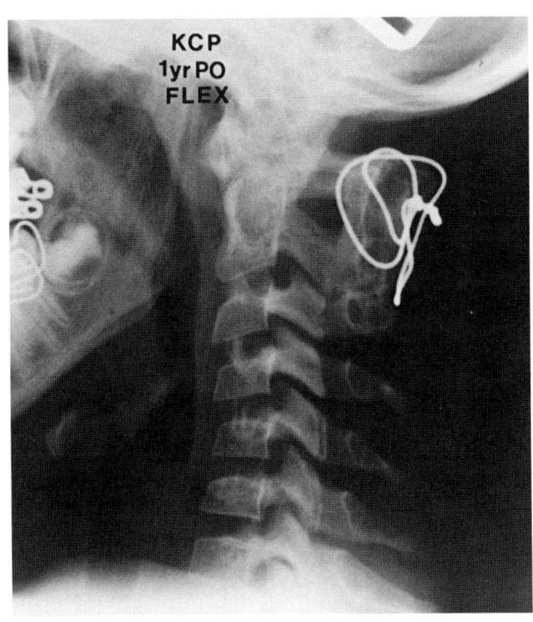

Figure 1–85

1.12 Posterior Iliac Bone Graft

There are many needs for autogenous bone in orthopaedic surgery. Because the commonest need for large amounts of bone is in spinal surgery, the technique will be described here. It should be recognized that when the requirements are for small amounts of bone, a much smaller incision can be used or the bone may be more easily obtained from another location. There are two ways to expose the posterior iliac crest during spinal surgery: through the same incision or a separate incision.

Figure 1–86. If the spinal incision is confined to the thoracic region it may be preferable to use a separate incision over the posterior iliac crest. In this case there are two important considerations given to placement of the incision. The first is that it should not cut the cluneal nerves and vessels, and the second is that it should give the surgeon the most direct access to the area of the crest that has the largest amount of bone. This area is the bone adjacent to the sacroiliac joint and the sciatic notch. An incision that follows the top of the iliac crest violates both of these considerations. The incision illustrated is an oblique incision that is centered over the posterosuperior iliac spine. Some surgeons prefer an incision that crosses the posterosuperior iliac spine at 90 degrees to the one illustrated; they think that the former incision gives a better cosmetic result.

Figure 1–87. If the incision for the spinal procedure extends into the lumbar spine, it is easiest to continue that incision down to the sacrum and expose the posterior iliac crest from the midline incision. This is done by dissecting on top of the lumbodorsal fascia laterally until the posterosuperior iliac spine can be palpated.

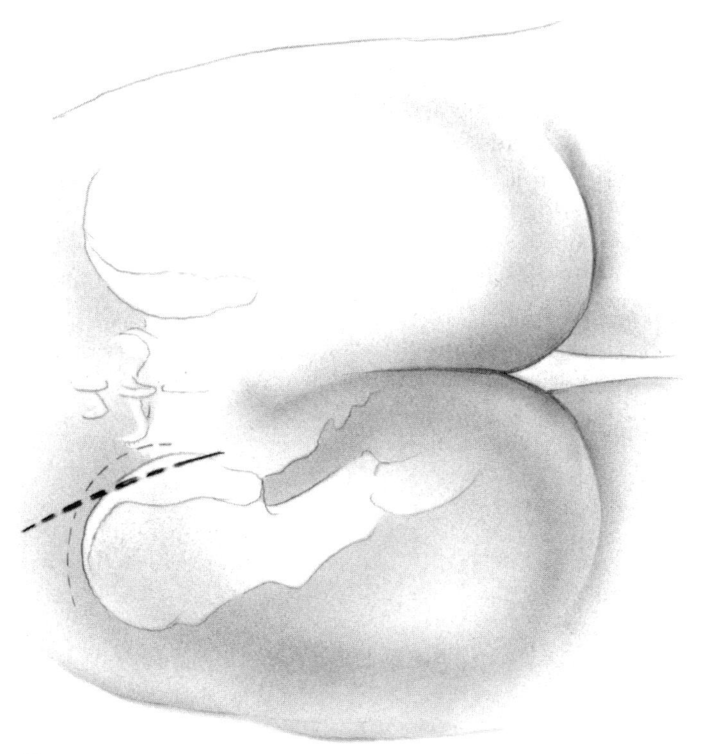

Figure 1–86

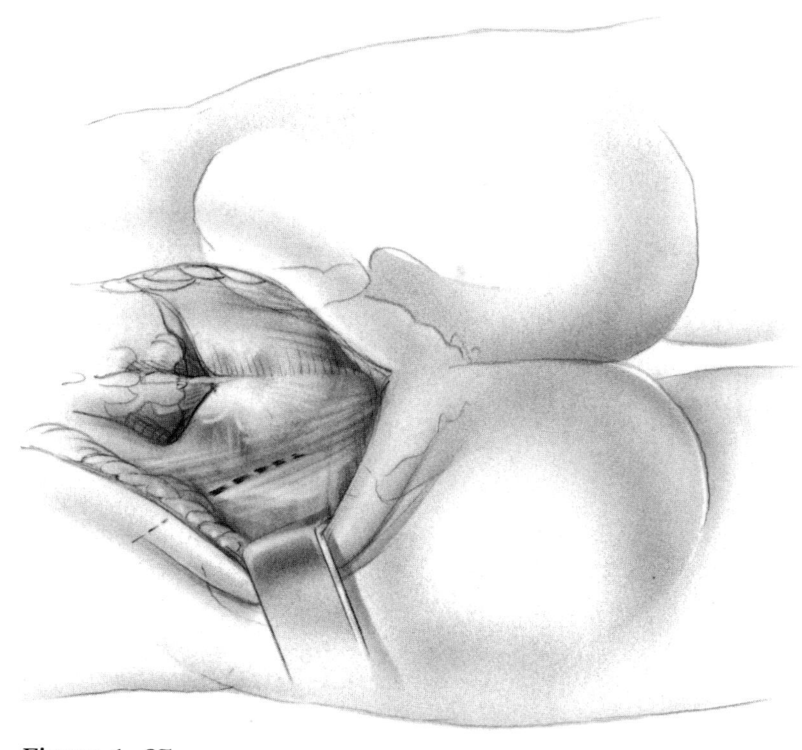

Figure 1–87

Figure 1–88. Although the posterosuperior iliac spine lies directly beneath the fascia, the remainder of the iliac apophysis is hidden. Superiorly the iliac crest curves anteriorly with the abdominal muscles inserting from above and the abductor muscles inserting from below while the cluneal vessels and nerves run over the top. To expose this region of the apophysis, a small incision is made in the lumbodorsal fascia just cephalad to the posterosuperior iliac spine. A finger is then inserted along the top of the iliac crest as it curves anterior, creating an interval between the insertion of the two muscle groups. The cluneal nerves and vessels will lie in the tissue above the finger.

Figure 1–89. With a long narrow retractor such as a small Meyerding inserted in the plane that has been created, the surgeon can visualize and palpate the iliac apophysis as it curves anterior, making its division easy while the cluneal nerves and vessels are safely retracted. Inferiorly the apophysis is covered by the attachment of the gluteal muscles. A small portion of this muscle is divided with the cautery by proceeding directly caudal from the posterosuperior iliac spine. Care should be taken not to cut too far caudal because this is both unnecessary and will result in excessive bleeding. The apophysis can be split with the cautery to lessen the bleeding, but a sharp knife should then be used to continue the cut down to the bone. The cautery will often fail to cut all the way to the bone, making it difficult to begin the subperiosteal dissection.

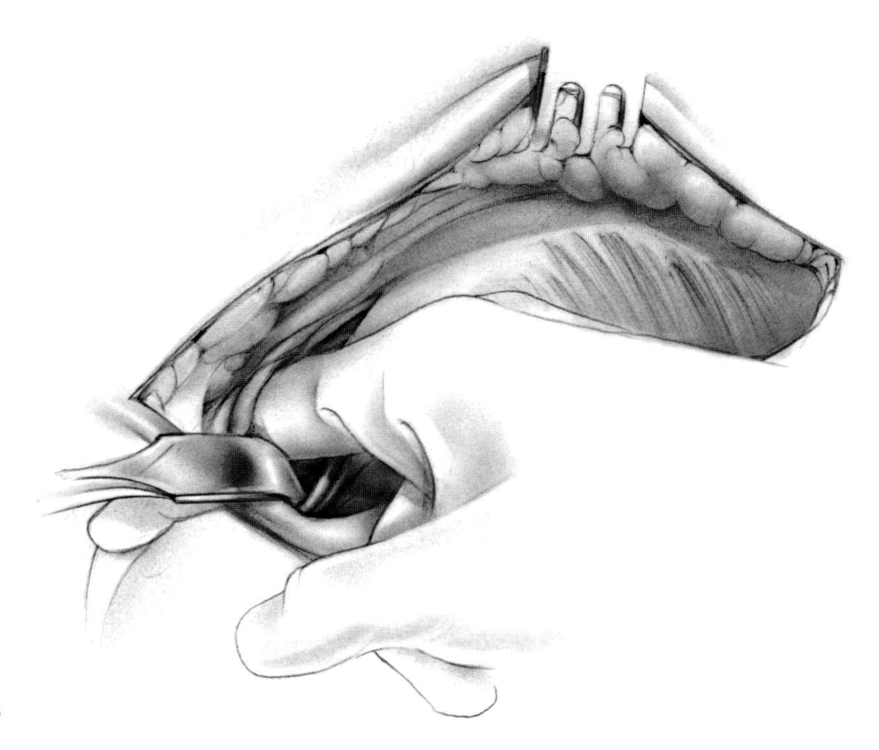

Figure 1–88

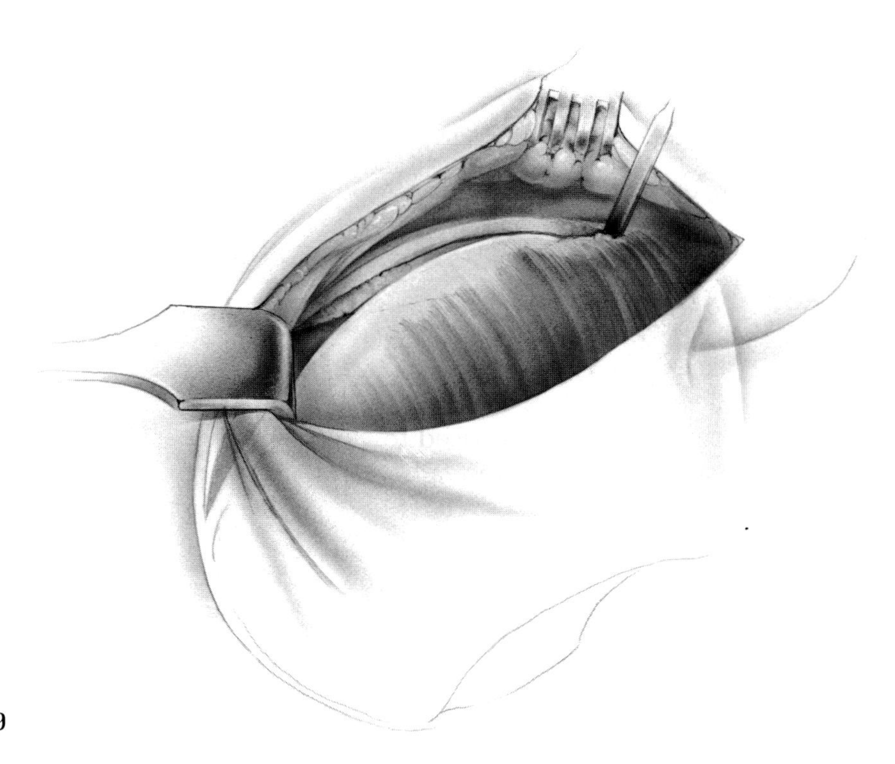

Figure 1–89

Figure 1–90. The subperiosteal dissection should completely expose the outer table of the iliac crest as shown. Care should be taken to expose the sciatic notch without plunging into it with the periosteal elevator. Many large veins and arteries run immediately beneath the fascia that covers the gluteal muscles in this region; if these muscles are cut, bleeding is often difficult to control. Of greater significance is the superior gluteal artery and veins that also course through the sciatic notch along with the sciatic nerve. If these vessels are cut, they will have to be controlled through an abdominal approach.

Figure 1–91. After the outer table is exposed, the cortical bone is removed. Insertion of a large Viboch iliac retractor facilitates this. This can be done in strips as illustrated or as one large piece to be cut into smaller pieces later. A small rim of bone may be left at the sciatic notch for safety. Because this is the thickest region of cancellous bone, however, the removal of the cortex should come as close to the notch as possible.

Figure 1–92. After the cortical bone is removed, the cancellous bone is harvested separately. The softness of this bone often tempts the surgeon to push the gouge rather than strike it with a mallet. It is much safer to advance the gouge by striking it, however. In this manner, control will be much better, and the potential for an uncontrolled plunge with the gouge lessened. After the cancellous bone is completely removed down to the inner table, a paste made from Gelfoam powder is rubbed into the raw bony surface, and the wound is packed tightly with lap sponges. At the completion of the operation, the lap sponges are removed. If there remains any significant bone bleeding, it can be controlled with bone wax. The closure of the wound is in layers: the apophysis; the fascial tissue over the apophysis, which is continuous caudally with the fascia over the gluteal muscles; the lumbodorsal fascia; and the skin. A drain is not necessary unless the crest has been approached from the midline, leaving a potential dead space under the skin.

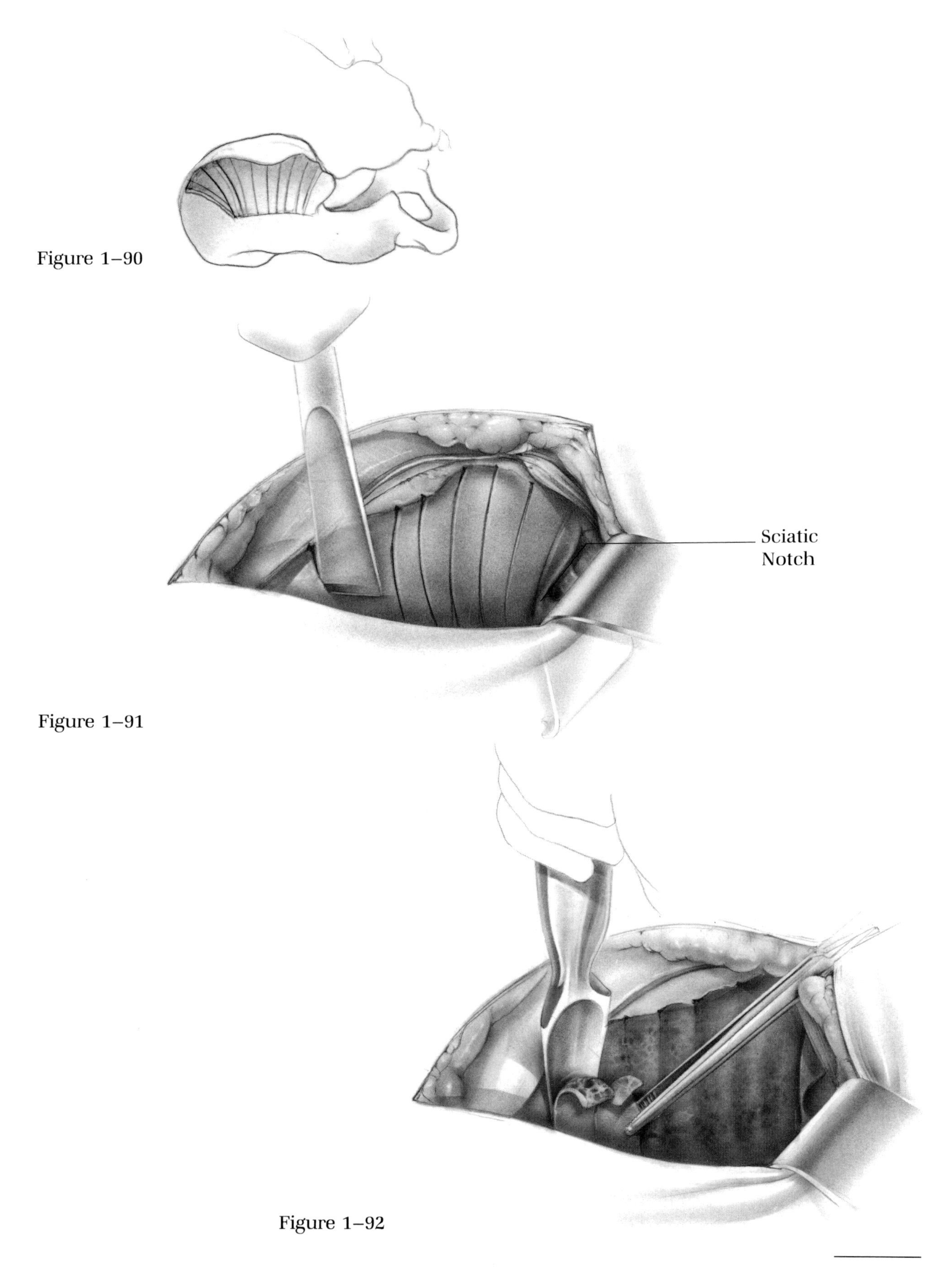

Figure 1–90

Figure 1–91

Figure 1–92

1.13
Release of Sternocleidomastoid Muscle

Figure 1–93. The incision should be placed in a skin crease a short distance above the clavicle. Because the skin is mobile and can be moved (not stretched) from medial to lateral the incision can be small, running from the lateral border of the sternal head to the midportion of the clavicular head.

Figure 1–94. The platysma muscle should be identified as a separate and distinct layer so that it may be repaired at the time of closure. This helps to preserve the contour of the neck and avoids an unsightly depression as a result of the resected sternocleidomastoid muscle.

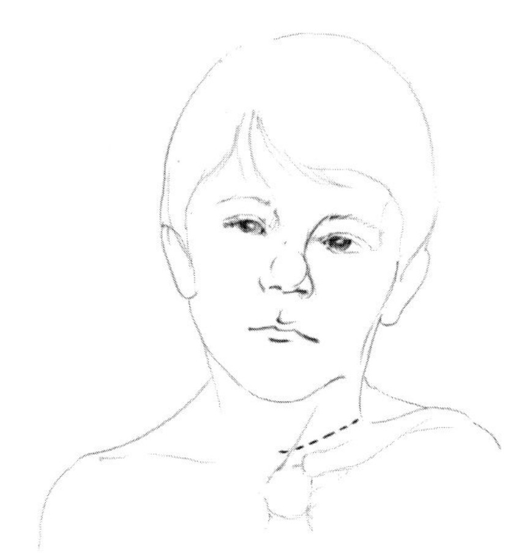

Figure 1–93

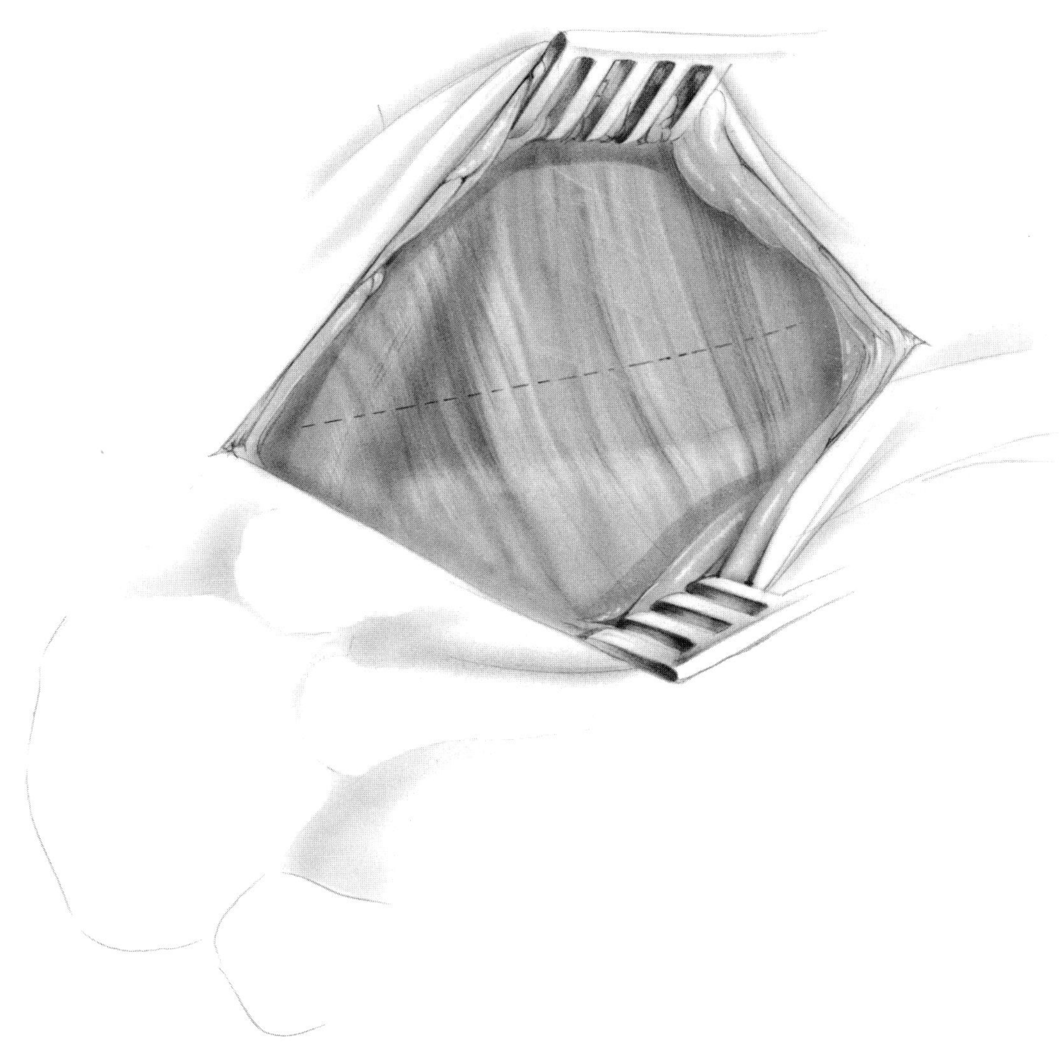

Figure 1–94

Figure 1–95. Beneath the platysma muscle the sternal and clavicular head of the sternocleidomastoid muscle can usually be identified as distinct structures. In some cases the clavicular head will be thin and seem of little importance. Failure to divide it will usually result in disappointment. Although the sternocleidomastoid muscle is separated from the deeper venous and arterial structures by a fascial layer, the muscle is usually very adherent and should be separated from this fascial layer with care. When isolated, the muscle can be divided with a low cautery current close to the clavicle in its tendinous portion.

Figure 1–96. Because the sternocleidomastoid muscle is adherent to the surrounding fascia, it is not sufficient merely to divide it. Rather it should be dissected free for a distance of approximately 2 cm, and the portion that is freed should be resected. In accomplishing this the adherence of the muscle to the investing fascia will be appreciated. If this dissection is not done, the severed muscle ends will lie in close proximity after the platysma muscle is repaired and recurrence is likely.

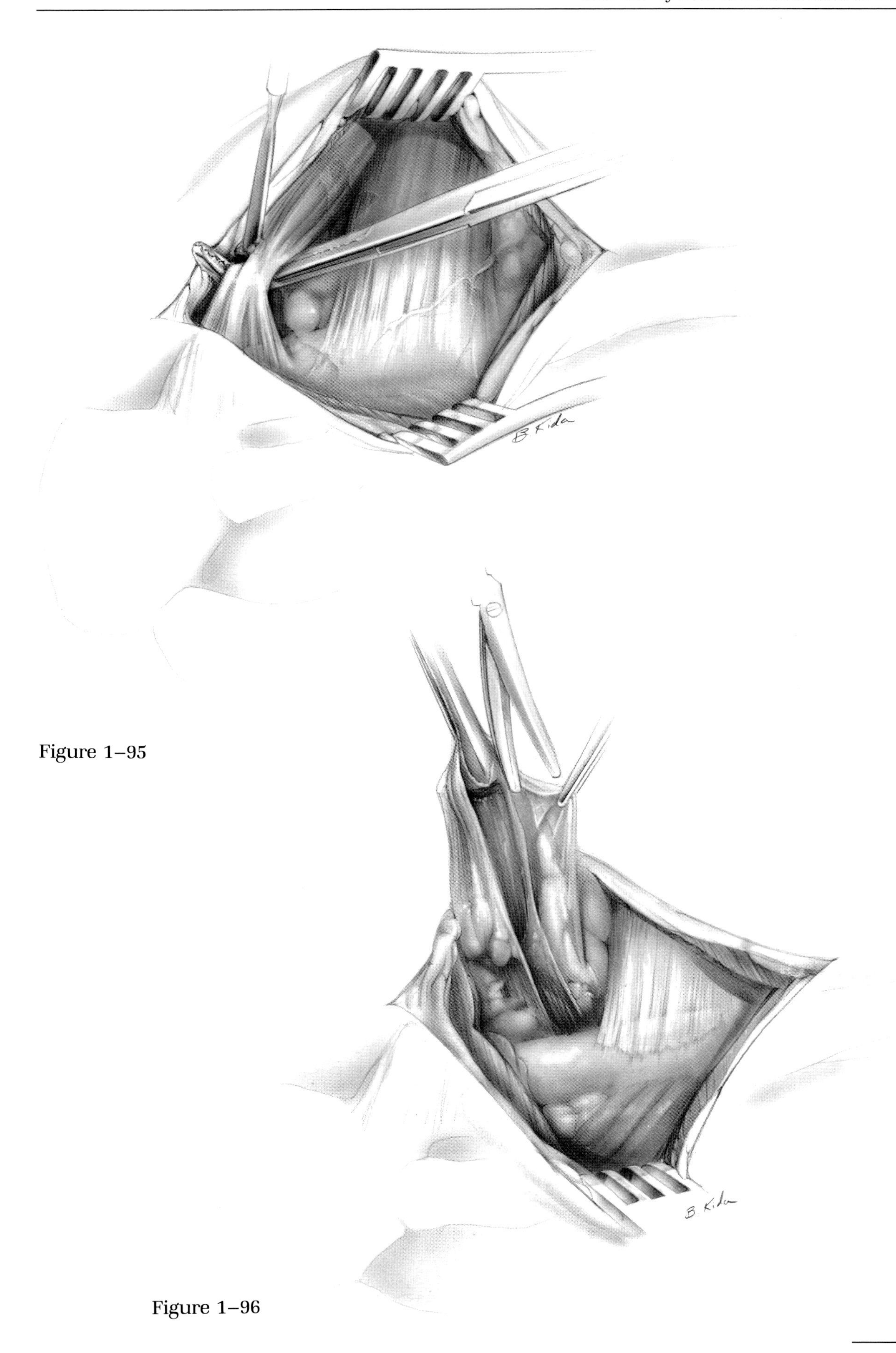

Figure 1–95

Figure 1–96

Figure 1–97. Next the clavicular head is divided. If the anesthesiologist is asked to turn the head toward and tilt it away from the operative side, the tightness of this structure will become apparent. It is divided, dissected free, and resected in the same manner as the sternal head. This is usually much easier, however, because the sternal head is usually the most involved. After both heads have been divided, the head is moved in the direction described earlier, while the operative area is inspected and palpated for any remaining tight structures. Often deep fascial bands will be identified and should be divided. The wound is inspected for bleeding, irrigated, drained with a small Silastic drain, and then closed in layers with particular attention to the platysma muscle.

Figure 1–98. Two modifications to the method described are frequently used. The first of these is a "Z" lengthening of the sternal head of the sternocleidomastoid muscle. This is done in an effort to preserve the normal contour that this muscle provides to the neck. Although it can be easily accomplished, it may risk recurrence and in the author's experience has not been necessary if the platysma muscle is repaired properly.

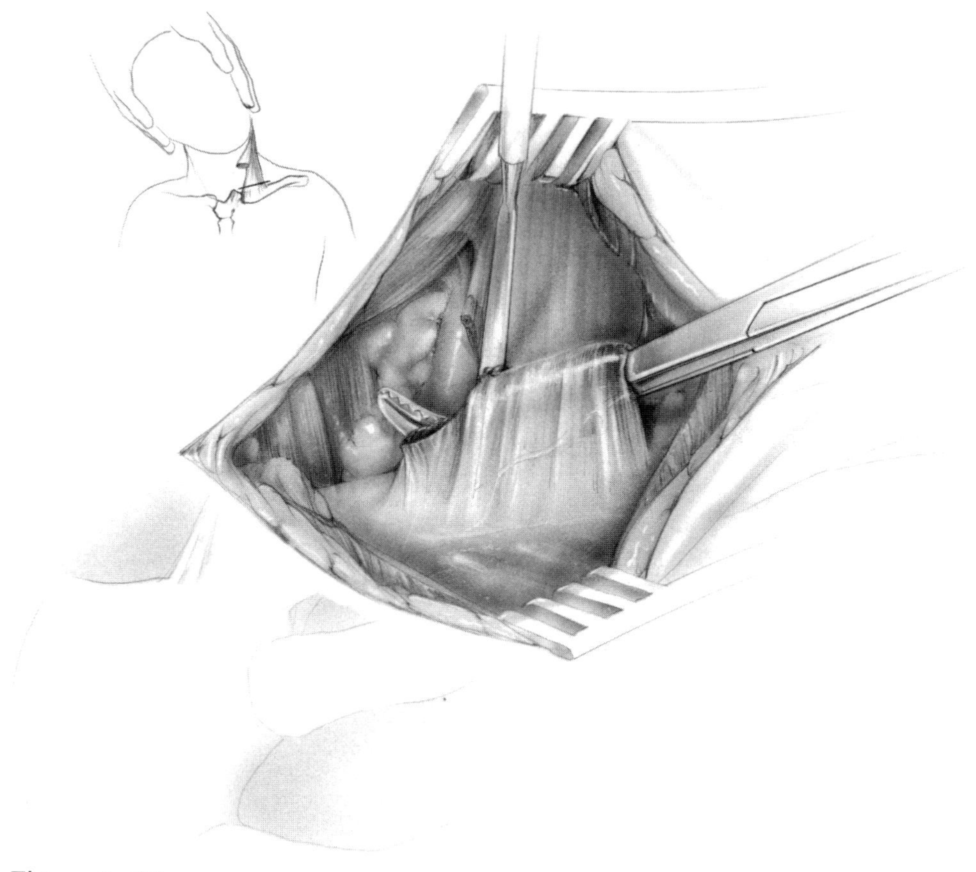

Figure 1–97

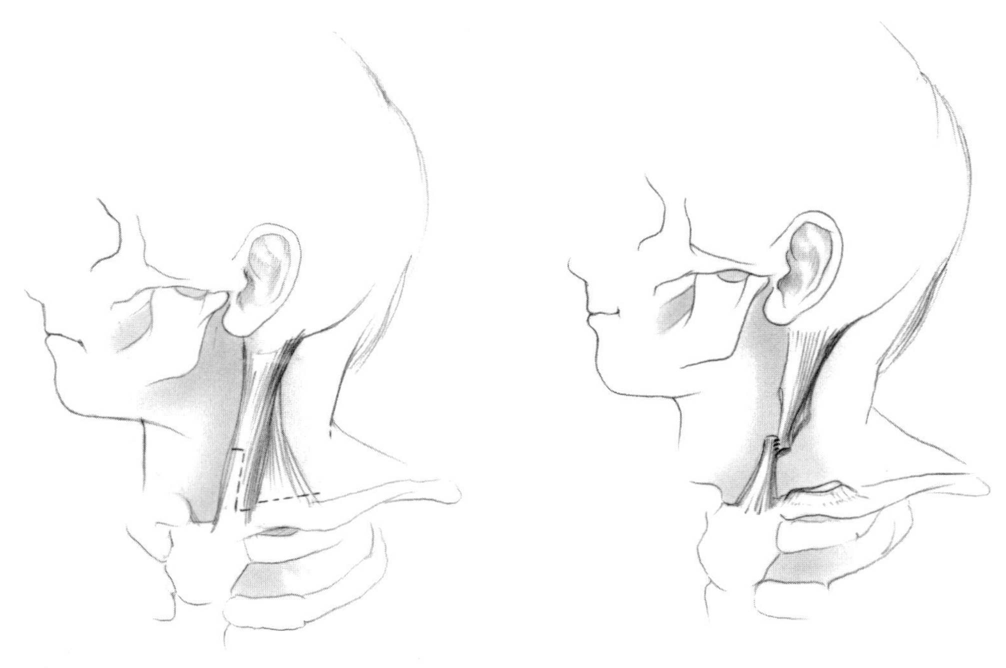

Figure 1–98

Figure 1–99. The second technique is the bipolar release. This is advocated in an effort to secure a more complete release. The author has never noticed a restriction of motion after release and suspects that it may be found necessary if the muscle is not dissected free of the investing fascia as described.

POSTOPERATIVE CARE

The drain is removed the morning following surgery, and the patient is discharged from the hospital. At 1 week stretching exercises are resumed and continued for 3 months. Collars and orthotic devices have not proved useful in the postoperative management.

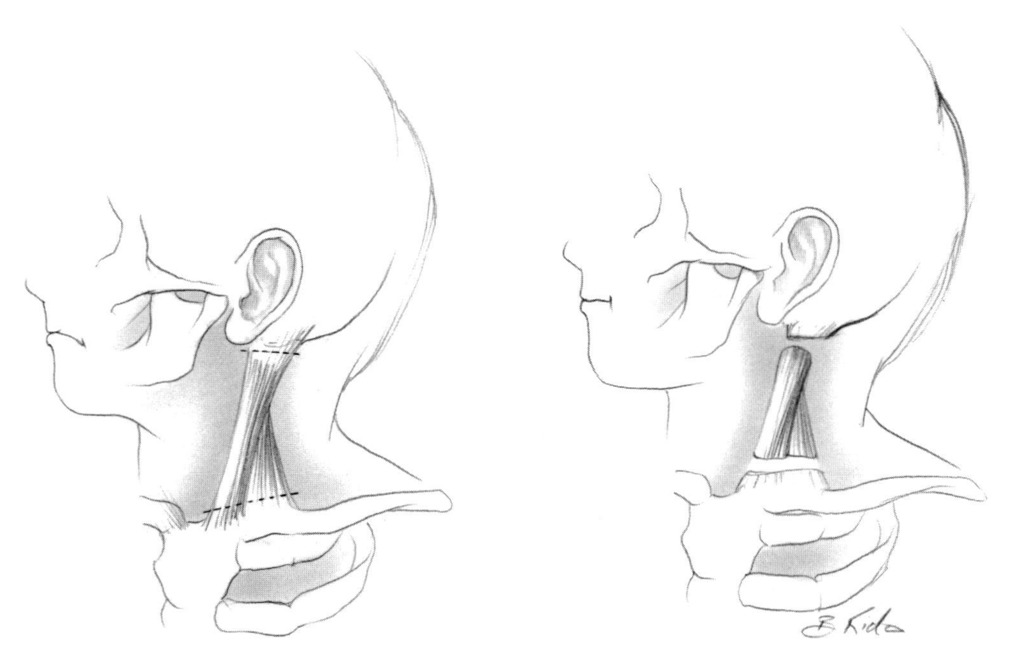

Figure 1–99

CHAPTER TWO
THE PELVIS AND HIP

2.1
Anterior Drainage of the Septic Hip

Drainage of septic arthritis of the hip is a procedure that few orthopaedic surgeons will be able to avoid because it is an emergency procedure. The controversy is not whether or not to drain a septic hip surgically, but whether to approach the hip anteriorly or posteriorly. There are several sound reasons to prefer an anterior approach, although this is not to say that a posterior approach is wrong or cannot be done well.

The transverse anterior incision in the skin is cosmetically superior to a posterior incision. The anterior approach provides a distinct anatomic landmark, the anterosuperior iliac spine, which is not the case in the chubby buttocks of an infant with a septic hip. The same is true deep where distinct anatomic intervals are separated rather than a large muscle being split in a region where the sciatic nerve may be accidentally encountered. Finally, and perhaps most important, it is preferable that the incision be placed in the anterior capsule. The hip will usually be treated in some degree of flexion whether it be in traction or a cast. This, plus the natural tendency of the hip to flex and dislocate posteriorly, dictates that the incision is best in the anterior capsule. There is no need for "gravity drainage" with modern methods of suction or suction-irrigation. In addition, one may question the wisdom of having a rubber drain communicate from the buttocks to the hip joint.

Figure 2–1. The patient is placed in the lateral decubitus position as for most other procedures on the hip. The incision, placed about a thumb's breadth beneath the anterosuperior iliac spine, can be smaller and more transverse than that used for other major hip procedures because it is not necessary to expose the outer table of the ilium.

Figure 2–2. The interval between the sartorius and tensor muscles is identified and separated up to the anterosuperior iliac spine. If necessary the periosteum can be elevated from the outer table of the ilium in the region of the anterosuperior iliac spine; however, after some experience with this approach, this will usually not be necessary.

Figure 2–3. At the base of the exposure between the sartorius and tensor muscles is the rectus muscle. In this area, close to the anterosuperior iliac spine, its tendinous portion can be identified. A periosteal elevator can be used to separate the fatty tissue covering this tendon. The lateral border of this tendon with its muscular origin is freed and retracted medially.

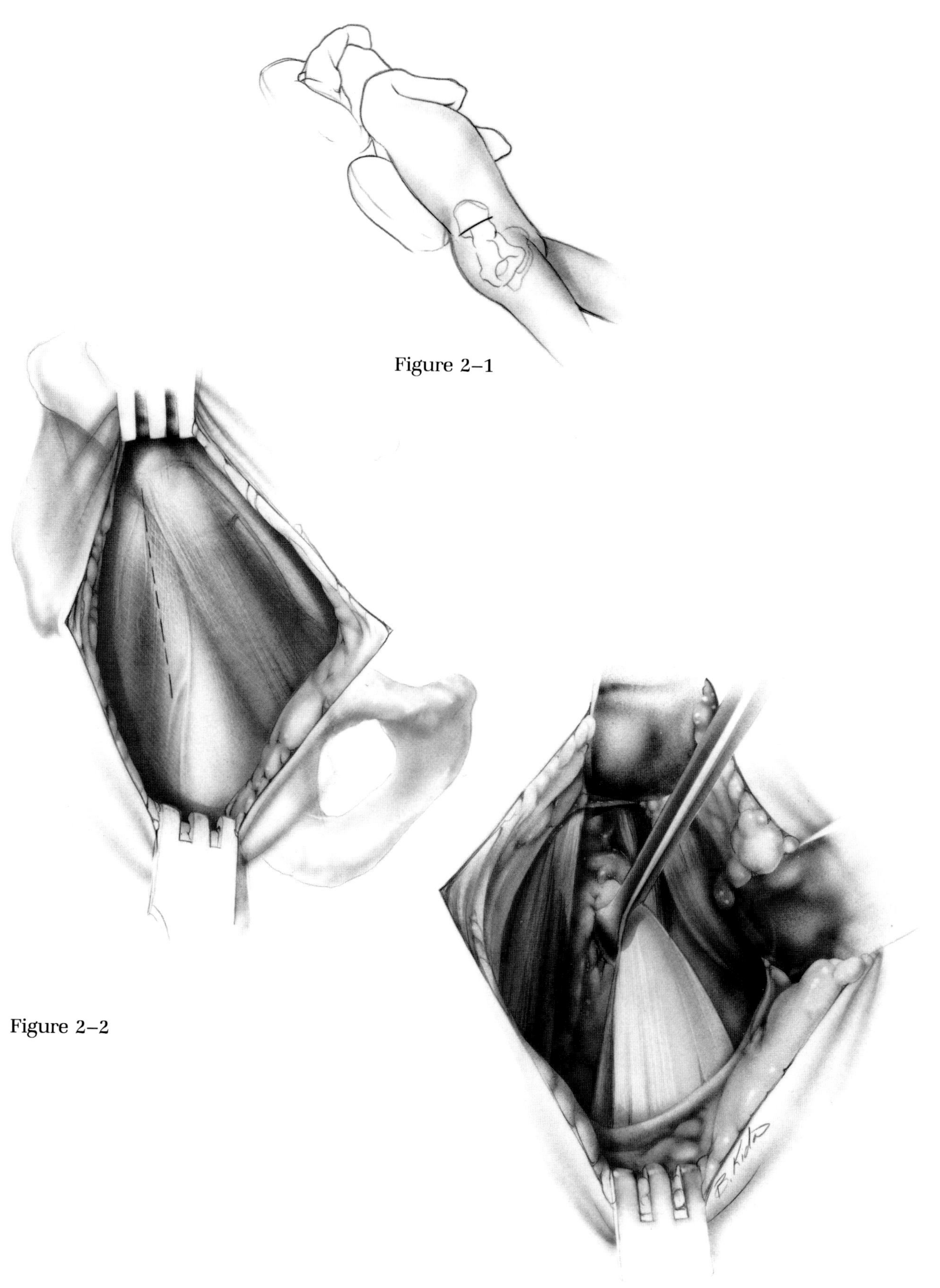

Figure 2–1

Figure 2–2

Figure 2–3

Figure 2–4. The hip capsule now lies in the base of the field. It will be covered by the precapsular fatty tissue, which may be quite thick and edematous in the septic hip. This can also be separated with a periosteal elevator exposing the hip capsule itself. A cruciate incision is now made in the capsule, exposing the femoral neck and part of the femoral head. This will provide adequate access for inspection and irrigation of the joint.

Figure 2–5. A small red rubber catheter, with the multiple perforations at the tip cut off, is passed around the femoral neck and into the various recesses of the joint to provide thorough irrigation. Inspection should assure that there are no fibrinous clots of inflammatory material remaining in the joint. Often these will have to be removed with a forceps when present.

After complete irrigation and debridement, and placement of drains and irrigation if desired, the muscles are allowed to fall back together, and the deep fascia and skin are closed.

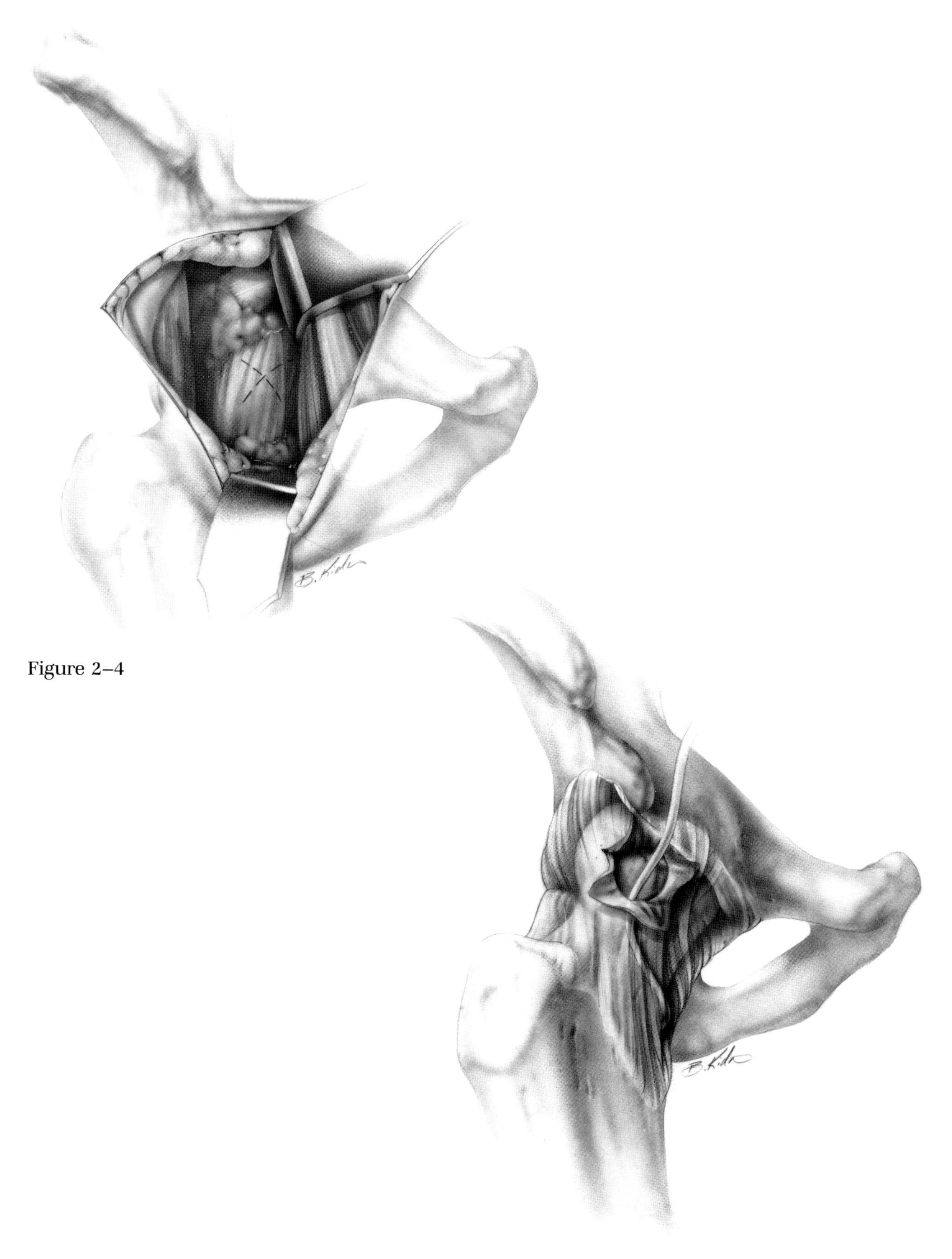

Figure 2–4

Figure 2–5

POSTOPERATIVE CARE

There are many options for care after the drainage and debridement depending on the surgeon's preferences and the circumstances of the case. The author's preference is to use suction-irrigation with physiologic solution. This provides a continuous debridement of the joint. The patient is placed in split Russell's traction initially while intravenous antibiotics are administered. The irrigation tube is switched to suction at 12 to 24 hours after surgery, and both it and the drain are removed 12 to 24 hours after that. If the hip is subluxated or dislocated it is often desirable to achieve a closed reduction at the time of wound closure and place the patient directly into a spica cast. It is the author's preference to treat all children with septic arthritis of the hip in a single-leg spica cast for 3 weeks to avoid any late subluxation secondary to capsular laxity. If the cast is not applied at the time of surgery, it is applied before discharge.

2.2 Anterior Approach to a Congenitally Dislocated Hip

The anterior approach to open reduction of congenital dislocation of the hip is the classic method. It has the advantage of exposing the capsule and both the superior and inferior aspects of the acetabulum allowing the surgeon to address all possible obstructions to reduction as well as perform a capsulorrhaphy to hold the femoral head in the acetabulum. The only disadvantage is the technical experience and expertise that is necessary to avoid all of the pitfalls that can lead to failure.

Figure 2–6. The patient is placed in the full lateral position with the affected hip up. A sand bag is placed behind the back, not extending to the buttocks. The leg is prepared and draped from the toes to the rib cage past the midline both ventrally and dorsally. The patient is then allowed to roll back on the sand bag, placing the hip in an obliquely elevated position with the buttocks free.

The incision can be either transverse or oblique. It is centered 2 to 2.5 cm below the anterosuperior iliac spine. This will permit the same exposure as the classic Smith-Petersen incision with a far better cosmetic result. The incision is carried down through the superficial fascia, and as this is done the skin is pulled up over the iliac crest so that the crest will be exposed. A finger is then used to pull the inferior edge of the wound distal, elevating a flap over the interval between the sartorius and tensor muscles.

Figure 2–7. The sartorius-tensor muscle interval is identified by palpating the depression between these two muscles just distal to the anterosuperior iliac spine (ASIS). A small stab wound is made through the fascia, and a scissors is used to open this interval from the ASIS to the distal extent of the exposure, staying toward the tensor muscle to avoid the lateral femoral cutaneous nerve. The nerve can be identified proximally and care taken to keep it medial.

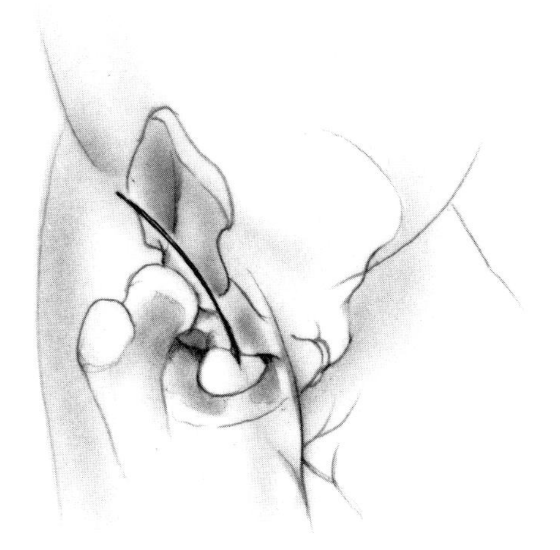

Figure 2–6

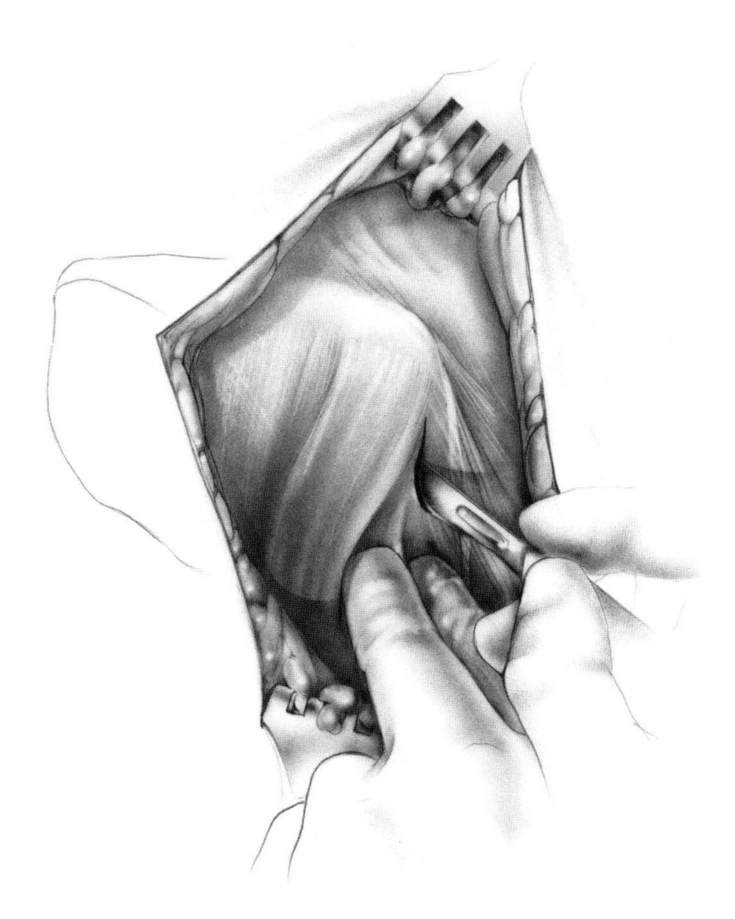

Figure 2–7

Figure 2–8. The sartorius-tensor interval is easily separated by gentle blunt dissection with a Cobb periosteal elevator, pulling the sartorius muscle and the fat that is found in this interval medial and the tensor muscle lateral. The rectus muscle forms the floor of this interval. At the inferior extent of the wound, passing deep between the sartorius and tensor muscles, the ascending branch of the medial circumflex artery and its accompanying veins should be identified and divided. If this interval is not opened beyond these vessels there will be insufficient exposure to reach the inferior aspects of the acetabulum. Proximally this interval needs to be opened to the anterosuperior iliac spine.

Figure 2–9. The retractors are now shifted to expose the iliac crest, and the iliac apophysis is split open down to the bone. The periosteum is elevated off of the outer table, pulling the tensor and the abductors laterally. Bleeding is controlled with cautery and bone wax, and a sponge is packed tightly into the proximal extent of the wound between the abductor muscles and the outer table of the ilium to provide retraction. Elevating the periosteum from the inner table of the ilium aids in the exposure and is necessary if an iliac osteotomy is to be performed.

The straight and reflected heads of the rectus muscle can be identified by a combination of sharp and blunt dissection. The reflected head of the rectus can be followed around the superior capsule by dividing the periosteum off the ilium. This helps to expose the superior capsule. The rectus muscle is then divided at its conjoined tendon and retracted distally. All that now remains to expose the capsule is to divide and clean the pericapsular fat and fibrous tissue from the capsule. This is best done by dividing it sharply down to the actual capsule and then using a combination of cautery current and dissection with a sharp periosteal elevator.

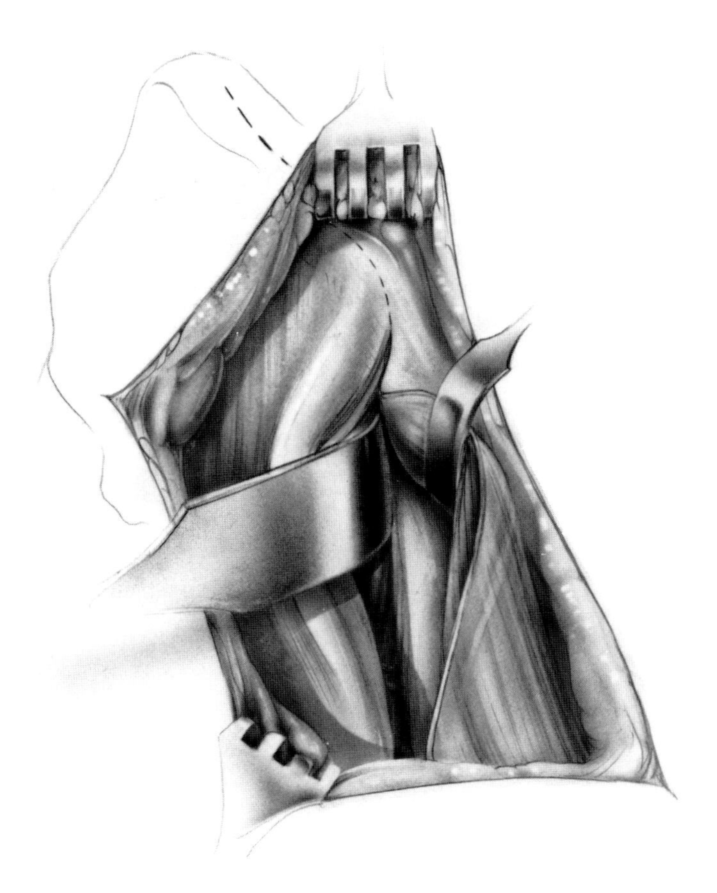

Figure 2–8

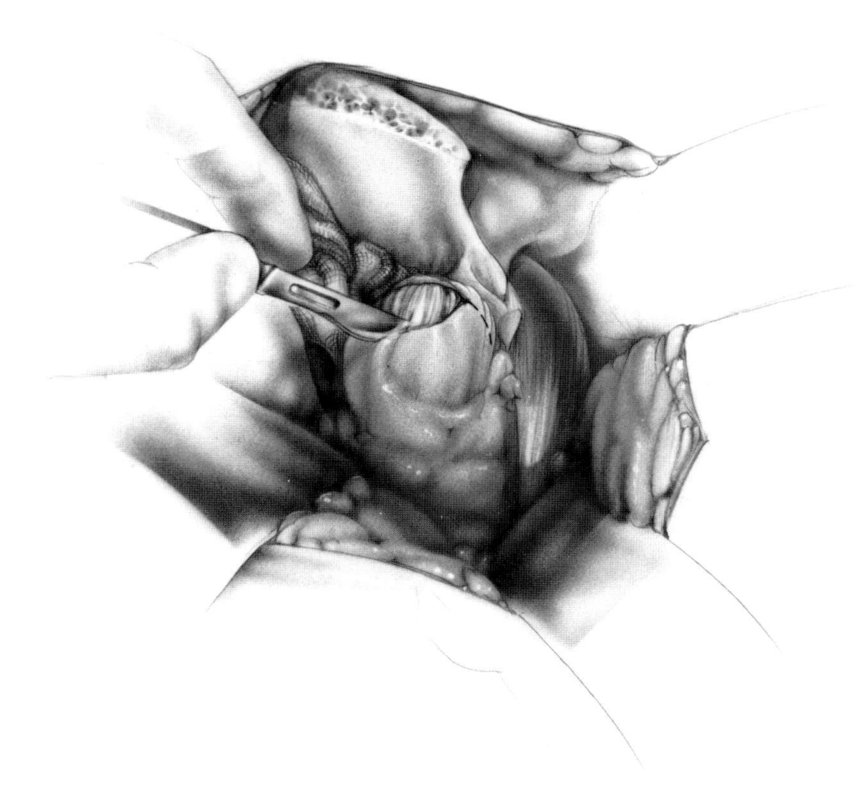

Figure 2–9

Figure 2–10. If the hip has been dislocated for any length of time there will be a false acetabulum, and the capsule will be adherent to it. It is essential that the capsule be stripped off of the ilium down to the true acetabulum, exposing this false acetabulum. This is done with the periosteal elevator and will leave a rough area of bone after the adherent capsule has been elevated. When seen from inside the capsule it is remarkable how much the surface of this false acetabulum resembles the true acetabular cartilage. Unfortunately, many hips have been "reduced" into this false acetabulum.

Before proceeding it is important to be sure that the capsule has been adequately exposed. Inferiorly the capsule should be exposed to its insertion into the bottom of the acetabulum. This will lie beneath the superiorly displaced iliopsoas tendon. If this is not done it will be difficult to divide the transverse acetabular ligament. Superiorly the capsule should be exposed around to the posterior aspect. If this is not accomplished it will be difficult to obliterate the redundant capsule, which is part of the capsulorrhaphy.

Figure 2–11. It is essential that the psoas tendon be divided to allow the hip to be reduced without tension that could result in avascular necrosis or redislocation. Because the proximal femur is superiorly displaced, the iliopsoas will also be superiorly displaced. It can be easily identified as it crosses the pubic ramus just medial to the anteroinferior iliac spine. Cutting the periosteum that was elevated off of the inner table of the ilium will expose the iliac portion of this muscle, making identification of the psoas tendon easier. The tendon will be found on the underside of the muscle and is drawn into view by the use of a right-angled clamp (*inset*). The tendon fibers are divided, leaving the muscle intact. Some care should be used in identifying the tendon because the femoral nerve lies nearby.

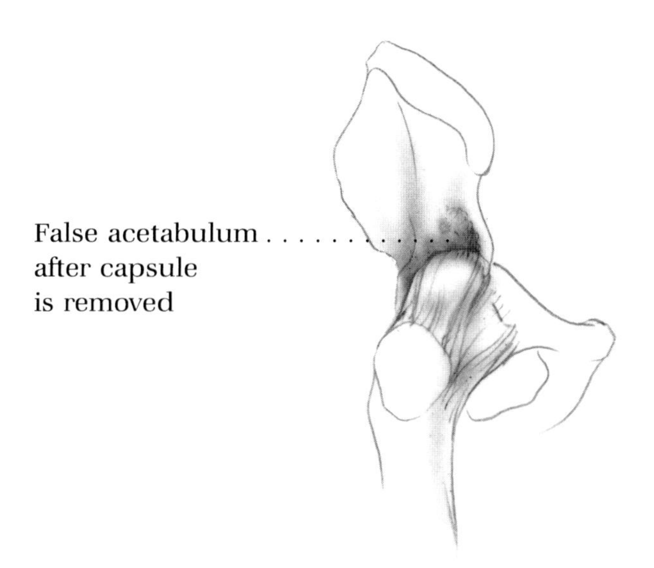

Figure 2–10

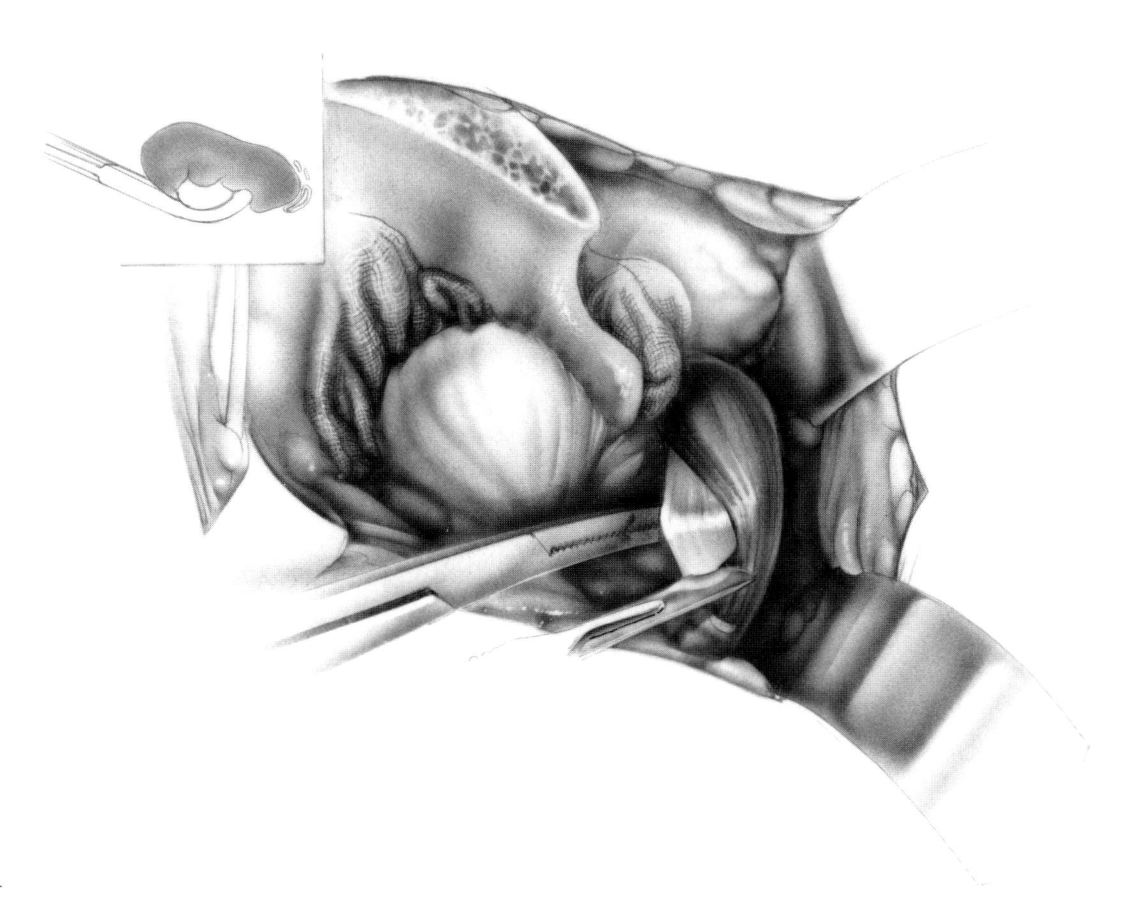

Figure 2–11

Figure 2–12. The proper placement of the incisions in the capsule is important to the capsulorrhaphy. The first incision is parallel to the acetabular rim, extending from the most inferior aspect of the acetabulum to the posterosuperior aspect. A transverse incision is then made in the capsule over the femoral neck. This cut will divide the capsule into a superior and inferior part. The ligamentum teres, if present, is identified and sectioned from the femoral head. It is followed down to the inferior acetabulum and excised. It provides an excellent guide to the inferior acetabulum and leads to the transverse acetabular ligament, which can be palpated as a sharp band. This should be divided because it will limit the size of the acetabulum and prevent the femoral head from contacting the medial wall of the acetabulum.

Figure 2–13. The femoral head should now reduce easily into the acetabulum. Sutures of a strong nonabsorbable material will be used to repair the capsule. They should be placed first on the acetabular side with the femoral head retracted laterally to expose the inferior and medial acetabular wall better. These sutures are placed medially beyond the acetabulum into the periosteum for a strong grip. They are then placed in the capsule to suture it in the manner illustrated.

The purpose of the repair is to suture the capsule in such a way that the femoral head is pulled both inferiorly and medially. The key to this is to suture the end of the vertical cut in the capsule (*A*) to the pubis inferior and medial to the anteroinferior iliac spine. The redundant portion of the capsule superior to this vertical cut is excised, thus obliterating the redundant portion of the capsule. The resulting cut edge will now lie along the acetabular margin where it is sutured.

After the capsulorrhaphy is completed the reduction can be checked by a portable radiograph. It should not be necessary to hold the hip in place or resort to the use of transfixing wires: The capsular repair should hold the femoral head securely in the acetabulum. The wound is closed. A one-leg spica cast is applied with the hip in approximately 30 degrees of flexion, 20 degrees of abduction, and 15 degrees of internal rotation.

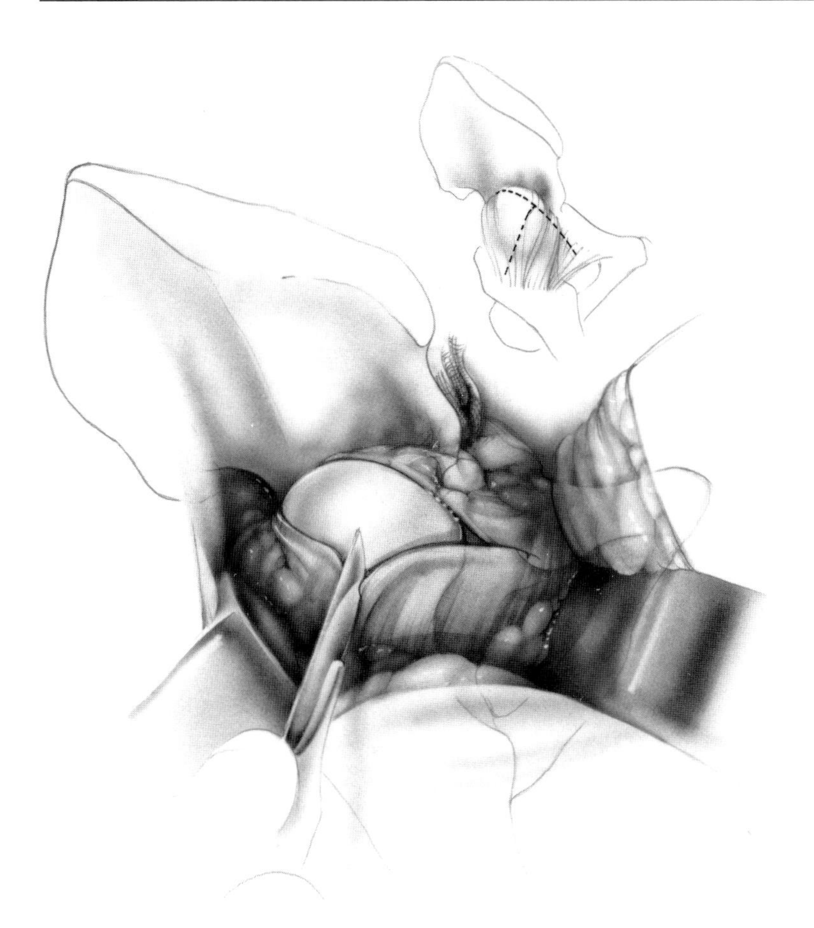

Figure 2–12

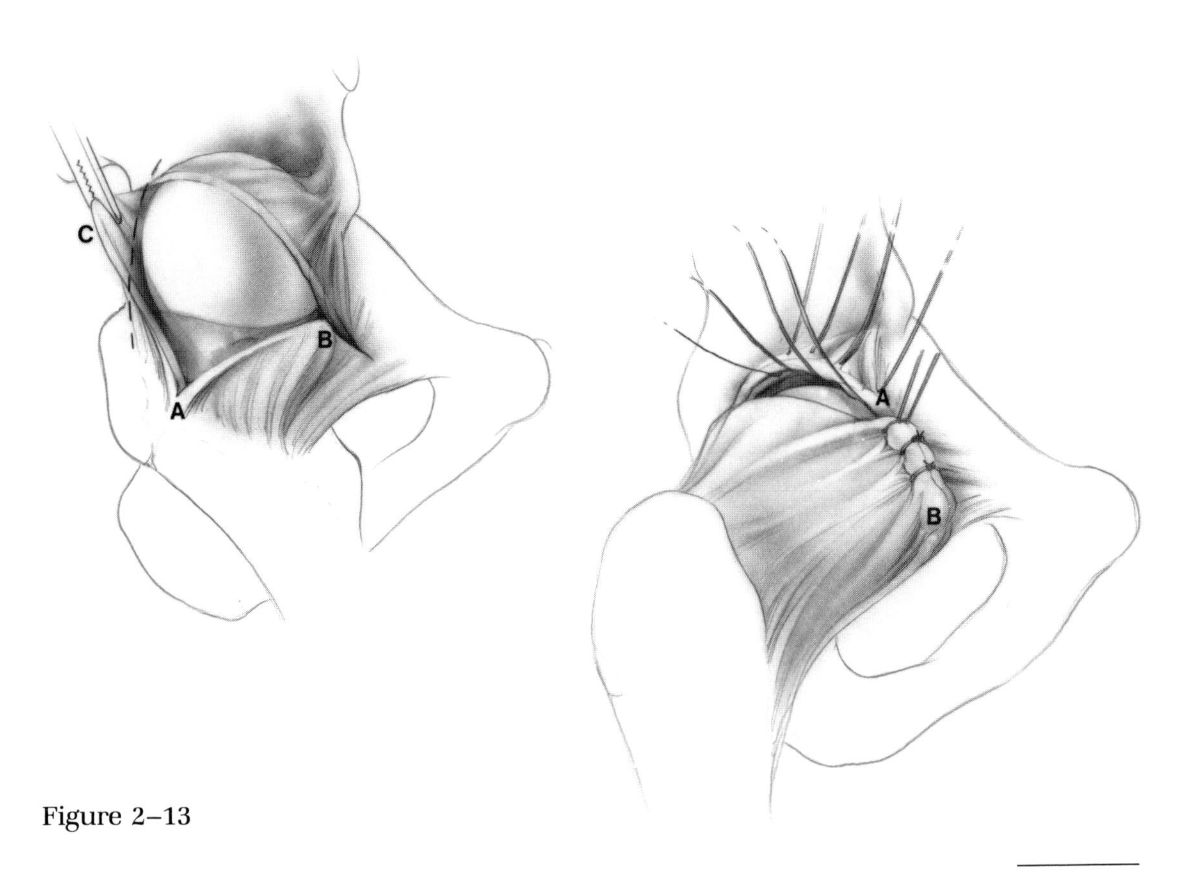

Figure 2–13

POSTOPERATIVE CARE

Although it is less difficult to care for a patient in a one-leg spica, the parents should be familiar with the routine care of their child and the cast. The patient is usually ready for discharge 2 to 3 days after surgery. The cast is left in place for 6 weeks. It is then removed and the reduction monitored with an anteroposterior radiograph. A cylinder cast is then applied to each leg with the knee bent about 15 degrees, and a bar is secured to these casts to maintain abduction. The patient may then start to sit and crawl. These casts are removed in 4 weeks. Further bracing should not be necessary as the soft tissues will have healed sufficiently to hold the reduction. Ambulation is started. The abduction contracture will gradually resolve.

2.3 Medial Approach to a Congenitally Dislocated Hip

The medial or anteromedial approach to the reduction of a congenitally dislocated hip was initially reported in the American literature by Ludloff in 1913.[1] Not until 10 years after the report of Mau et al in 1971[2] and Ferguson in 1973[3] did this procedure receive wide usage in the United States. Although the indications for this procedure are not universally agreed on,[4] it is generally indicated in younger children under 18 months of age who fail closed reduction. In principle the operation is designed to remove certain obstacles to closed reduction, *eg*, a tight iliopsoas tendon, a constricted capsule, and the transverse acetabular ligament. Unlike the anterior approach, a capsulorrhaphy is not possible, and it is difficult or impossible to deal with the cranial structures, *eg*, the labrum.

There are several variations on the medial approach. The most common approach and the one described here is between the pectineus muscle anteriorly and the adductor longus and brevis muscles posteriorly. Ferguson passed between the adductor longus and brevis muscles anteriorly, and the gracilis and adductor magnus muscles posteriorly. Weinstein and Ponseti[5] use a more anterior approach than either of these, going between the neurovascular bundle anteriorly and the pectineus muscle posteriorly.

Figure 2–14. A transverse incision 3 to 4 cm in length and 1 cm distal to the groin crease is made with two thirds of the incision superior to the adductor longus tendon. This incision is similar to that used to release the adductors in cerebral palsy.

Figure 2–15. The fascia along the superior border of the adductor longus is opened, and this muscle is isolated and divided close to its insertion on the pelvis and retracted distally.

Figure 2–16. The cut muscle is retracted distally, exposing the adductor brevis muscle in the inferior part of the wound and the pectineus muscle in the superior part of the wound. The branches of the anterior obturator nerve can be seen on the surface of the adductor brevis muscle. Blunt dissection follows this nerve beneath the pectineus muscle.

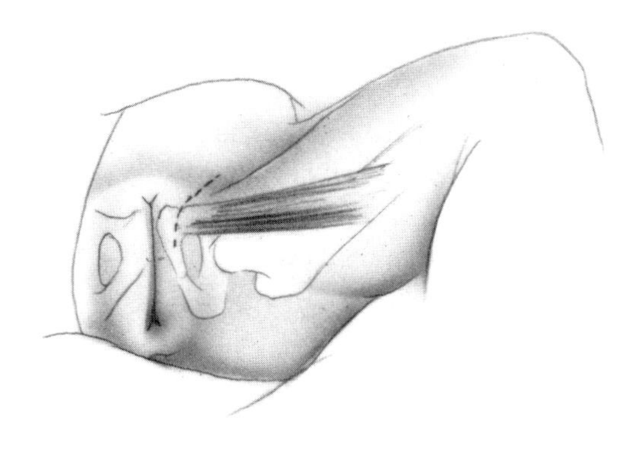

Figure 2–14

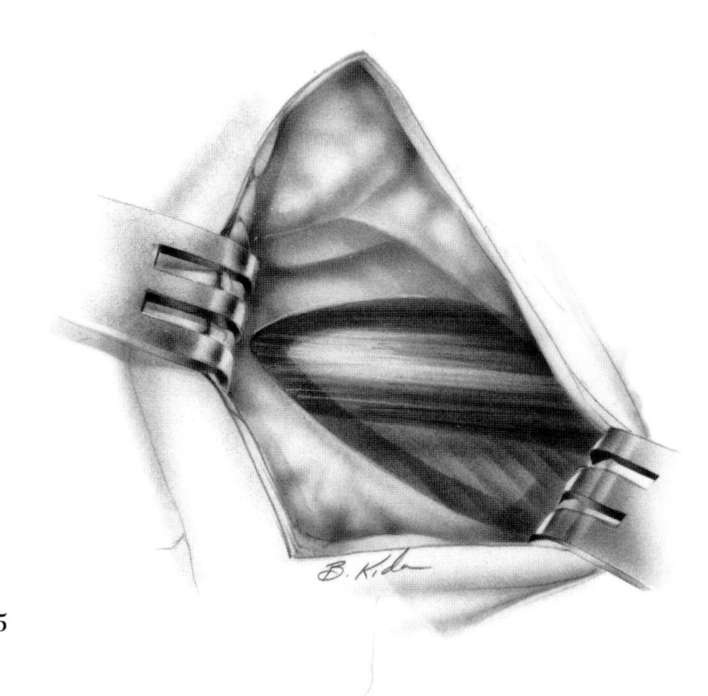

Figure 2–15

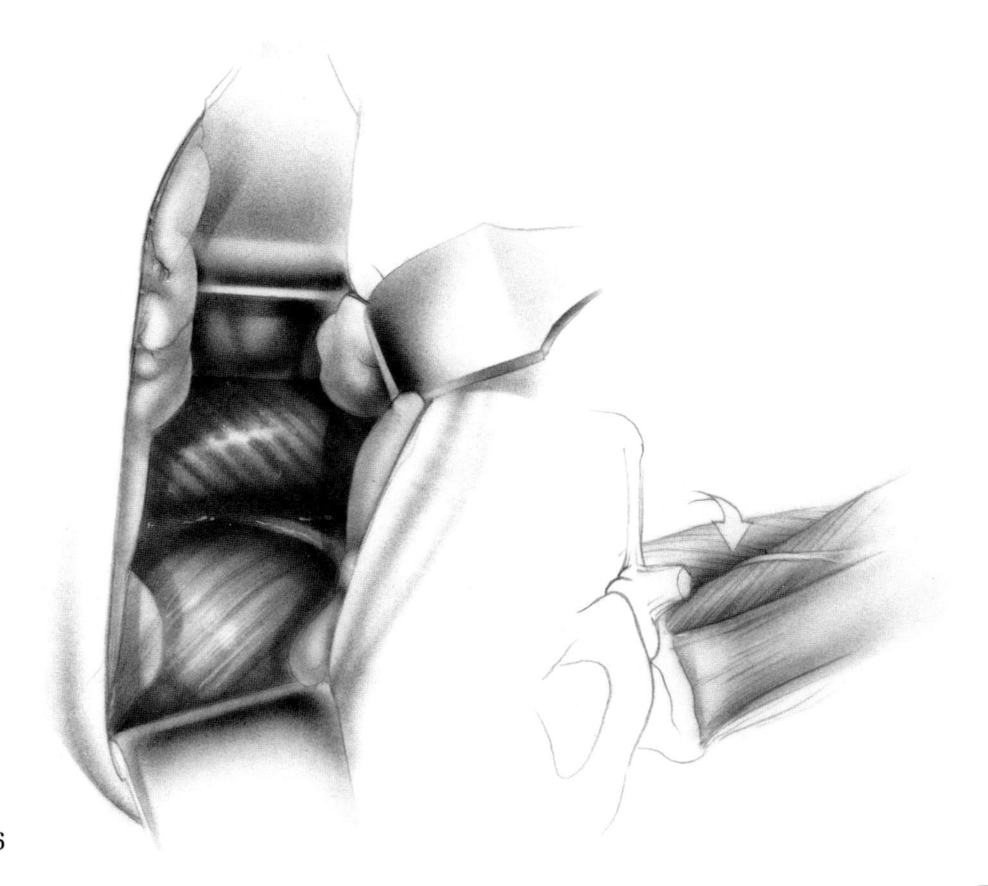

Figure 2–16

Figure 2–17. The posterior border of the pectineus muscle is freed proximally to its insertion on the pelvis as well as distally. This step is essentially the same as that in performing an iliopsoas tenotomy through the medial approach, except that more proximal dissection is required. A retractor is placed beneath the pectineus muscle, retracting it superiorly. The lesser trochanter and the iliopsoas tendon can be felt but not easily seen. This is because the tendon is surrounded by a fascial layer that must first be opened. Once the tendon is visualized, it can be pulled into the wound with a right-angled clamp and sharply divided.

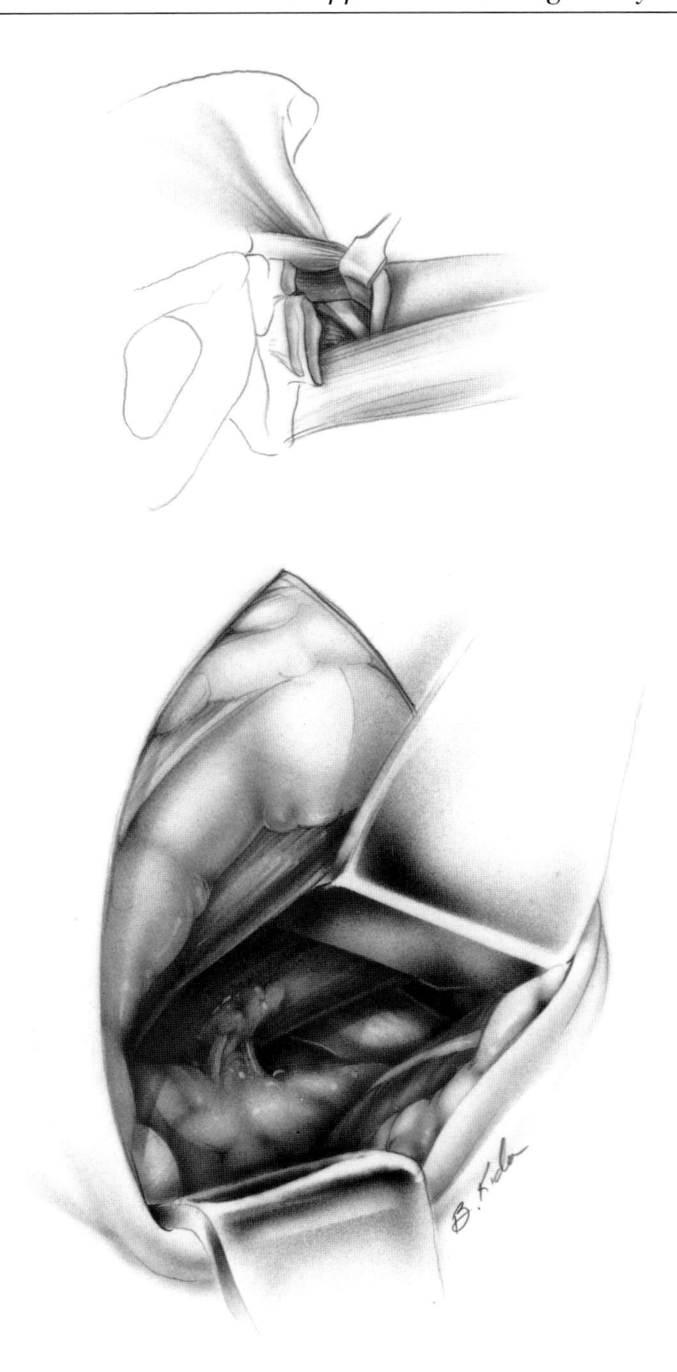

Figure 2–17

Figure 2–18. After the iliopsoas tendon is divided, it only remains to clear the precapsular fat from the capsule. This is accomplished with blunt dissection. A small branch of the medial circumflex artery will be seen crossing the capsule inferiorly. This can be dissected free and occasionally spared, although its ligation has not resulted in an increase in avascular necrosis.[5]

Figure 2–19. The capsule is now cut open in the direction of the femoral neck. The transverse acetabular ligament is readily identified and may be sectioned. The ligamentum teres can be seen. Additional release of the capsule can be performed if necessary, but in most cases the hip will be seen to reduce easily into the acetabulum.

The hip should be reduced and held in various postions to determine the best position for postoperative immobilization. This is because it will not be possible to perform a capsulorrhaphy to hold the hip in place. This will be accomplished as in closed reduction by the cast. It is particularly important to note what degree of flexion causes the hip to subluxate inferiorly. Finally, the deep fascia and skin are closed.

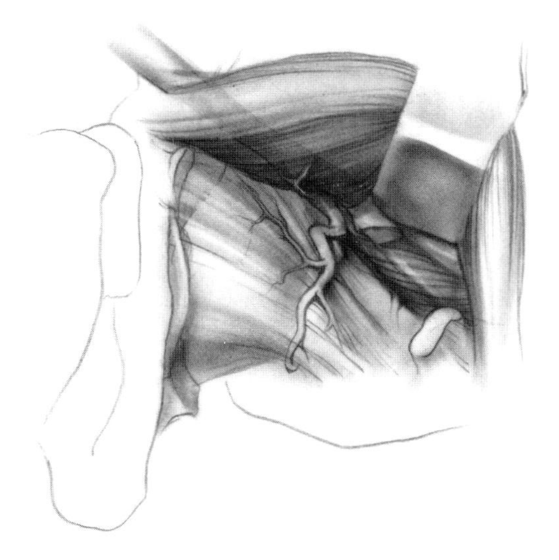

Figure 2–18

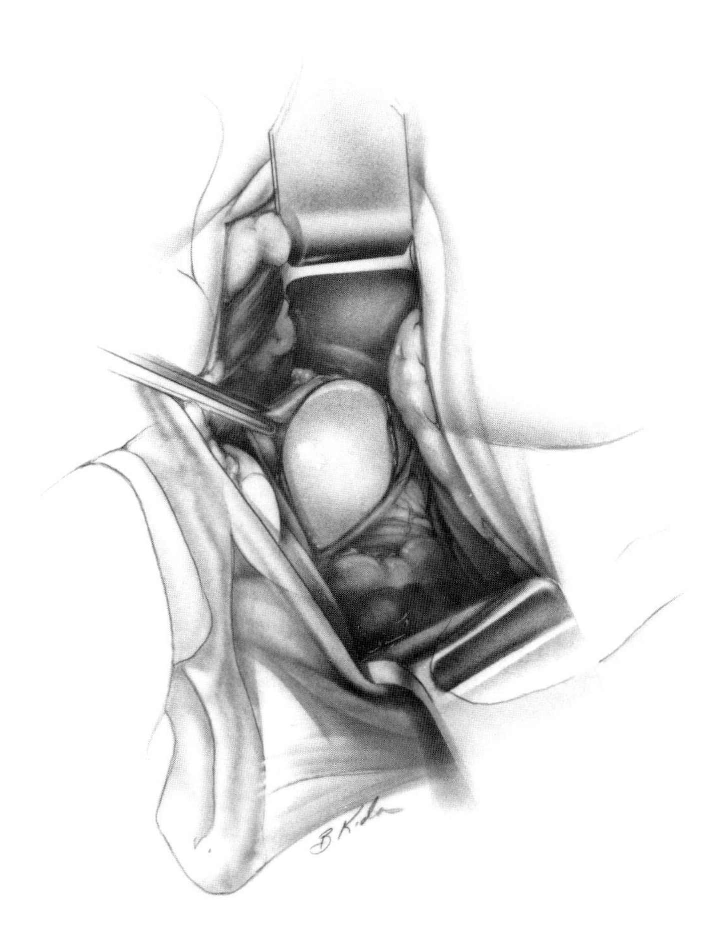

Figure 2–19

POSTOPERATIVE CARE

A one-and-one-half spica cast (double spica cast if both hips are opened) is applied while the patient is still under anesthesia. The hip is placed in the position that was determined best by inspection. This will usually be similar to the human position of Salter that is used in closed reduction but with somewhat less flexion.

The patient should be maintained in the cast for the same time the surgeon would use had a closed reduction been performed. This will vary considerably on the age of the child and the surgeon's reliance on methods of abduction splinting other than the spica cast. Development of the lateral edge of the acetabulum is a useful sign of a stable reduction.

REFERENCES

1. Ludloff K. The open reduction of the congenital hip dislocation by an anterior incision. Am J Orthop Surg 1913;10:438.
2. Mau H, Dorr WM, Henkel L, Lutsche J. Open reduction of congenital dislocation of the hip by Ludloff's method. J Bone Joint Surg 1971;53A:1281.
3. Ferguson SB Jr. Primary open reduction of congenital dislocation of the hip using a median adductor approach. J Bone Joint Surg 1973;55A:617.
4. Herring JA. Congenital dislocation of the hip. In: Morrissy RT, ed. Lovell and Winter's pediatric orthopaedics, 3rd ed. Philadelphia: JB Lippincott, 1990:836.
5. Weinstein SL, Ponseti IV. Congenital dislocation of the hip. J Bone Joint Surg 1979;61A:119.

2.4 Salter's Innominate Osteotomy

In 1961 Salter described an operation based on a new principle: redirection of the entire acetabulum as a unit. This was accomplished by performing a transverse osteotomy of the ilium just above the acetabulum, and opening the osteotomy anterolaterally by hinging and rotating the acetabular segment on the symphysis pubis.[1] It was designed to preserve the normal acetabular structures and shape while at the same time correcting the abnormal anterior and lateral facing of the acetabulum seen in late cases of congenital dislocation of the hip. It is probably the most widely used and written about pelvic osteotomy in the treatment of congenital dislocation of the hip. Unfortunately it is also the most poorly performed and misapplied because of the apparent ease with which it can be performed. The judgment involved in the application of Salter's osteotomy and its proper technical execution are not easy.[2] The prerequisites, contraindications, and potential errors are all well described.[3] Among the most obvious and frequent errors is the failure to obtain a concentric reduction before performing the osteotomy.

The patient is positioned as for open reduction of the hip through the anterior approach, and the same incision and approach are used. If an open reduction of the hip is not to be performed at the same time, it is not necessary to expose the hip capsule.

Figure 2–20. The inner and outer table of the ilium are exposed. The periosteum is carefully elevated from the sciatic notch with a curved periosteal elevator, *eg,* one of the Crego elevators. A right-angled forceps is then passed from medial to lateral while the finger of the other hand is used to push the periosteum down and away from the sciatic notch on the outer table. A Gigli saw is then grasped in the forceps and pulled through the sciatic notch (***Figure 2–20A***).

Retractors are placed in the sciatic notch on each side of the ilium to provide wide retraction and protection of the soft tissues. The osteotomy is performed with the Gigli saw, which emerges at or just above the anteroinferior-superior iliac spine. While using the Gigli saw the hands should be spread as far apart as possible and constant tension kept on each end of the Gigli saw, or else there will be a tendency for it to bind (***Figure 2–20B***).

The bone graft that will be used to hold the osteotomy site open is taken from the anterior iliac crest. This can be done with a bone-biting forceps in young children but is facilitated with a power saw in older children (***Figure 2–20C***).

At this point it is imperative to perform an intramuscular tenotomy of the iliopsoas as described in the anterior approach to the congenitally dislocated hip.

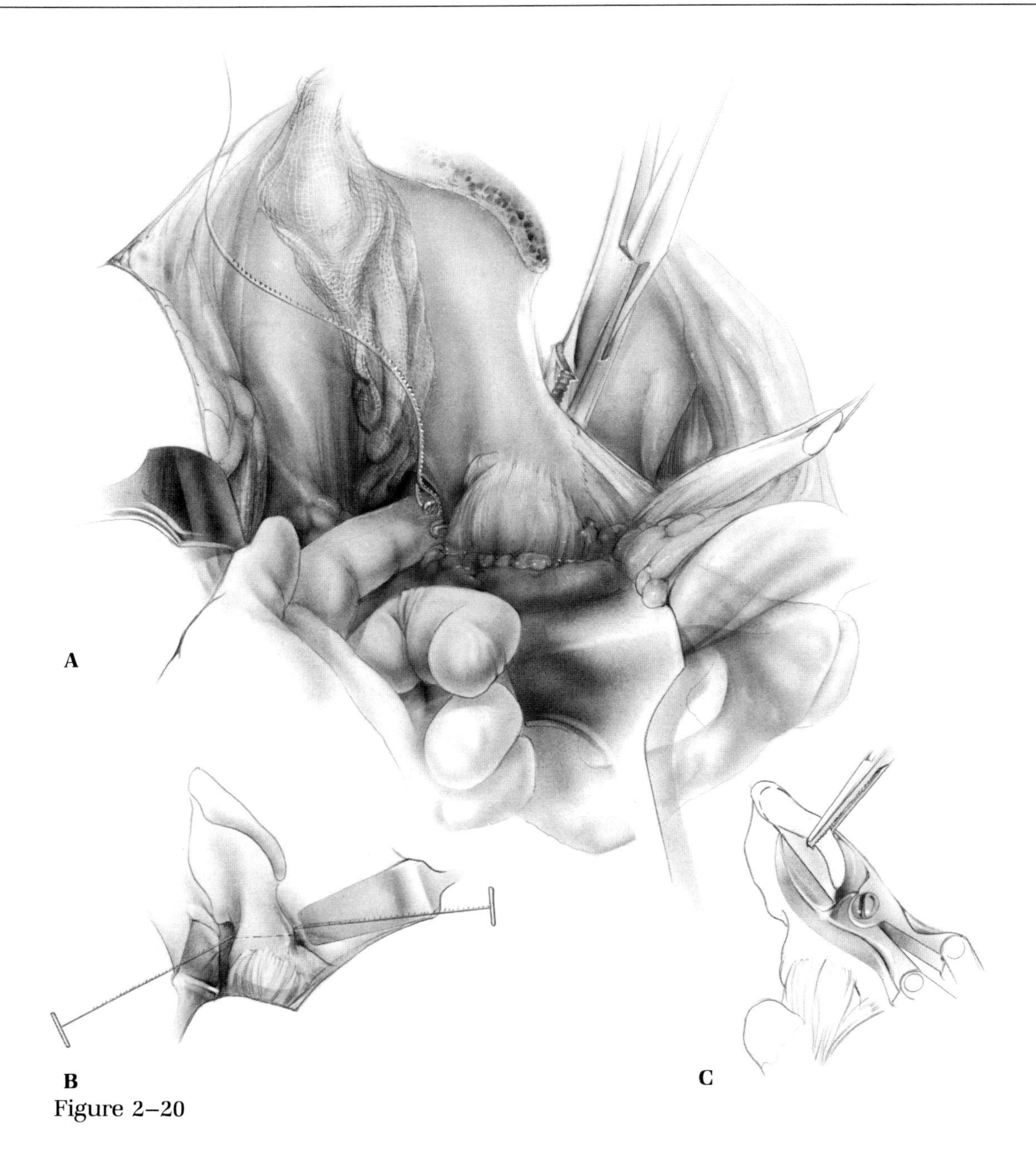

Figure 2–20

Figure 2–21. Towel clips are used to grasp the two fragments. The proximal fragment is grasped and held not to help pull open the osteotomy site but rather to stabilize the pelvis. Any upward movement of this fragment will create spurious correction and create the appearance of a high iliac crest simulating a leg-length inequality. The distal fragment is grasped as far posterior and as close to the hip capsule as possible so that there is not a tendency to break off a piece of bone (***Figure 2–21A***).

If the hip capsule has not been opened the leg can be used to produce the desired correction in the acetabulum. This is done by placing the foot on the opposite knee in the "figure 4" position. Pushing down on the knee will produce the desired rotation although perhaps not the desired degree (***Figure 2–21B***). If the capsule has been opened the towel clip grasping the distal fragment is used to rotate this fragment downward in line with the ilium (***Figure 2–21C***). It is this rotation that will account for the difference in shape of the obturator foramen, which is seen on the postoperative radiograph.

At the same time this fragment, which probably slipped posterior after the osteotomy, should be pulled forward. The bone graft is tailored to fit tightly in the gap that has been created in the osteotomy, and it is inserted. This graft should be relatively stable once inserted. This can be tested by pulling on the graft with a Kocker clamp. It is important that after the graft is inserted the posterior aspect of the osteotomy is closed and the distal fragment not be displaced posteriorly relative to the proximal fragment. Kalamchi has suggested a modification, placing a notch in the posterior cut surface of the proximal fragment and inserting the posterior edge of the distal fragment into the notch.[4] This tends to increase stability and help to avoid posterior displacement of the distal fragment.

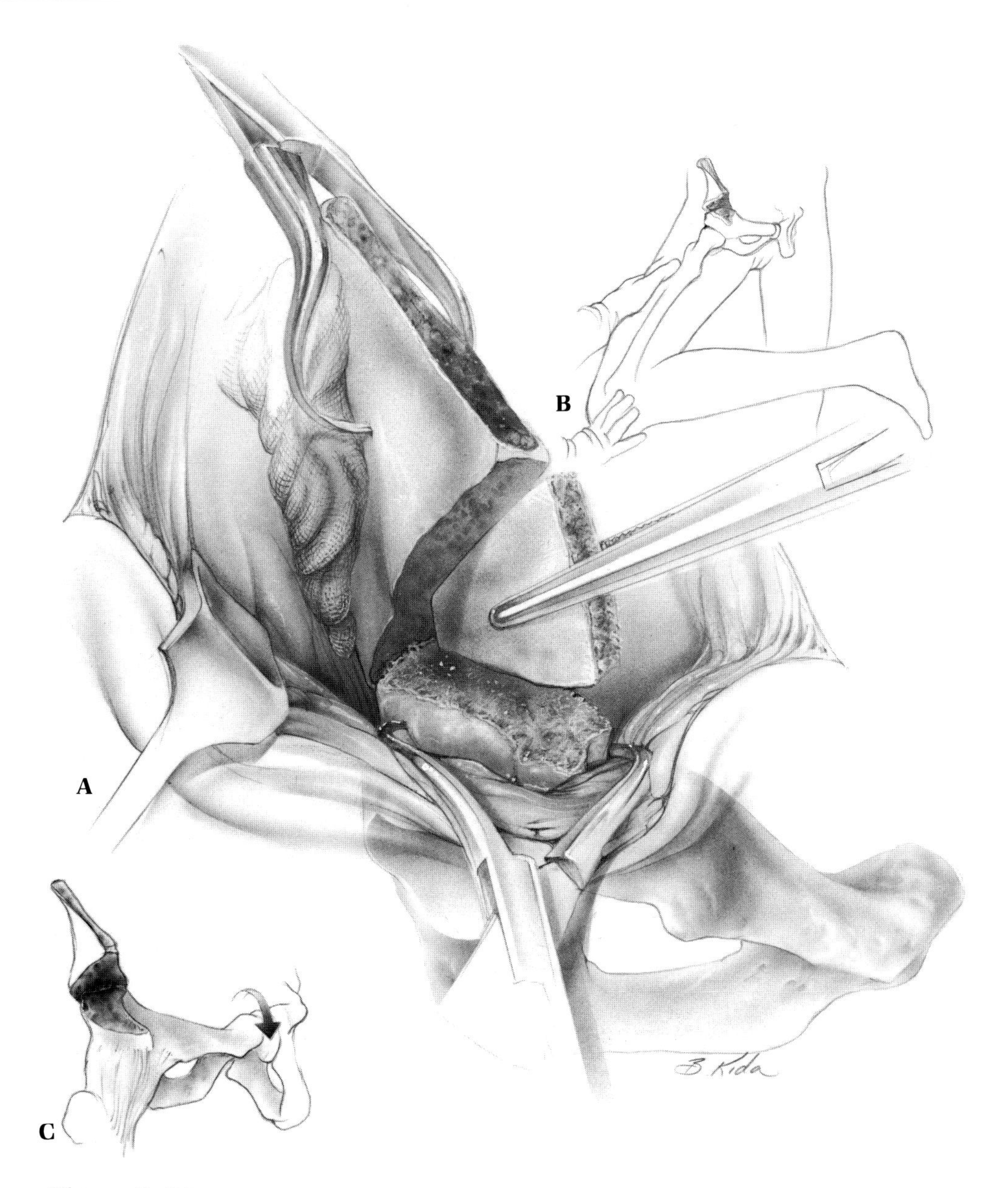

Figure 2–21

Figure 2–22. Although the graft should be secure it will not be secure enough to leave without fixation. Two heavy threaded Kirschner wires should be used. Smooth or thin wires should not be used. These wires are passed from the proximal fragment into the distal fragment (***Figure 2–22A***). In the distal fragment they should lie medial and posterior to the acetabulum (***Figures 2–22B, C***) and this will determine their starting point in the proximal fragment. There is a danger of passing one of the wires into the hip joint when the capsule has not been opened as in the treatment of acetabular dysplasia. This plus the fact that properly placed pins will appear to penetrate the hip joint on the postoperative radiograph makes it imperative that the surgeon has a good grasp of the pelvic anatomy, and that he or she also carefully moves the hip to feel and listen for crepitus. Following this the wound is closed. A drain is usually not necessary if only an innominate osteotomy has been performed, as the bleeding from the bone is not unusual.

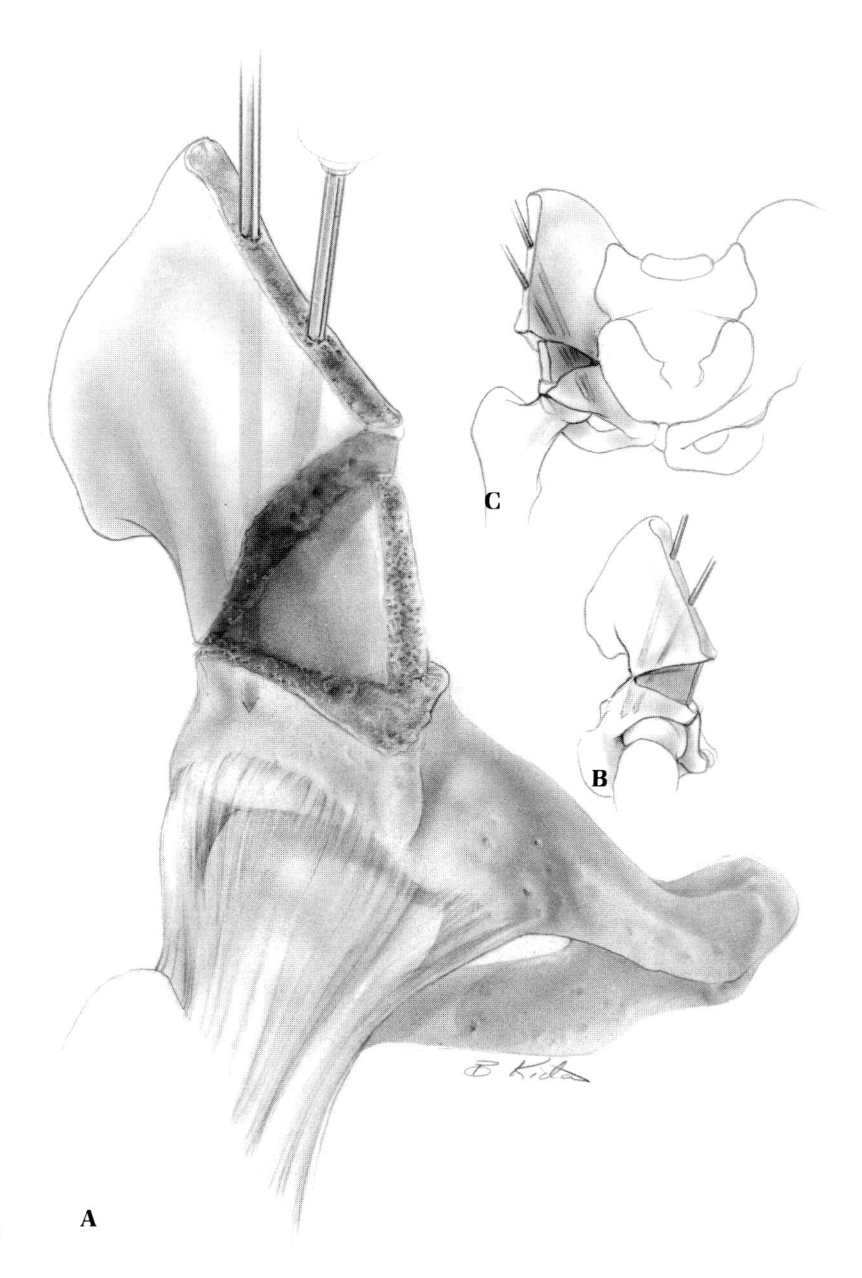

Figure 2–22

Figure 2–23. MP is a 2 + 10-year-old female in whom there have been no signs of acetabular remodeling 18 months following closed reduction of a congenitally dislocated hip (***A***) In addition there is excessive femoral anteversion. It was decided to correct these problems with an innominate osteotomy as described by Salter.

Six weeks after the osteotomy certain features are noted (***B***). The posterior aspect remains closed, and posterior displacement of the distal fragment was avoided. The pins could have been inserted further, continuing down into the ischium behind the hip capsule. Also there was more lateral than anterior rotation achieved as evidenced by only a slight asymmetry of the obturator foramen.

At 6 + 1 years of age the resulting containment is good as evidenced by the development of the hip (***C***).

POSTOPERATIVE CARE

Immobilization will depend on the circumstances. In older children and teenagers who are deemed reliable with a three-point partial weight-bearing crutch gait, no immobilization and early ambulation can be permitted. Young or untrustworthy children should always be immobilized for 6 weeks before weight bearing is permitted. If an open reduction has been performed at the same time the hip will be immobilized in accordance with the treatment for that procedure.

REFERENCES

1. Salter RB. Innominate osteotomy in the treatment of congenital dislocation and subluxation of the hip. J Bone Joint Surg 1961;43B:518.
2. Gallien R, Bertin D, Lirette R. Salter procedure in congenital dislocation of the hip. J Pediatr Orthop 1984;4:427.
3. Salter RB. Specific guidelines in the application of the principle of innominate osteotomy. Orthop Clin North Am 1972;3:149.
4. Kalamchi A. Modified Salter osteotomy. J Bone Joint Surg 1982;64A:183.

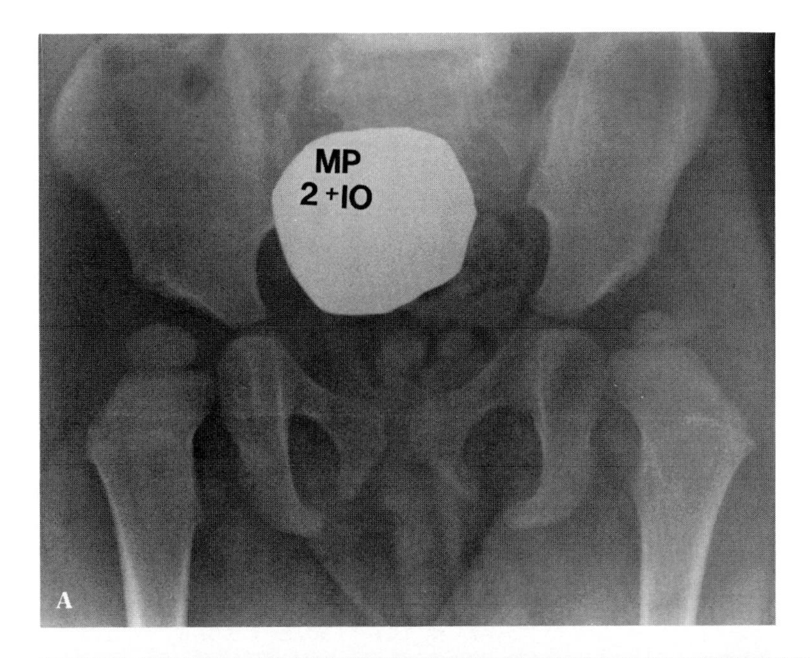

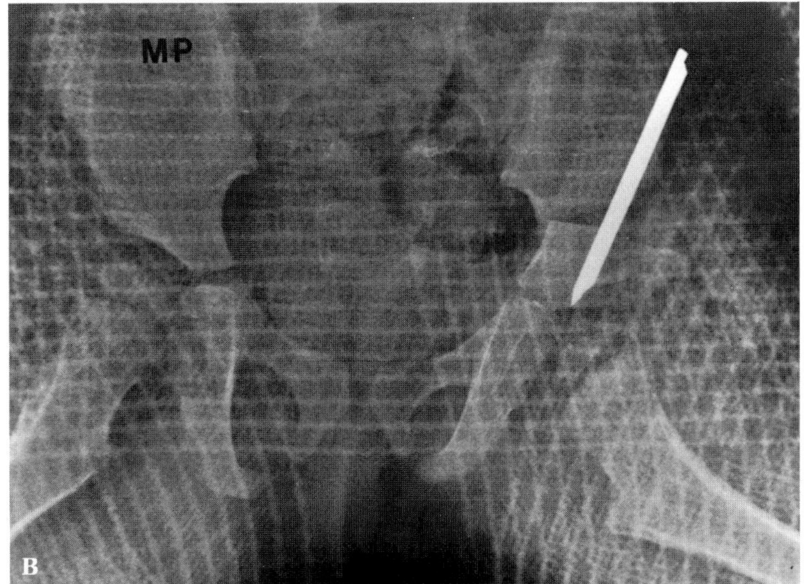

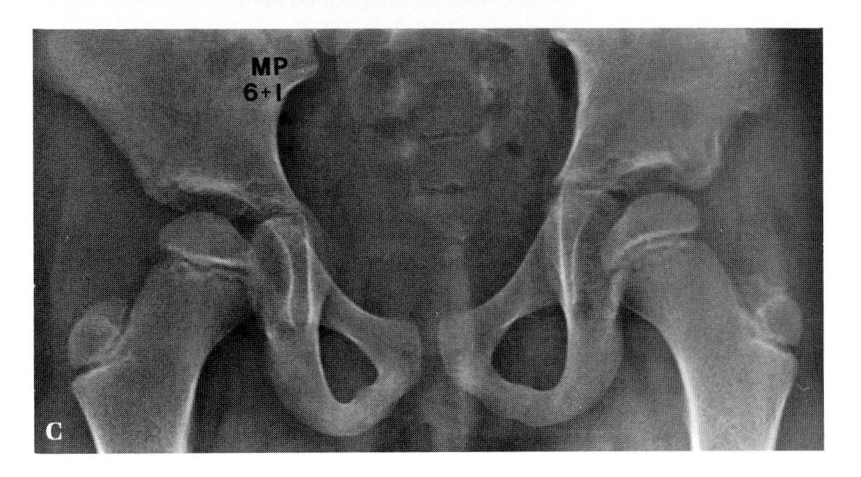

Figure 2–23

2.5 Transiliac Leg Lengthening

Millis and Hall have proposed a modification of Salter's innominate osteotomy to increase the length of the lower limb.[1] This procedure will find its ideal indication in the patient who has an acetabular dysplasia associated with the ipsilateral shortening of the leg of 2 to 2.5 cm.

Figure 2–24. The innominate osteotomy of Salter is performed. Unlike the procedure described by Salter, however, opening of the posterior aspect is required rather than prohibited. It is this opening or distraction between the two fragments that produces the lengthening of the lower extremity. If correction of the acetabular dysplasia is also desired the distal fragment must also be rotated. This is accomplished by a combination of forces: distally directed pressure to prevent the proximal fragment from moving cephalad, manual distraction of the limb, and rotation of the distal fragment. The distraction is held with a spreader. Time should be spent to allow the tissues to stretch. The distraction may occur during 20 to 30 minutes depending on the desired amount of distraction and the patient's age.

The graft that is shaped to hold the osteotomy open will not be triangular as in the classic Salter osteotomy, but rather quadrangular with the width above the hip joint equal to the amount of lengthening achieved, and the wider anterior portion holding the rotation of the distal fragment. This graft will be under extreme tension and requires at least two heavy threaded Kirschner wires to hold it in place. Because of this lengthening it is imperative that an iliopsoas tenotomy be performed as described for the anterior approach to open reduction of the dislocated hip.

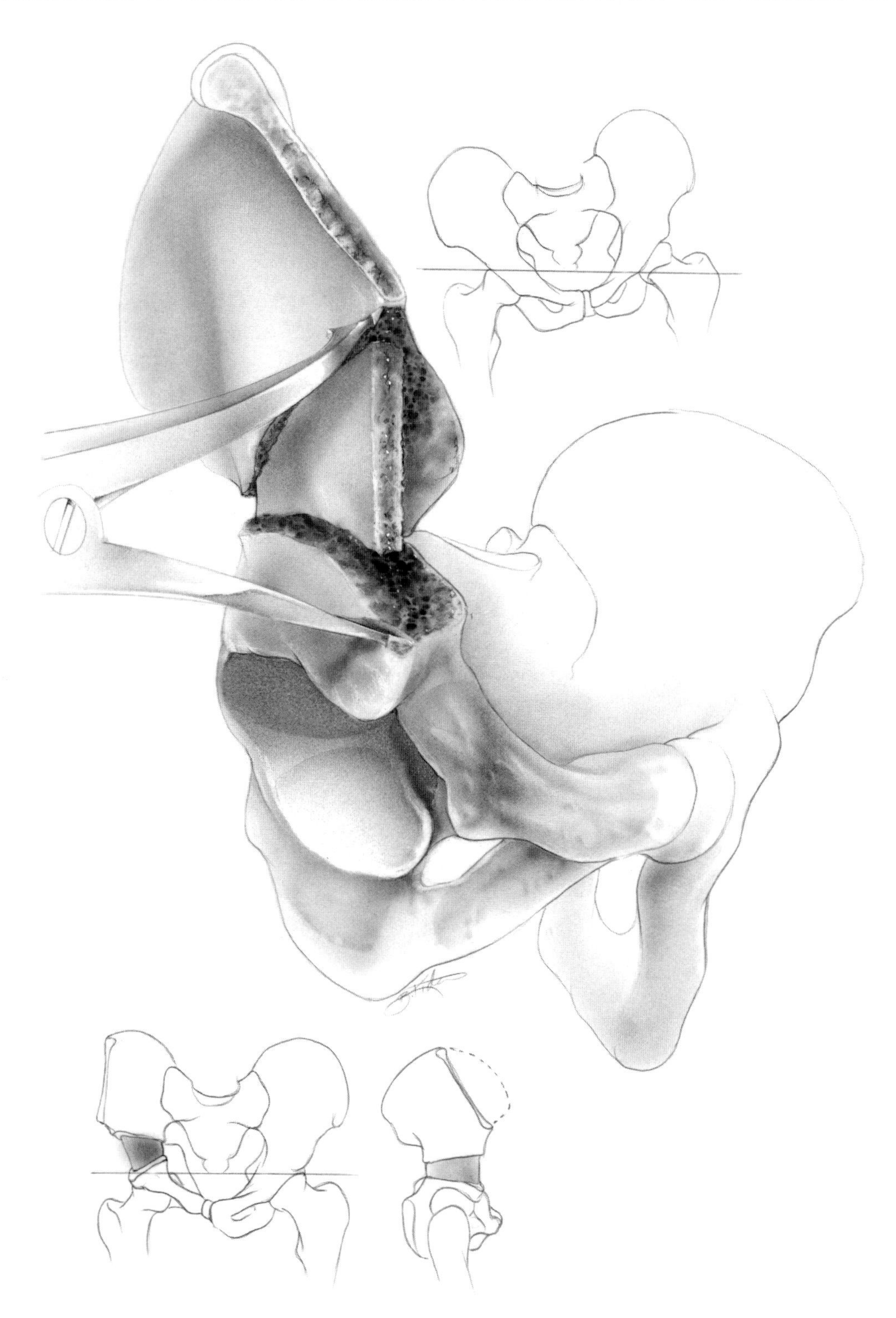

Figure 2–24

Figure 2–25. The radiographs of a patient 6 weeks after a transiliac leg lengthening of 3 cm show the wide distraction of the posterior aspect of the osteotomy. Also notice the increased number of pins used for fixation. (Courtesy of Michael Millis, MD.)

POSTOPERATIVE CARE

The patients are placed in a balanced suspension with traction on the leg and the hip flexed. Range of motion of the hip is started the day after surgery. When the patient has gained sufficient motion, usually 4 to 5 days after surgery, ambulation with three-point touch-down weight bearing is begun. The patient is protected with crutches for a minimum of 3 months. The pins should not be removed until there is radiographic evidence of solid healing. This will usually take 6 to 12 months depending on the age of the patient.

REFERENCE

1. Millis MB, Hall JE. Transiliac lengthening of the lower extremity. J. Bone Joint Surg 1979;61A:1182.

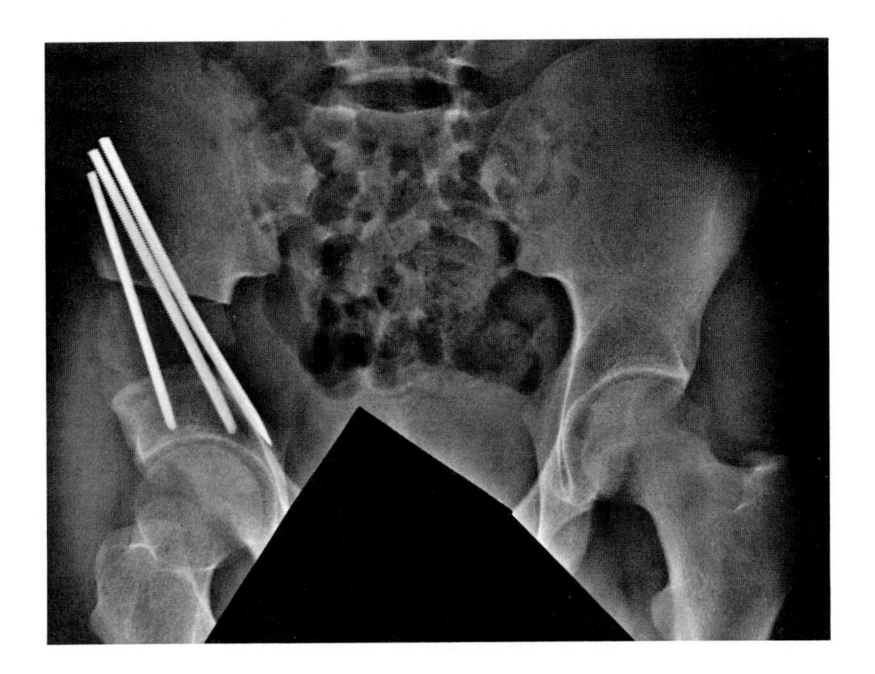

Figure 2–25

2.6
Pemberton's Innominate Osteotomy

The pericapsular osteotomy was conceived of by Pemberton to address two problems that he saw in the older child with subluxation or dislocation of the hip: The acetabulum was not only "shallow," but was facing forward and lateral; in the dislocating hip the femoral head was usually small in relation to the acetabulum, whereas in the subluxating hip the acetabulum was large relative to the femoral head. The osteotomy was designed to hinge in the acetabulum through the flexible triradiate cartilage. He also noted that the direction of coverage obtained could be varied depending on the direction of the osteotomy of the ilium.[1,2]

Today the eclectic surgeon will recognize the value of this procedure in the subluxating or dislocated hip with an acetabulum that is relatively large in relation to the femoral head, eg, the subluxating hip or in some of the neurogenic dislocating hips. At the same time this can be a disadvantage if there is not a relative size discrepancy between the acetabulum and femoral head. The ability to vary the direction of the coverage is an additional advantage especially when more lateral than anterior coverage is desired. A final advantage is that the bone graft is stable without additional pins, obviating the need for subsequent pin removal.

The prerequisites for the operation are that there be a concentric reduction of the hip and that the triradiate cartilage be open to the extent that it is sufficiently mobile. In normal children the triradiate cartilage is sufficiently mobile until the age of 7 or 8 years of age. In children with severe cerebral palsy or myelomeningocele in whom the author often finds this a useful operation, mobility in the triradiate cartilage may be present until 10 years of age or later.

A combination of the Pemberton and Salter osteotomies has also been described, which has come to be called the Pember-Sal osteotomy.[3] As described, the osteotomy continues past the triradiate cartilage into the body of the ischium: It does not break through into the sciatic notch. The author sees this term most often used to describe an osteotomy in which the surgeon has not stayed within the ilium but rather has broken into the sciatic notch before reaching the triradiate cartilage. When this occurs correction will be limited.

As in all acetabular redirections the matter of incongruity must be considered. Although minor degrees of incongruity between the acetabulum and the femoral head will remodel, the extent of this process will depend on the age of the child. It is probably wise to apply the criteria that Salter uses for his innominate osteotomy for the best results.

The patient is placed in the same position as for open reduction of the hip joint through the anterior approach, and the same incision and approach are used.

Figure 2–26. After the iliac apophysis is split, both the inner and outer tables of the ilium are exposed subperiosteally sufficient to expose the sciatic notch on both sides. It is not necessary to expose the capsule of the hip joint unless an open reduction is to be performed at the same time. Likewise, it is not necessary to divide the combined head of the rectus femoris muscle. Although Pemberton did not recommend division of the psoas tendon, it may be advisable to do this as in Salter's innominate osteotomy.

The osteotomy is planned depending on the direction in which coverage is needed. If more anterior coverage is desired, the plane of the osteotomy is more transverse (***Figure 2–26A***). If lateral coverage is desired, the plane of the osteotomy will be inclined more laterally (***Figure 2–26B***). Once this is determined a small $\frac{1}{4}$-in osteotome can be used to outline the osteotomy by cutting the cortex of the inner (***Figure 2–26C***) and outer (***Figure 2–26D***) table.

The osteotomy is begun about 1 cm above the anteroinferior iliac spine and proceeds posteriorly, keeping about 1 to 1.5 cm away from the attachment of the joint capsule. As the osteotome proceeds posteriorly and then inferiorly through the outer table, it will disappear from site in the soft-tissue attachments behind the posterior aspect of the capsule; there will be a strong tendency for the osteotome to cut into the sciatic notch (***Figure 2–26C***). Care in exposing the sciatic notch as far inferior as possible will make this error easier to avoid by visualizing that portion of the ilium that lies between the sciatic notch posteriorly and the capsule of the hip joint anteriorly. It is not possible, necessary, nor advisable, however, to expose this down to the triradiate cartilage. The same problem exists when cutting the cortex of the inner table but not to the same extent. No capsule is present, so it is sufficient to stay slightly anterior to the sciatic notch (***Figure 2–26D***).

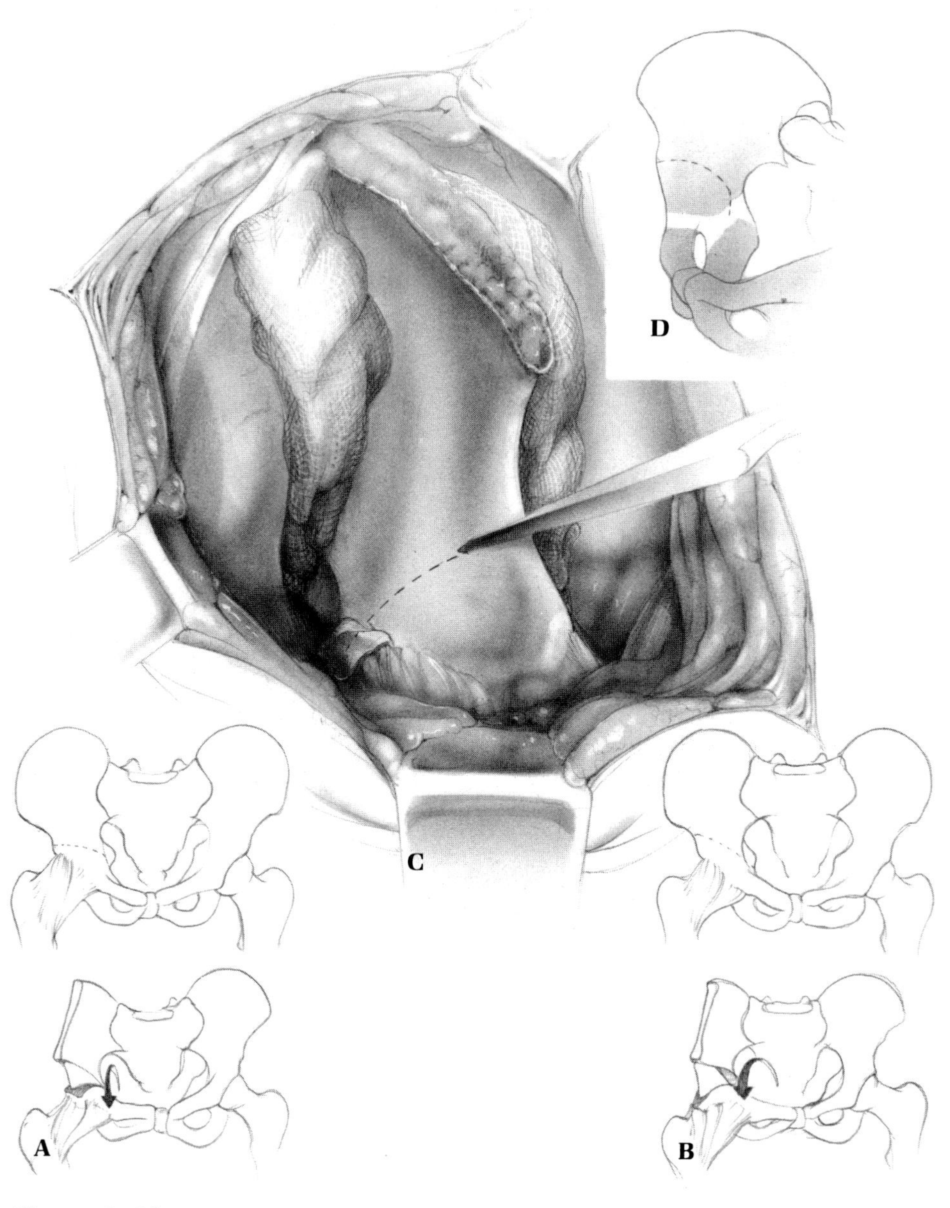

Figure 2–26

Figure 2–27. After both the inner and outer cortex of the ilium are divided as far as can be visualized, a wider curved osteotome is used to connect these two cuts. As this osteotome proceeds posteriorly it will become apparent that it will not be able to make the sharp turn inferior to avoid cutting into the sciatic notch. At this point an osteotome with a right-angled curve, available on special order from Zimmer,* is inserted into the osteotomy. This can be made easier by prying down on the acetabular roof with an osteotome and inserting a small lamina spreader to hold the osteotomy apart. The special osteotome is used to complete the cut into the triradiate cartilage. It will not be possible to visualize the tip of the osteotome as it completes the osteotomy. It is not necessary and usually will not be possible to visualize the triradiate cartilage unless the acetabulum is levered down excessively. When the osteotomy is complete, the acetabular roof can be levered down into the desired position and held there with a lamina spreader.

*Zimmer Co., Warsaw, Indiana.

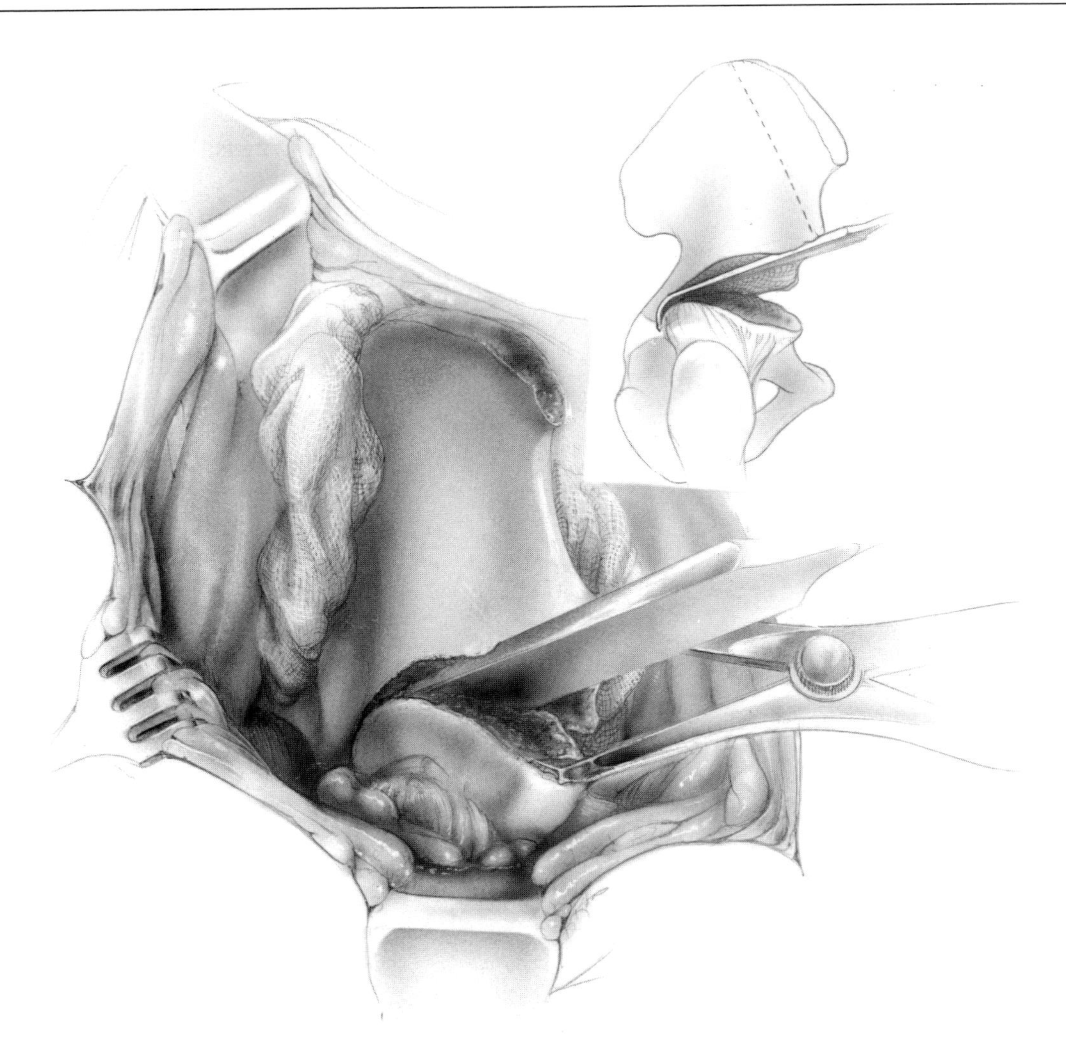

Figure 2–27

Figure 2–28. Grooves are prepared in the cancellous surface on each side of the osteotomy to provide secure fixation of the bone graft. This can be done with a curette. A triangular wedge of bone is cut from the anterior iliac crest. It should be larger than the gap it is designed to span because it will be recessed into the cancellous bone. Once in place the bone graft should be secure and stable, and this can be verified by attempting to dislodge the graft. The wound is closed in a routine manner.

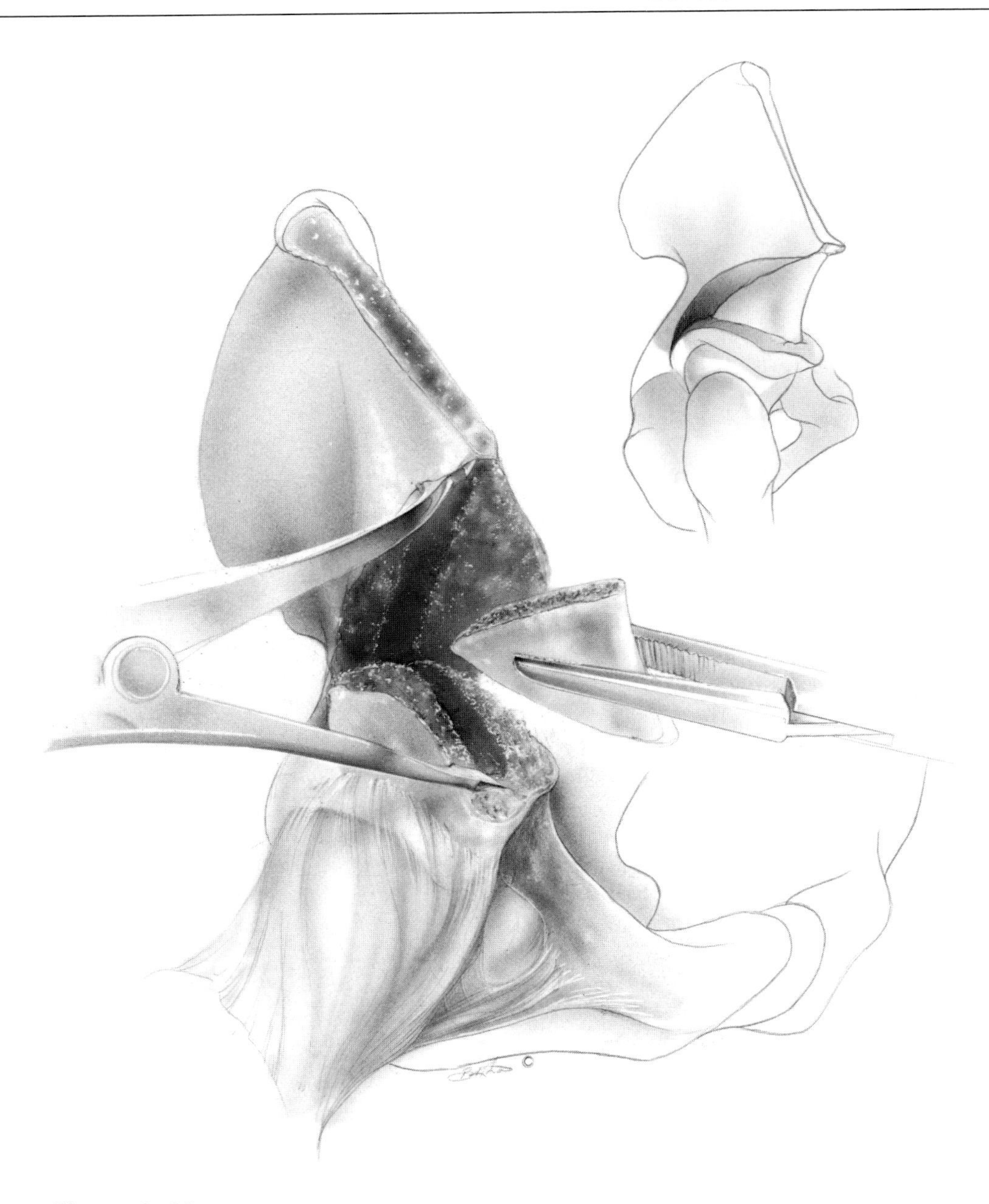

Figure 2–28

Figure 2–29. JB is a 4-year-old boy who had an open reduction, femoral shortening and rotation, and Pemberton osteotomy for spastic dislocation. A radiograph immediately after surgery demonstrates the osteotomy extending into the triradiate cartilage and not breaking into the sciatic notch (***Figure 2–29A***). Radiographs 6 weeks (***Figure 2–29B***) and 6 months (***Figure 2–29C***) demonstrate the rapid healing and the excellent containment of the femoral head.

POSTOPERATIVE CARE

Because of the usual age at which this osteotomy is performed the patient is immobilized in a single-leg spica cast. The length of immobilization will depend on what other procedures were done but usually 6 weeks of immobilization is sufficient to allow protected weight bearing and physical therapy to regain motion.

REFERENCES

1. Pemberton PA. Pericapsular osteotomy of the ilium for treatment of congenital subluxation and dislocation of the hip. J Bone Joint Surg 1965;47A:65.
2. Pemberton PA. Pericapsular osteotomy of the ilium for the treatment of congenitally dislocated hips. Clin Orthop 1974;98:41.
3. Perlik PC, Westin WG, Marafioti RL. A combination pelvic osteotomy for acetabular dysplasia in children. J Bone Joint Surg 1985;67A:842.

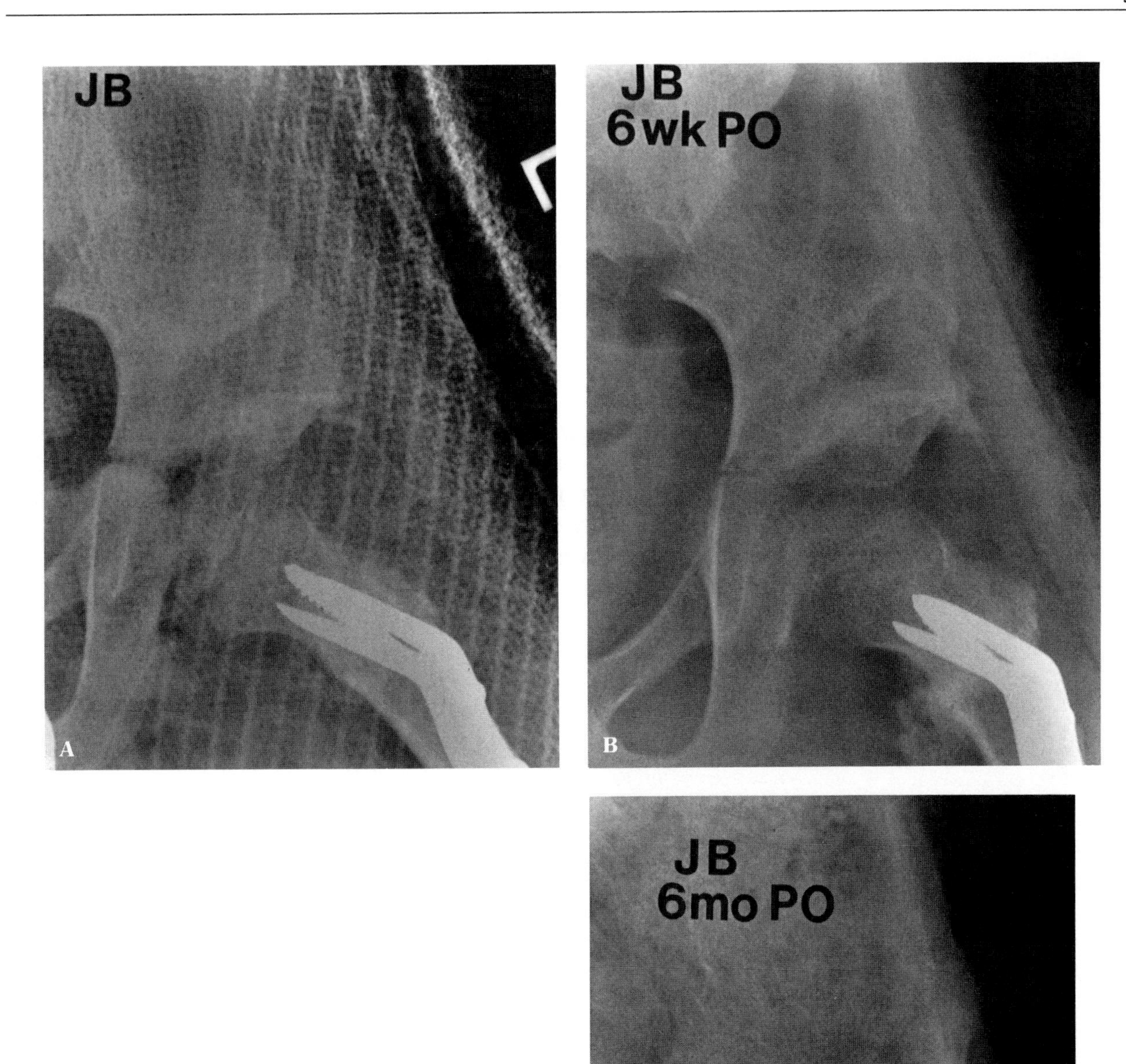

JB
6mo PO
C

Figure 2–29

2.7 Dega's Innominate Osteotomy

Although not well described in the English literature until recently,[3] the Dega pericapsular osteotomy[1] is gaining wider usage, particularly in the treatment of hip dislocation in cerebral palsy where posterior coverage is of primary importance.

Dega illustrated the osteotomy as extending from the lateral cortex above the acetabulum toward the inner wall of the ilium behind the acetabulum. This is similar to the osteotomy described by Albee early in this century.[2] The results have been discussed by Mubarak et al.[3] This differs from the pericapsular osteotomy of Pemberton in that only the lateral cortex of the ilium is cut as opposed to both the inner and outer cortices. Thus, in the Dega osteotomy all of the coverage is directed lateral, whereas in the Pemberton osteotomy the coverage is anterolateral. Unlike the Pemberton osteotomy, this osteotomy need not extend into the triradiate cartilage. The advantage is that coverage is enhanced even in the most posterior aspect of the acetabulum. Even the Chiari osteotomy cannot provide this extreme posterior coverage because the osteotomy cannot stay in contact with the most posterior aspects of the hip capsule.

Figure 2–30. The exposure of the ilium is the same as for the Salter osteotomy. Soft-tissue release, open reduction, and femoral osteotomy may all be performed at the same time to gain the concentric reduction of the femoral head, which is a prerequisite for the Dega osteotomy.

The osteotomy is begun about 1.5 cm above the acetabulum on a line that extends from the anteroinferior iliac spine to the sciatic notch. The cortex is completely divided with a straight osteotome along the desired line.

Figure 2–31. Then using a combination of straight and curved osteotomes, the osteotomy is deepened heading medially and caudally behind the acetabulum. This cut must proceed between the medial wall of the ilium and the medial wall of the acetabulum. This can be monitored on an image intensifier. The osteotomy does not have to be carried to the triradiate cartilage as illustrated here; however, this will increase the mobility of the acetabular fragment (***Figure 2–31A***).

Next, a Kerrison rongeur is used to remove the cortex both anteriorly and posteriorly as it extends around to the medial iliac wall. This is essential to allow the fragment to bend freely (***Figure 2–31B***).

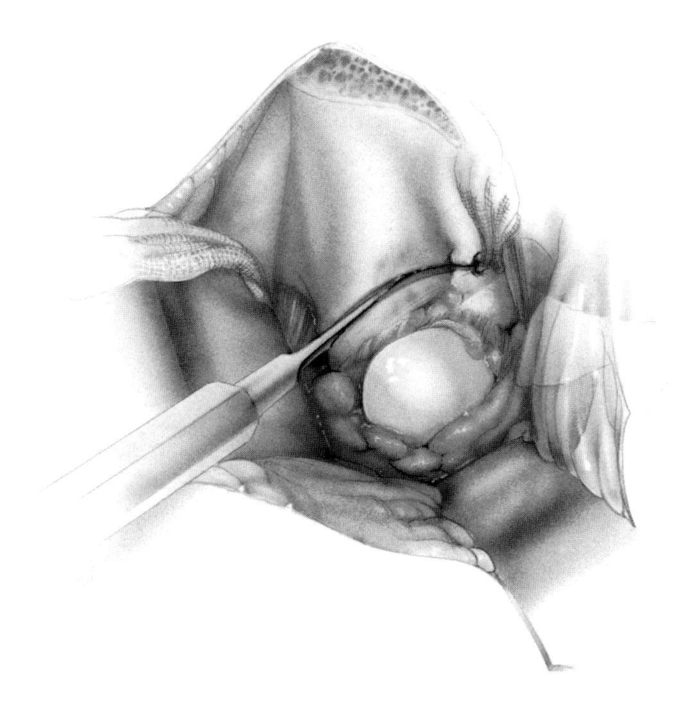

Figure 2–30

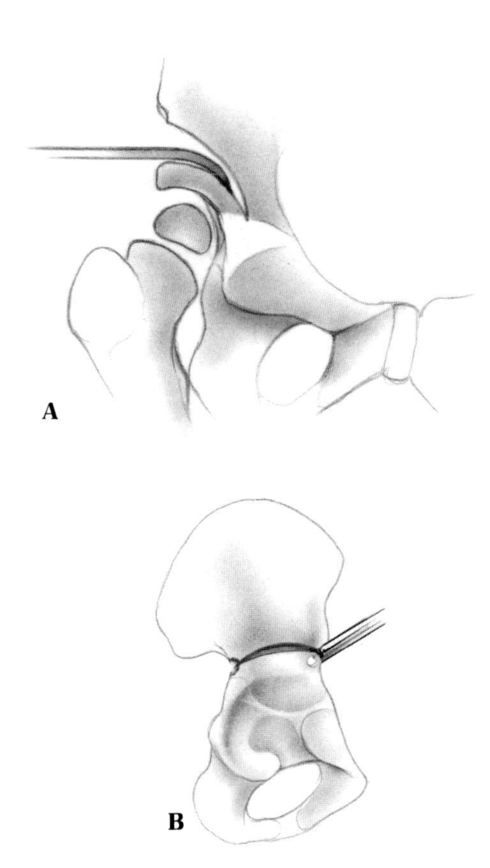

Figure 2–31

Figure 2–32. When the osteotomy is completed, the superior aspect of the acetabulum can be hinged downward by prying with a broad curved osteotome and inserting a small lamina spreader.

Figure 2–33. A piece of the ilium in the region of the antero-superior iliac spine is removed, and three tricortical triangular pieces of bone are fashioned. These are wedged securely in the osteotomy site, which is held open with a lamina spreader. It should be verified that the desired amount of coverage has been obtained, and that the grafts are secure. No internal fixation is necessary. The wound is closed.

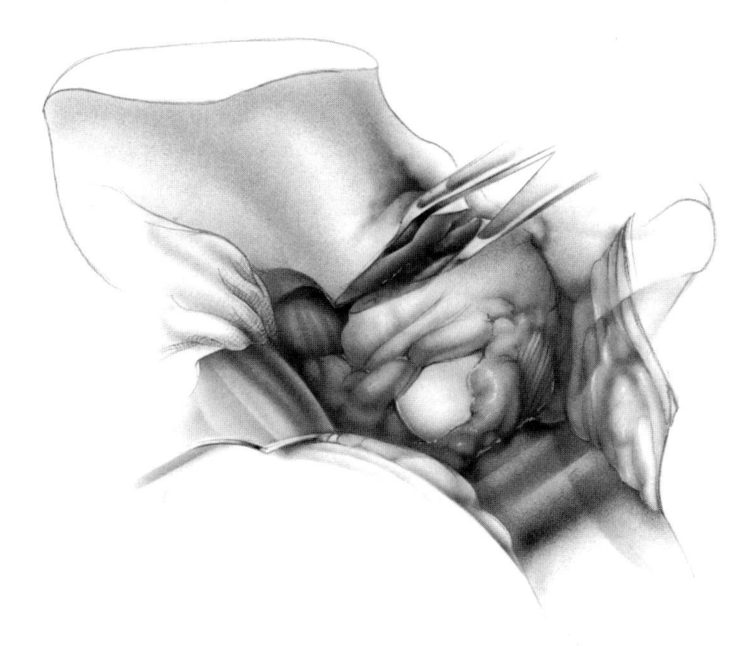

Figure 2–32

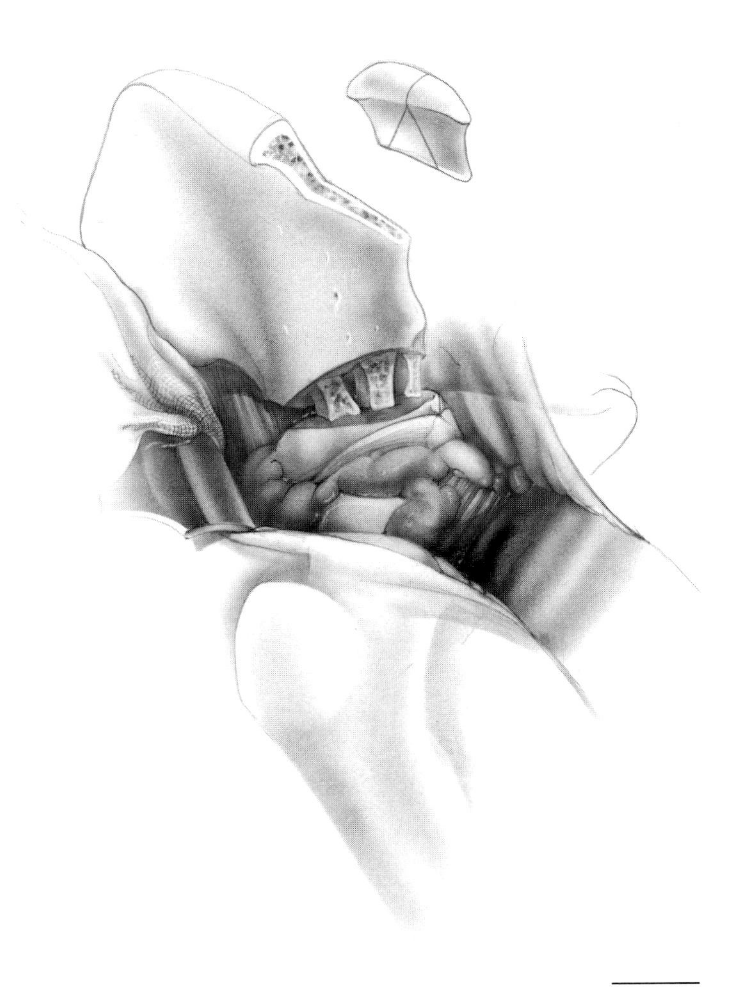

Figure 2–33

Figure 2–34. Illustration of a dislocated hip in a young boy with spastic cerebral palsy (***Figure 2–34A***). Note the significant acetabular dysplasia. The image obtained with the image intensifier during the Dega osteotomy shows the direction of the cut (***Figure 2–34B***). It appears that the osteotomy has cracked into the triradiate cartilage. The osteotomy is healed in 2 months, and the coverage excellent (***Figure 2–34C***). (Courtesy of Scott Mubarak, MD.)

POSTOPERATIVE CARE

After wound closure a hip spica cast is applied—either one leg or one and one half legs depending on the surgeon's preference. This should be maintained until healing, noted by radiograph, which usually takes 6 to 8 weeks depending on the age of the patient.

REFERENCES

1. Dega W. Osteotomis trans-iliakalna w leczeniu wrodzonej dysplazji biodra. Chir Narz Ruchu Orthop Pol 1974;38:601.
2. Albee FH. The bone graft wedge: its use in the treatment of relapsing, acquired, and congenital dislocation of the hip. NY Med J 1915;102:433.
3. Mubarak SJ, Mortensen W, Katz M. Combined pelvic (Dega) and femoral osteotomies in the treatment of paralytic hip dislocation. Orthop Trans 1987;11:456.

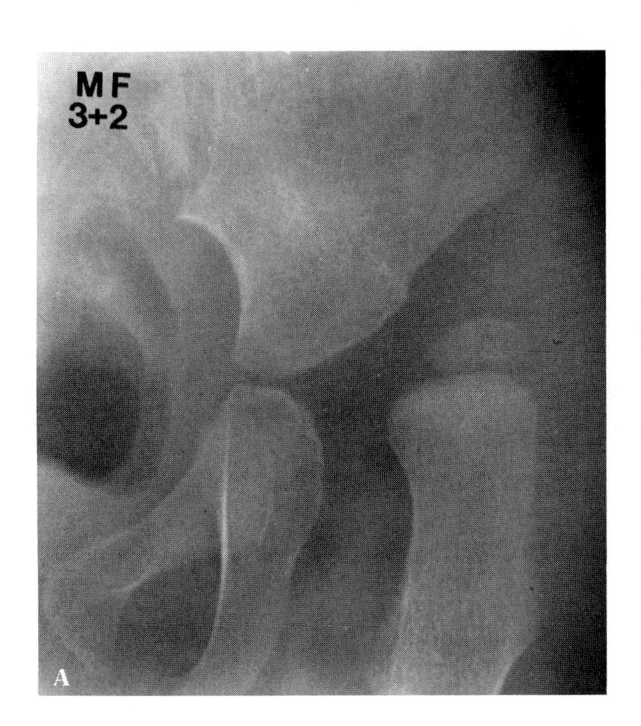

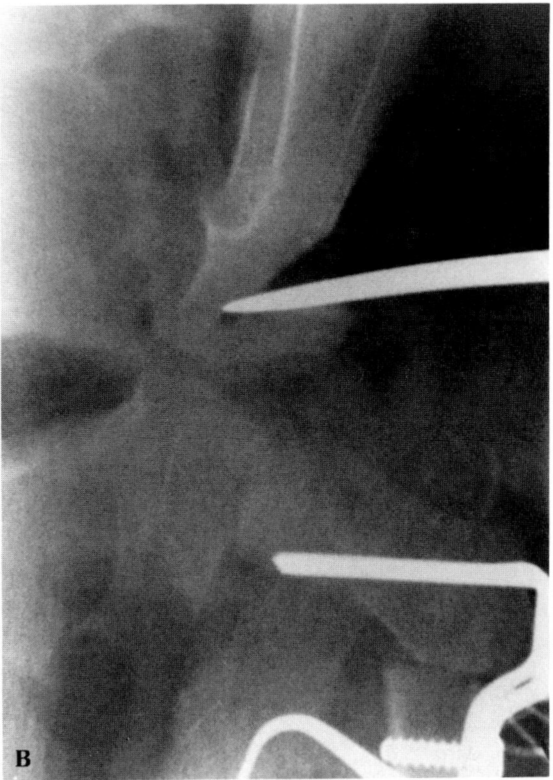

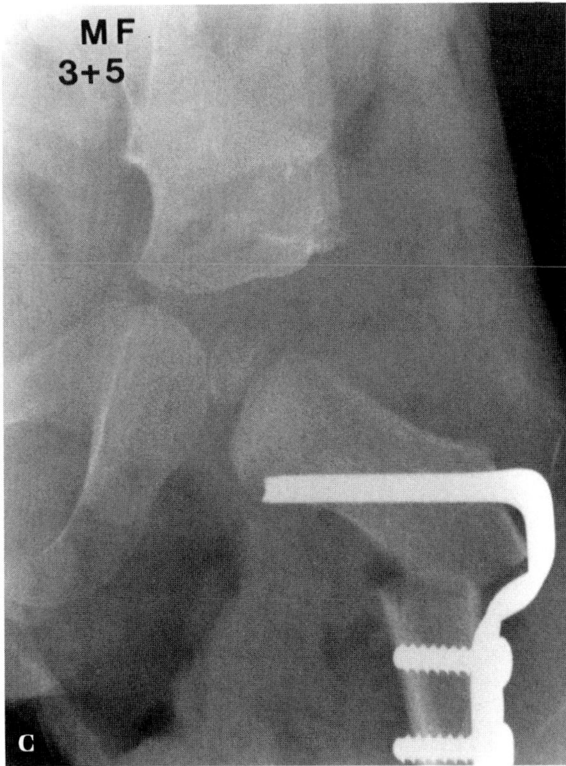

Figure 2–34

2.8 Steel's Innominate Osteotomy

The triple innominate osteotomy of the pelvis divides the iliac bone as in the Salter osteotomy while additionally dividing the pubic bone and ischial bone. It is a reconstructive procedure because it uses the articular cartilage and subchondral bone of the acetabulum. In this respect it is like the osteotomies of Salter and Pemberton. It differs from these osteotomies, however, in that there is no hinge; the acetabular fragment is completely free. This permits a greater degree of mobility in obtaining anterior or lateral coverage.

Like the Salter and Pemberton osteotomies, a prerequisite for the triple innominate osteotomy is that the femoral head and the acetabulum will be congruous after the osteotomy is completed. It is indicated when this condition can be met but when adequate containment of the femoral head cannot be achieved with either the Salter or Pemberton osteotomy. Preoperative traction or femoral osteotomy with or without shortening may all be used to ensure a concentric reduction of the femoral head.

The operation as originally described by Steel used a separate incision in the buttocks to divide the ischium while dividing the pubic ramus through the same incision that is used to divide the iliac bone.[1] Dividing the ischium is difficult because the surgeon is "standing on his head" while an assistant must hold the leg up, and the pubic ramus is difficult to reach from the transverse incision anteriorly. Some surgeons have adapted the approach used by LeCoeur[2] in his osteotomy to divide both the ischium and pubis through a groin incision similar to that used in adductor myotomy or proximal hamstring release. Both of these approaches will be described.

Figure 2–35. In the operation as described by Steel, the entire leg and buttocks area are prepared and draped free. The operation starts with a transverse incision about 1 cm cephalad from the natal crease (***A***). This incision is deepened down to the gluteus maximus muscle. It is important to gain a wide exposure in all directions at this point, or the remainder of the exposure will be difficult. The medial border of the gluteus maximus muscle is identified and freed, allowing the muscle to be retracted laterally exposing the muscle attachments to the ischial tuberosity.

The biceps femoris and the semitendinous muscles insert with a common tendon. The tendinous insertion of the semimembranous muscle lies lateral to this and the sciatic nerve lateral to the semimembranous insertion. If the long head of the biceps femoris is dissected free and detached, the interval between the semitendinous and semimembranous muscles can be identified (***B***). This interval is the ideal site for the osteotomy of the ischium. It is best to expose this osteotomy site sufficiently so that at least 1 cm of bone can be removed. This will ensure that no periosteum is holding the bone ends together, a situation that may limit mobility of the fragment. In addition, it will allow some medial displacement of the acetabular fragment, which tends to be lateralized with this procedure.

The ischial ramus is dissected subperiosteally. It is usually not possible to stay subperiosteal all the way around, but care must be taken to remain in close proximity to the bone. A curved kidney pedicle forceps or retractor, *eg*, a wide curved Crego elevator is passed around the ischium and out through the obturator foramen to elevate the obturator muscles, and protect the internal pudendal vessels and nerve (***C***). The initial cut is made with an osteotome that approximates the width of the ischium. It is directed laterally and posteriorly. A rongeur can also be used to remove this bone. When this is completed the wound is closed.

Figure 2–36. An oblique incision is made, and the innominate bone is exposed as in the Salter osteotomy. The osteotomy of the pubis requires a medial exposure of the pubic ramus that taxes the limits of the incision. A major pitfall in this exposure is that the surgeon will feel that the exposure is far enough medial and begin the osteotomy only to find it extending into the anteromedial acetabulum. It is important that the pectineal tubercle be identified and the pectineus muscle be reflected off of it. The osteotomy should be medial to this pectineal tubercle. As for the ischium, a curved forceps or retractor is passed around the pubic ramus superiorly and out of the obturator foramen inferiorly while staying in contact with the bone. The osteotome is directed medially to cut the pubic ramus. A rongeur can also be used here to create the osteotomy.

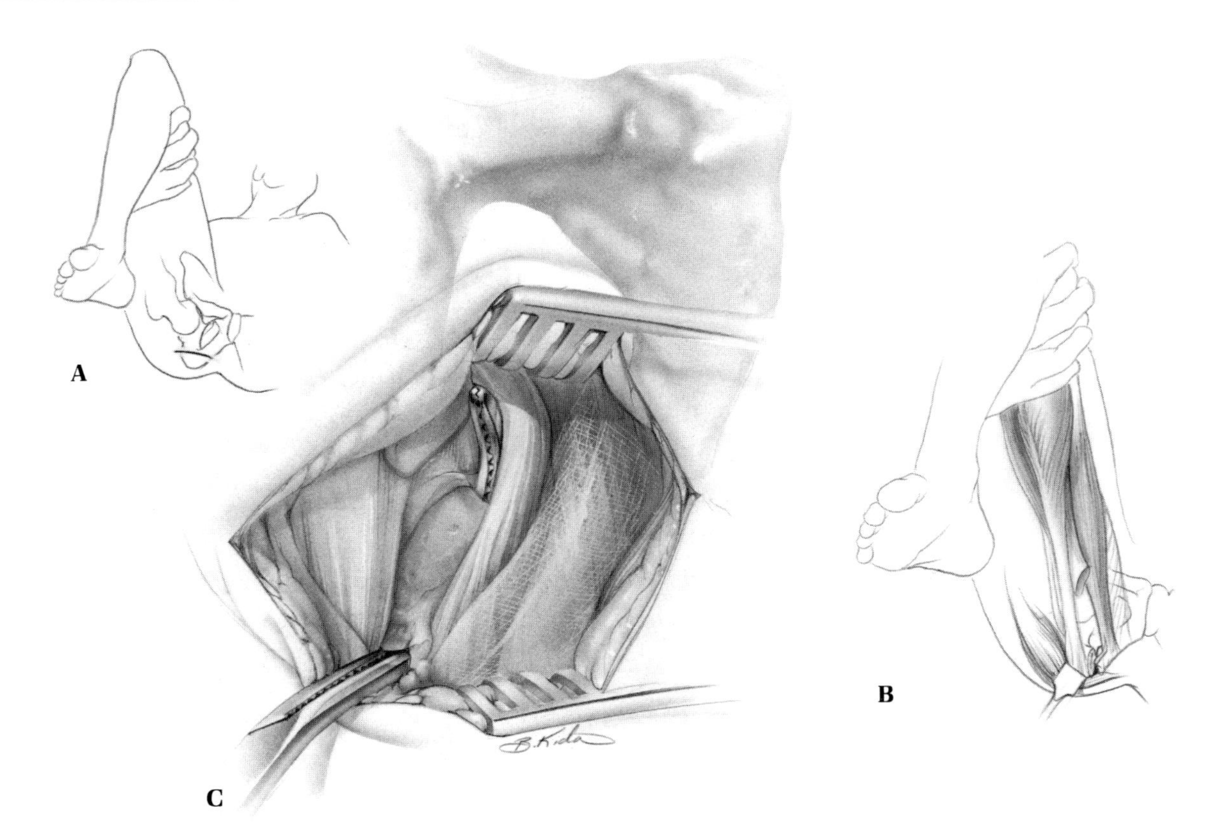

Figure 2–35

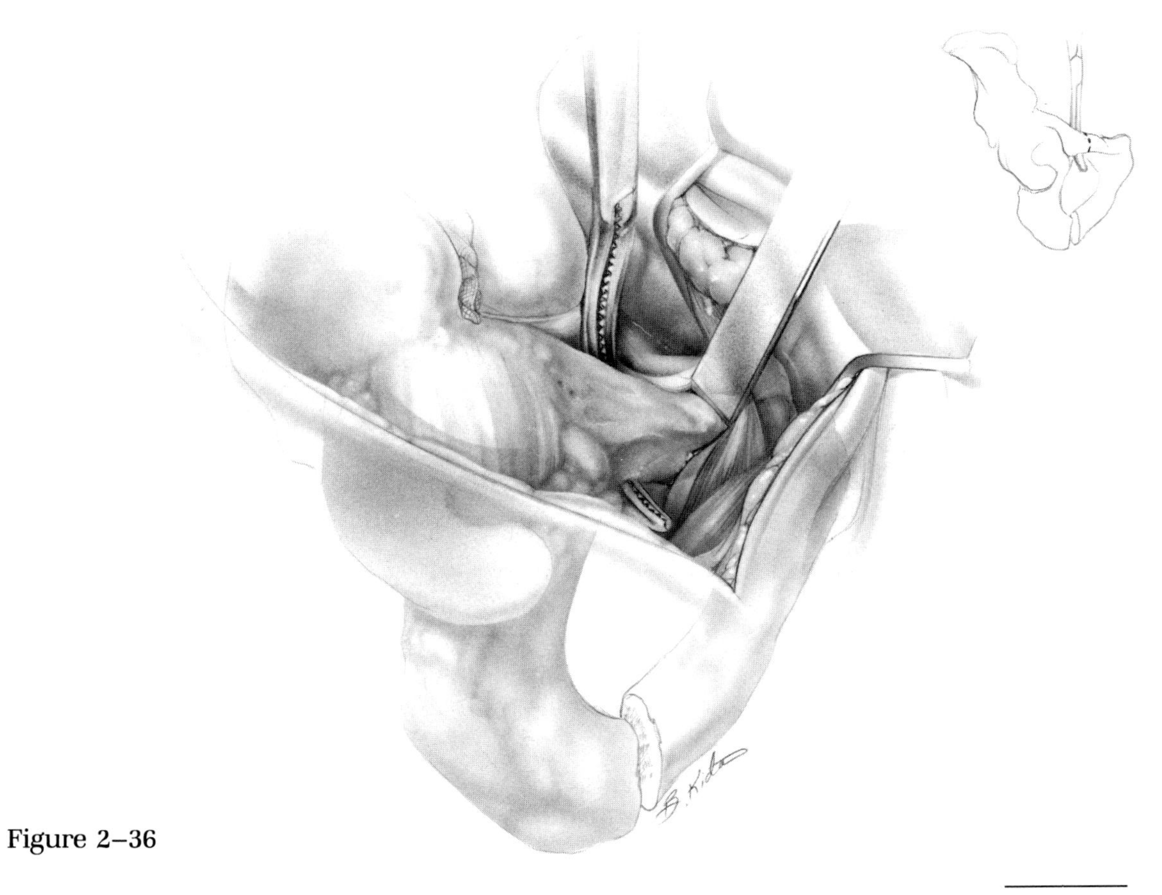

Figure 2–36

Figure 2–37. There now remains only one of the three osteotomies, that of the iliac bone. This is accomplished exactly as described for the Salter osteotomy.

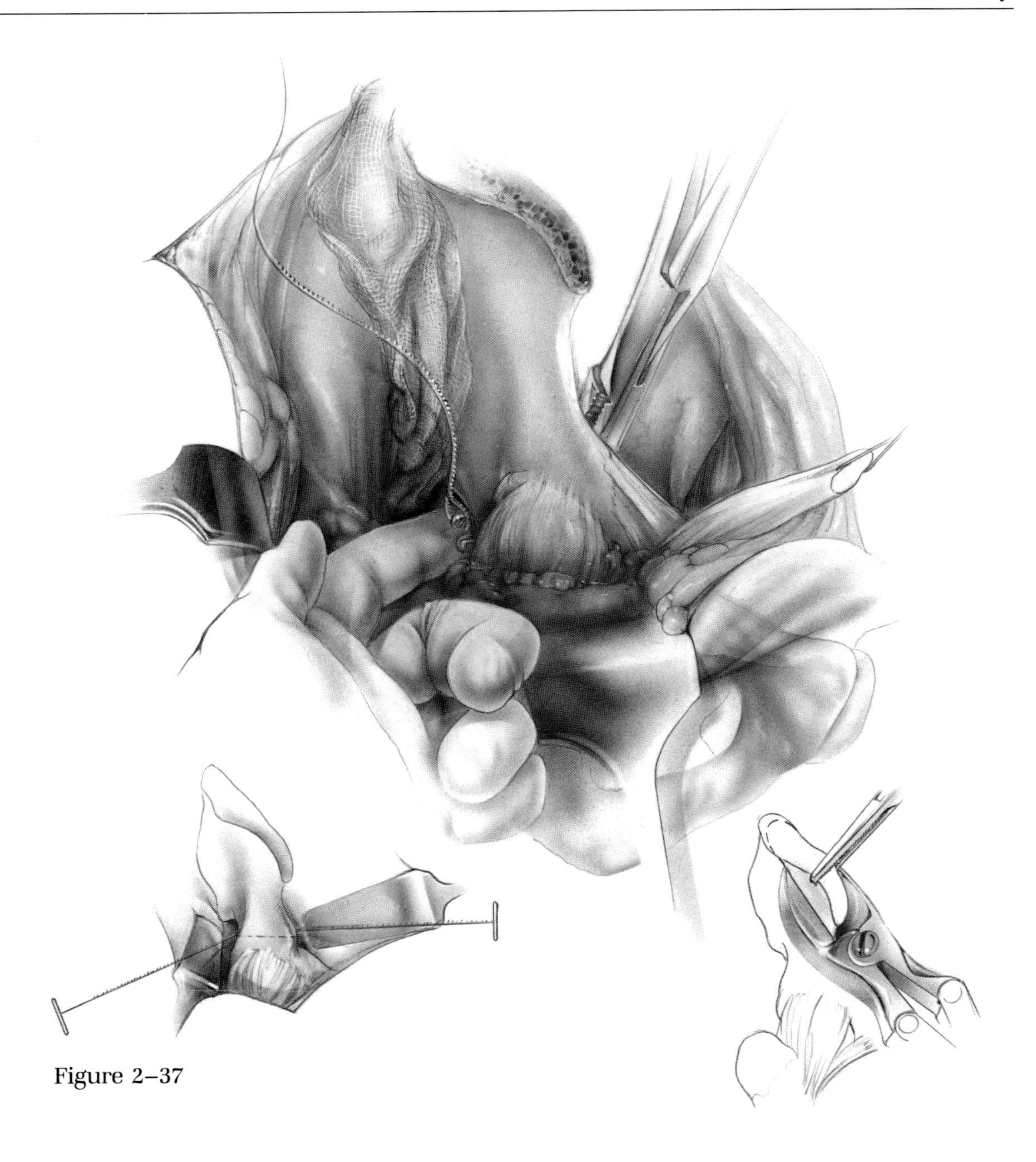

Figure 2–37

Figure 2–38. An alternative exposure to divide the pubic and ischial ramus is through a groin approach. The incision is transverse. It is placed approximately 1 cm from the groin crease starting 2 cm anterior to the adductor longus tendon and extending back to the posterior border of the gracilis muscle (***Figure 2–38A***). The adductor longus tendon is isolated and retracted posteriorly. The pectineus muscle, which lies superior to the adductor longus tendon is identified, and its border is dissected free up to its insertion on the pubis. The anterior branch of the obturator nerve lies deep in this interval between the adductor longus and pectineus, and should be protected. The femoral vessels and nerve lie just lateral to the pectineus muscle. This approach places the surgeon medial to the pectineal tubercle without strenuous retraction as is needed when this area is approached from the transverse iliac incision. At this point a subperiosteal dissection of the pubic ramus is accomplished. A suitable curved forceps, retractor, or elevator is placed around the back side of the pubic ramus after the periosteum and obturator muscle origins are elevated. An osteotome cutting toward the protecting forceps completes the osteotomy.

Figure 2–39. The next part of the exposure is similar to that for proximal hamstring release but must be accomplished through a wider exposure. The gracilis is separated from the crural fascia and its posterior border identified. The adductor magnus muscle will lie deep and anterior to this posterior border. The interval between the posterior border of the gracilis and the adductor magnus muscles anteriorly and the proximal insertion of the hamstrings posteriorly is opened. It will require sharp dissection to open this interval sufficiently.

Once the insertion of the hamstrings into the ischium is visualized, exposure is carried superiorly along the ramus of the ischium. Here the periosteum is incised and elevated. A forceps is passed around the ischium to protect the structures beneath, and an osteotome is used to divide the ischial ramus.

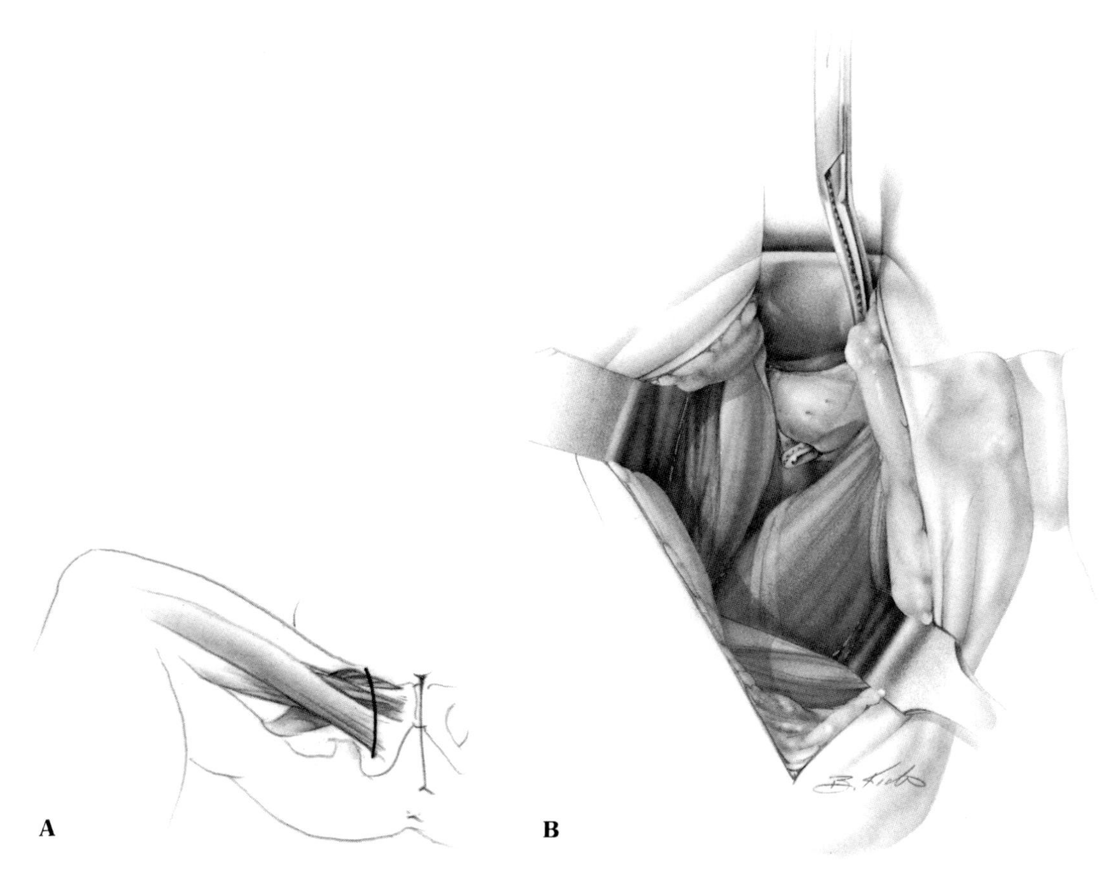

Figure 2–38

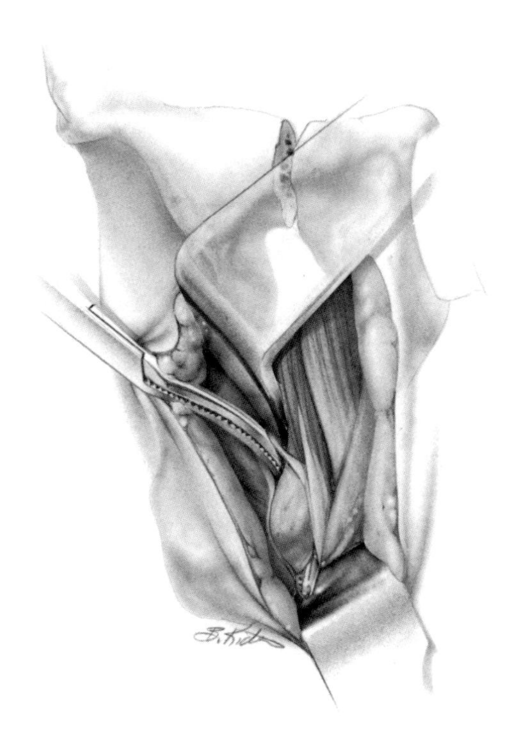

Figure 2–39

Figure 2–40. With the acetabular fragment now completely mobile, the fragment is grasped with a towel clip in the same manner as for a Salter osteotomy. It should be possible to rotate it freely as far anteriorly and laterally as desired. Care should be taken to gain only the correct amount of coverage because excessive rotation, especially anteriorly, could block motion. Unlike the Salter osteotomy, a lamina spreader can be used to separate the osteotomy in the iliac bone. This is because the fragment is free and will not exert excessive upward pressure on the sacroiliac joint. When the desired correction is obtained, a bone graft from the anterior crest of the ilium is fashioned to fit in the gap in the iliac osteotomy. This osteotomy site is then fixed with two $\frac{5}{32}$-in threaded Kirschner wires or two screws. Because of the amount of displacement and the resulting configuration of the osteotomy site both may be placed from below, or one from below and one from above. The osteotomy of the ischium and the pubis are not fixed. The wound is closed, and a drain is used at the surgeon's discretion.

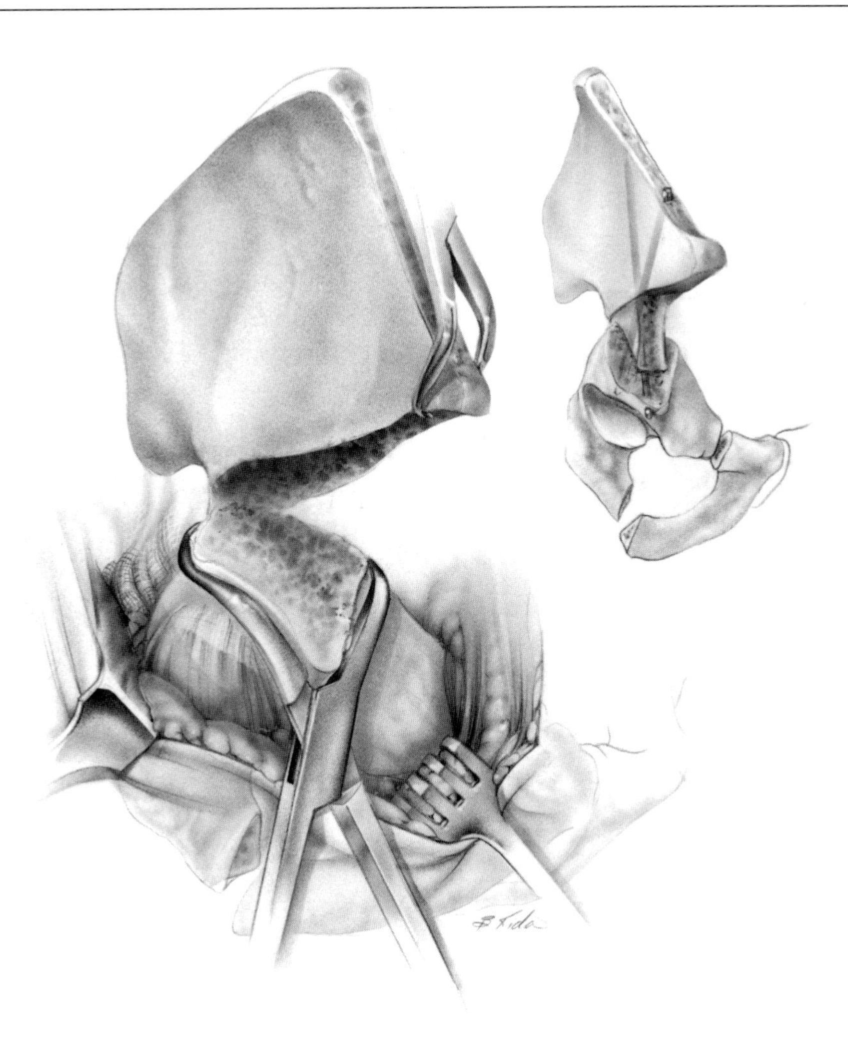

Figure 2–40

Figure 2–41. TW is a 13 + 2-year-old female who presented with a history of 6 months of increasing right hip pain. She was treated for congenital dislocation of the right hip at 3 months of age with a closed reduction. She has type II avascular necrosis and acetabular dysplasia of the right hip (***Figure 2–41A***). She was treated with a triple innominate osteotomy fixed with two $\frac{5}{32}$-in threaded pins (***Figure 2–41B***). Five years postoperatively, she remains asymptomatic and with good radiographic containment of the hip (***Figure 2–41C***).

POSTOPERATIVE CARE

The patient is usually placed in a spica cast. In a more reliable patient this can be a single-leg spica. In older patients who are reliable with crutches and in whom the fixation is secure, balance suspension may be used immediately after surgery until motion and comfort are restored, and then a partial weight-bearing crutch gait begun. The healing time for this osteotomy depends on the age of the patient, but for the same age is generally longer than the Salter osteotomy. Young children may be healed in 8 weeks, whereas it may take 12 weeks or longer in young adults.

REFERENCES

1. Steel HH. Triple osteotomy of the innominate bone. J Bone Joint Surg 1973;55A:343.
2. Le Coeur P. Correction des defauts d'orientation de l'articulation coxxo-femorale par osteotomie de l'isthme iliaque. Rev Chir Orthop 1965;51:211.

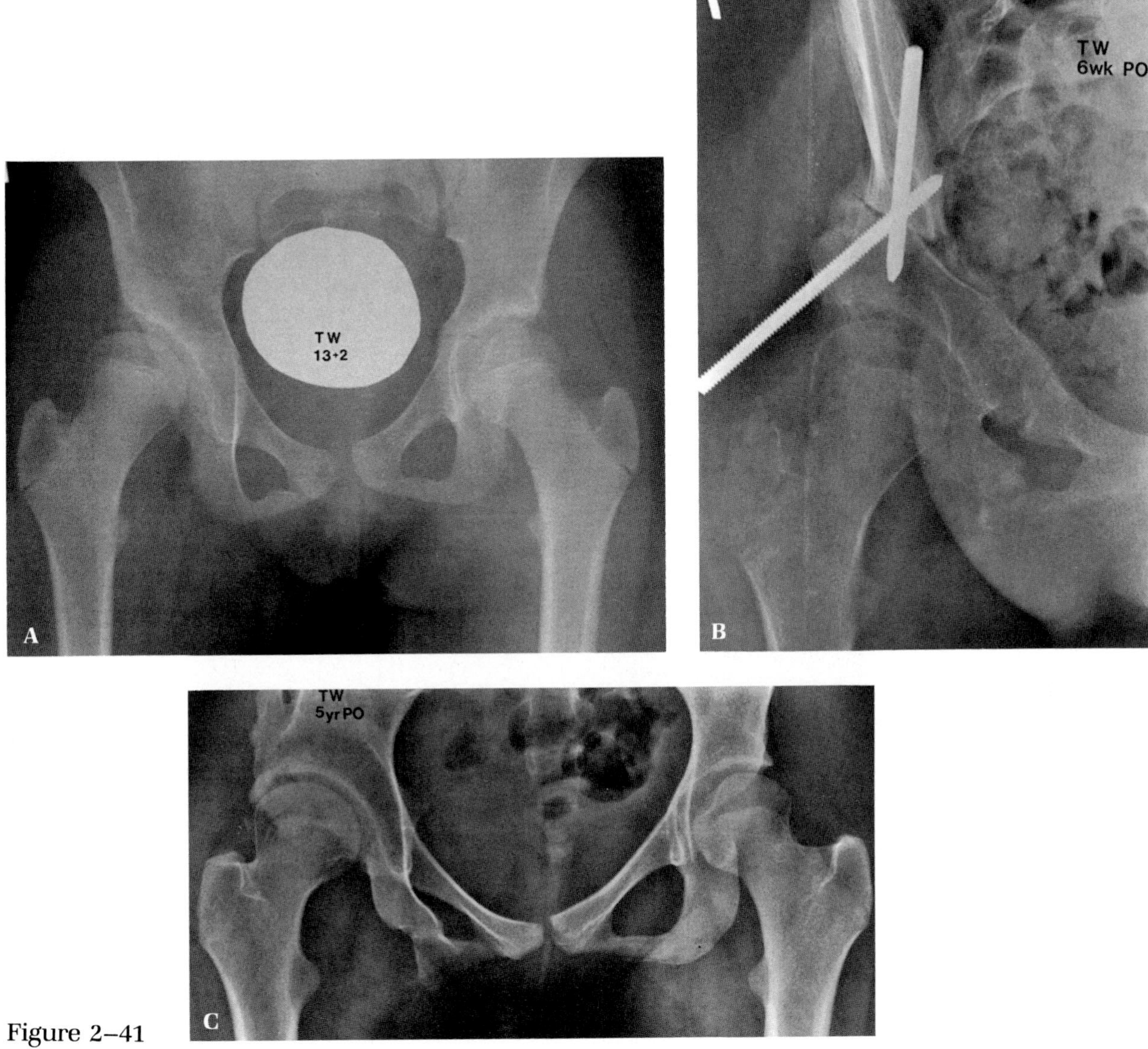

Figure 2–41

2.9 Chiari's Innominate Osteotomy

Unlike those operations that redirect the acetabular cartilage and subchondral bone and can be called reconstructive procedures, the Chiari medial displacement osteotomy is a salvage procedure in that it uses the cancellous bone of the ilium with interposed hip joint capsule as the material to contain the femoral head and bear weight. It accomplishes this by a single osteotomy through the ilium just above the hip joint capsule with medial displacement of the hip joint and its capsule under the superior iliac fragment.

The operation is primarily indicated in the older patient with a subluxated hip who is experiencing pain and in whom one of the reconstructive procedures that redirects the acetabulum is not possible. It is not necessary to achieve a concentric reduction of the femoral head to perform this procedure. Because coverage is dependent on the width of the ilium at the site of the osteotomy this procedure is less successful in young children, especially those with myelomeningocele and other paralytic conditions that result in a small thin pelvis. It has also been recognized that the width of the ilium is not sufficient to achieve adequate coverage in many cases of subluxation. This has led to the use of bone graft to augment the lateral coverage.[1–3] Because so much of the anterior femoral head is uncovered by the ilium in most cases, a strong case can be made for always augmenting a Chiari osteotomy in this fashion.

The operation has become popular for the adolescent and young adult with subluxation of the hip and pain because it does not require reduction of the hip and gives excellent pain relief in most series. It has a biomechanical advantage in that it medializes the hip and thus reduces the force through the hip joint. This also shortens the abductor lever arm, however, and can produce increased gluteal weakness and consequent limp. The biggest problem with the operation is that it appears deceptively easy to perform, and the postoperative radiographs may not accurately reflect the amount of coverage obtained.[4]

The incision and exposure of the ilium are the same as described for the Salter osteotomy. Although Chiari did not expose the inner wall of the ilium, this adds no morbidity to the procedure while it increases the safety and aids in orientation.

Figure 2–42. The placement of the osteotomy is critical to the success of the operation. If it is too high it will not provide coverage for the hip, and if it is too low there will not be sufficient capsule between the femoral head and ilium. Therefore, it is important that the superior aspect of the hip capsule be well exposed from anterior to posterior. In addition it is necessary to know where the roof of the acetabulum lies. This may be difficult in many subluxated hips because of a thickened capsule. In some cases it may be necessary to thin this capsule.

Also critical is the direction of the osteotomy. Proceeding from lateral to medial, the osteotomy should incline cephalad about 10 degrees (***Figure 2–42A***). This permits the inferior fragment containing the hip joint to displace medially while providing better contact of the superior fragment against the lateral capsule.

These two critical points, the location of the acetabular roof and the direction of the osteotomy, can be verified by drilling a small guide wire from lateral to medial in the estimated direction of the osteotomy at the proposed site of the osteotomy, and viewing this with a radiograph or image intensifier.

The osteotomy as originally described by Chiari was straight from anterior to posterior. Common usage has modified this to produce a dome-shaped osteotomy that will more closely conform to the hip capsule after displacement. This is easily accomplished in the anterior and midportion of the osteotomy but cannot be achieved posteriorly (***Figure 2–42B***).

The author's preference is to cut the lateral cortex first (***Figure 2–42C***) and then cut the medial cortex (***Figure 2–42D***). This allows the surgeon excellent orientation. These cuts in the cortex are not extended into the sciatic notch because splintering of this posterior cortex may impinge on the sciatic nerve. The cuts in the lateral and medial cortex are then connected, leaving only the posterior cortex of the sciatic notch intact.

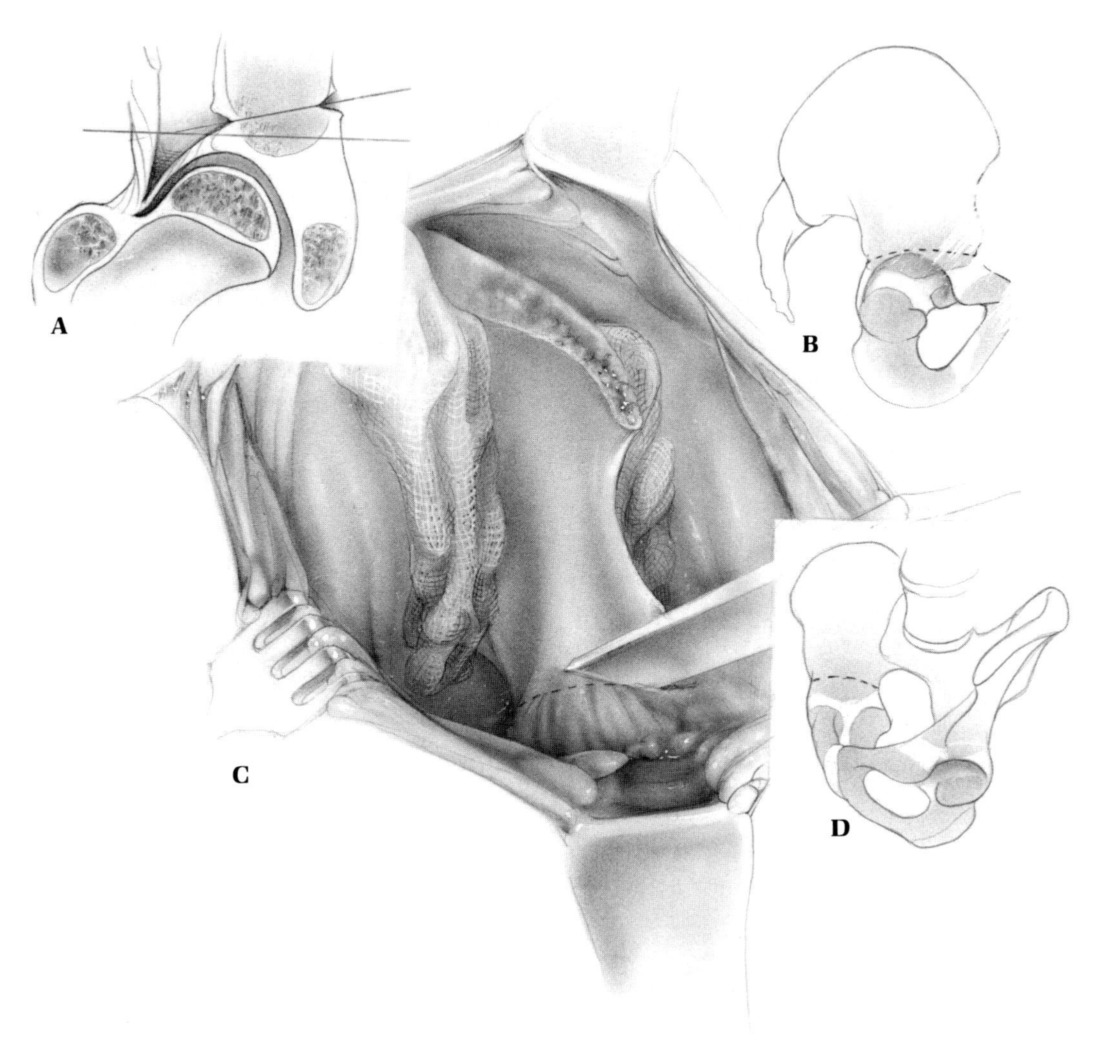

Figure 2–42

Figure 2–43. A Gigli saw is passed through the sciatic notch as described for the Salter osteotomy. This is used to complete the osteotomy.

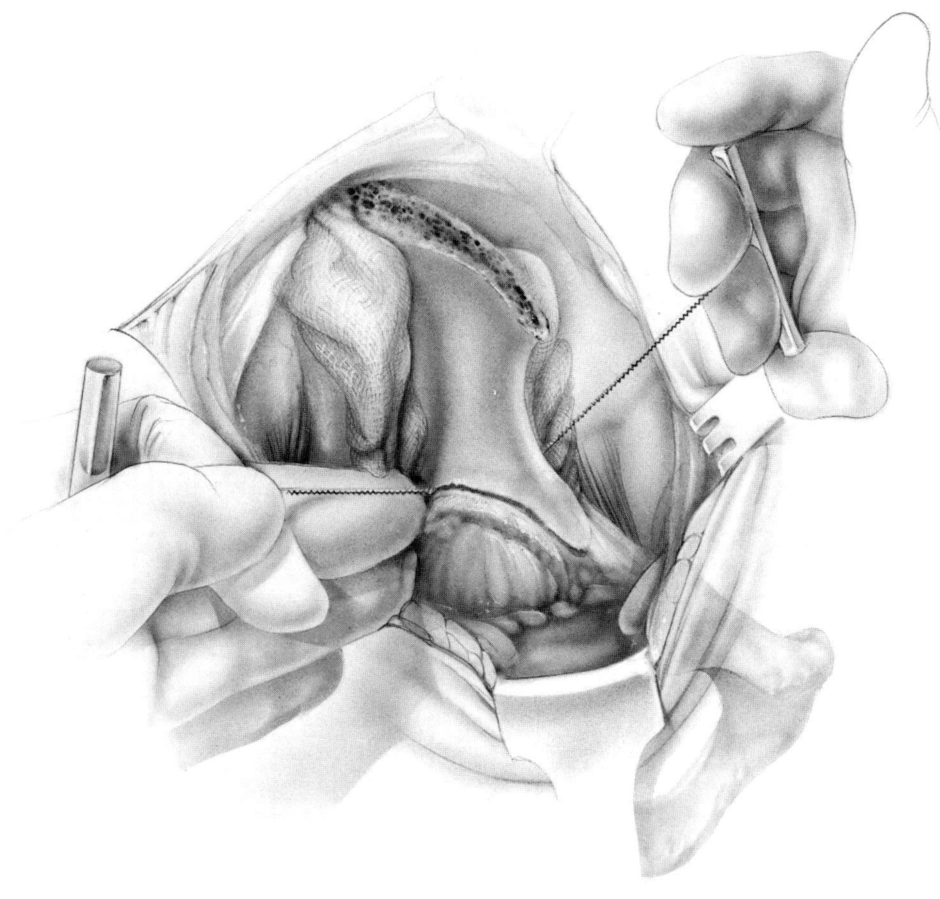

Figure 2–43

Figure 2–44. With the osteotomy complete the distal fragment is displaced medially (***Figure 2–44A***). A common error at this point is to hinge the osteotomy on a posterior tether. This will result in only the anterior aspect displacing. Without careful inspection of the posterior aspect of the osteotomy this may go unnoticed, and it will not be reflected on postoperative radiographs.

The osteotomy can usually be displaced by abducting the leg (***Figure 2–44B***). If the osteotomy has been properly performed it should move easily with this maneuver. Further displacement can be achieved with direct pressure over the greater trochanter. There is a tendency for the inferior fragment with the hip joint to displace posteriorly. This should probably be avoided because it may increase the pressure on the sciatic nerve. Posterior displacement will, however, increase the amount of coverage because the ilium is wider in its posterior aspect than its anterior aspect (***Figure 2–44C***).

How much displacement is advisable is a matter of debate, with some saying that there should be no more than 50% displacement.

Such admonitions do not account for the variable width of the ilium, which is thin in cross-section anteriorly and wide posteriorly. It is certainly possible and often advisable to achieve 100% displacement at the midportion of the osteotomy over the dome of the hip joint. If this much displacement is achieved it should be secured with strong fixation to prevent further displacement and supplemented with bone graft to avoid delayed or non-union.

Healing may be slow, especially if the patient is older and the displacement greater. In these circumstances it is best to fix the osteotomy with two or three strong screws, which can be left in place for several months without bothering the patient. In cases in which more rapid healing is anticipated, heavy threaded pins can be used and left subcutaneously for easy removal.

Figure 2–45. It is often necessary to augment the coverage obtained with the Chiari osteotomy. This is especially true anteriorly where the ilium is thin. An excellent method for accomplishing this coverage has been described.[1,2] An appropriate size piece of corticocancellous bone is removed from the inner table of the ilium. This is placed in the osteotomy site before fixation. The screws or pins used for fixation then transfix this graft. Additional cancellous bone graft is then added over this graft and is held in place by the periosteum and muscles when the wound is closed.

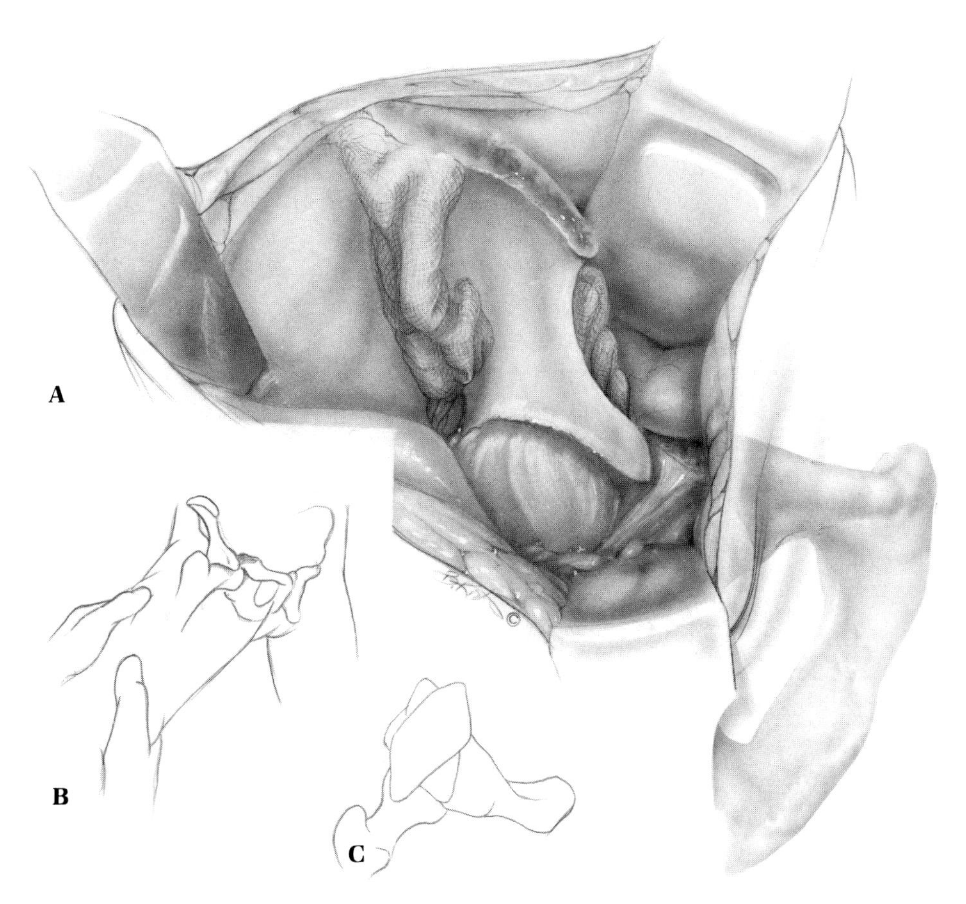

Figure 2–44

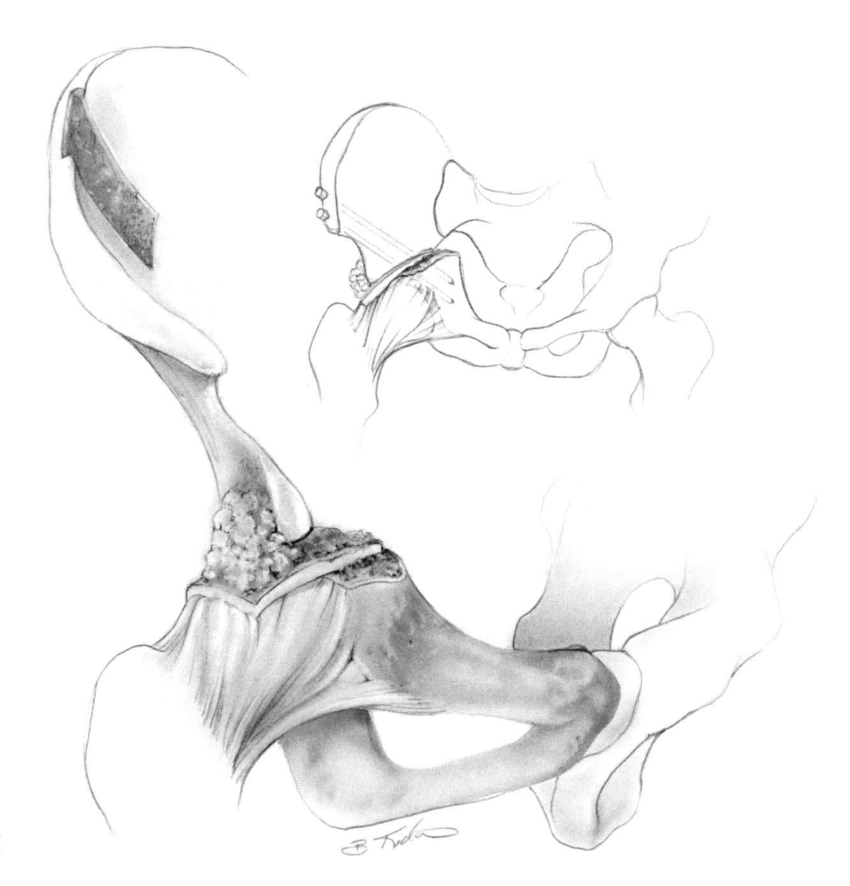

Figure 2–45

Figure 2–46. The radiograph of a 16-year-old girl with severe and painful dysplasia as a result of congenitally dislocated hip (***Figure 2–46A***). The anteroposterior radiograph postoperatively demonstrates the coverage (***Figure 2–46B***). This can be misleading on the true anteroposterior view, however, because the posterior aspect of the ilium is rotated outward. Four years after the surgery the hip is well contained and the patient asymptomatic (***Figure 2–46C***). (Courtesy of Michael Millis, MD.)

POSTOPERATIVE CARE

It is not necessary to place the older reliable patient in a cast. The osteotomy has a high degree of intrinsic stability, which if supplemented with strong internal fixation will permit a partial weight-bearing crutch gait. Crutches should be continued until both radiographic evidence of healing is seen and the patient has rehabilitated the abductor muscles. If a spica cast is used in the younger child it should be continued until radiographic evidence of union is present, and the pins are removed. This will usually be 8 to 12 weeks.

REFERENCES

1. Fernandez DL, Isler B, Muller M. Chiari's osteotomy: a note on technique. Clin Orthop 1984;185:53.
2. Bailey TE, Hall JE. Chiari medial displacement osteotomy. J Pediatr Orthop 1985;5:635.
3. Betz RR, Kumar SJ, Palmer CT, MacEwen GD. Chiari pelvic osteotomy in children and young adults. J Bone Joint Surg 1988;70A:182.
4. Benson MKD, Evans DC. The pelvic osteotomy of Chiari: an anatomical study of the hazards and misleading radiographic appearances. J Bone Joint Surg 1976;58B:164.

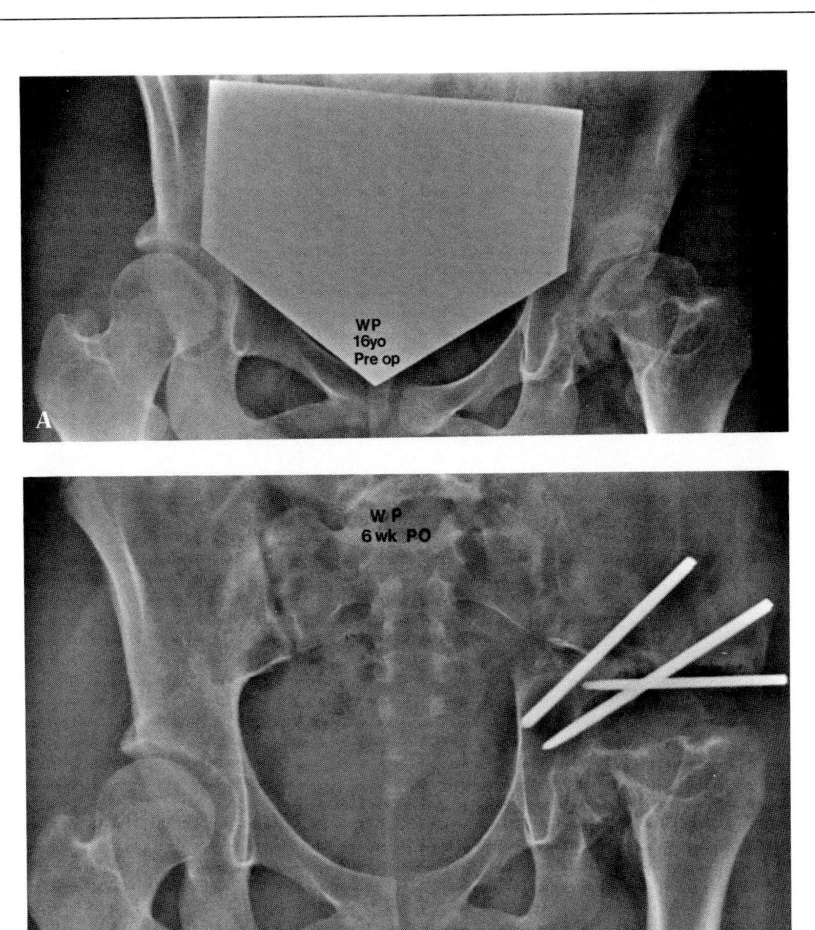

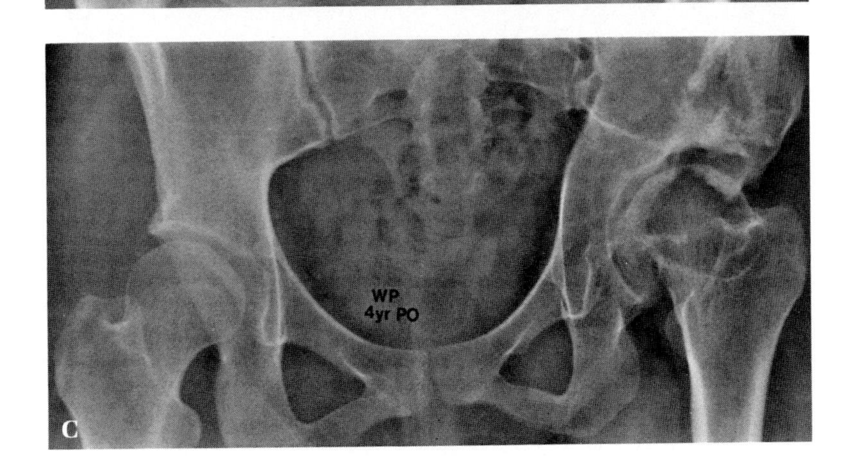

Figure 2–46

2.10
Staheli's Shelf Procedure

Various procedures for creating a shelf of bone to augment a deficient acetabulum were first performed in the last century. In its various forms it remained the main method of treating the dysplastic acetabulum until procedures that redirected or displaced the acetabulum became popular. During the past 20 years the popularity of the shelf procedures waned because of the popularity of the newer osteotomies and the poor technical performance of the shelf procedures.[1]

The primary goal in the creation of an acetabular shelf, as in any of the acetabular procedures, is to increase the load-bearing area between the femoral head and the acetabulum, or increase the stability of the hip. The shelf procedures, like the Chiari osteotomy, are salvage procedures because they use bone over capsule rather than articular cartilage and subchondral bone for the increased area. Although this at first may seem less than ideal, there are certain circumstances in which a salvage procedure is the only choice.

The indications for the slotted acetabular augmentation are the same as for any shelf procedure: hips with asymmetric incongruity. The operation should not be done in a hip with spheric congruity in which acetabular redirection is more appropriate. The operation is not ideal when the capsule must be opened, although, like the Chiari, it can be performed.

The slotted acetabular augmentation developed by Staheli is a shelf procedure in which a slot in the ilium is created for the bone graft. This aids in the correct and secure placement of the graft.[2] The amount of coverage can be calculated by determining the length of the graft that is necessary to create the desired center-edge angle.

The exposure for the operation is done the same as for the anterior approach for the open reduction of congenital dislocation of the hip. Larger teenaged children can be done on a fracture table if the surgeon chooses. The outer table of the ilium and the entire superior capsule must be clearly visualized. The inner table of the ilium does not have to be exposed.

Figure 2–47. During the exposure the reflected head of the rectus tendon should be identified, dissected free from the capsule, and divided in its middle leaving it attached anteriorly and posteriorly. This will be used to secure the grafts in place. If it is not present, flaps can be created from the thickened capsule, which will serve the same purpose.

The most important part of the surgery is to identify the correct location for the slot. It should be placed at the exact acetabular edge. The surgeon will have to determine if this is to be the true or false acetabulum based on which affords the greatest stability and congruity. The acetabulum can be identified by a small incision in the capsule or by inserting a probe. In the subluxated and dysplastic hip the capsule will usually be thickened and adherent to the ilium, causing the surgeon to place the slot and hence the graft too high. The correct location should be radiographically verified by placing a guide pin into the ilium at the presumed acetabular edge. In some cases it may be necessary to thin the capsule to permit the graft to be placed in the proper location.

After the correct location is verified, a $\frac{5}{32}$-in drill is used to make a series of holes at the edge of the acetabulum. These holes should be drilled to a depth of about 1 cm. These holes should extend far enough anteriorly and posteriorly to provide the necessary coverage.

Figure 2–48. A narrow rongeur is then used to connect these holes and thus produce the slot. The floor of this slot should be the subchondral bone of the acetabulum, and it should be level with the capsule.

The bone graft is obtained from the outer table of the ilium. Starting at the iliac crest corticocancellous and then cancellous strips of bone are removed. In the region above the slot the decortication should be very shallow so as to aid the incorporation of the graft without disrupting the integrity of the slot. It may be necessary in some neuromuscular patients to use bank bone.

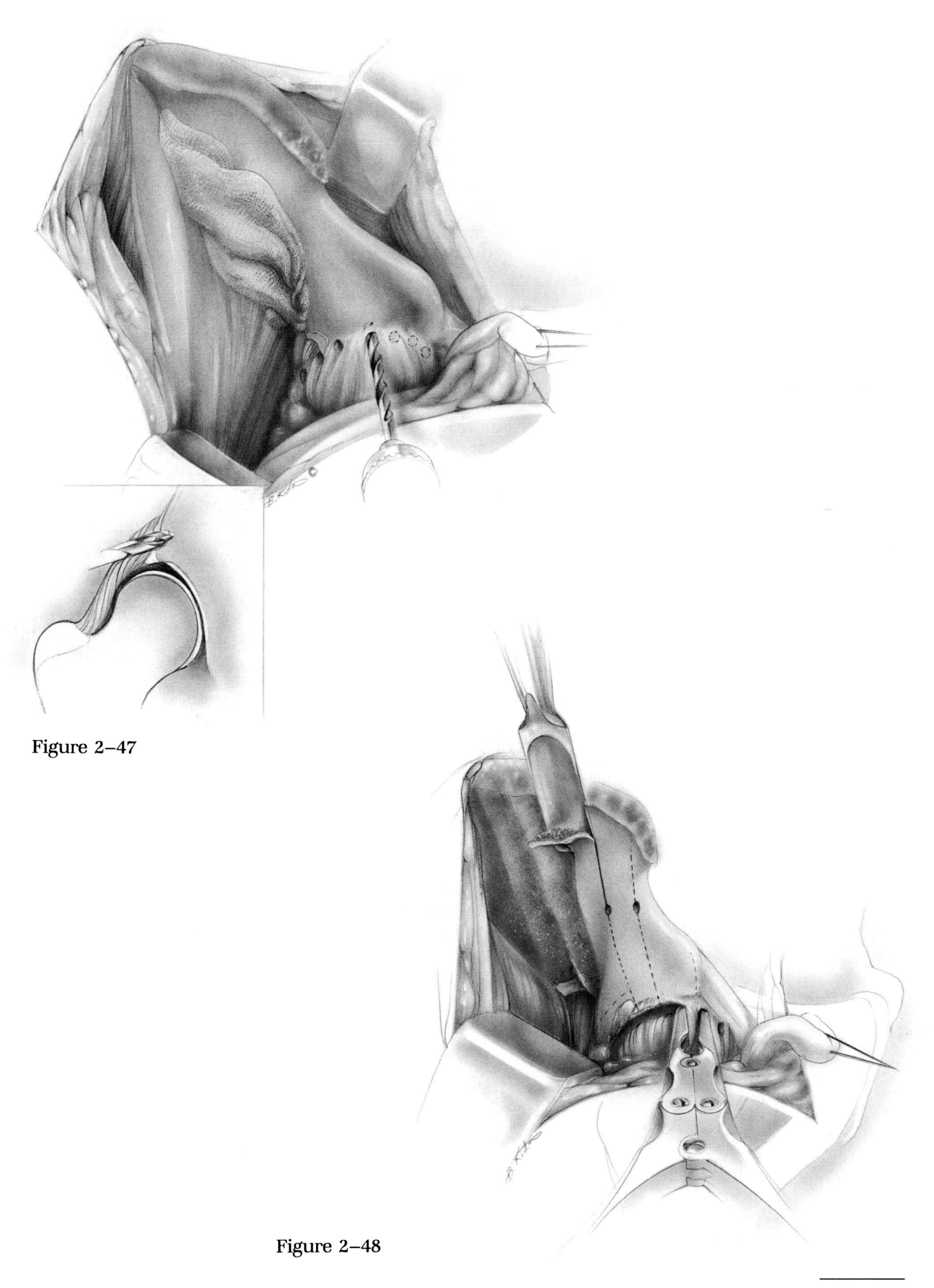

Figure 2–47

Figure 2–48

Figure 2–49. The cancellous grafts are cut in strips 1 cm wide and of appropriate length to provide the desired amount of lateral coverage. These are placed in the slot extending out over the capsule. A second layer of cancellous strips are then placed at 90 degrees to the first strips of graft. It is important that the grafts not extend too far lateral or anterior in the quest for spectacular radiographic coverage of the hip as this could result in a loss of motion.

Figure 2–50. The reflected head of the rectus tendon is then sutured together holding the grafts in place. The remaining bone is cut into small pieces and placed over the previously placed graft. This will be held in place by the abductor muscles when the wound is closed.

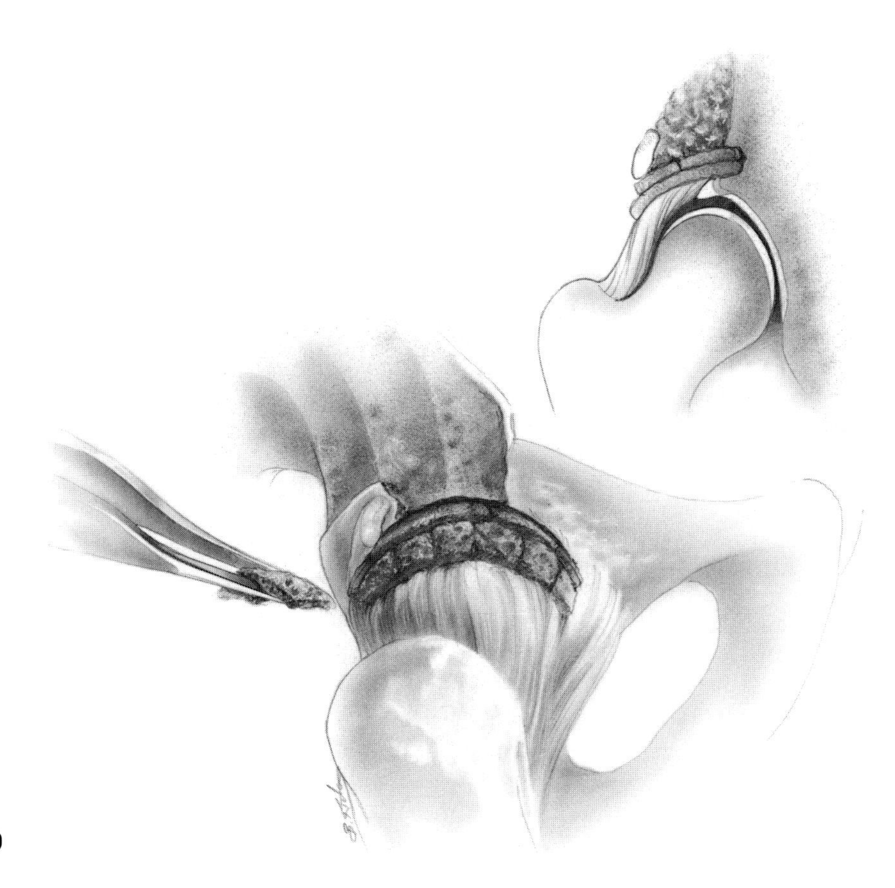

Figure 2–49

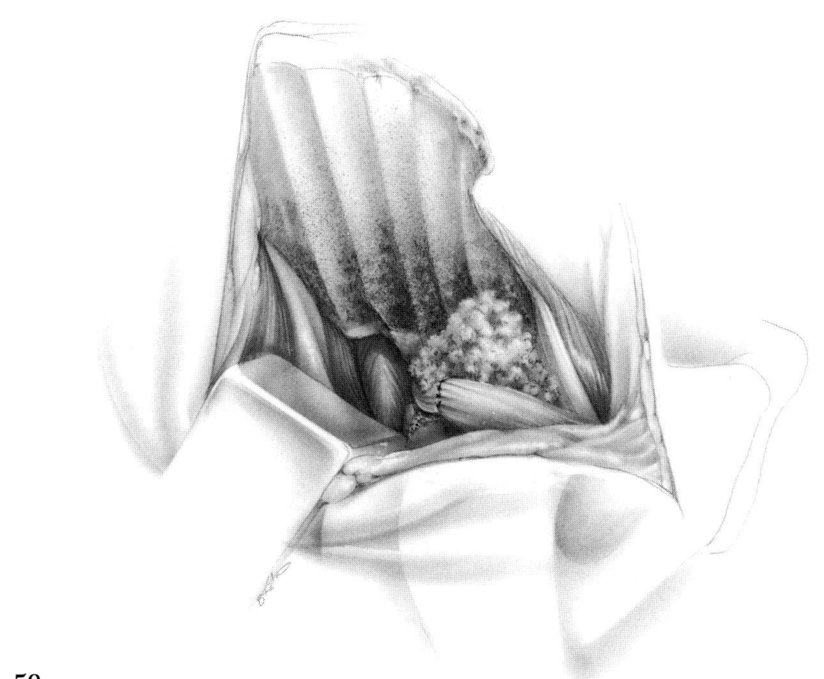

Figure 2–50

Figure 2–51. Acetabular dysplasia in a 17-year-old woman that resulted from treatment of congenital dislocation of the hip with subsequent type II avascular necrosis of the femoral head (***Figure 2–51A***).

The radiograph taken 6 weeks after a slotted acetabular augmentation demonstrates the large amount of graft that is used (***Figure 2–51B***).

Eighteen months after surgery good incorporation of the graft with a strong shelf is demonstrated (***Figure 2–51C***). Note the remaining hole in the graft where the reflected head of the rectus tendon was repaired. (Courtesy of Lynn T. Staheli, MD.)

POSTOPERATIVE CARE

The patient is placed in a single-leg spica cast with the hip in the position of 15 degrees abduction, 20 degrees flexion, and neutral rotation. The cast can be removed in 6 weeks and radiographic assessment of graft incorporation made. Reliable patients may begin partial weight bearing. In less reliable patients weight bearing may be permitted in a walking spica. It usually takes 4 months for complete graft incorporation.

REFERENCES

1. White RE, Sherman FC. The hip-shelf procedure: a long-term evaluation. J Bone Joint Surg 1980;62A:928.
2. Staheli LT. Slotted acetabular augmentation. J Pediatr Orthop 1981;1:321.

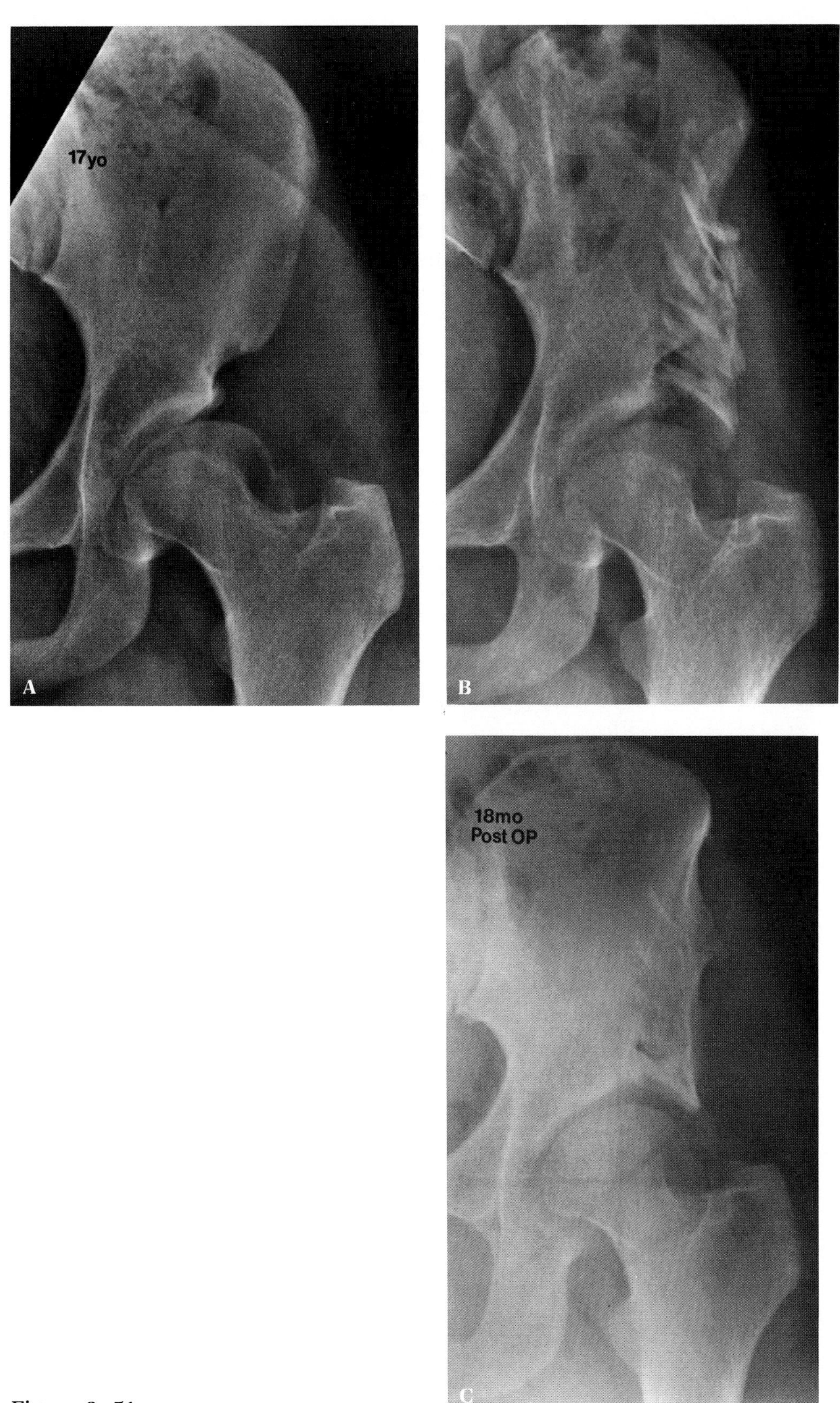

Figure 2–51

2.11
Arthrodesis of the Hip Joint

Despite advances in total joint arthroplasty, arthrodesis of the hip joint remains the best option for the adolescent or young adult with destruction of the joint and pain. Despite the limitations imposed by hip arthrodesis, this will probably remain true until technologic advances have convincingly solved the problem of loosening in total joint arthroplasty, especially in young active patients.

Most long-term studies have demonstrated that most patients are satisfied with the results of hip joint arthrodesis and lead active lives without hip pain.[1,2] From such studies, however, it is also apparent that many patients will develop back pain and knee pain with radiographic signs of osteoarthritis decades after the arthrodesis. Today these problems are being solved with conversion to total hip arthroplasty.[3,4] This does not necessarily negate the value of hip arthrodesis, because at the time of conversion patients will be more suitable candidates for total joint arthroplasty and will be able to take advantage of several decades of technology improvement.

The relevant message from these studies for the surgeon performing a hip arthrodesis on a young patient is twofold. First, as much of the normal architecture of the hip as possible should be preserved so that total joint arthroplasty can be accomplished. This rules out the use of the cobra plate or other methods that alter the normal anatomy. Second, the position of the leg in relation to the pelvis is important in the development of late back and knee symptoms. Specifically, any abduction of the hip should be avoided.

A technique that has proved successful is that described by Thompson[5] and evaluated by Price and Lovell.[6] It uses an intertrochanteric osteotomy to relieve the effect of the long-lever arm of the leg on the arthrodesis and allow accurate positioning of the leg after the drapes are removed.

Figure 2–52. The hip is approached as for the Salter osteotomy. It is important that the hip capsule be widely exposed because dislocation of the diseased hip is difficult and requires an extensive capsulectomy. Both the inner and outer tables of the ilium should be exposed subperiosteally.

Figure 2–53. The femoral head is dislocated by adducting, externally rotating, and extending the leg. This will dislocate the femoral head anteriorly into the wound. Because of the amount of flattening of the femoral head, especially in cases of avascular necrosis, it is not usually possible to use a reaming cup to recreate the ideal rounded shape of the femoral head, which is often seen in diagrams of hip arthrodesis. Rather, curved osteotomes or gouges should be used to remove the remaining articular cartilage and dead avascular bone, accepting the more flattened surface that will result. The surface, regardless of its shape, should be bleeding bone.

Figure 2–54. Flexion and internal rotation of the leg will now displace the femoral head posterior to the acetabulum. Because access to the acetabulum will be somewhat restricted and it will not be deformed, a reaming tool is ideal to remove the cartilage and subchondral bone. It is usually not necessary to alter the resulting shape of the acetabulum, as the femoral head can be moved into the most congruous position. Usually, this is abduction.

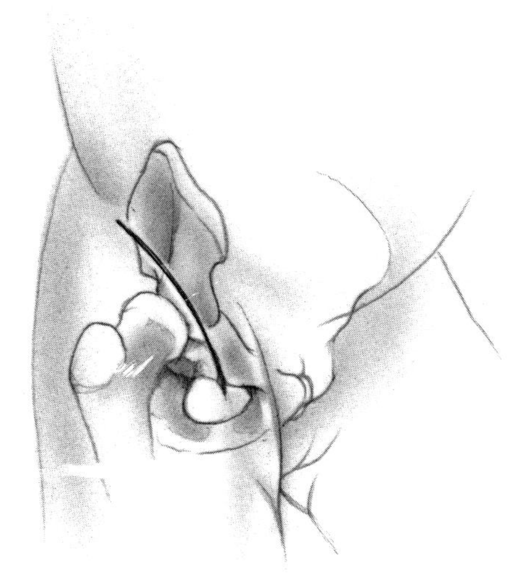

Figure 2–52

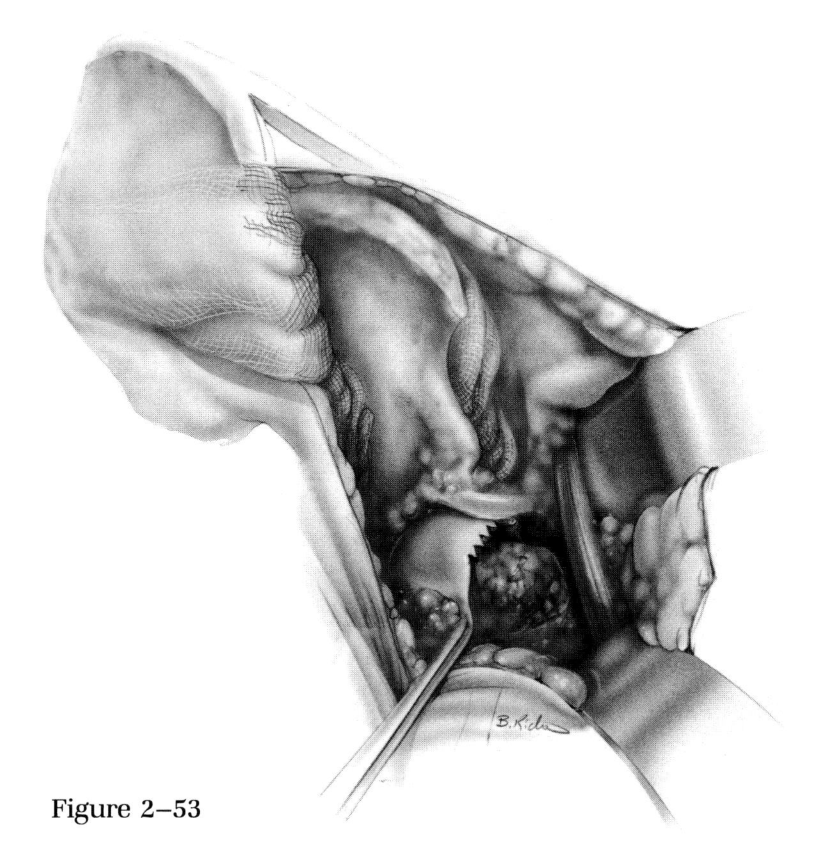

Figure 2–53

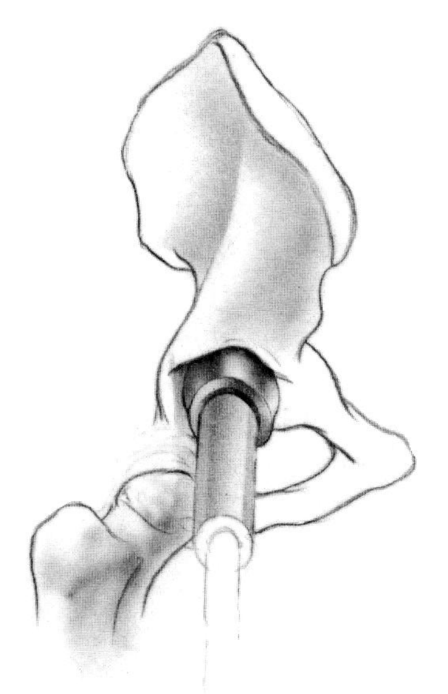

Figure 2–54

Figure 2–55. After the femoral head is placed in the desired position, one or two large, long, and strong screws with washers are directed from the inner side of the ilium, through the acetabulum, and into the femoral head and neck.

Figure 2–56. Using osteotomes or an oscillating saw, a trough is cut into the superior aspect of the ilium, just above the acetabulum and lateral to the iliopubic eminence, extending down onto the femoral neck. This should be as wide as the anterior portion of the iliac crest and about 1.5 cm deep to accommodate a tricortical piece of graft, which is taken from the anterior iliac crest. This graft is then wedged into place and may be secured by two screws. Cancellous bone can be removed from the exposed surface of the iliac crest with a curette and packed into the acetabulum around the femoral head.

Figure 2–57. An osteotomy of the femur is now performed just above the lesser trochanter. The surgeon may prefer to perform this step before fixing the femoral head to the ilium. If this is done, a large Steinmann pin should be drilled into the femoral head fragment so that it can be controlled. Performing the osteotomy at this stage ensures that sufficient but not excessive mobility is achieved at the osteotomy site to allow proper positioning of the leg in the cast.

The osteotomy can be performed through a small anterolateral incision, which splits the fibers of the tensor fascia muscle to reach the proximal femur. The periosteum is cut in the direction of the bone and is elevated with a curved Crego periosteal elevator. The less periosteal disruption that is created, the more stable the osteotomy will be. Multiple drill holes are made, and the osteotomy is completed with an osteotome. In the author's experience this results in quicker union than the use of the oscillating power saw, an important factor because rigid internal fixation is not used. The limb is now moved to ensure that sufficient mobility is present at the osteotomy site.

With time the distal fragment, the femoral shaft, will tend to displace posteriorly. This will present a difficult situation regarding stem placement if revision to total joint arthroplasty is needed in the future. This can be avoided by placing a drill hole through the anterior cortex on each side of the osteotomy and passing a heavy strong suture through the holes. This is tied loosely enough to permit flexion and some extension, and abduction and adduction at the osteotomy site while preventing any significant posterior displacement. The use of the anterolateral incision gives the surgeon a better exposure for this step than the traditional lateral incision.

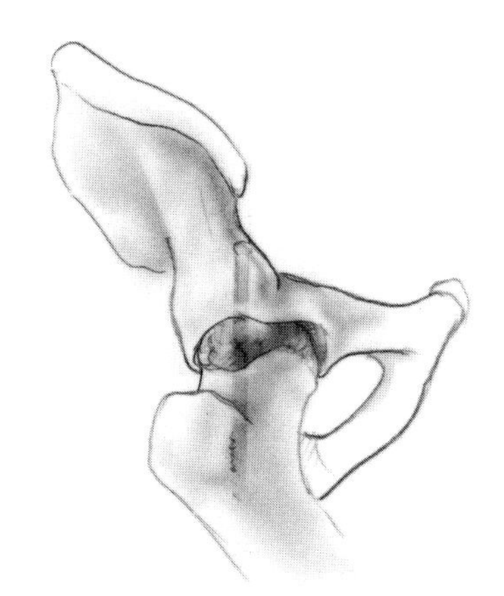

Figure 2–55

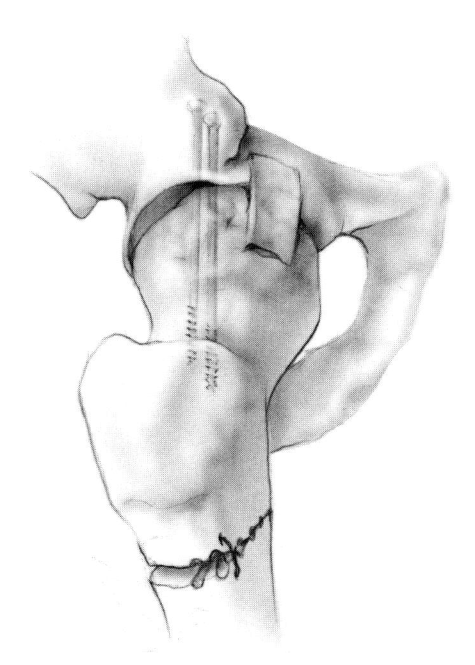

Figure 2–56

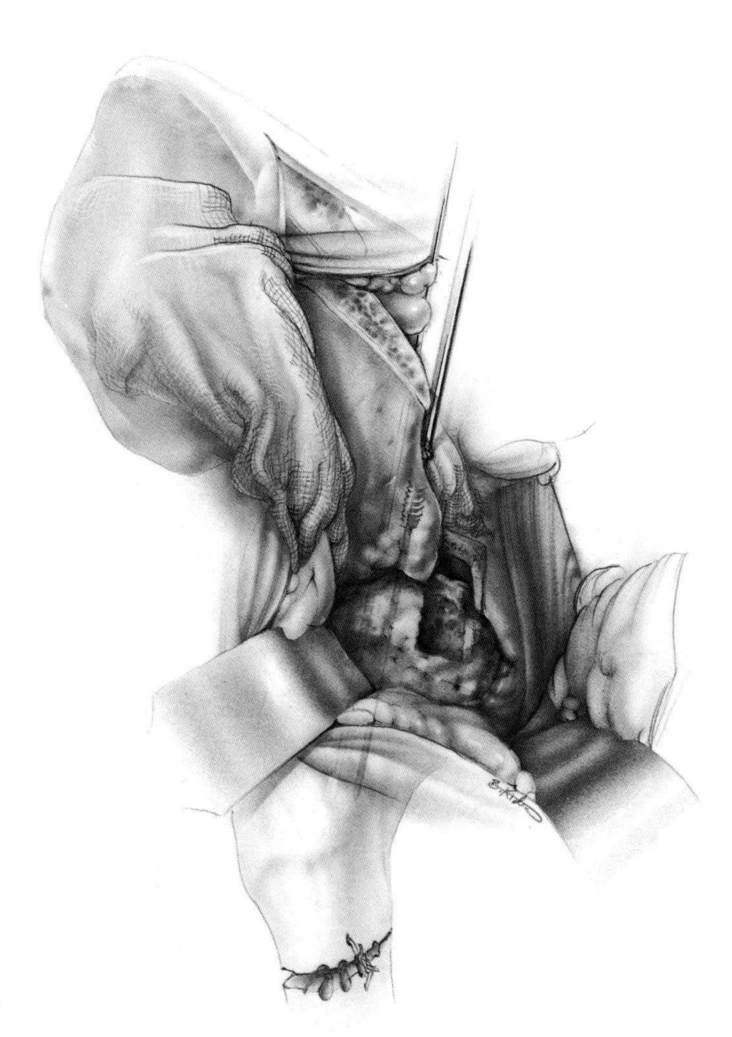

Figure 2–57

Figure 2–58. After the wounds are closed the patient is moved to a fracture table for application of a spica cast. This is a critical stage in the operation because it will determine the position of the leg relative to the pelvis, the importance of which has already been discussed. The best position for the leg is 30 degrees of flexion, 0 degrees of abduction, and 0 to 5 degrees of external rotation. In most situations the correct amount of flexion will be achieved by keeping the unoperated leg parallel to the floor and elevating the operated leg about 10 degrees. The resulting pelvic tilt as evidenced by the lumbar lordosis will result in approximately 30 degrees of hip flexion. Because of the dressings and the fact that the anterosuperior iliac spine is missing on the operated side, it is difficult to be sure of the degree of abduction. Because of its importance the degree of abduction should be verified by radiographic control. This is made easier by the use of a large, metal "T" square and an image intensifier.

The initial spica cast should include the entire leg and the foot if the knee is not bent, so that rotation of the osteotomy site is controlled. It is wise to verify the position of the limb radiographically again after cast placement.

Figure 2–59. Radiographs of a hip arthrodesis 3 months (***Figure 2–59A***) and 6 months (***Figure 2–59B***) after surgery for avascular necrosis secondary to slipped capital femoral epiphysis illustrate the delayed healing that can occur at the osteotomy site when it is created with a power saw. In this case the graft was wedged tightly into place and screws were not used to secure it.

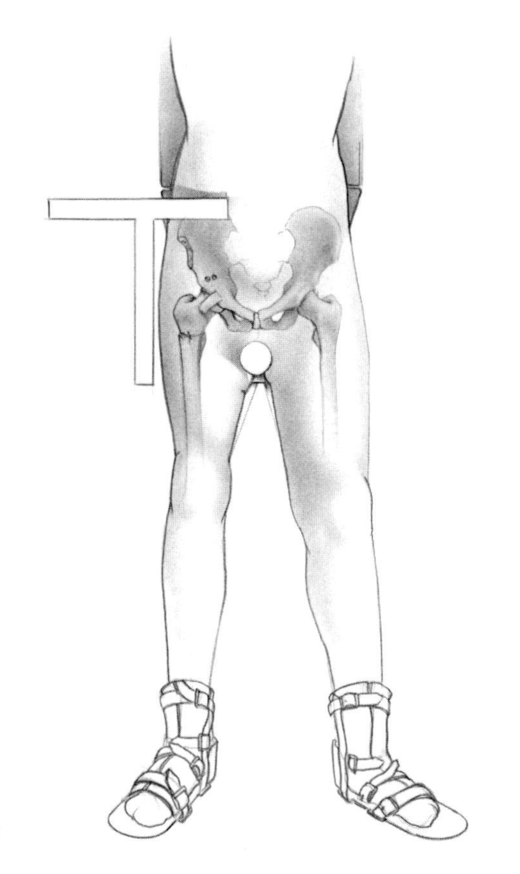

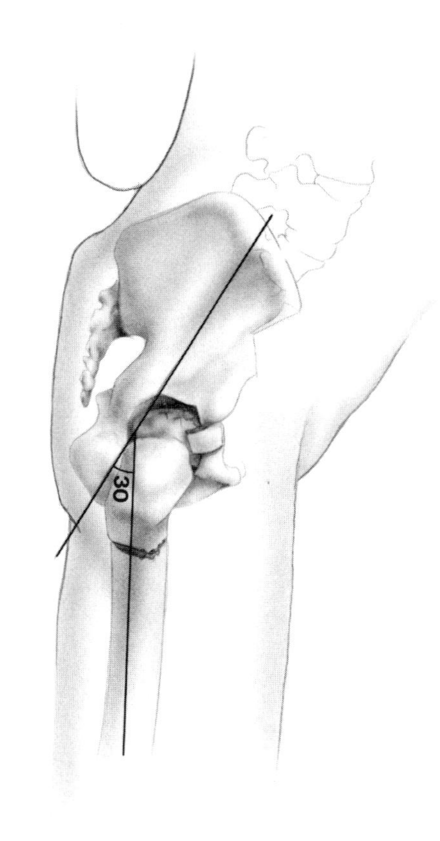

Figure 2–58

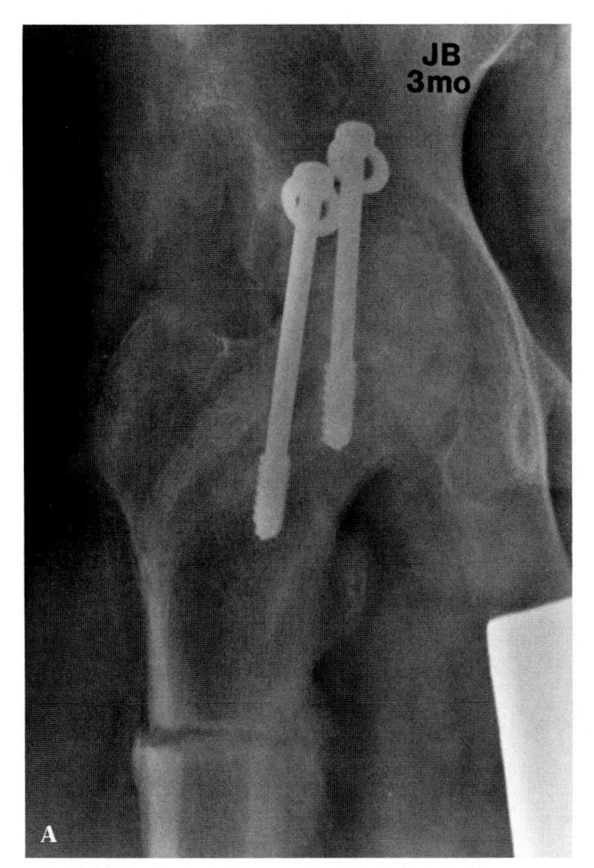

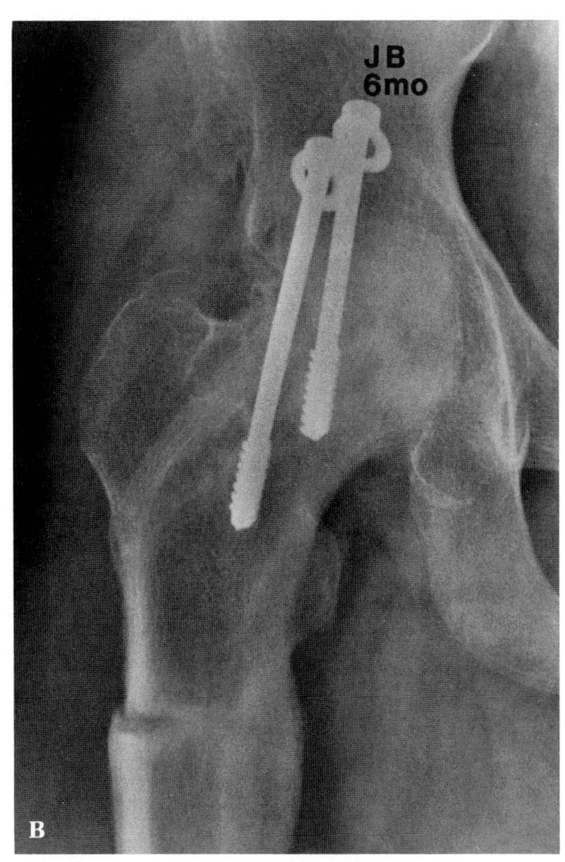

Figure 2–59

POSTOPERATIVE CARE

Depending on the surgeon's confidence in the internal fixation of the hip, the spica cast's immobilization of the femoral osteotomy, and the patient's ability to follow instructions, the patient may be mobilized on crutches or kept at bed rest. Bed rest is the usual result after examination of these questions. When early radiographic signs of healing are noted at the osteotomy site, usually by 6 weeks, the cast can be altered to allow knee motion and the patient mobilized on crutches. This is important to avoid permanent knee stiffness in these patient who will depend on full function of adjacent joints for full function. The cast is discontinued when there is radiographic evidence of union between the femoral head and the ilium. This usually takes 12 weeks.

REFERENCES

1. Sponseller PD, McBeath AA, Perrich M. Hip arthrodesis in young patients: a long-term follow-up study. J Bone Joint Surg 1984;66A:853.
2. Callaghan JJ, Brand RA, Pedersen DR. Hip arthrodesis: a long-term follow-up. J Bone Joint Surg 1984;67A:1328.
3. Brewster RC, Coventry MB, Johnson EW Jr. Conversion of the arthrodesed hip to a total hip arthroplasty. J Bone Joint Surg 1975;57A:27.
4. Lubhan JD, Evarts CM, Feltner JB. Conversion of ankylosed hips to total hip arthroplasty. Clin Orthop 1980;153:146.
5. Thompson FR. Combined hip fusion and subtrochanteric osteotomy allowing early ambulation. J Bone Joint Surg 1956;38A:13.
6. Price CT, Lovell WW. Thompson arthrodesis of the hip in children. J Bone Joint Surg 1980;62A:1118.

2.12
In Situ Fixation of Slipped Capital Femoral Epiphysis

Since the 1950s the commonest method of treatment for slipped capital femoral epiphysis (SCFE) has been in situ fixation with threaded pins of one type or another. The treatment of SCFE has recently undergone several changes as a result of that experience.[1] Chondrolysis may be related to persistent pin penetration of the joint, which goes unrecognized on the radiographs; avascular necrosis may be caused by disruption of the lateral epiphyseal arteries within the femoral head by the pins or a drill that enters the superior aspect of the femoral head. This means that the surgeon must know where the tip of the fixation device is within the femoral head. It thus becomes apparent that in situ fixation of a SCFE is a radiographic technique, because no incision, no matter the placement or size, can show the surgeon where the tip of the fixation device is within the femoral head.

Figure 2–60. The development of strong cannulated screws has allowed significant improvement in both the safety and ease of in situ fixation for SCFE. Because the strength of one screw seems sufficient for the treatment of a chronic SCFE and two screws for an acute SCFE, there is little need for any fixation device to be placed outside of the central axis of the femoral head. In addition, the cannulated aspect allows the screws to be inserted percutaneously, thus decreasing the postoperative morbidity.

Figure 2–61. The patient is placed on a fracture table with the image intensifier placed between the legs. It is important to verify that the subchondral bone of the femoral head as well as the physeal plate can be visualized in both the anteroposterior and lateral plane. The operation should not begin until this is achieved.

The most difficult problem is the lateral view. In many cases this is due to the angle of the x-ray beam relative to the femoral head. This is not solved by abducting or adducting the leg because the femoral head and neck will remain in almost the same position. Rather both the base of the image intensifier and its angle to the hip will have to be varied. In cases of obese patients and older, less powerful image intensifiers, there may not be adequate power to obtain a good image. In such cases the image intensifier is positioned for the anteroposterior view on the opposite side of the patient, and a portable radiographic machine is positioned between the legs for lateral radiographs taken on conventional radiographic film.

In the illustration the x-ray tube is positioned above the table, which is necessary because of the difficulty in positioning the machine for the lateral view. It would reduce the radiation scatter to the operating personnel to have this part of the machine below the table on the anteroposterior view and pointing away from the operating personnel on the lateral view.

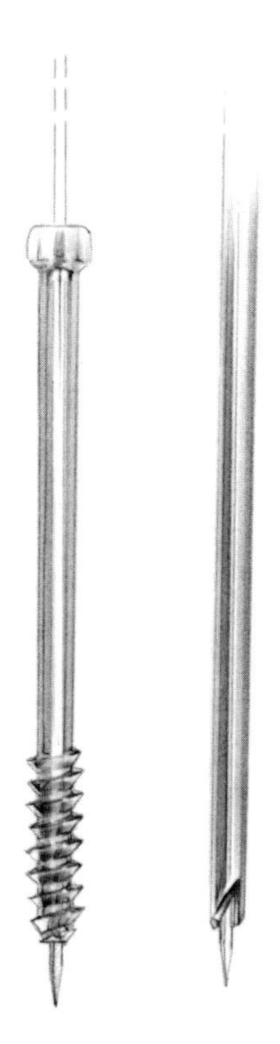

Figure 2–60

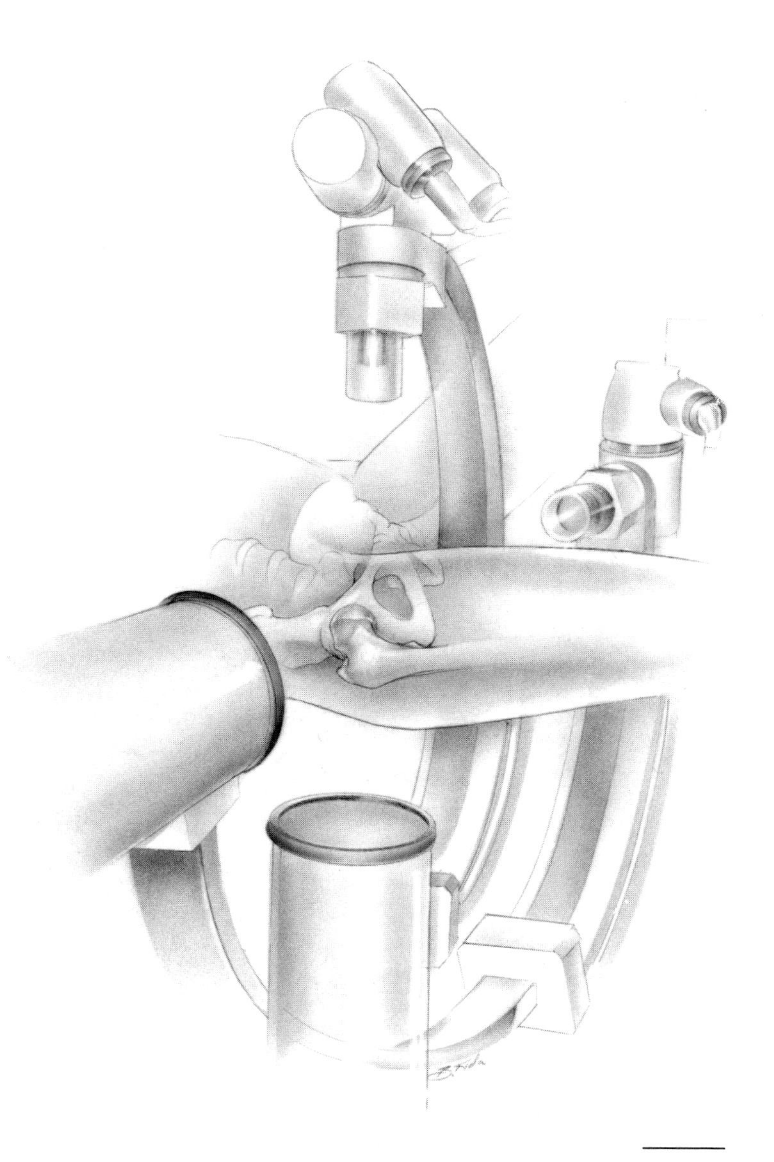

Figure 2–61

Figure 2–62. The next step is to pass a guide wire percutaneously down to the femoral neck. First, the exact location and angle of the femoral neck can be identified by lying a second guide wire over the femoral neck on the anterior thigh under radiographic control. This permits more accurate placement of the percutaneous guide wire. At this point the percutaneous guide wire shows the correct placement of the screw on the anteroposterior view. The surgeon, however, will still not know if it is aimed posteriorly in the correct direction to enter the midpoint of the femoral head. This determination is best left to the next step because this guide wire is not fixed in the bone and will tend to move. After a little experience and understanding the anatomy of a slipped capital femoral epiphysis, it becomes surprisingly easy to judge this posterior inclination of the percutaneous guide pin and the screw correctly.

Figure 2–63. With the percutaneous guide wire in the correct position over the femoral neck, and in what the surgeon estimates to be the correct degree of posterior tilt to enter the center of the femoral head, the cannula with the guide pin is inserted through a stab wound near the percutaneous guide wire. This is pushed down to the bone and its position checked on the image intensifier to be sure it is in the desired position. This is then drilled into the femoral neck.

This should proceed easily until either cortical bone or the epiphyseal plate is encountered. At this point the drill will be more difficult to advance and should be stopped. The position can again be confirmed on the anteroposterior view and should be in the center of the femoral neck (***Figure 2–63A***). The C arm is then moved to the lateral position and the direction of the cannula visualized on the lateral view.

If it is not heading for the center of the femoral head on this view (***Figure 2–63B***), a second cannula and guide wire assembly is inserted using the one that is already inserted as a guide (***Figure 2–63C***). It should be in the same plane relative to varus and valgus, but either its starting point on the femoral neck, its angle, or both should be altered so that it enters the center of the femoral head and is perpendicular to the physeal plate. If a second cannula is necessary its position should again be verified on the anteroposterior image, because if it is inserted in a few degrees more of valgus it could enter the superior aspect of the femoral head. It is important that no bending stress be placed on this assembly in an effort to change its direction because this will make it difficult to withdraw the cannula and leave the guide wire in place.

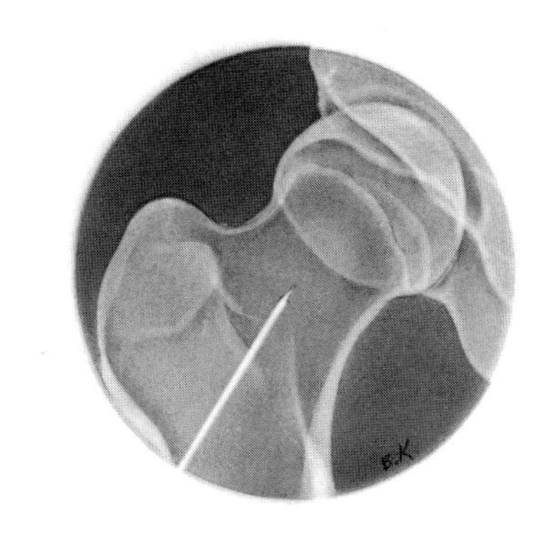

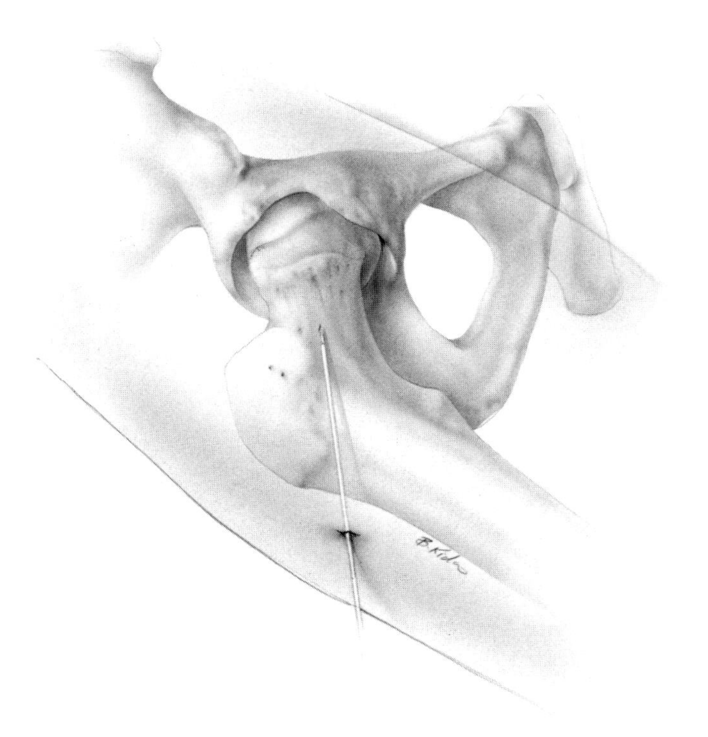

Figure 2–62

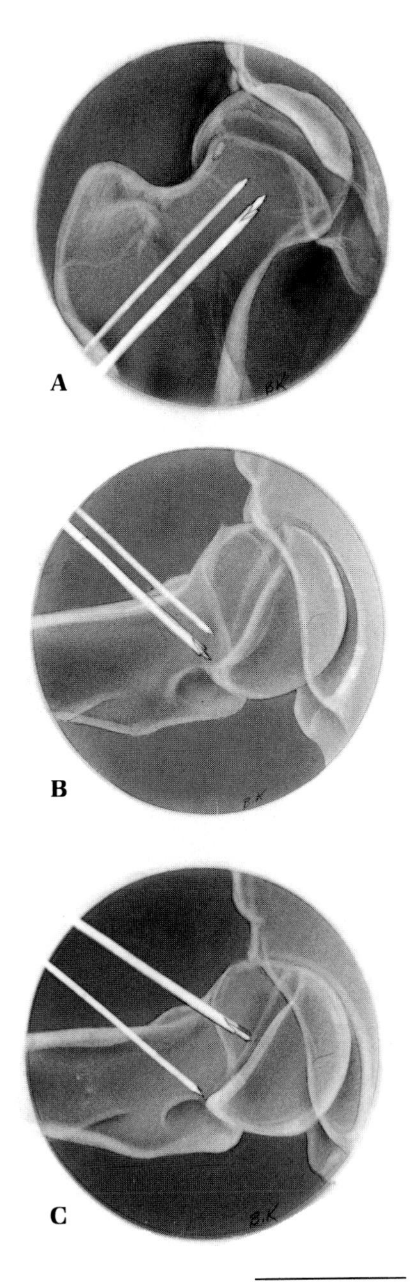

Figure 2–63

Figure 2–64. When the proper placement and direction of the cannula and guide assembly is achieved, it can be drilled across the physeal plate. This should be monitored on the lateral view. The anteroposterior view will not accurately portray the true placement of the screw in relation to the joint surface because it is passing posteriorly and is not perpendicular to the plane of the radiograph. When the tip of the guide wire within the cannula is in the desired location (the center of the femoral head and at least 5 mm from the subchondral bone), the cannula is removed. Care should be used here so as not to withdraw the guide pin at the same time. This can happen if the cannula and guide wire assembly was bent during insertion.

Figure 2–65. When the cannula is withdrawn, a second guide wire (of equal length to the one that is in the bone) is inserted alongside the first guide wire down to the bone. The difference between the two is the length of the screw.

Figure 2–66. The correct length screw is then inserted over the guide wire and its position monitored on the lateral view. Although the author has not had a single case of screw penetration using the method of insertion described, it is comforting to check for screw penetration before leaving the operating room. The leg is removed from traction and put through a range of motion to confirm under the image intensifier as recommended by Moesley. It is important to recognize that this method of seeking screw penetration has a significant limitation. Unless the screw can be aligned perpendicular to the plane of the x-ray beam, it will not be 100% accurate. Because of the lack of internal rotation in the hip with a slipped capital femoral epiphysis, this may be difficult to achieve.

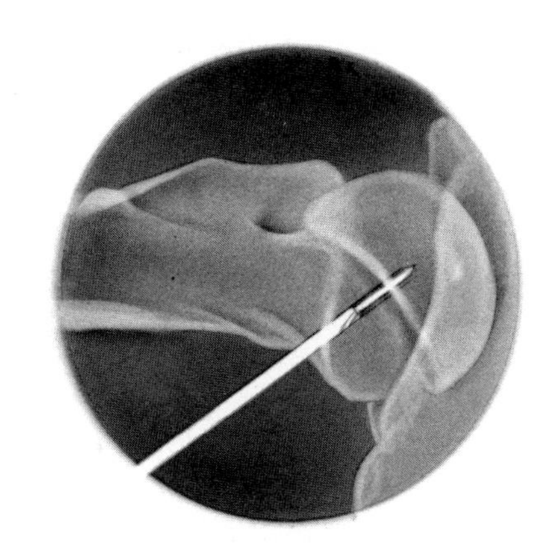

Figure 2–64

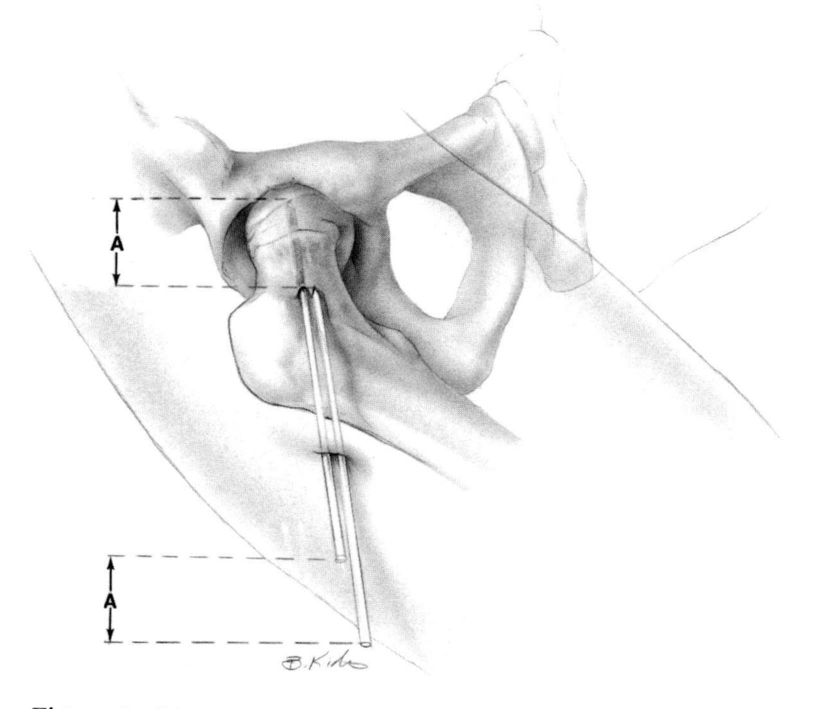

Figure 2–65

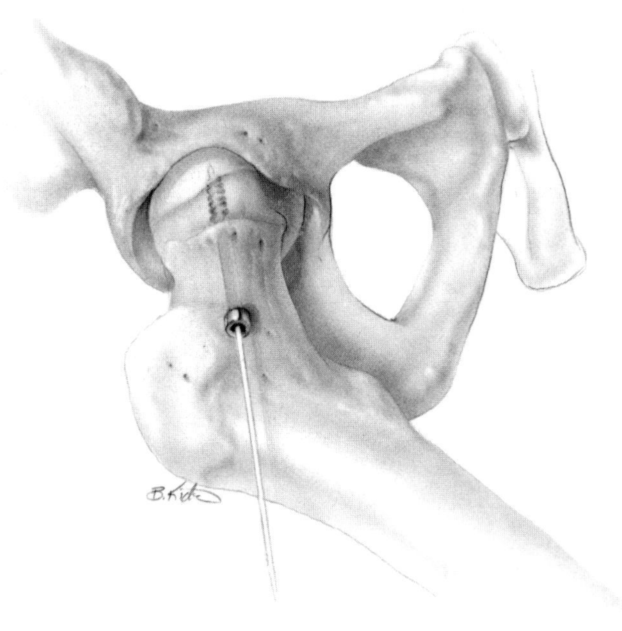

Figure 2–66

Figure 2–67. Radiographs of a 13-year-old boy whose complaint is limp and pain in the knee for 3 months (***Figures 2–67A, B***). Klein's line, drawn on the right hip, does not appear abnormal on the left hip. The frog lateral radiograph (***Figure 2–67B***), however, demonstrates slight irregularity and widening of the physis, and no overlap of the epiphysis on the metaphysis typical in a mild chronic slipped capital femoral epiphysis. An anteroposterior and lateral radiograph were obtained 1 day following percutaneous in situ fixation with a single screw (***Figures 2–67C, D***). Notice on the true lateral radiograph (***Figure 2–67D***) how far posterior the femoral head is actually displaced. The screw is almost perfectly located in the central axis of the femoral head. On the anteroposterior radiograph (***Figure 2–67C***) the screw is slightly below the central axis of the femoral head. Notice the position on the anterior femoral neck where the screw must start to remain in the central axis of the displaced femoral head.

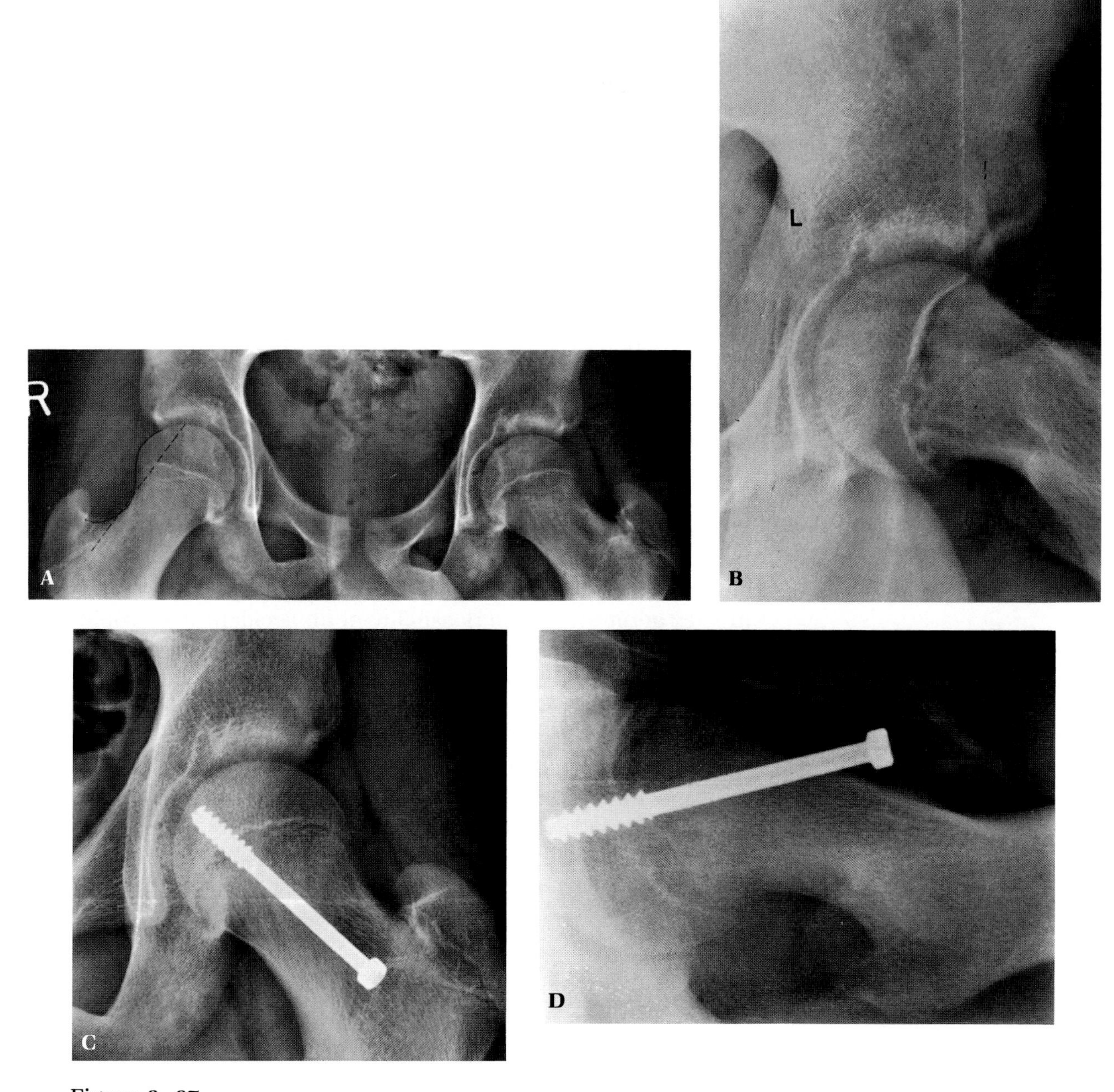

Figure 2–67

POSTOPERATIVE CARE

Patients are started on a three-point partial weight-bearing crutch gait as soon as their recovery from anesthesia permits. This is usually the next morning, although some patients may be discharged the day of surgery. Crutches are discontinued as soon as the patient can walk comfortably. This is usually 1 week in cases of chronic slip. In those with a severe acute slip that is reduced, it may be best to continue crutches for a longer time. In such cases the author recommends 6 weeks, but without discomfort compliance is difficult to gain.

The patients are given instructions about the same symptoms, particularly anterior thigh or knee pain, developing in the opposite hip, and the need for prompt return. They are seen routinely every 3 months and progress monitored with an examination for range of motion and synovitis, and anteroposterior radiographs.

When radiographs demonstrate physeal plate closure the screw can be removed. The reasons for screw removal are not absolute, and the morbidity can be considerable if the device used for fixation is not designed with removal in mind. Reasons given for removal are the possible need for hip reconstruction in later adult life or the possibility of an accident that would cause fracture of the femoral neck and screw fracture. The cannulated screw used by the author has presented no difficulty in removal. It is achieved as an outpatient under general anesthesia. A guide wire is passed down the center of the screw under radiographic control and the screwdriver inserted over the wire into the screw head. The screws back out easily. Occasionally, the head of the screw will be covered by bone, and this can be cleared with a small periosteal elevator, which is passed percutaneously to the screw.

REFERENCE

1. Morrissy RT. Slipped capital femoral epiphysis. In: Morrissy RT, ed. Lovell and Winter's pediatric orthopaedics, 3rd ed. Philadelphia: JB Lippincott, 1989:892–896.

2.13 Open Epiphysiodesis of Slipped Capital Femoral Epiphysis

The original procedure of open bone graft epiphysiodesis for the treatment of slipped capital femoral epiphysis was originally described by Ferguson and Howorth.[1] Subsequent experience with this procedure has been limited to the hands of a few, but is characterized by a striking absence of the complications of avascular necrosis and chondrolysis.[2–4] The possible reasons for this low complication rate in contrast to the historical rate of complications for in situ pin fixation have been discussed.[5]

The philosophy underlying this procedure is that closure of the growth plate is the best way to prevent further slipping. This is accomplished by open reaming and curettement of the growth plate and femoral head followed by the insertion of corticocancellous bone grafts.

Figure 2–68. The capsule of the hip joint and the outer table of the ilium are exposed as for a Salter osteotomy or anterior open reduction of the hip. It is not necessary to expose the inner table of the ilium but is important to obtain good exposure of the hip capsule. The anterior capsule will be opened with an incision parallel to and 1 cm from the acetabular margin. The second incision extends at right angles from this incision over the anterior femoral neck.

Figure 2–69. The hip joint is now exposed. Inspection will show the articular surface of the femoral head to be displaced posteriorly, the amount of displacement depending on the severity of the slip. The capsule may be slightly adherent to the anterior femoral neck as a result of the healing callus and inflammation. An adequate amount of the femoral neck and the articular surface of the femoral head should be visualized by the surgeon so that he or she is properly oriented to the anatomy. This will be important to the proper performance of the operation.

Next the periosteum over the anterior neck is incised in a cruciate fashion and is elevated exposing the bone. This should be placed in a location that will allow the hollow mill drill to cross perpendicular to the epiphyseal plate.

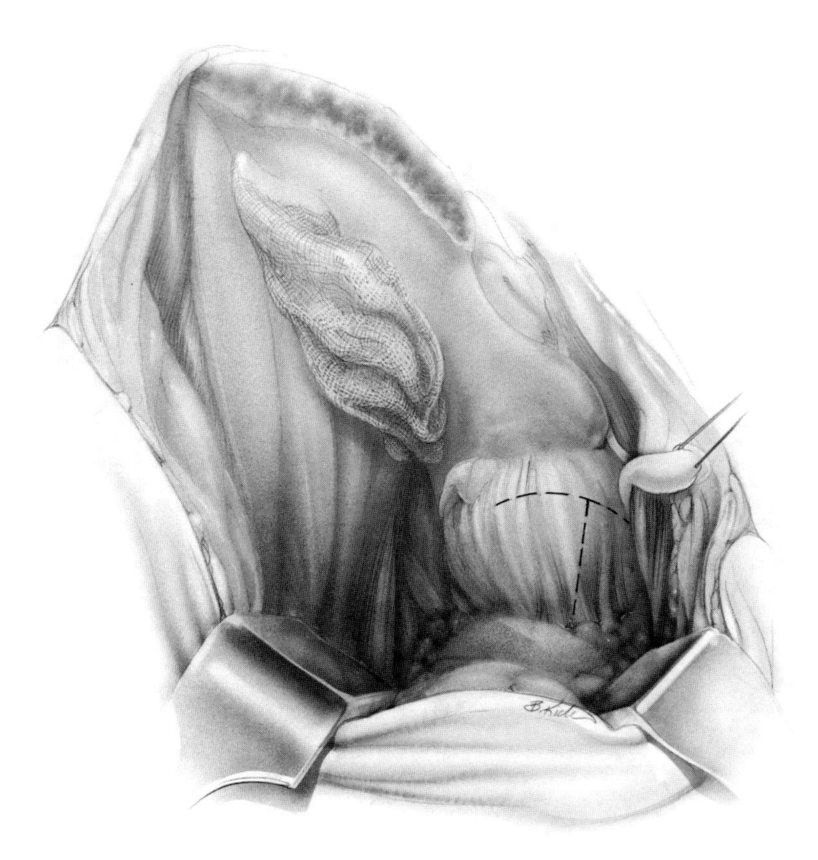

Figure 2–68

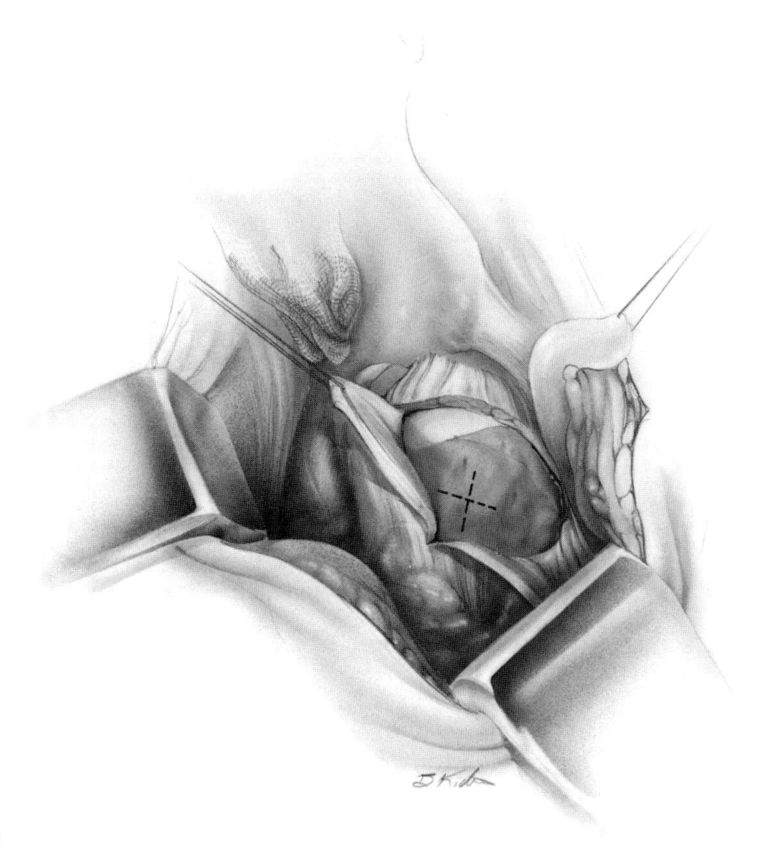

Figure 2–69

Figure 2–70. A guide wire is inserted, and its proper placement in the center of the femoral head and at a safe distance from the articular surface is verified by an anteroposterior and frog lateral view on the image intensifier. When the proper direction is verified the hollow mill is drilled through the anterior cortex of the femoral neck, across the physeal plate, and into the femoral head.

Figure 2–71. The hole in the cortex can be enlarged with a curette, which can also be used to remove additional physeal plate (***Figure 2–71A***). The hollow mill is then angled in multiple directions (***Figures 2–71B, C***) to enlarge the hole. This is important to allow the placement of grafts of sufficient strength to give some stability temporarily to the epiphysis.

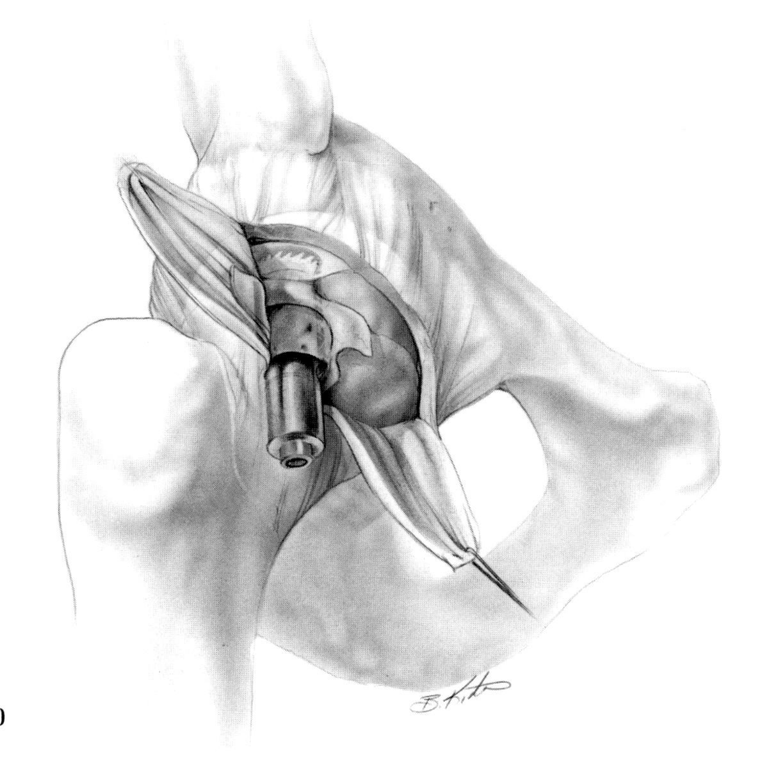

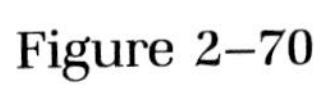

Figure 2–70

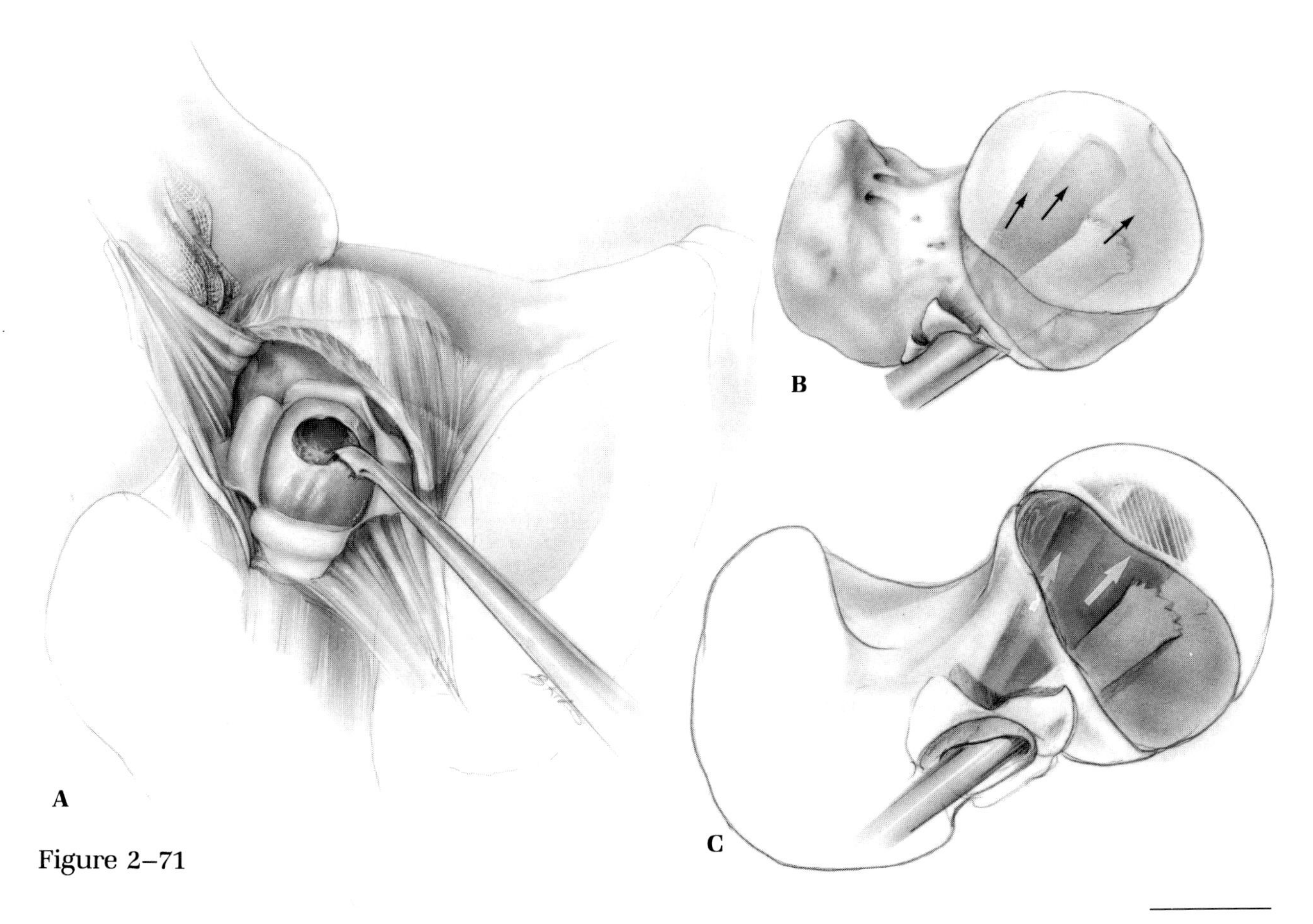

Figure 2–71

Figure 2–72. Three or four corticocancellous strips of bone are removed from the outer table of the ilium. This is preferable to several small matchstick-sized pieces because the larger grafts will possess more strength. These grafts are then driven into the hole and their location verified. The periosteum, capsule, and the wound are closed.

POSTOPERATIVE CARE

A drain may be used at the discretion of the surgeon, but there should be no dead space and little bleeding at the conclusion of the procedure. Those series reporting no further slipping after grafting used a spica cast for immobilization until healing was complete in 8 to 12 weeks. More recently there have been reports of not using a cast but only crutch protection with an incidence of further slipping in a few patients.[6]

REFERENCES

1. Ferguson A, Howorth B. Slipping of the upper femoral epiphysis. JAMA 1931;97:1867.
2. Heyman C, Herndon C. Epiphysiodesis for early slipping of the femoral epiphysis. J Bone Joint Surg 1954;36A:539.
3. Heyman C, Herndon C, Strong J. Slipped femoral epiphysis with severe displacement: a conservative operative treatment. J Bone Joint Surg 1957;39A:293.
4. Melby A, Hoyt W, Weiner D. Treatment of chronic slipped capital femoral epiphysis by bone graft epiphysiodesis. J Bone Joint Surg 1980;62A:119.
5. Morrissy RT. Slipped capital femoral epiphysis. In: Morrissy RT, ed. Lovell and Winter's pediatric orthopaedics, 3rd ed. Philadelphia: JB Lippincott, 1989:896.
6. Weiner DS, Weiner S, Melby A, Hoyte WA Jr. A 30-year experience with bone graft epiphysiodesis in the treatment of slipped capital femoral epiphysis. J Pediatr Orthop 1984;4:145.

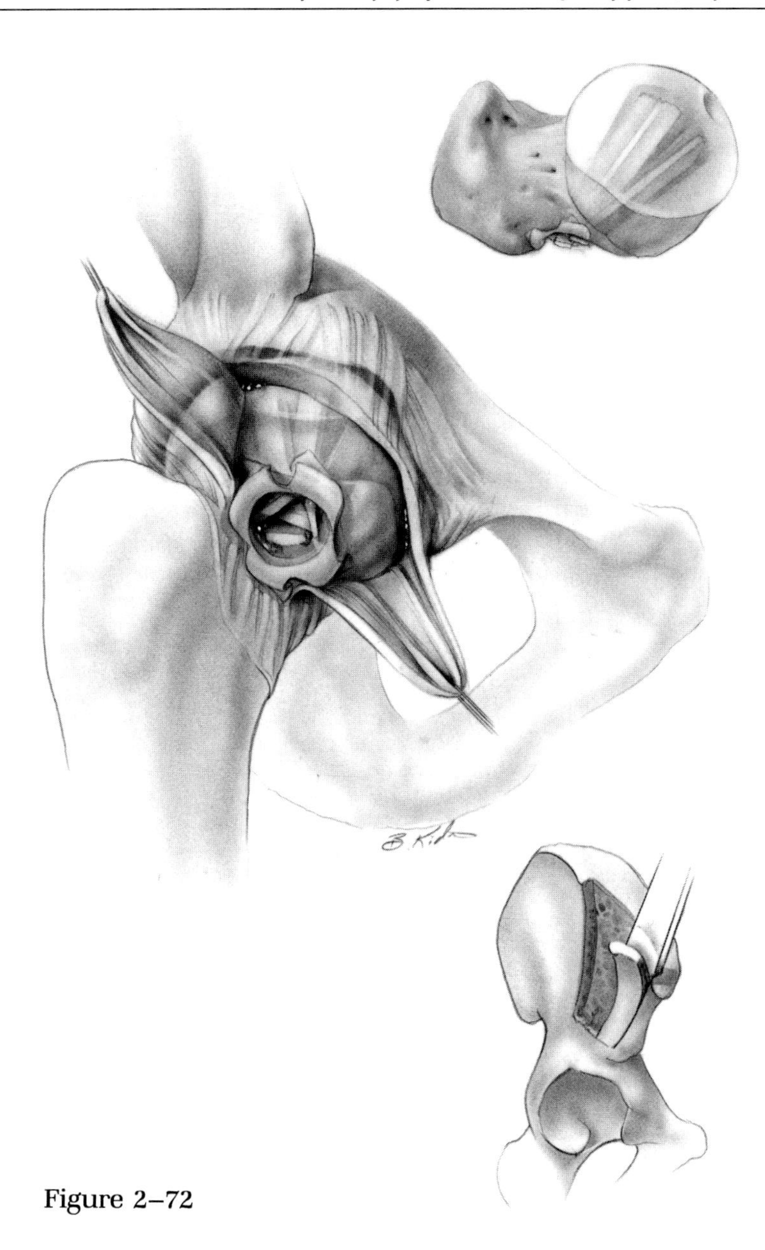

Figure 2–72

2.14 Adductor and Iliopsoas Release

Adductor myotomy is one of the oldest and today most commonly performed operations in children with spastic cerebral palsy. Here the operation is described in conjunction with iliopsoas tenotomy because the two procedures are often indicated in the same patient and can be performed through the same incision. The indications for these procedures are well discussed by Rang.[1] It is important to recognize that simply because these operations are described together does not mean that they all need to be performed in every patient. For many ambulatory children with spastic diplegia, release of the adductor longus and gracilis muscles is all that will be necessary, whereas in a dependent sitter all of the components described including iliopsoas tenotomy and proximal hamstring release may be necessary.[2]

Although anterior branch obturator neurectomy was a routine part of this procedure in the past, its value is in question and it is usually not considered necessary today. If the adductor brevis muscle is not to be sectioned, anterior branch obturator neurectomy should not be done because it will denervate this muscle. If all of the muscles supplied by this nerve are cut and retract sufficiently, what is the value in cutting the nerve? The posterior branch of the obturator nerve should not be cut since it will denervate the adductor magnus, removing all of the adductors and resulting in unopposed abduction.

Figure 2–73. The patient is draped so that the perineum is isolated and both legs are free. The incision may be either longitudinal over the tight tendinous portion of the adductor longus muscle, or as illustrated transverse, centered over the adductor longus tendon about one finger breadth distal to the groin crease. This transverse incision is opened down to the deep fascia.

Figure 2–74. A sponge is placed over the index finger, and this is then pulled proximal and distal along the adductor longus tendon, exposing the deep fascia overlying it. This fascia is in turn opened longitudinally, exposing the adductor longus muscle and tendon. This will permit the deep fascia to be closed in a direction 90 degrees to the superficial fascia and skin providing for a tighter wound closure.

Figure 2–75. The tendon of the adductor longus is easily isolated in the proximal part of the wound and can be cut close to its attachment to the pelvis. If the surgeon wishes to perform an anterior branch obturator neurectomy, this common trunk can be found deep to the adductor longus between the pectineus muscle superiorly and the adductor brevis muscle inferiorly.

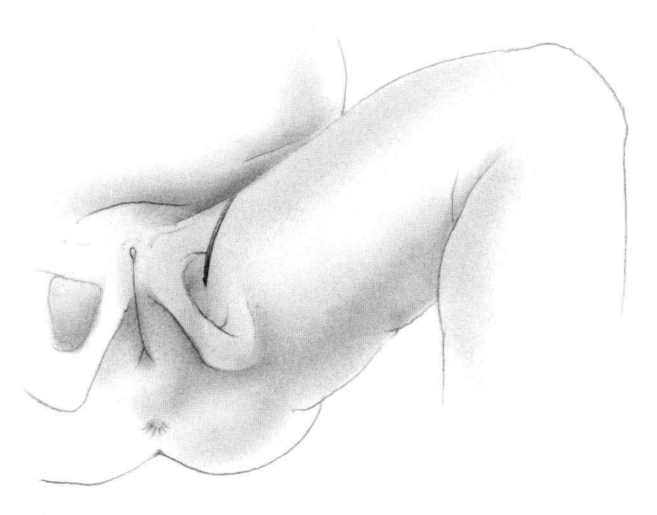

Figure 2–73

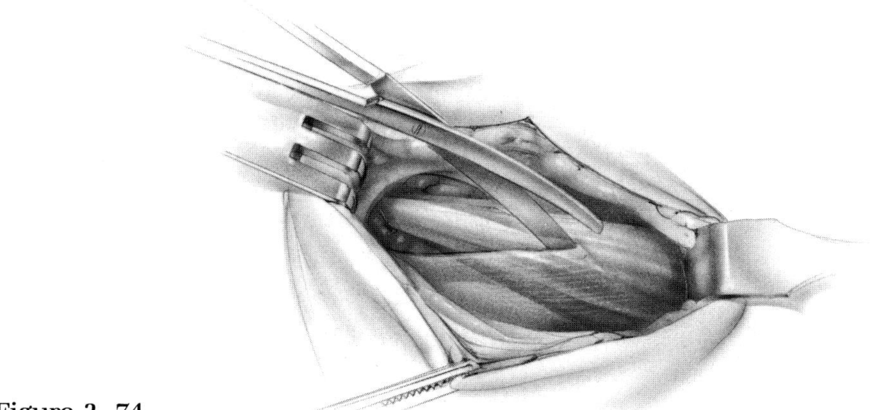

Figure 2–74

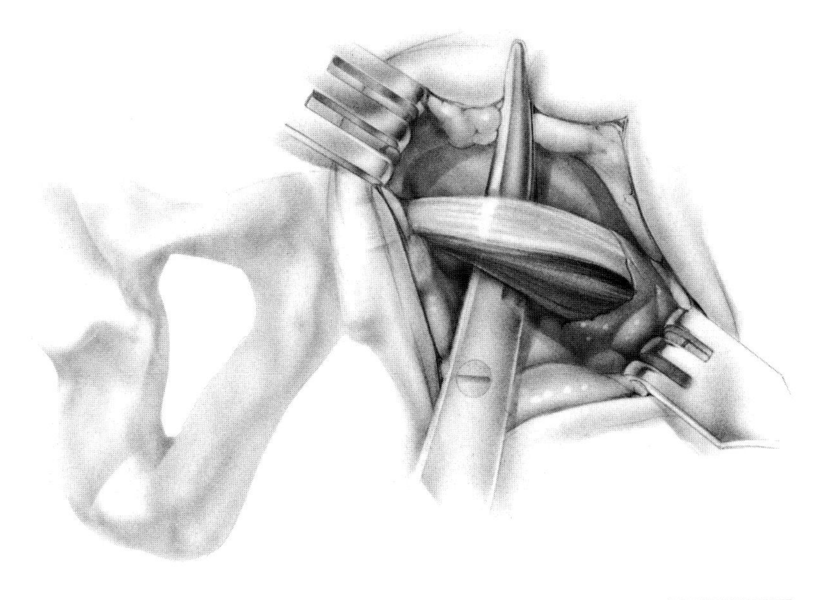

Figure 2–75

Figure 2–76. Lying below the adductor longus tendon is the adductor brevis. A retractor pulling the pectineus superiorly helps in visualizing the full extent of this large muscle. Some branches of the anterior obturator nerve can usually be seen coursing over the upper or side of this muscle. If desired each of these branches to the adductor longus, adductor brevis, and gracilis muscles can be identified by stimulating them and then dividing them. It is easiest at this point to leave the adductor brevis muscle and first divide the gracilis muscle (*dotted line*).

The gracilis muscle is, as its name implies, a long thin muscle that is found medial to the adductor brevis muscle. It is easily isolated by dissecting posteriorly between it and the deep crural fascia by spreading with a scissors. The inner aspect of the muscle is now identified and separated from the adductor brevis muscle in the same manner. Abducting the leg and straightening the knee helps to both identify the entire extent of this muscle and to cut it. Two long retractors are placed, one on either side of the muscle, and it is then divided close to its attachment to the pelvis.

Figure 2–77. It is now relatively easy to divide the adductor brevis if this is the operative plan. Although many surgeons make a fetish of passing an instrument behind this muscle before beginning to divide it, this can be difficult and cause unnecessary trauma if the muscle is large. Much of this muscle can first be divided with the cautery current leaving a much smaller posterior part that is easier to isolate and then divide. Behind this muscle lies the adductor magnus muscle. It will be covered by a layer of fascia, beneath which the posterior branch of the obturator nerve that supplies this muscle can be seen. It is important that this nerve not be injured or all adduction will be lost.

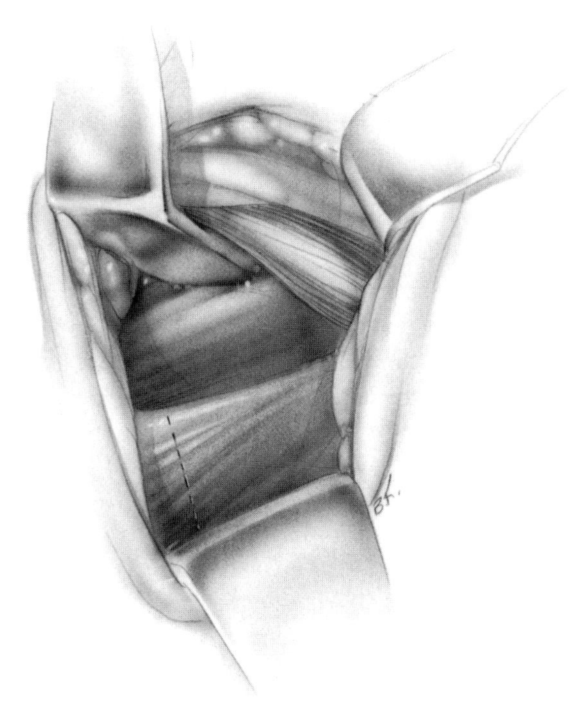

Figure 2–76

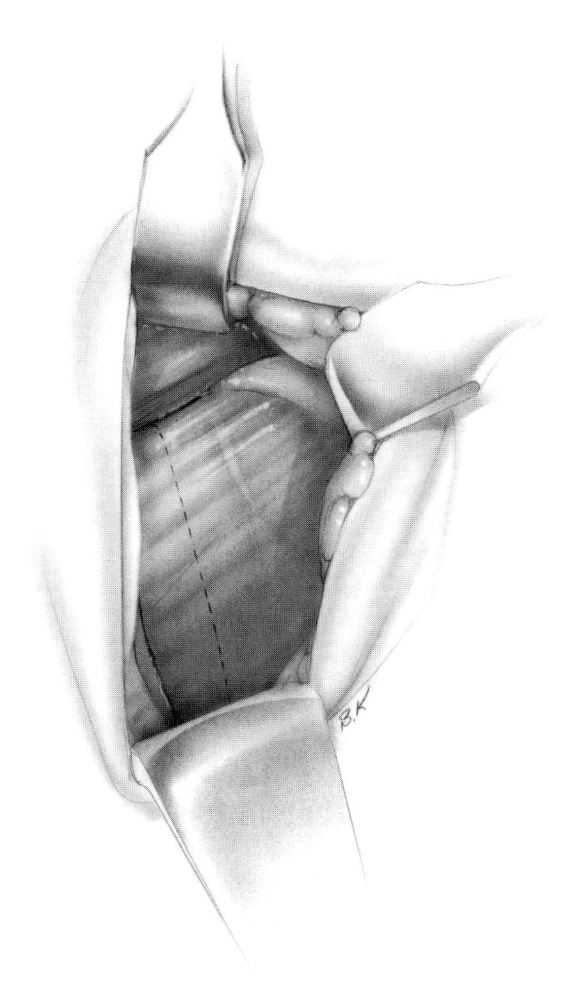

Figure 2–77

Figure 2–78. If it is desired to divide the iliopsoas tendon it can be done at this time. The surgeon should constantly consider the orientation of the pelvis, femur, and direction of the psoas tendon, because it is easy to become confused at this stage (***Figure 2–78A***). The leg should be held in about 70 degrees of flexion, 20 to 30 degrees of abduction, and slight internal rotation to make the exposure easier.

A long right-angled retractor is placed under the pectineus muscle, which is retracted superiorly (***Figure 2–78A***) while blunt dissection with the index finger identifies the lesser trochanter. A common error here is to go too far proximal and mistake the bulge of the inferior portion of the femoral head for the lesser trochanter. When the lesser trochanter is identified it should also be possible to palpate the psoas tendon coming off of the lesser trochanter if the surgeon is properly oriented.

To expose the tendon it will be necessary to open the sheath that surrounds it by sharp dissection with a knife or scissors. This will usually provide a glimpse of the tendon, which can be pulled into better view with a right-angled clamp (***Figures 2–78B, C***). It can then be sharply divided with a knife.

Note the cut ends of the adductor longus, adductor brevis, and gracilis (***Figure 2–78A***). The large posterior muscle remaining intact is the adductor magnus. Just posterior to this are the proximal insertions of the hamstrings.

The wound should be inspected for bleeding and any that is found controlled. It is much easier, however, to accomplish hemostasis at each step. It is important to minimize hematoma formation in the dead space that is inevitable. The deep fascia is closed with a running suture, and the deep crural fascia is closed with an interrupted suture. This will give a tight wound closure without puckering of the skin. This skin can be closed with a running subcuticular suture and the dressing applied.

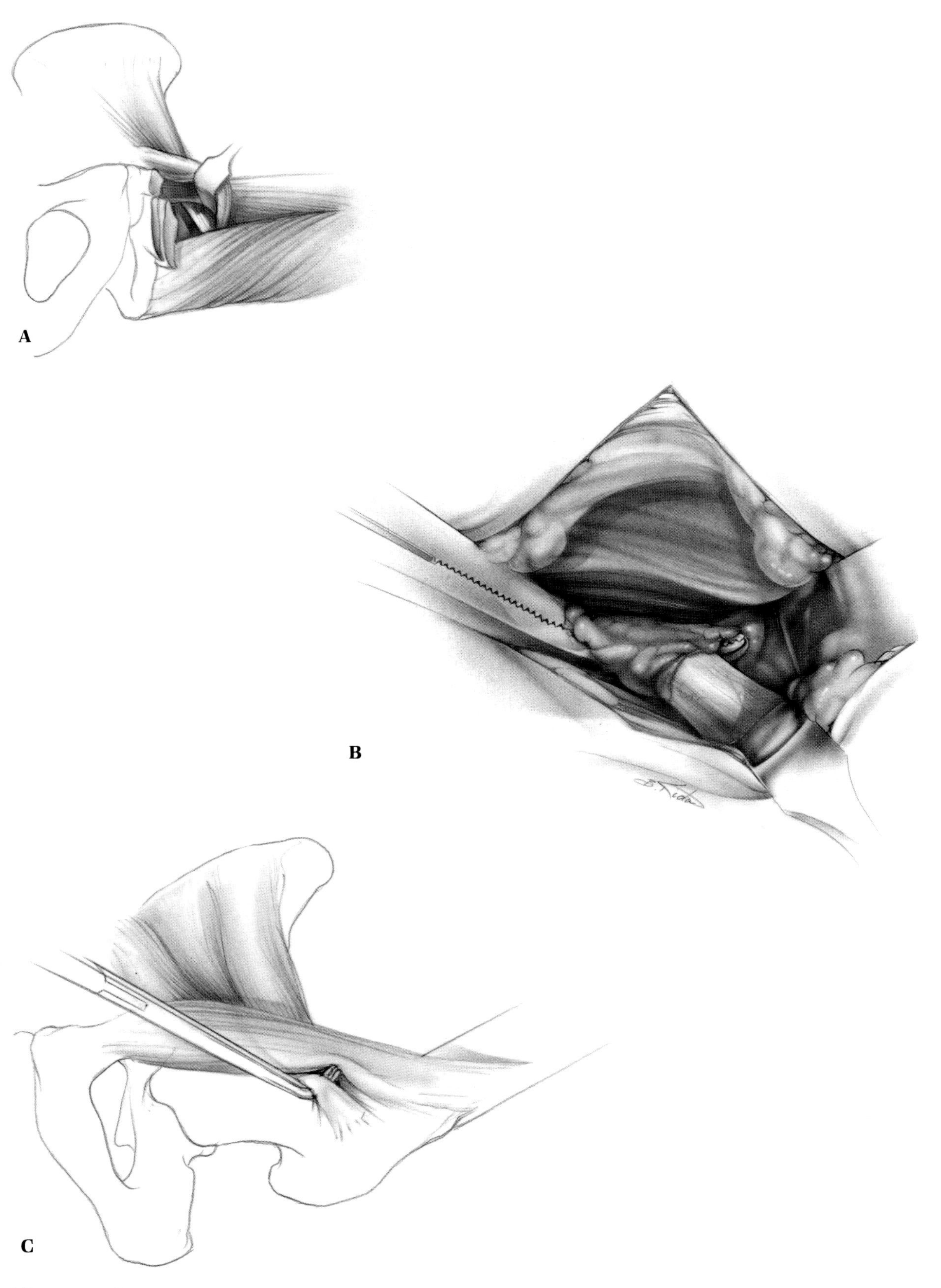

Figure 2–78

POSTOPERATIVE CARE

Whether a spica cast or double-long leg casts with an abduction bar is used is a matter of preference among surgeons. A spica cast is believed by some to provide more rigid immobilization and better correction of the hip flexion contractures and may give greater comfort immediately postoperatively. The author, however, thinks that the extra difficulties in care do not warrant a spica cast. In addition, it is difficult to eliminate the hip flexion in a spica cast because it is almost impossible to control the lumbar lordosis. It is probable that the hip flexion can be dealt with more effectively by prone positioning after the acute pain has subsided. In addition, these patients seem to have less stiffness after cast immobilization when they are permitted some motion in the long leg casts.

The amount of abduction does not have to be excessive, and combined abduction of 70 degrees is probably sufficient. More abduction only increases the postoperative pain. Casts are maintained in place for 4 to 6 weeks. After removal of the casts a short course of physical therapy is definitely beneficial to speed the patient's return to his or her preoperative activity level.

In the first 24 to 36 hours after surgery patients will experience episodes of severe spasm and pain as they jerk awake from sleep. This has been impossible to eliminate completely with narcotics or other medication. The parents should be forewarned of this and the fact that it will pass. It is possible that continuous epidural anesthesia will alleviate this, but its effectiveness and safety has not yet been proved.

REFERENCES

1. Rang M. Cerebral palsy. In: Morrissy RT, ed. Lovell and Winter's pediatric orthopaedics, 3rd ed. Philadelphia: JB Lippincott, 1989:490.
2. Bleck E. Orthopaedic management in cerebral palsy. Philadelphia: JB Lippincott, 1978:289.

2.15
Adductor Transfer

Transfer of the hip adductor origins posterior to the ischium was first reported by Stephenson and Donovan in 1969.[1] The design of the operation resulted from their belief that the function of this group of adductor muscles (adductor longus, adductor brevis, and gracilis) was hip flexion, internal rotation, and adduction, all of which conspired to create the troublesome problems seen in the hip in spastic cerebral palsy, and that their transfer would eliminate them as a source of the trouble. In the 31 patients presented they noted no bad effects and thought that gait was improved in many. Root and Spero have also commented on the beneficial effect on gait.[2] Unfortunately they did not use quantitative assessment of preoperative and postoperative gait; presumably the adductor brevis was released along with the adductor longus and the gracilis muscles.

Because it is recognized that some degree of adduction is necessary for efficiency in gait the real comparison of the effect on gait should be between transfer of the adductor origins and release of the adductor longus and gracilis muscles only, leaving the brevis intact.[3] Studies that have compared adductor release with transfer have not shown to be any different in preventing or correcting subluxation of the hip when radiographic criteria are used to show the effectiveness of these procedures.[4,5]

The approach to the adductors is the same as described for adductor myotomy with the following exceptions: The origins of the muscles must be isolated at their attachment to the bone, and the area of the ischium posterior to the gracilis muscle must be exposed.

Figure 2–79. The origin of the adductor longus muscle is first separated from its attachment using the cautery current. The anterior branch of the obturator nerve is next identified between the adductor brevis and pectineus muscle so that it can be protected. Next the entire origin of the adductor brevis is removed from the bone. Here it is necessary to cut the muscle directly off of the bone to preserve some strong tissue that will hold a suture.

Figure 2–80. The gracilis is now easy to identify and can be cut close to the bone with the cautery current preserving its tendinous origin. Blunt finger dissection will expose the ischium posteriorly, just lateral to the insertion of the adductor magnus muscle.

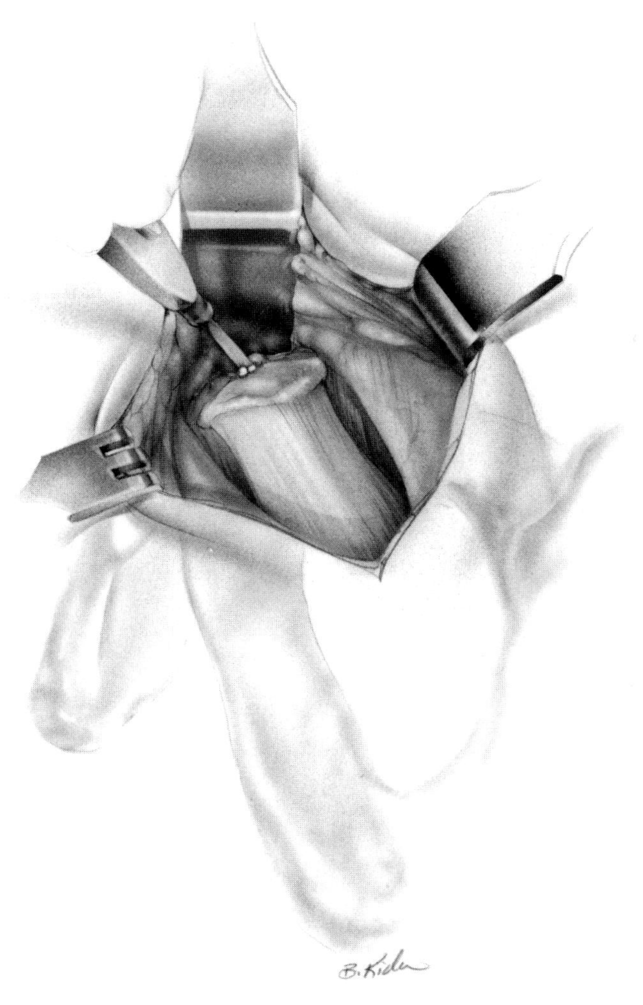

Figure 2–79

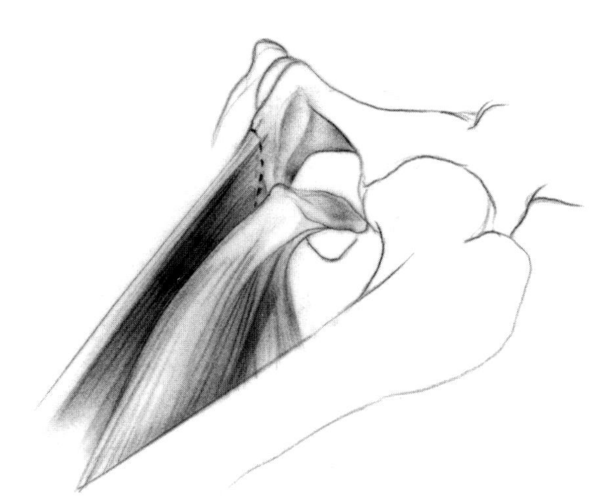

Figure 2–80

Figure 2–81. The three muscles, the adductor longus, the adductor brevis, and the gracilis, are all pulled together by two strong absorbable sutures, which are then passed through the periosteum of the ischium and tied. The wound is then closed as in adductor myotomy.

POSTOPERATIVE CARE

The patient is held in a double spica cast for 6 weeks. Following this procedure the amount of abduction will be less than for adductor release to avoid tension on the repair; 25 degrees of abduction in each hip is sufficient.

REFERENCES

1. Stephenson CT, Donovan MM. Transfer of hip adductor origins to the ischium in spastic cerebral palsy. J Bone Joint Surg 1969;51A:1040.
2. Root L, Spero CR. Hip adductor transfer compared with adductor tenotomy in cerebral palsy. J Bone Joint Surg 1981;63A:767.
3. Bleck EE. Orthopaedic management in cerebral palsy. Philadelphia: JB Lippincott, 1987:286.
4. Schultz RS, Chamberlain SE, Stevens PM. Radiographic comparison of adductor procedures in cerebral palsied hips. J Pediatr Orthop 1984;4:741.
5. Reimers J, Poulsen S. Adductor transfer versus tenotomy for stability of the hip in spastic cerebral palsy. J Pediatr Orthop 1984;4:52.

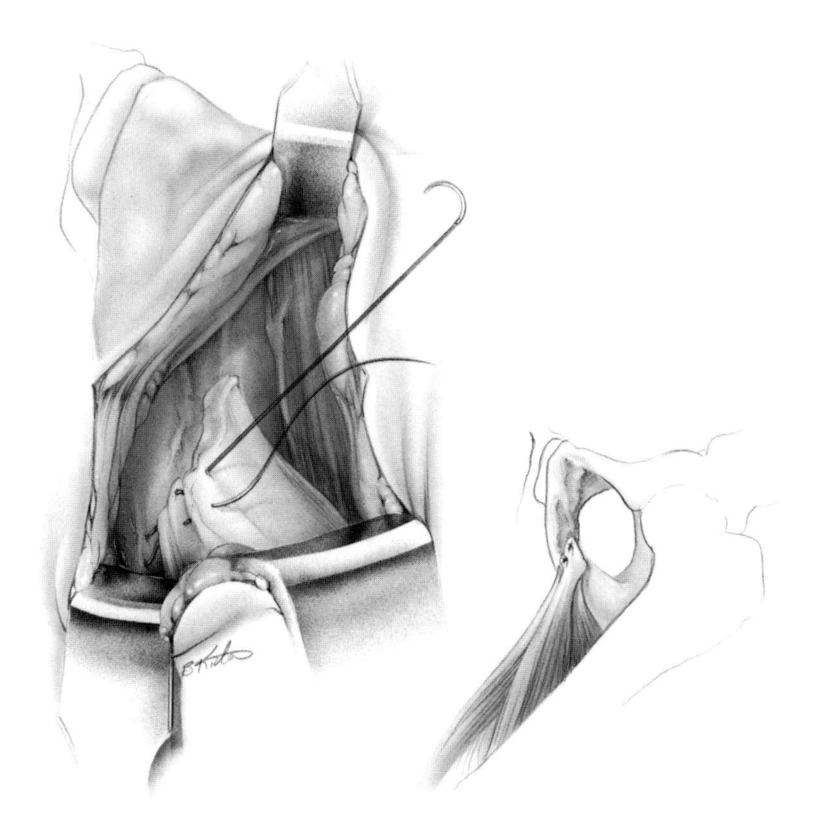

Figure 2–81

2.16
Proximal Hamstring Release

Seymour and Sharrard[1] were the first to describe a proximal release of the hamstring tendons in patients with cerebral palsy. They and subsequent authors who have found this a suitable technique describe performing this operation with the patient prone and the incision placed either lateral to the ischial tuberosity or in the natal crease.[2,3] Bell[4] reported performing this operation through an anterior approach, which has several advantages. Release of the adductor muscles and iliopsoas can be performed at the same time and straight leg raising can be tested to be certain that the preoperative goals are achieved.

Rang[5] has succinctly summarized the indications for this operation as well as the complications. The proximal lengthening is mainly indicated in the total-body–involved patient in conjunction with adductor myotomy and iliopsoas tenotomy for subluxating hip or difficulty in sitting because of tight hamstrings. It may also be the operation of choice in patients with a short stride length. Release of the proximal hamstrings may result in forward tilt of the pelvis with subsequent lordosis of the spine. This complication can be avoided by correction of any hip flexion contracture before release of the hamstrings.

Figure 2–82. The patient is placed supine with a small folded towel or sand bag under the sacrum. The legs are draped free so that they can be moved through a full range of motion. The incision used is the same as for adductor tenotomy. The author prefers a transverse incision placed 1 cm distal to the groin crease starting at the adductor longus tendon and extending posteriorly (***Figure 2–82A***). The incision does not have to be excessively long because the skin is quite mobile in this region, and the incision can be shifted anterior and posterior without unduly stretching the skin.

In the illustration the gracilis muscle is seen divided, exposing the adductor magnus muscle, which lies deep to it. The posterior border of the adductor magnus is identified, and the fascia along its posterior border is opened (***Figures 2–82B, C***). This fascial compartment should be opened sharply for an adequate distance so the surgeon does not find himself or herself in a deep dark hole.

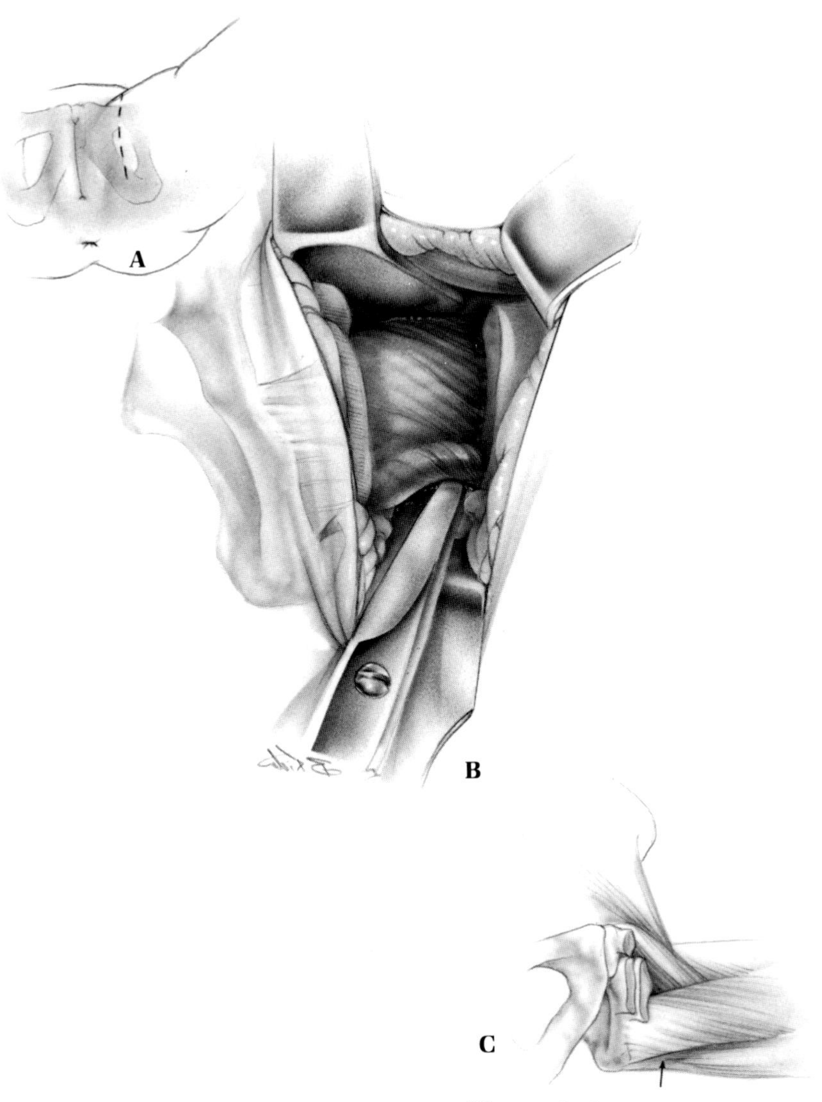

Figure 2–82

Figure 2–83. Retractors are placed to pull the adductor magnus anterior and lateral, and open the interval on its posterior surface. At this point the origins of the hamstring tendons can be palpated. Straight leg raising will demonstrate their tightness. The most medial tendon of origin is that of the semitendinosus muscle followed by the semimembranosus muscle and the biceps femoris muscle. These muscles need not be identified separately as they will seem to have a common tendinous origin from the ischial tuberosity. The sciatic nerve will lie anterior and slightly lateral to these muscles. The surgeon should be comfortable that he or she has identified the sciatic nerve by palpation. It does not become so tight as the hamstrings when straight leg raising is performed, and unlike the hamstring tendons, it extends proximal to the ischial tuberosity.

Figure 2–84. With the adductor magnus retracted anterior and lateral, a finger is inserted to palpate the sciatic nerve, elevate it, and push it laterally. An assistant then performs straight leg raising to place the tendons of origin of the hamstrings under tension, and the surgeon divides them by directing the knife posteriorly. The degree of correction and adequacy of the release can be assessed by the straight-leg–raising test.

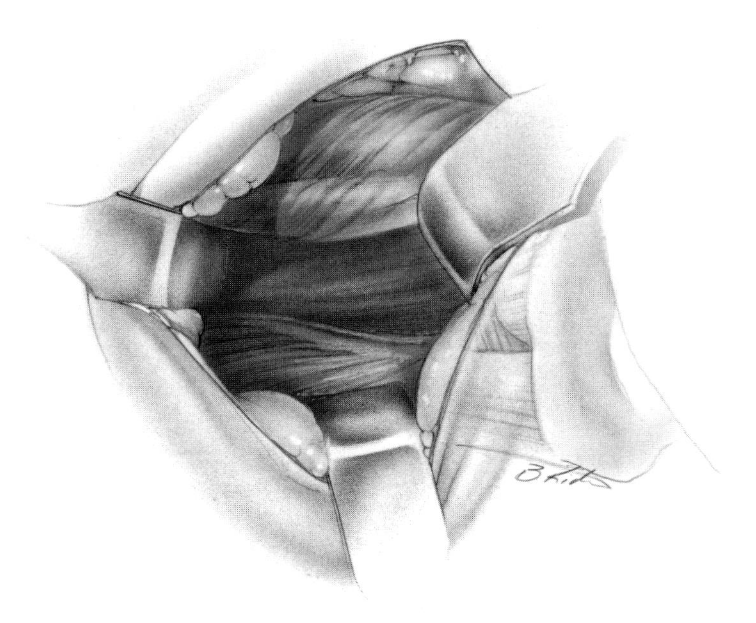

Figure 2–83

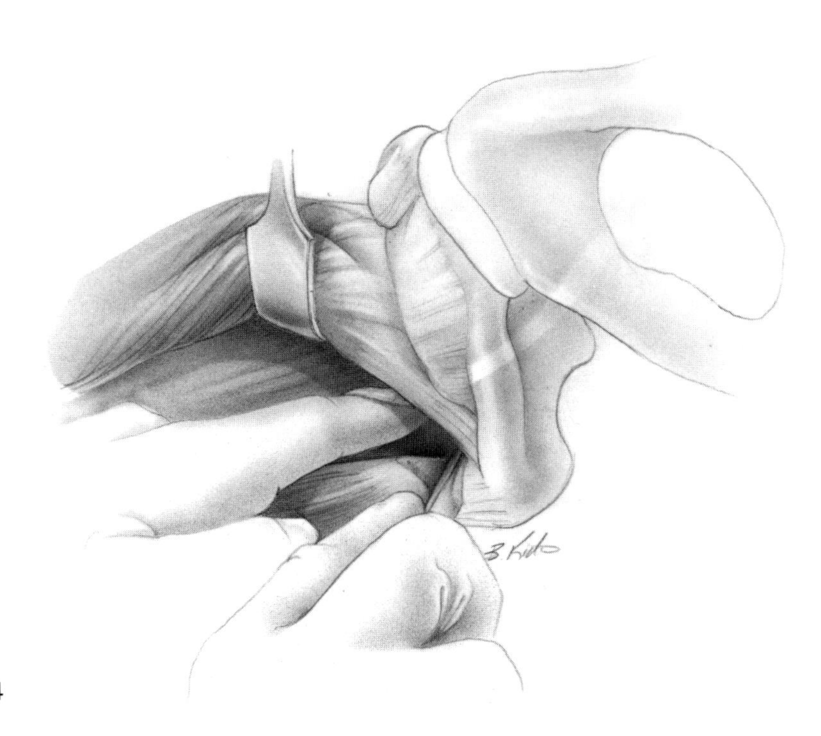

Figure 2–84

POSTOPERATIVE CARE

The legs are immobilized in long leg casts with the knees straight but not hyperextended and a bar between the legs to maintain the desired degree at abduction. Therapy should be instituted as soon as the acute pain and spasm of the surgery subside. It consists simply of having the child begin sitting. If the iliopsoas tendon has been sectioned because of associated hip flexion contractures, sitting should be alternated with prone lying. Six weeks of immobilization is sufficient, and at that time the casts are removed while the therapy is continued.

REFERENCES

1. Seymour N, Sharrard JW. Bilateral proximal release of the hamstrings in cerebral palsy. J Bone Joint Surg 1968;50B:274.
2. Reimers J. Contracture of the hamstrings in spastic cerebral palsy: a study of three methods of operative correction. J Bone Joint Surg 1974;56B:102.
3. Drummond DS, Rogala E, Templeton J, Cruess R. Proximal hamstring release for knee flexion and crouched posture in cerebral palsy. J Bone Joint Surg 1974;56A:1598.
4. Bell M. Proximal hamstring release-anterior approach. J Bone Joint Surg 1973;55B:661.
5. Rang M. Cerebral palsy. In: Morrissy RT, ed. Lovell and Winter's pediatric orthopaedics, 3rd ed. Philadelphia: JB Lippincott, 1989:492.

CHAPTER THREE
THE FEMUR

3.1
Planning an Intertrochanteric Osteotomy

MECHANICAL CONSIDERATIONS

Intertrochanteric osteotomy is probably the commonest operation performed around the child's hip. It is used in a variety of conditions: congenital dislocation of the hip, acetabular dysplasia, Perthes's disease, congenital coxa vara, post-traumatic problems, and so forth. In addition, it is a deceptively easy operation to perform. This results in little attention being given to the details of the osteotomy and often even less attention to the preoperative planning that is essential.

An intertrochanteric osteotomy may have one or several components to it. Among these are varus, valgus, extension, flexion, rotation, shortening, medialization, lateralization, and transfer of the trochanter. The indications for each of these components is found in a careful analysis of the physical examination and the preoperative radiographs. It is important for the surgeon to recognize that altering the varus inclination of the femoral neck will have profound effects on the abductor lever arm as well as the forces across the knee joint. Thus, in a particular circumstance, a varus osteotomy may require both greater trochanter transfer to restore the articulotrochanteric distance as well as medialization of the femoral shaft to maintain an equal weight distribution through the medial and lateral compartments of the knee. An analysis of all of the different permutations of intertrochanteric femoral osteotomy is beyond the scope of this discussion but has been well discussed in other publications.[1–4]

For most of the intertrochanteric osteotomies in children in which the remainder of the limb is in normal alignment, it is usually sufficient to account for the following relationships in planning:

Varus osteotomy results in genu varum and requires medial displacement of the femoral shaft to restore normal alignment to the leg.

Valgus osteotomy results in genu valgum and requires lateral displacement of the femoral shaft to restore normal alignment to the leg.

A varus intertrochanteric osteotomy in the normal hip of greater than 25 degrees may need trochanteric transfer to maintain normal abductor muscle function. If a varus intertrochanteric osteotomy is performed in a hip with an already decreased articulotrochanteric distance, a proximal physeal growth arrest as frequently seen in Perthes's disease, or in conjunction with a medial displacement pelvic osteotomy (*eg*, a Chiari), the need for transfer of the greater trochanter is greater.

A valgus intertrochanteric osteotomy will lengthen the leg and increase the pressure on the femoral head (just as a varus osteotomy will shorten the leg). Release of tight muscles or shortening of the bone should be considered.

PREOPERATIVE PLANNING

Preoperative planning in the detail described here is not usually necessary for an intertrochanteric varus osteotomy in a 2-year-old child undergoing reduction of a congenitally dislocated hip. It is essential for intertrochanteric osteotomies in the older child, however, because the mechanical effects will be greater, the potential for remodeling less, and derangements more complex.

After clinical considerations, planning begins with a preoperative anteroposterior view of the pelvis and both hips. The normal hip should be taken in internal rotation to see the normal neck shaft angle. If there are other mechanical alterations in the alignment of the limb, a full-length radiograph from the hips to the ankles with the patient standing should be obtained on a 36-in cassette. This will permit the surgeon to examine both the effect of the intertrochanteric osteotomy on the alignment of the limb as well as the need for additional osteotomies. Depending on the circumstances, additional radiographs with the limb in various positions can be obtained to determine the range of motion of the femoral head in the acetabulum as well as the best position for congruity. In some difficult cases this is best done with an arthrogram. In the author's opinion, the degree of anteversion is best determined functionally by the rotation of the hip in extension rather than by radiographic means. This is because the surgeon may be misled into correcting the radiographically determined amount of rotation, only to find that the hip will not have sufficient internal rotation postoperatively.

The actual process of planning the osteotomy has been well described by Muller.[5] This can be done on transparent paper or radiographic film. Two drawings are made on two separate sheets of paper or film.

Figure 3–1. The first drawing traces the exact outline of the femoral head and proximal shaft and the acetabulum. A dotted line (**a**) is drawn down the axis of the femoral shaft and a second solid line (**b**) is drawn perpendicular to **a** just above the lesser trochanter. This will be the line of the osteotomy.

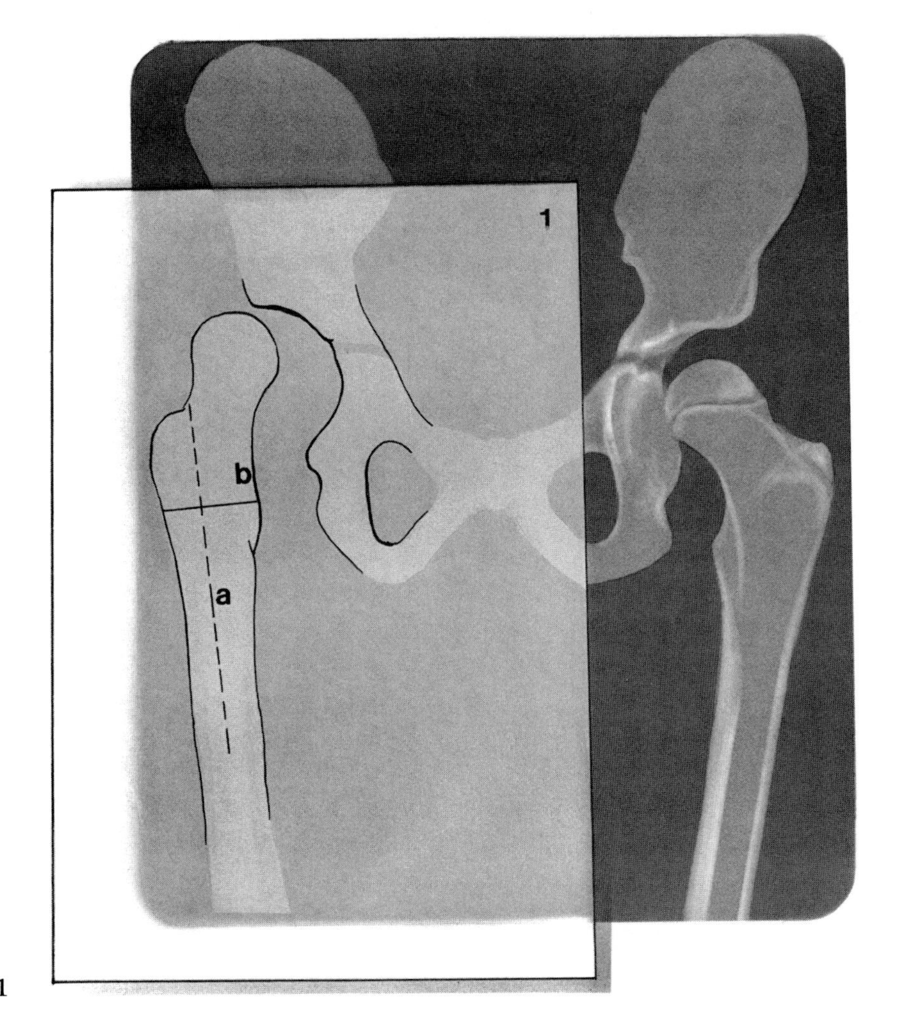

Figure 3–1

Figure 3–2. The second drawing, on a separate sheet of paper, traces the outline of the acetabulum. Again, draw in line the axis of the femoral shaft (**a**).

Figure 3–3. Superimpose the second drawing on the first one. Turn the drawings until the femoral head on the first drawing is in the desired relationship to the acetabulum of the second one. Now draw in the proximal femur down to the osteotomy line (**b**) along with the new femoral axis (**a′**) and the line of the osteotomy (**b**). The amount of varus that is needed to produce the desired result is found by measuring the angle between the original femoral axis (**a**) and the new femoral axis (**a′**).

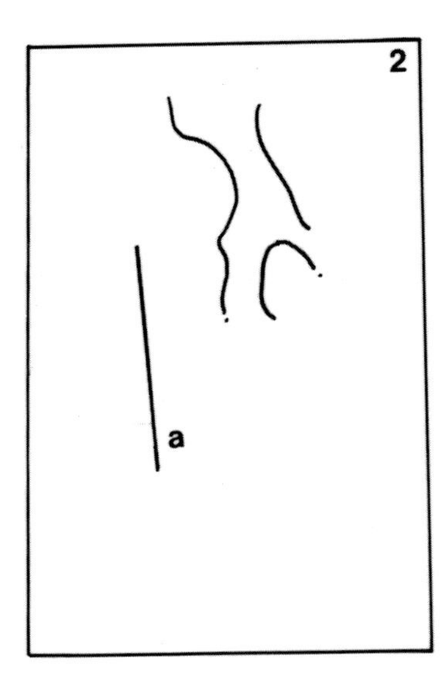

Figure 3–2

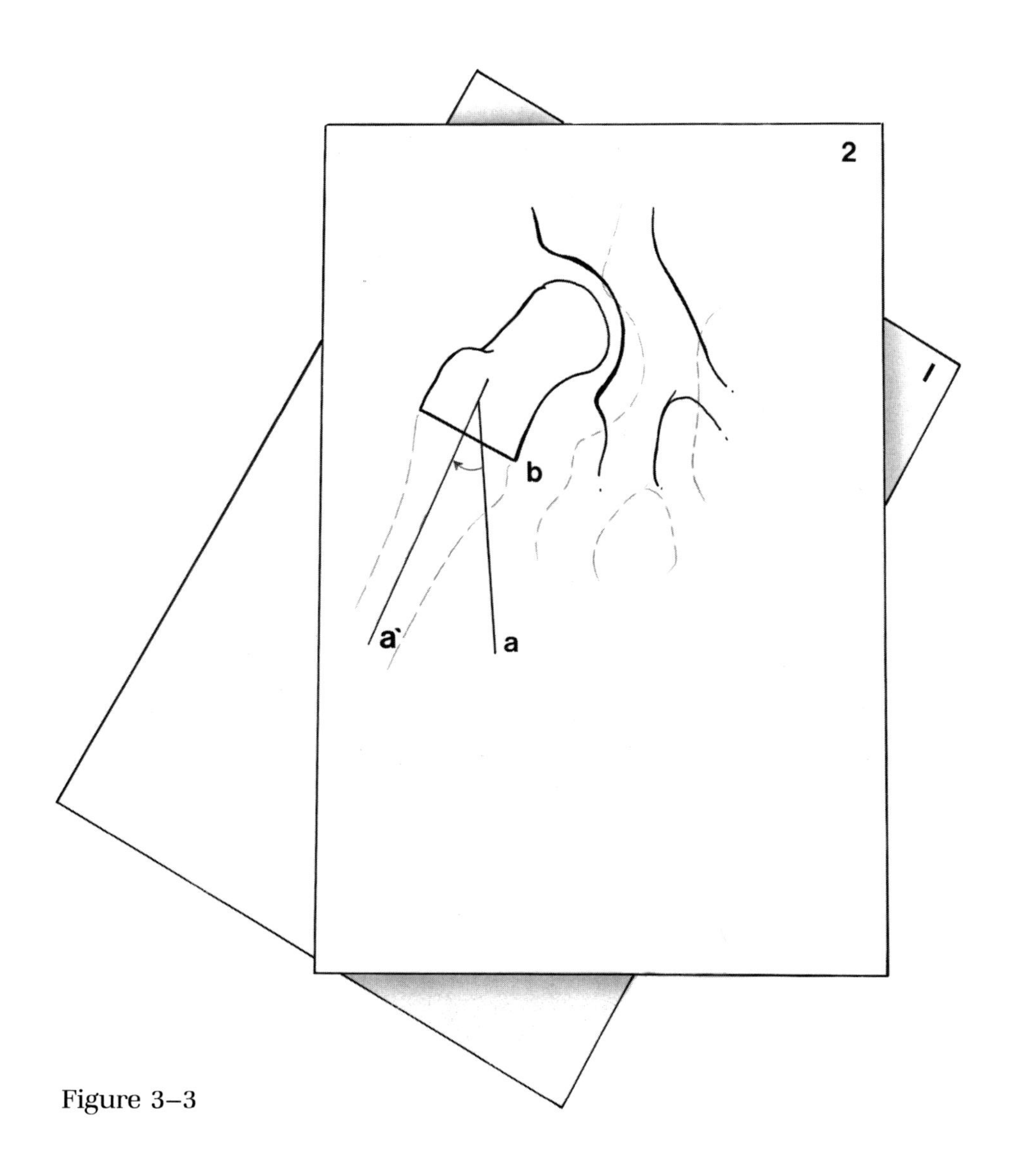

Figure 3–3

Figure 3–4. Now superimpose the two drawings, lining up the femoral axis (**a**) of each. Slide the second drawing up and down until the intersection of **a**′ and **b** of the second drawing intersects with line **b** on the first drawing. At this point draw line **b**′ perpendicular to the axis of the femoral shaft (**a**). This is now the definitive osteotomy line. The wedge that lies below the definitive osteotomy line (**b**′) is the wedge that will be resected. Because the femoral axis had remained superimposed, the correct amount of medial displacement is accounted for, and there is no change in the alignment of the leg.

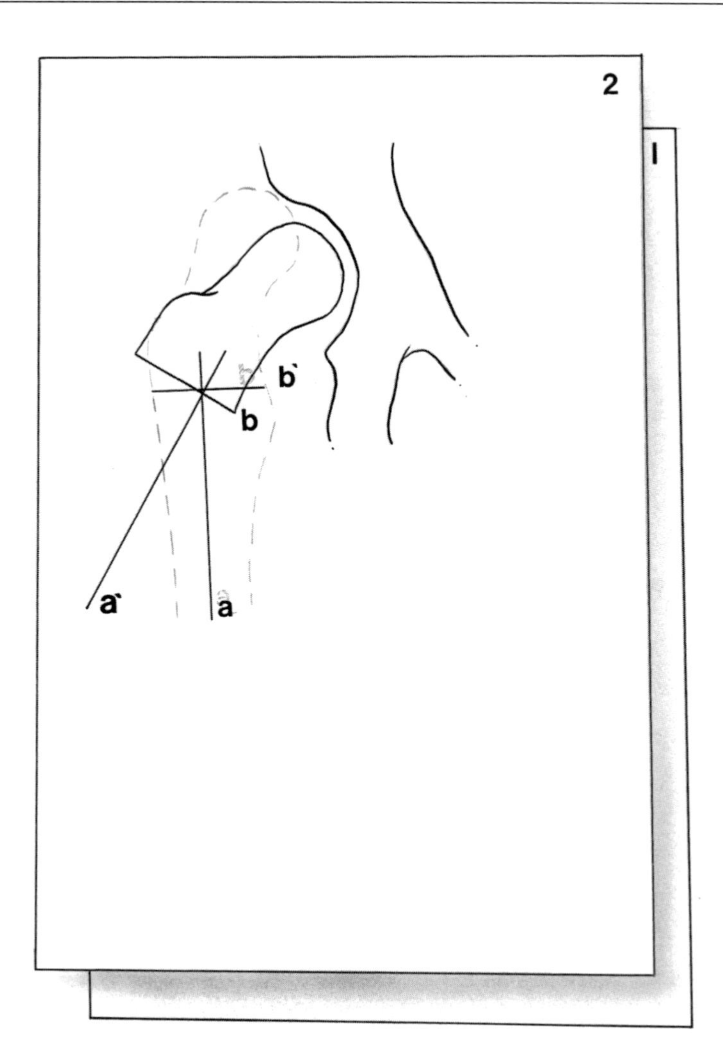

Figure 3–4

Figure 3–5. Draw in the distal part of the femur below the osteotomy line. If blade plates are used as a means of internal fixation, the insertion point of the chisel is now determined. For the adult-sized plate, this will be approximately 12 to 15 mm proximal to the osteotomy site. For the juvenile and adolescent plates, this distance will be less and can be determined from transparent templates or measurement from the desired size plate. On this same drawing, the correct amount of displacement can also be measured, and the correct plate selected. Finally the desired length of the blade can be measured and the blade plate drawn in. This should now represent what the postoperative radiograph will look like.

Figure 3–6. The amount of shortening that the osteotomy produces can be determined directly from the drawings. Align the femoral axis (**a**) of both drawings and superimpose the acetabular joint line of each. The amount of shortening produced is the distance between the osteotomy line (**b**) of the first drawing and the definitive osteotomy line (**b'**) of the second drawing.

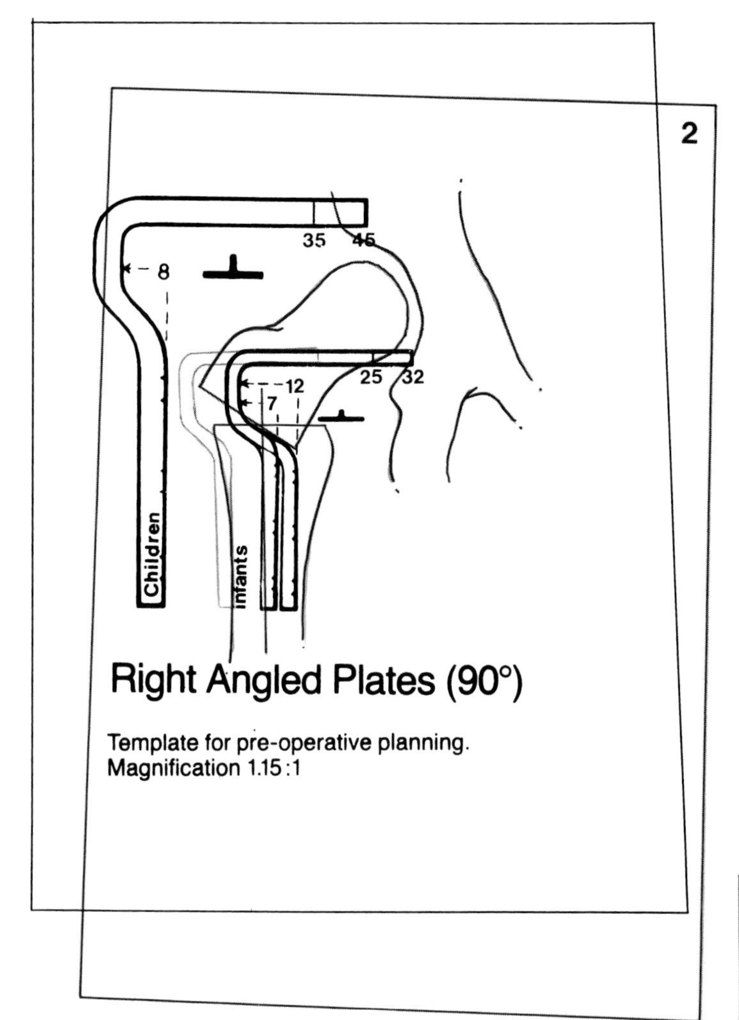

Figure 3–5

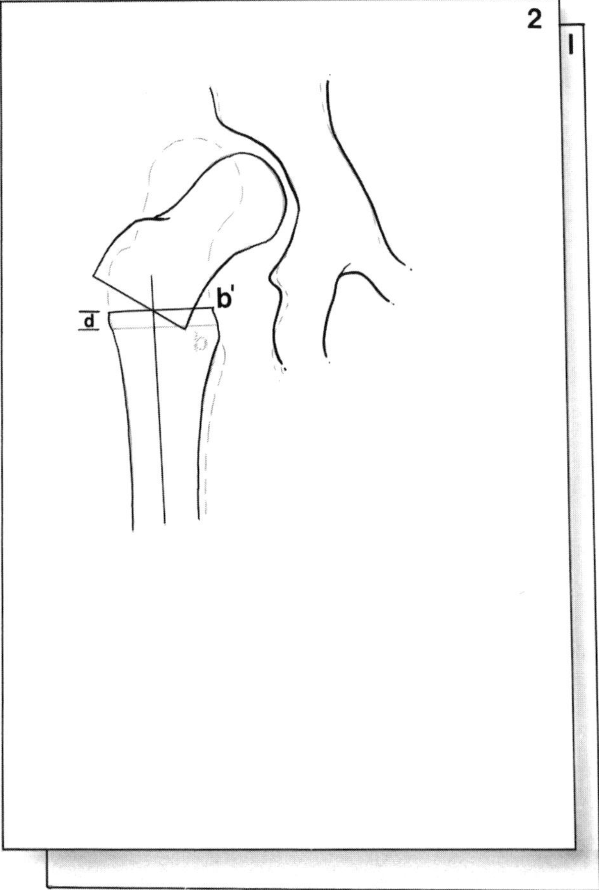

Figure 3–6

REFERENCES

1. Pauwels F. Biomechanics of the locomotor apparatus. Berlin: Springer-Verlag, 1980.
2. Pauwels F. Biomechanics of the normal and diseased hip. Berlin: Springer-Verlag, 1976.
3. Schatzker J. The intertrochanteric osteotomy. Berlin: Springer-Verlag, 1984.
4. Oest O. Special diagnostic and preoperative planning of corrective osteotomies. In: Hierhlozer G, Muller KH, eds. Corrective osteotomies of the lower extremity after trauma. Berlin: Springer-Verlag, 1985:29–37.
5. Muller M. Intertrochanteric osteotomies in adults: planning and operating technique. In: Cruess RL, Mitchell NS, eds. Surgical management of degenerative arthritis of the lower limb. Philadelphia: Lea & Febiger, 1975:53–64.

3.2 Proximal Femoral Varus Osteotomy in Children Using a 90-Degree Blade Plate

As the child becomes older or larger there is a need for both increased precision in the performance of the osteotomy and increased strength or rigidity of the fixation. For these reasons the author prefers to use the AO blade plates. Although their use may seem difficult to the novice, careful preoperative planning and a little experience will give the surgeon a degree of control and security that is not possible with most other methods of fixation.

Figure 3–7. An intertrochanteric femoral osteotomy may be performed on either a fracture table or a regular operating table with a translucent top. The choice is the surgeon's. Many fracture tables will not accommodate small children or permit bilateral hip surgery, making the choice obvious. Conversely, the surgeon without an assistant may find it easier to place the larger adolescent patient on a fracture table to control the leg more easily. The patient should be positioned so that an anteroposterior view of the hip can be obtained on an image intensifier. This will be necessary to confirm the correct placement of the osteotomy and blade of the fixation device. For this purpose it can be positioned from the opposite side of the operating table when needed. The author has not found a lateral view necessary.

The incision should extend from the tip of the greater trochanter as far distal as necessary. The distal extent of the incision will depend on the fixation device used and the type of osteotomy; a shortening osteotomy requires a longer incision.

Figure 3–8. After the incision is deepened through the subcutaneous fat and fascia lata, two self-retaining retractors are placed beneath the fascia lata. The vastus ridge where the vastus lateralis muscle inserts is identified, and the cautery current is used to cut through this muscle. This cut in the vastus lateralis muscle should extend from the anterior femoral shaft posteriorly to the point where the insertion ends.

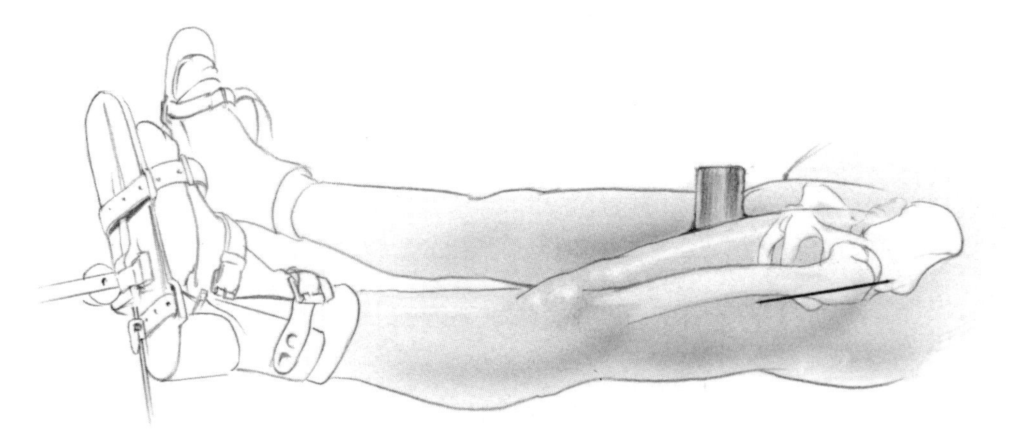

Figure 3–7

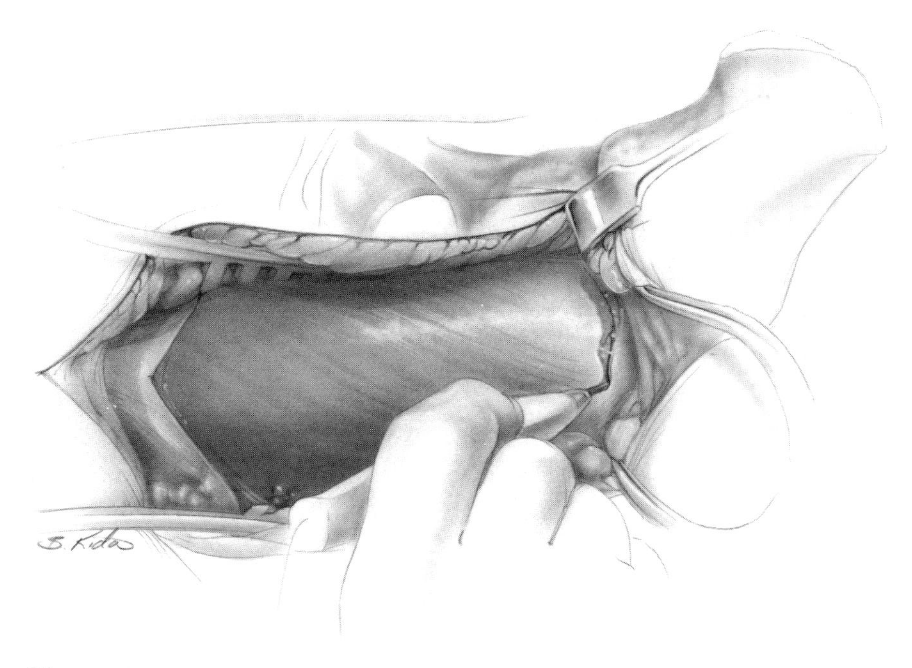

Figure 3–8

Figure 3–9. A sharp rake is used to pull the belly of the vastus lateralis muscle up, exposing its posterior attachment into the femur at the linea aspera. This muscle should be divided as close to this attachment as possible because all of the muscle posterior to the division will be denervated. It is not wise to cut the muscle at its attachment because two to three large vessels will be encountered coming around the posterior aspect of the femur to enter the muscle. Therefore, the muscle is divided about 1 cm anterior to its attachment. This can be done carefully with the cautery current or bluntly by pulling a periosteal elevator from cephalad to caudad, tearing the muscle and dividing the periosteum.

Figure 3–10. A periosteal elevator is used to elevate the entire quadriceps muscle group from the bone. In elevating the muscle from the medial side of the femur, care must be taken to stay subperiosteal. The use of a curved elevator (*eg*, a curved Crego elevator) is helpful in this regard. The same is true in elevating the attachments off the linea aspera; a sharp elevator or osteotome should be kept in close contact with the bone, even elevating small fragments of bone. This will reduce bleeding, which is greatest in this area. The amount of circumferential periosteal elevation that is done depends on the type of osteotomy to be performed. A varus osteotomy without rotation requires the least elevation, whereas a rotational osteotomy requires the most.

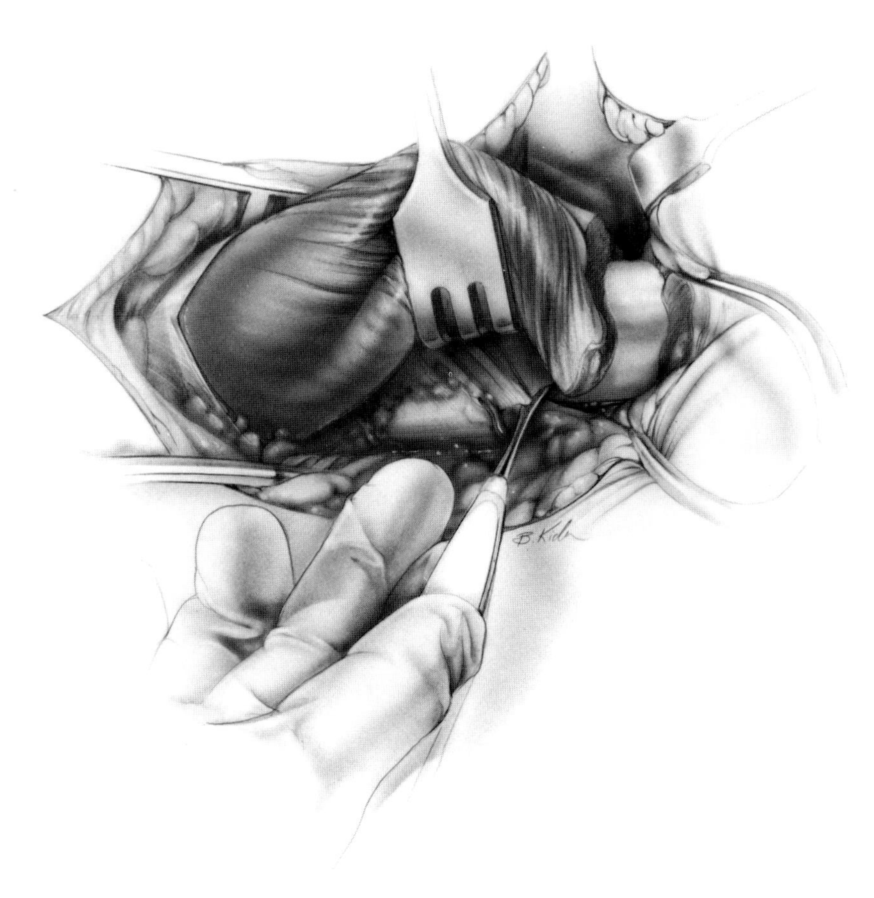

Figure 3–9

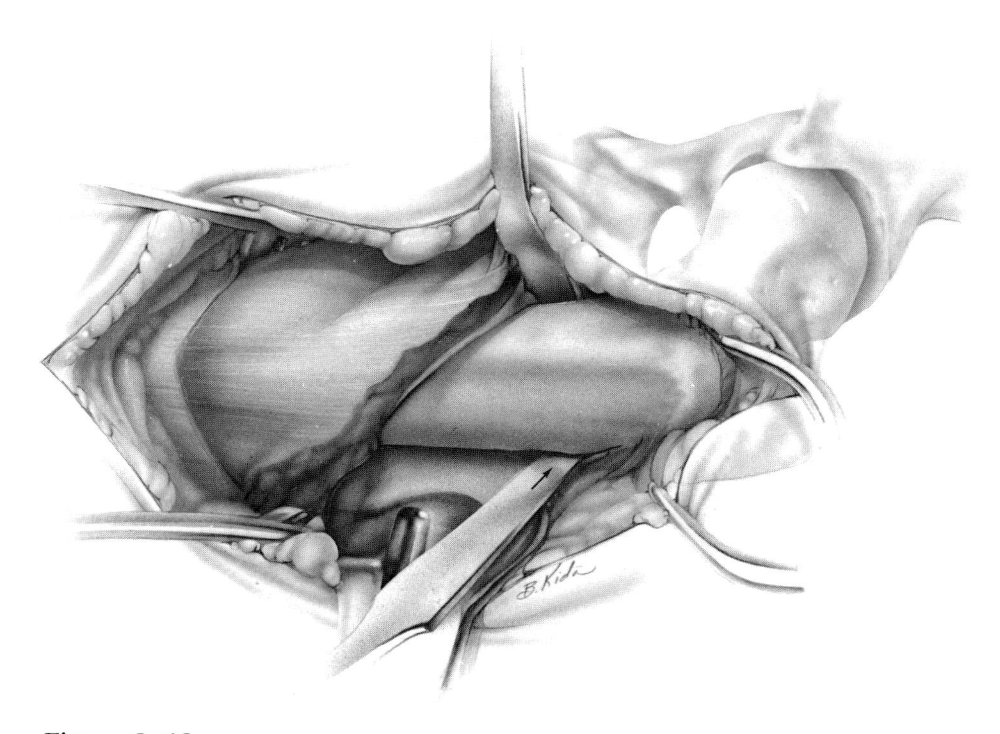

Figure 3–10

Figure 3–11. At the completion of the exposure it should be possible to visualize the anterior femoral shaft as it curves medially, including the inferior curve of the femoral neck. It should be possible to palpate both the lesser trochanter and the anterior femoral neck with a finger. This exposure allows accurate placement of the blade plate and the osteotomy without the excessive use of radiographs.

Figure 3–12. The first step after the exposure is to identify the correct placement of the osteotomy and determine the placement of the blade of the fixation device. First, a Kirschner wire (**a**) is passed on top of the femoral neck until it encounters the femoral head (***Figures 3–12A, B***). This determines the amount of anteversion of the femoral neck, an important bit of knowledge for the correct insertion of the blade.

The next step is to determine at what angle the blade should be inserted relative to the femoral shaft. The correct amount of angular correction will be achieved when the blade is attached to the femoral shaft, and this will in turn be determined by the angle at which the blade enters the femoral neck. If it is desired to create 30 degrees of varus with a 90-degree plate, then the blade should enter the femoral neck at a 60-degree angle to the femoral shaft. When the plate is attached to the femoral shaft, the amount of correction has to be 30 degrees if the blade was inserted correctly (***Figure 3–12C***).

In this example the template that had the 60-degree angle on it is selected and placed on the femoral shaft. A second Kirschner wire (**b**) is now drilled into the most cephalad portion of the femoral neck. The amount of anteversion in this wire will be guided by the first wire that was placed along the anterior femoral neck (**a**) and the amount of varus-valgus will be guided by the 60-degree angle on the template (***Figures 3–12A, B***). This wire will serve as the guide for the direction of the seating chisel and the blade. The Kirschner wire on the anterior femoral neck (**a**) can now be removed.

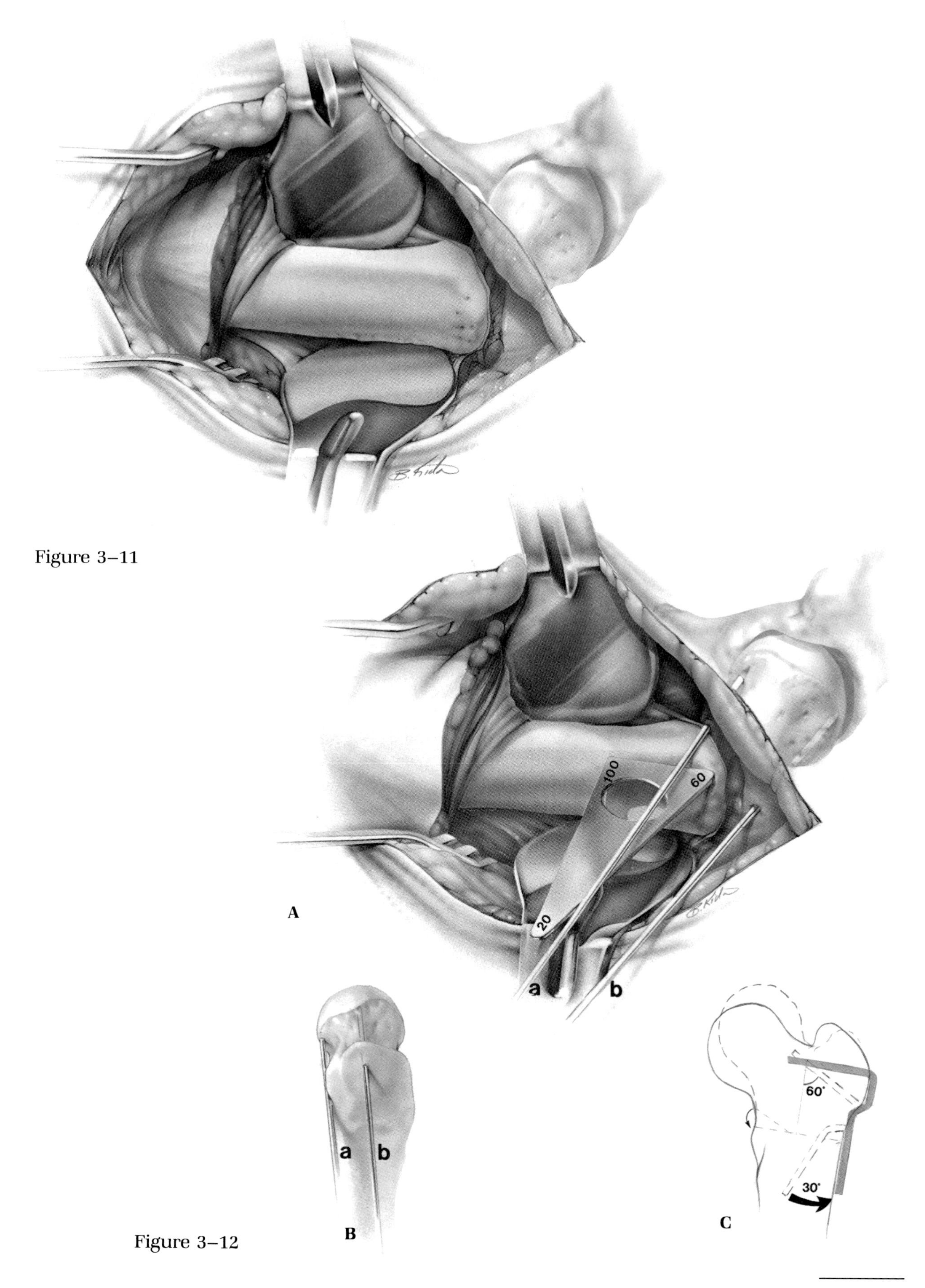

Figure 3–11

Figure 3–12

Figure 3–13. The next step is to mark the site of the osteotomy and insert the seating chisel. Palpate the lesser trochanter with a finger and drill a Kirschner wire (**c**) perpendicular to the femoral shaft into the center of the lesser trochanter. This should place the wire about 5 mm below the site for the osteotomy, which is just at the superior margin of the lesser trochanter. Keep this wire anterior so that it will not interfere with the seating chisel guide (***Figure 3–13A***).

In preparation for placement of the seating chisel, select the site where it will enter the bone. Its distance cephalad to the osteotomy will be determined by the size of the blade plate to be used. This will have been determined from the preoperative plan and can be confirmed by direct measurement of the plate. This distance is represented by **d** (***Figure 3–13B***).

It is important that the insertion point not be too far posterior, or the blade will cut out of the back of the femoral neck. Because the flat surface of the greater trochanter faces about 25 degrees more posterior than if it were perpendicular to the axis of the femoral neck and it lies posterior to the femoral neck, it is easy to make this mistake (***Figure 3–13C***). The shape of the greater trochanter should be ignored and the chisel inserted in line with the femoral neck. To achieve this it will seem that the chisel is starting rather far anteriorly on the greater trochanter.

With the correct insertion point selected, the correct chisel for the plate being used is selected. If the large adult plate is used, it is best to open the cortex of the femur before driving the chisel in, but with the use of the adolescent and child plates this is not necessary. The chisel guide is placed along the femoral shaft. This is essential to be sure that the plate will not lie anterior or posterior to the shaft after the plate is inserted. If flexion or extension is to be a part of the osteotomy, the angle that this guide forms either anterior or posterior to the femoral shaft will determine the amount of flexion or extension, respectively. If necessary, the rotation of the chisel can be controlled with the slotted hammer. The chisel is now driven into the femoral neck using both the chisel guide and the Kirschner wire (**b**) as a guide. The depth of the chisel is read from the scale on the bottom side and correlated with the preoperative plan. At this point an anteroposterior image may be obtained to check the placement of the seating chisel and the osteotomy site marked by the Kirschner wire (**c**).

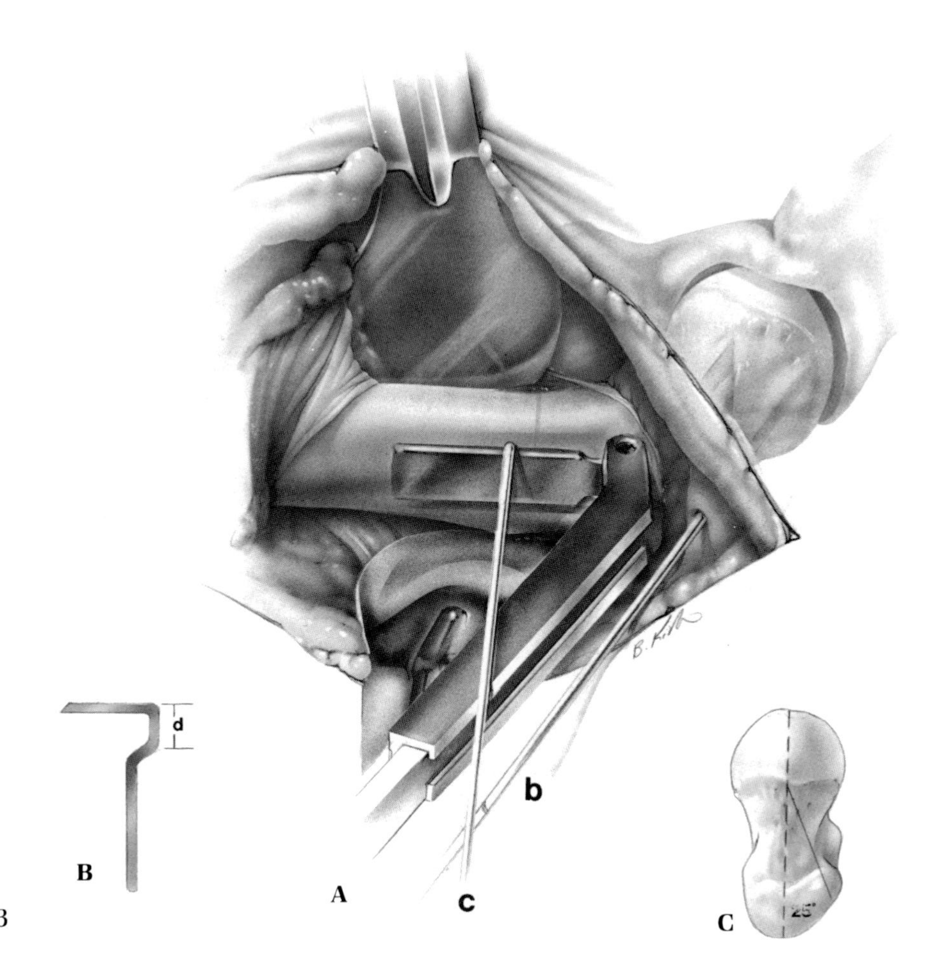

Figure 3–13

Figure 3–14. Before making the osteotomy cut, it is wise to score the anterior femoral shaft longitudinally with the saw to serve as a mark that will indicate if any rotation has occurred. If it is planned to rotate the osteotomy, pins can be placed as described in the rotational osteotomy of the proximal femur. The osteotomy is performed by making the first cut perpendicular to the femoral shaft. This cut should be just cephalad to the lesser trochanter (***Figures 3–14A, B***). The soft tissues are protected by placing two Bennett or similar retractors around the bone. An oscillating saw is used to cut the bone. Copious irrigation is used during the cutting to reduce heating of the bone.

After the first cut is completed, the seating chisel is used to tip the proximal fragment into varus. Beginning halfway across the bone, the desired wedge is removed from the medial side (***Figures 3–14A, B***). This completes the osteotomy.

Figure 3–15. The seating chisel is removed and the blade plate inserted. The blade should be started by hand and then softly tapped with a mallet to avoid starting a false channel. Once it is fully seated, it is held to the femoral shaft with a bone clamp. If it is desired to rotate the osteotomy, that is accomplished at this point. The plate is then fixed to the femoral shaft with the appropriate screws. The wound is closed by reattaching the vastus lateralis to its origin at the base of the trochanter and closing its fascia posteriorly. A drain is placed deep to the fascia lata, and it and the remainder of the wound is closed in a routine manner.

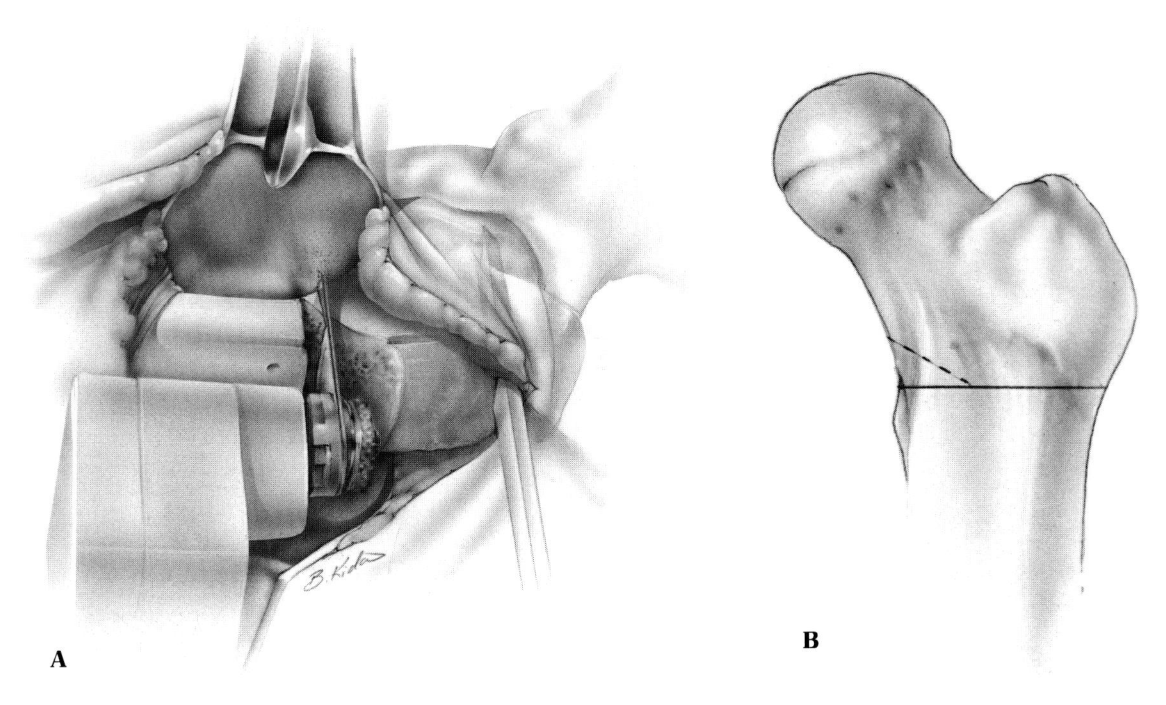

Figure 3–14

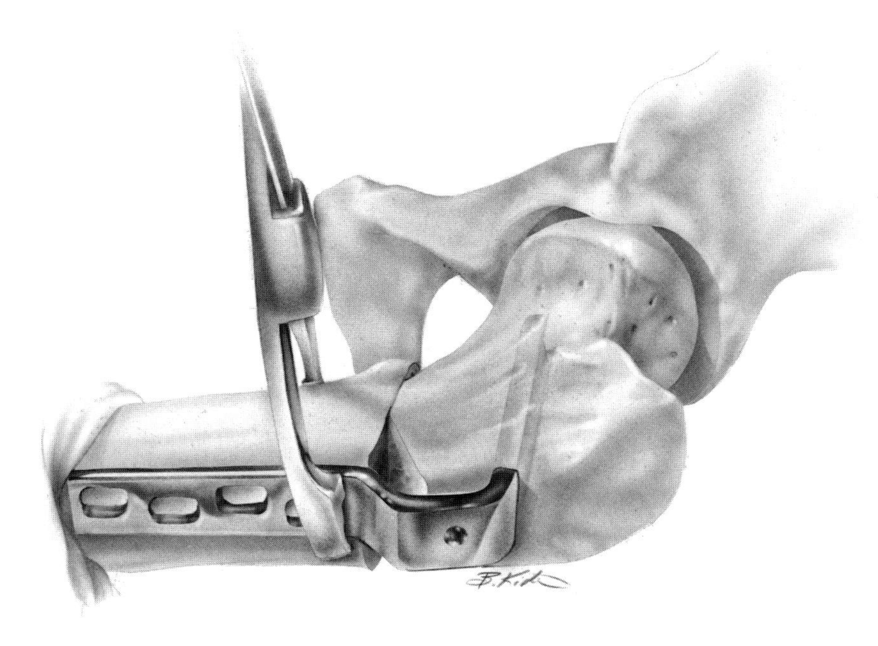

Figure 3–15

Figure 3–16. CP is a 14-year-old boy who presented with a painful hip 1 year after a motor vehicle accident in which he sustained an unrecognized posterior dislocation of the hip with a posterior acetabular fracture (***Figure 3–16A***). He was treated successfully with a varus and rotational osteotomy of the proximal femur, which eliminated the posterior subluxation and consequent synovitis. The fixation is strong enough to permit immediate, protected weight bearing (***Figure 3–16B***).

POSTOPERATIVE CARE

Subtrochanter osteotomies usually take 6 to 8 weeks to heal. The degree of immobilization or bed rest during this period is dependent on many factors: the size of the child and hence the strength of the plate that was used, the strength of the bone, the stability of the osteotomy, and the ability of the patient to cooperate with partial weight-bearing. The author's preference is to place small children in a one-leg spica cast at bed rest. Cooperative children in the age range of 8 to 12 years can usually be left out of a cast at bed rest or given the use of a wheel chair. In the adolescent group, the fixation is usually strong enough to permit a partial weight bearing crutch gait if the patient is cooperative. Full weight bearing is permitted in all age groups when there is radiographic evidence of bony union.

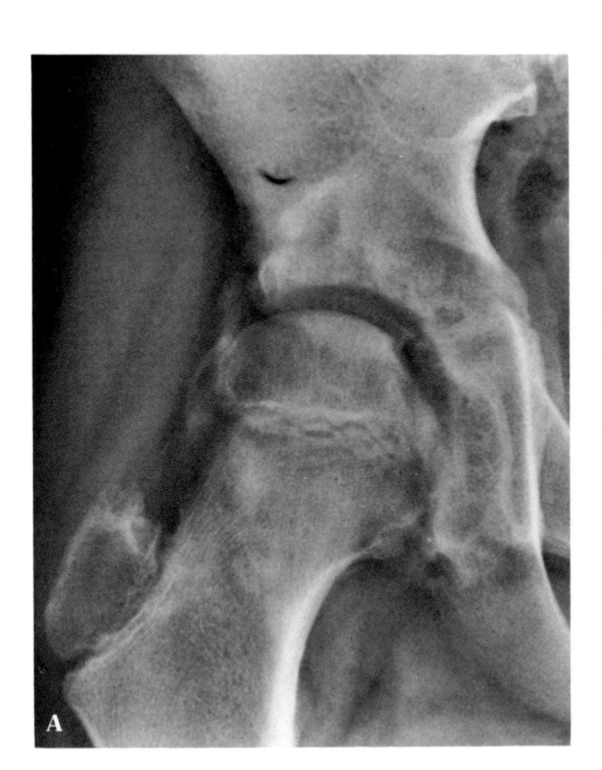

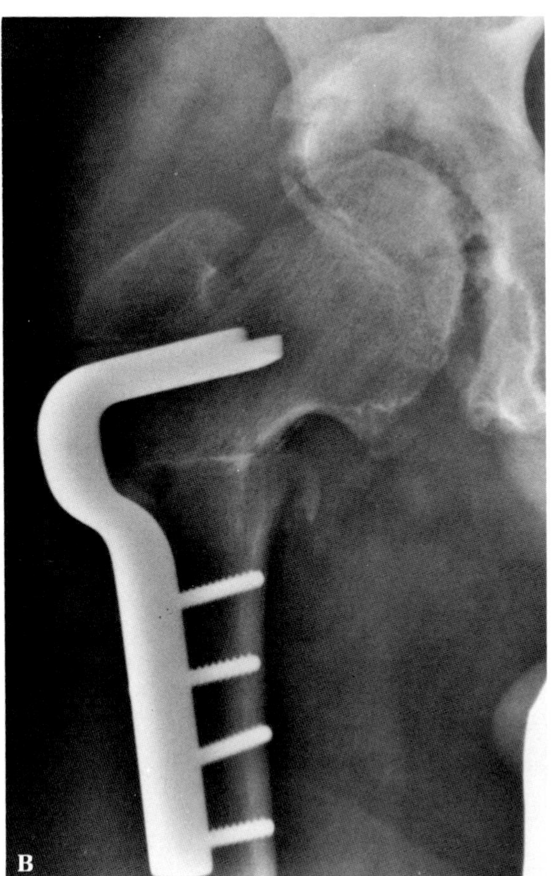

Figure 3–16

3.3
Proximal Femoral Osteotomy in Infants Using Altdorf Hip Clamp

The Altdorf hip clamp, designed by professor Heinz Wagner, is a 130-degree angled malleable blade plate. Wagner[1] has described the technique for using the plate, which greatly simplifies an intertrochanteric osteotomy.

The author finds this plate most useful in children younger than 5 to 6 years of age who are undergoing a femoral osteotomy in conjunction with treatment of congenital dislocation of the hip. However, it has been used in children up to 12 years of age.[2] Although this plate is designed for varus osteotomies, the fact that it can easily be bent makes it ideal for the treatment of developmental coxa vara in small children.

Figure 3–17. The Altdorf clamp is an angled blade plate of 130 degrees. The blade is bifurcated, and the entire plate is malleable. The plate comes in three sizes: 9, 10.5, and 12 mm wide, with different blade lengths. There are two oval holes on the side plate, which in the smaller two plates accommodate the 3.5-mm cortical screws and in the larger plate the 4.5-mm cortical screws. There is also a round hole proximal that is designed to accept a cancellous screw to hold the blade securely in the proximal fragment.

Figure 3–18. It is easiest to perform this operation on a regular flat radiolucent operating table. After the intertrochanter region of the femur is exposed, the leg is manipulated to place the femoral head and neck in the desired position. This can be ascertained by an image intensifier. A Steinmann pin heavy enough to control the proximal fragment is then drilled into the proximal fragment. This pin should start just below the epiphysis of the greater trochanter, be parallel to the floor, and perpendicular to the median plane of the body (***Figures 3–18A, B***). Whenever this pin is returned to this position after the osteotomy, the femoral head will be returned to the desired relationship with the acetabulum.

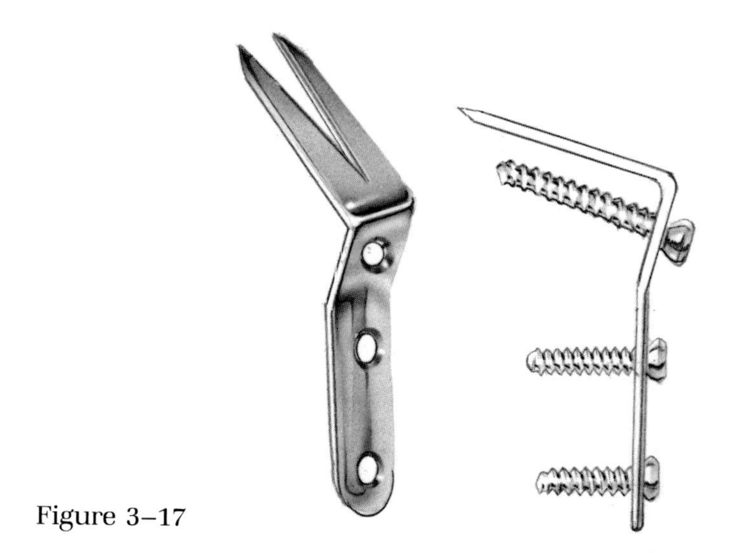

Figure 3–17

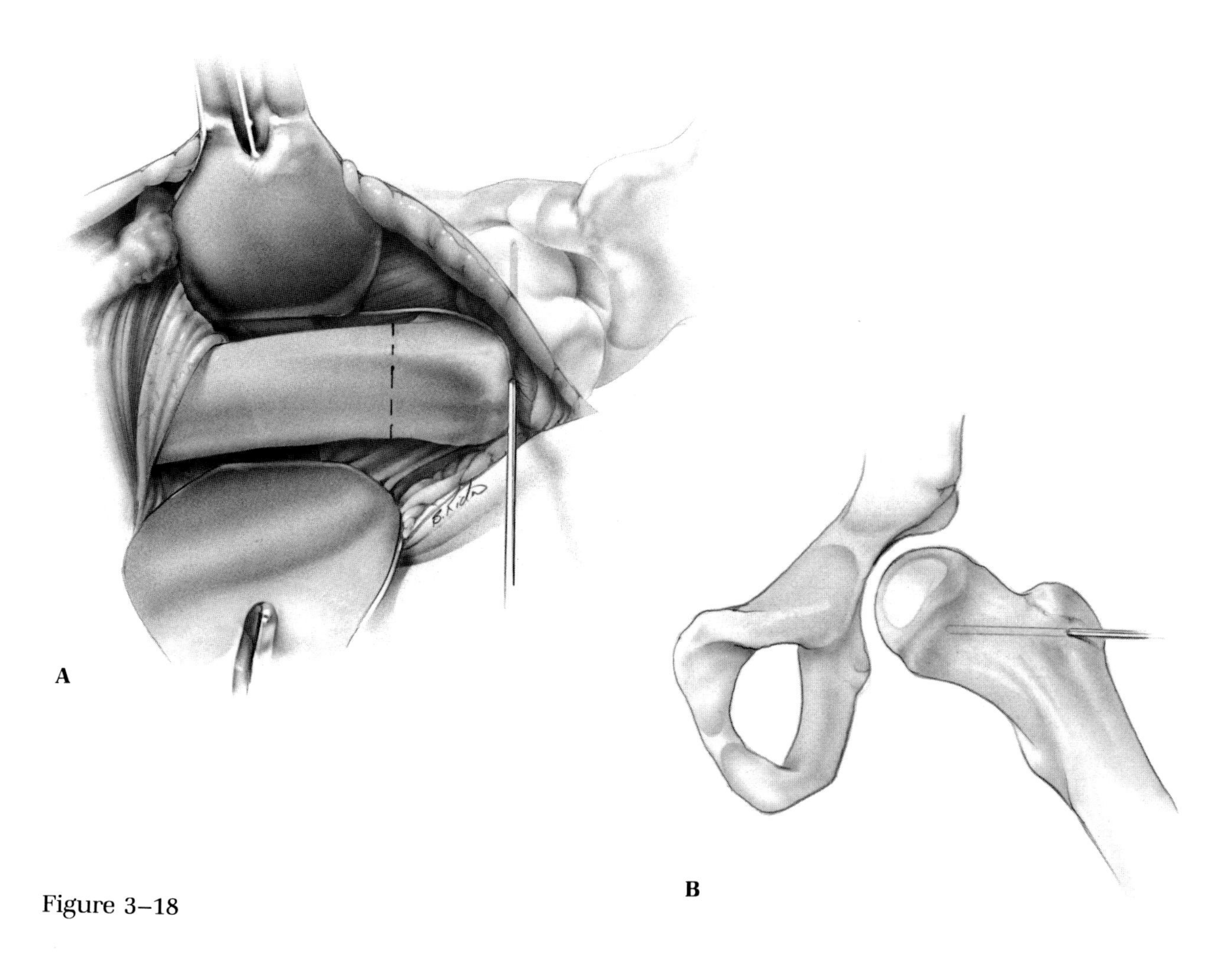

A

B

Figure 3–18

Figure 3–19. The osteotomy cut is then made parallel to this pin and just above the lesser trochanter. The leg is then placed in a neutral position relative to the body, and a medial portion of the distal fragment is removed perpendicular to the femoral shaft (***Figures 3–19A, B***). In small children, under 3 or 4 years of age, a single osteotomy cut perpendicular to the femoral shaft and just proximal to the lesser trochanter can be made. As the proximal fragment is tipped back up into the desired position and displaced medially, the spike it forms will tend to stabilize in the canal of the distal fragment (see ***Figure 3–21A***).

Figure 3–20. The angle of the Altdorf clamp is 130 degrees but can be bent with pliers to whatever angle the situation calls for. In most cases of varus osteotomy the 130-degree angle is ideal. The Altdorf clamp is designed to be pushed into the cut surface of the proximal fragment and not through the lateral cortex. To accomplish this the proper size clamp is grasped with the holding device.

Medial displacement is controlled by the point at which the splines of the clamp enter the proximal fragment. The more medial the splines enter the proximal fragment, the more medial the displacement that will be achieved. The amount of varus achieved depends on the angle the blade enters the femoral neck. To judge the angle for insertion of the blade, the fragments are held in the desired position while the splines are first pushed into the cancellous bone of the femoral neck and then impacted with a mallet.

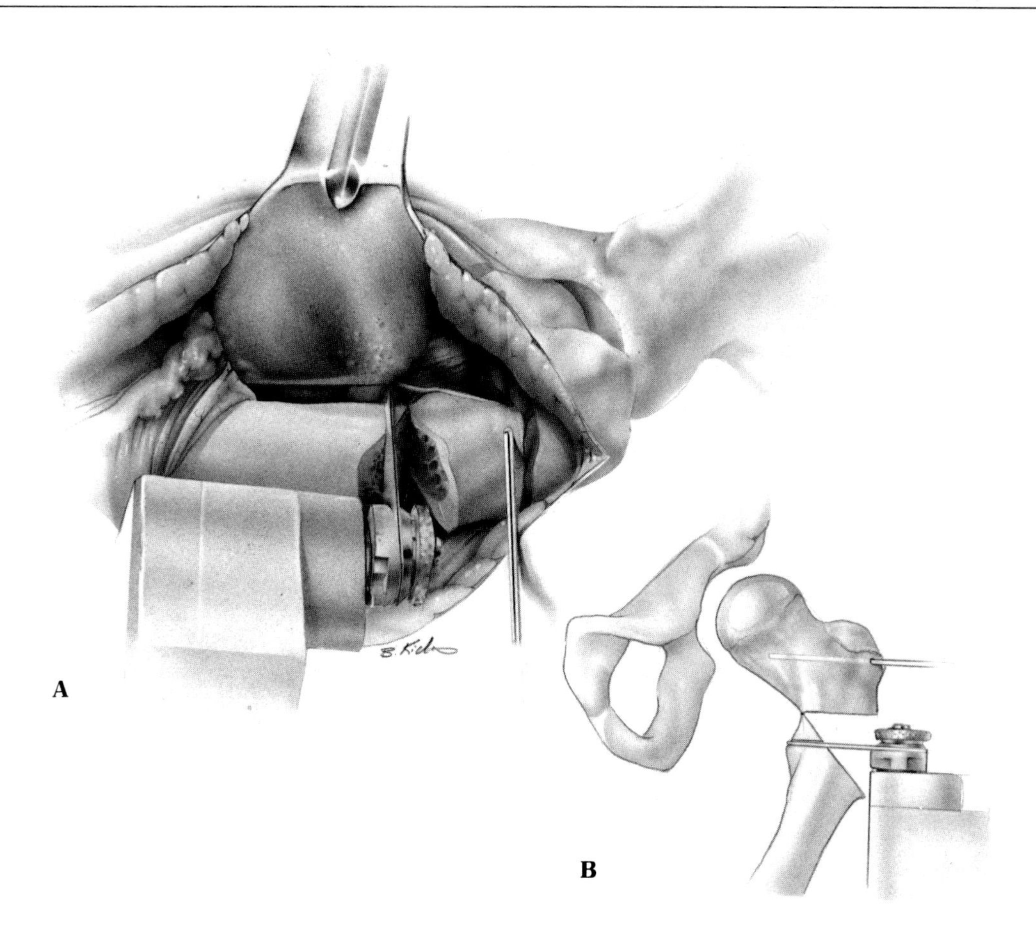

Figure 3–19

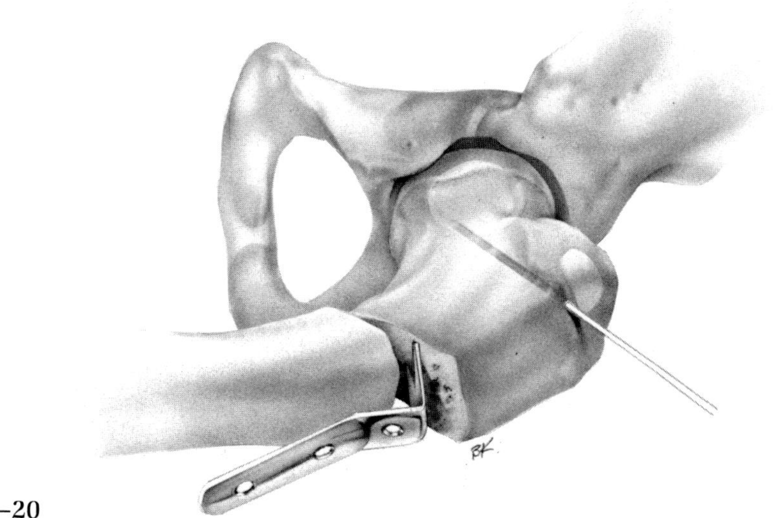

Figure 3–20

Figure 3–21. After the bifurcated blade is inserted, the osteotomy fragments are brought together in a position of slightly exaggerated medial displacement and slightly less varus than planned.

This should result in the distal tip of the plate touching the femoral shaft, but the proximal part of the plate will not be in contact with the shaft. The plate is first attached to the femoral shaft through the most distal screw hole (***Figure 3–21A***). Next the screw is placed in the middle hole on the plate. As this is tightened, it will pull the shaft laterally and push the proximal fragment into more varus, thus producing interfragmentary compression (***Figure 3–21B***).

Figure 3–22. Finally, a 4-mm cancellous screw is inserted through the proximal round hole into the proximal fragment. This screw should not be longer than the bifurcated blade to avoid penetrating the physeal plate.

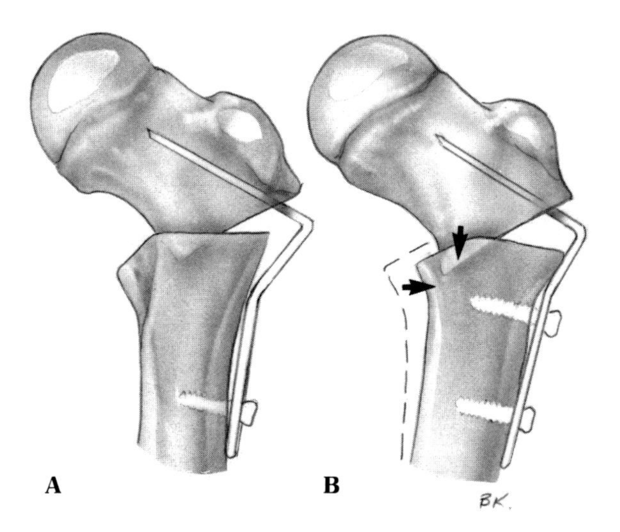

Figure 3–21

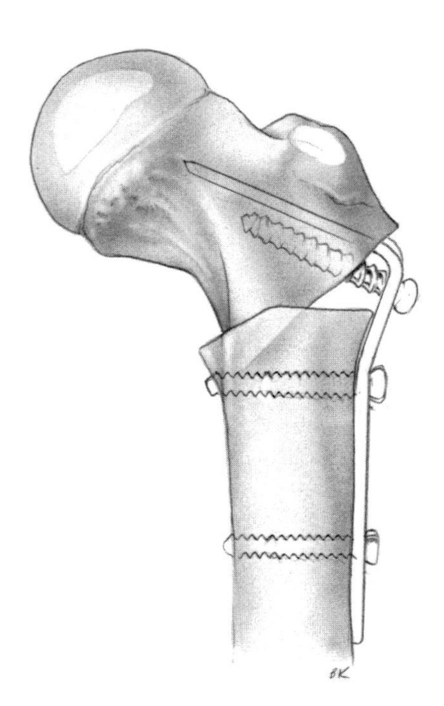

Figure 3–22

Figure 3–23. SC is a 2-year-old girl who underwent a closed reduction of the left hip at 3 months of age. Radiographs (***Figure 3–23A***) showed persistent widening of the joint and failure of the acetabulum to remodel. A varus and rotational osteotomy was performed. The position of the femur was ascertained interoperatively by image intensifier (***Figure 3–23B***). The position of the femoral head in relation to the acetabulum and the healing osteotomy is shown 6 weeks after surgery (***Figure 3–23C***).

POSTOPERATIVE CARE

The fact that this method of fixation is most often used in young children in combination with other procedures for congenital dislocation of the hip means that a cast will usually be required. In addition, the difficulty in executing this osteotomy to perfection, which is what produces the compression and stability (along with the malleable plate and only two screws for fixation), makes the author very uncomfortable without cast immobilization.

REFERENCES

1. Wagner H. Osteotomies for congenital hip dislocation. In: The hip: proceedings of the fourth open scientific meeting of The Hip Society. St. Louis: CV Mosby, 1976:45–66.
2. Alonso JE, Lovell WW, Lovejoy JF. The Altdorf hip clamp. J Pediatr Orthop 1986;6:399.

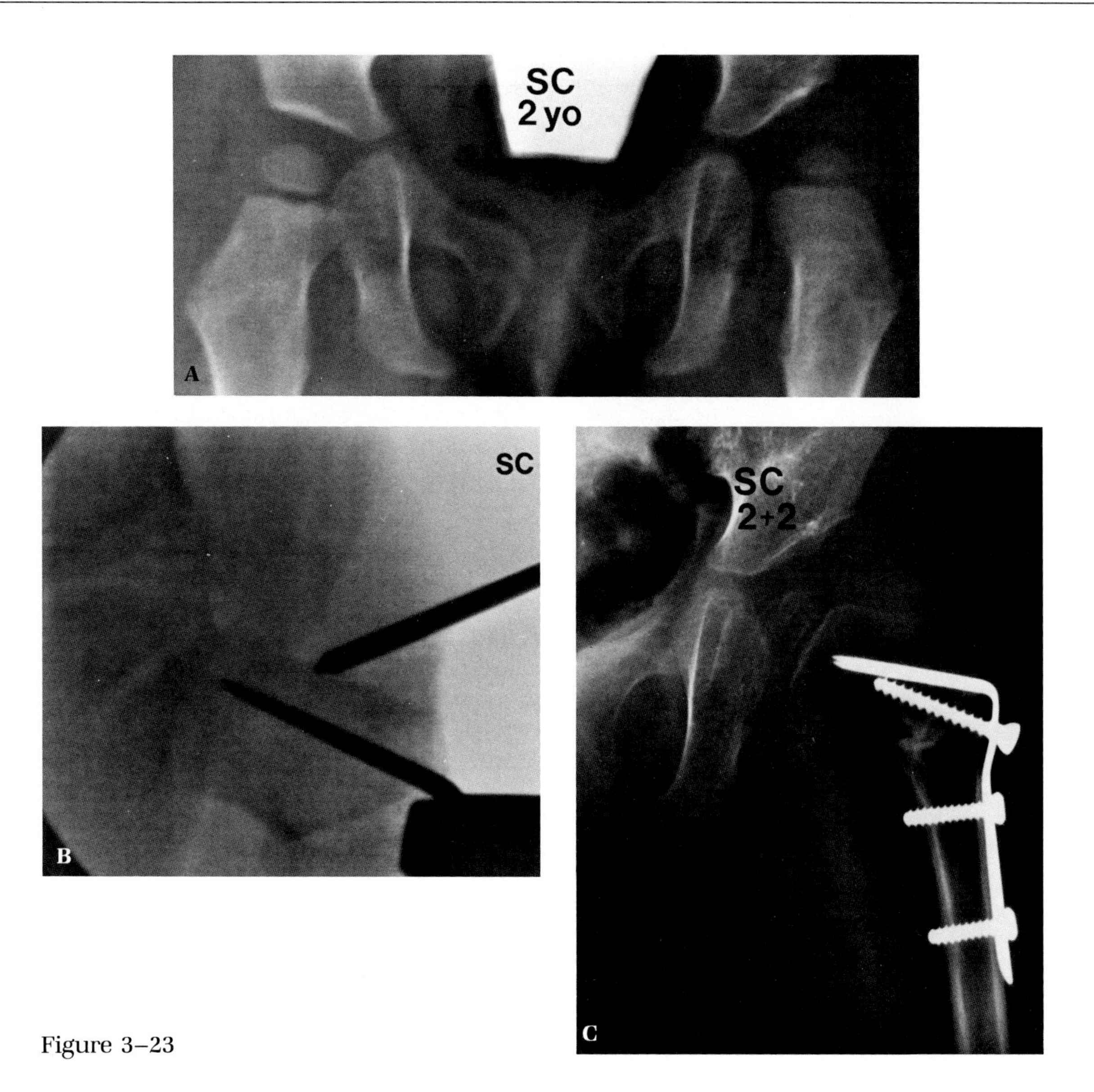

Figure 3–23

3.4
Proximal Femoral Rotational Osteotomy

Rotational intertrochanteric osteotomy is often done as an isolated procedure for the severe case of excessive femoral anteversion, but is more often done in conjunction with other procedures associated with congenital dislocation of the hip. The technique described here is for a pure rotational osteotomy; however, the technique is equally useful when rotation is needed in combination with a varus intertrochanteric osteotomy.

Precision in the amount of rotation at the osteotomy site is the single biggest problem in this osteotomy. There are several reasons for this. First, the hip has a limited arch of motion, and in some patients who need a rotational osteotomy this arch is less than usual. Any "overcorrection" may produce an opposite deformity. In addition, the surgeon will have a difficult time determining 30 degrees of rotation by the separation of two marks on the femoral shaft.

Figure 3–24. Crider and Leber[1] have described a geometric formula for determining the degree of rotation achieved by the distance between two marks on the femur. The formula states that the distance between the two marks (**L**) is equal to the radius of the bone at the osteotomy site (**R**) × the desired degrees of rotation (**Q**) × a constant (0.017). This formula assumes that the bone is a circle that is nearly true in the intertrochanteric area if the lesser trochanter is ignored. In addition, it is necessary to keep the central axis of both fragments aligned, something that is not so easy to accomplish in all cases.

Although the author thinks this is a good check, he has preferred to rely on a more direct method of determining rotation intraoperatively, namely the angular deviation of two pins.

Figure 3–25. The intertrochanteric region of the femur is exposed as previously described (see discussion on intertrochanteric osteotomy). For rotational osteotomies, it is necessary to strip the periosteum and in particular the attachments to the linea aspera for a considerable distance to maintain the alignment of the axis of both fragments during rotation (***Figure 3–25A***). If this is not done, the attachments will act as a tether, causing translation of the fragments as well as rotation (***Figure 3–25B***). This will decrease the contact between the cut surface of the bone, make fixation more difficult, and make it impossible to calculate the amount of rotation that has been achieved by inspecting marks on the bone.

Figure 3–26. After the exposure is completed, two heavy $\frac{5}{32}$-in smooth Steinmann pins are drilled into the anterior femoral shaft. One is placed above the proposed osteotomy site and one below (***Figure 3–26A***). They must be parallel (***Figure 3–26B***). They should engage the posterior femoral cortex. The reason for this and the heavy pins is that if they are placed far enough medially on the anterior surface of the femoral shaft to be out of the way, they will be subjected to a considerable bending force from the muscle. This could bend the pins, causing a miscalculation in the amount of rotation.

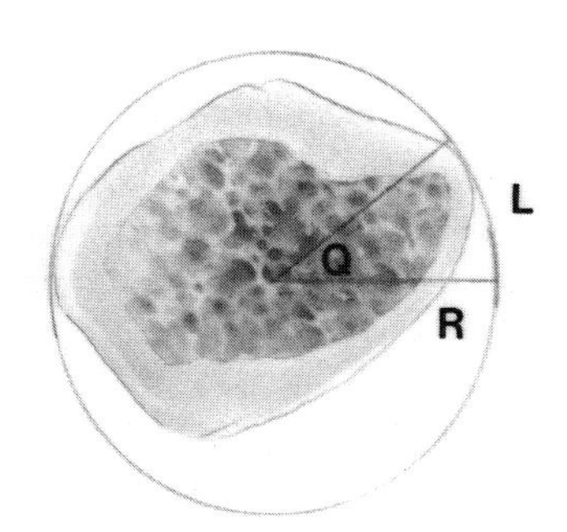

Figure 3–24

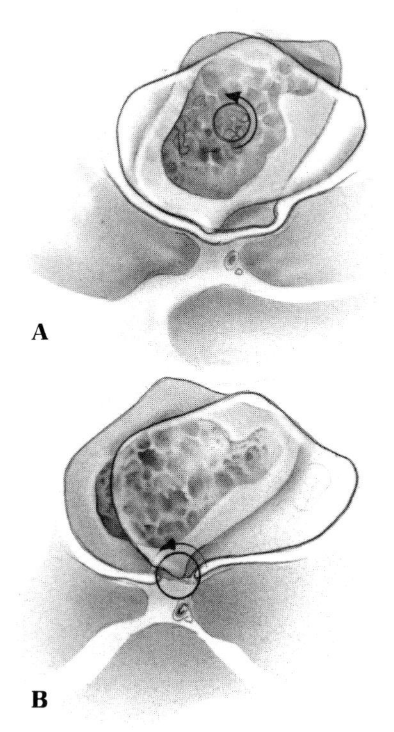

Figure 3–25

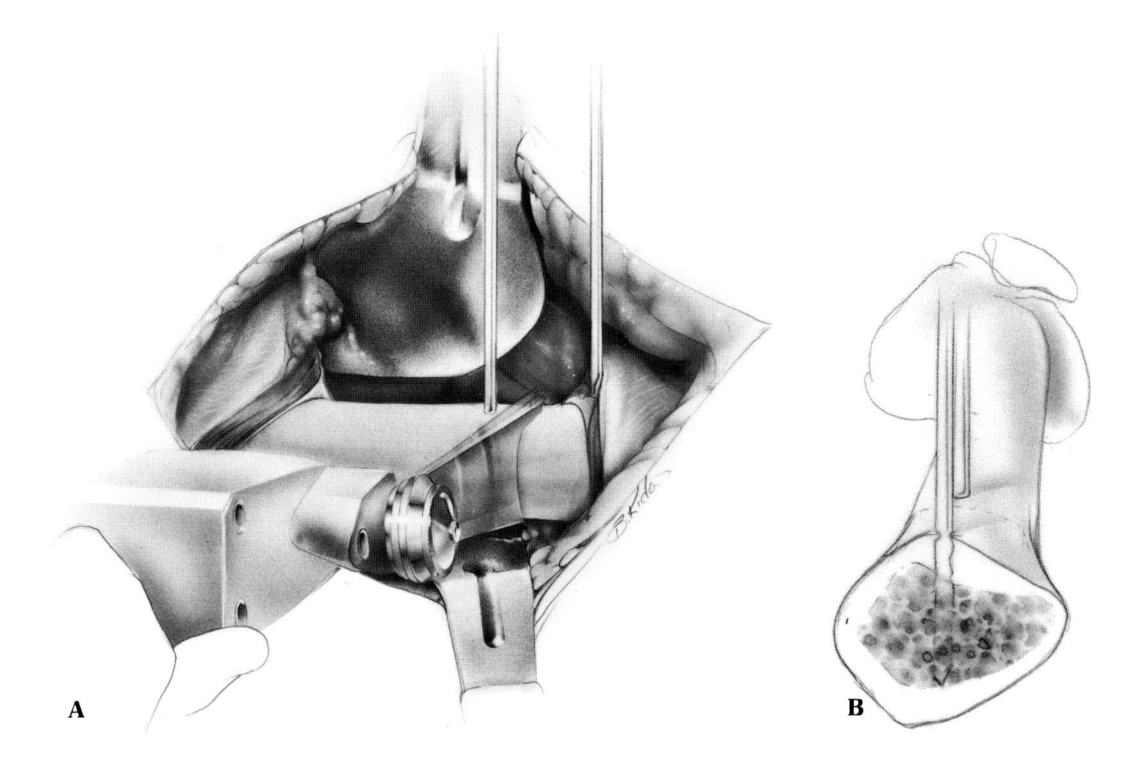

Figure 3–26

Figure 3–27. The next step is the insertion of the seating chisel. Because no angular correction is needed, the fixed 90-degree guide can be used. The chisel should be chosen to fit the plate that is to be used. In adolescents the condylar plate is ideal, but in smaller children a right-angled plate of appropriate size is used. A transverse osteotomy is performed at the level of the lesser trochanter.

Figure 3–28. While the proximal fragment is stabilized, the distal fragment is rotated, in this case externally to correct excessive femoral anteversion. The angle templates from the Synthes osteotomy set are used to judge the amount of angular rotation between the two Steinmann pins (***Figure 3–28A***). Looking from above or below makes it easier to judge the amount of rotation (***Figure 3–28B***).

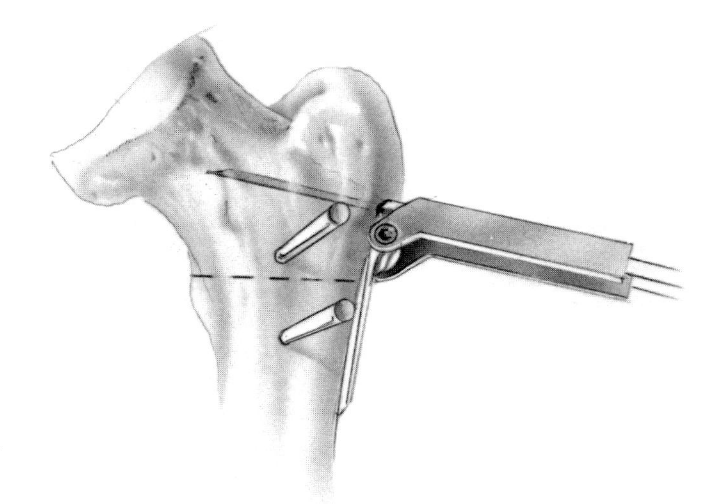

Figure 3–27

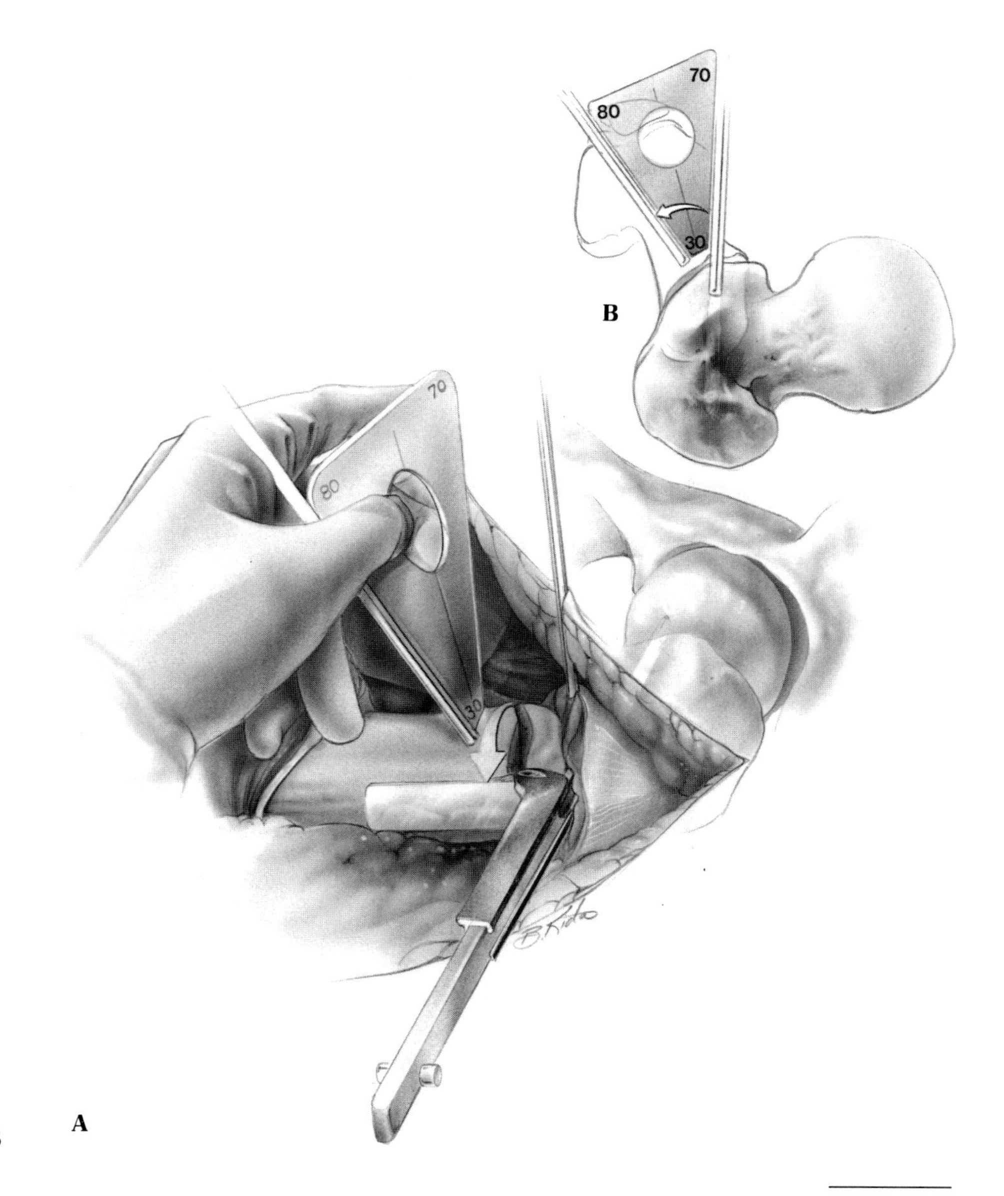

Figure 3–28 A

Figure 3–29. Because the amount of rotation is so critical, the surgeon may wish to check the rotation clinically. If this is attempted with only the clamp holding the plate, rotation of the distal fragment may occur undetected by the surgeon as he or she tests the extremes of internal and external rotation. Therefore, it is best to place one screw in the plate and then test the rotation. After the surgeon is satisfied that the new alignment is correct, all of the screws are placed to secure the plate, and the wound is closed over a drain.

Figure 3–30. BW is a 9-year-old boy who had 70 degrees of internal rotation and 5 degrees of external rotation when his hips were in extension. His rotational osteotomies were fixed with the 90-degree-angled plates (***Figure 3–30A***). Because the osteotomies do not require displacement, these plates remain slightly prominent and are not exactly ideal. GW is a 13-year-old female with a similar clinical picture who was large enough to permit the use of the condylar blade plates (***Figure 3–30B***). These are ideally suited to the contours of the proximal femur when no displacement is required.

POSTOPERATIVE CARE

The postoperative care does not differ from other intertrochanteric osteotomies. Cast, bed rest without cast, or protected ambulation is permitted, depending on the fixation used and the ability of the patient to cooperate with limited weight bearing. As healing proceeds, it is important to increase the therapy to strengthen the hip musculature, especially the abductors and the extensors. The patient's gait was the main reason the parents sought treatment, and when the patient continued to waddle and limp after discontinuing crutches, the parents became increasingly anxious about the success of the surgery.

REFERENCE

1. Crider RJ, Leber C. Accurate correction in rotational osteotomies. J Pediatr Orthop 1987;7:468.

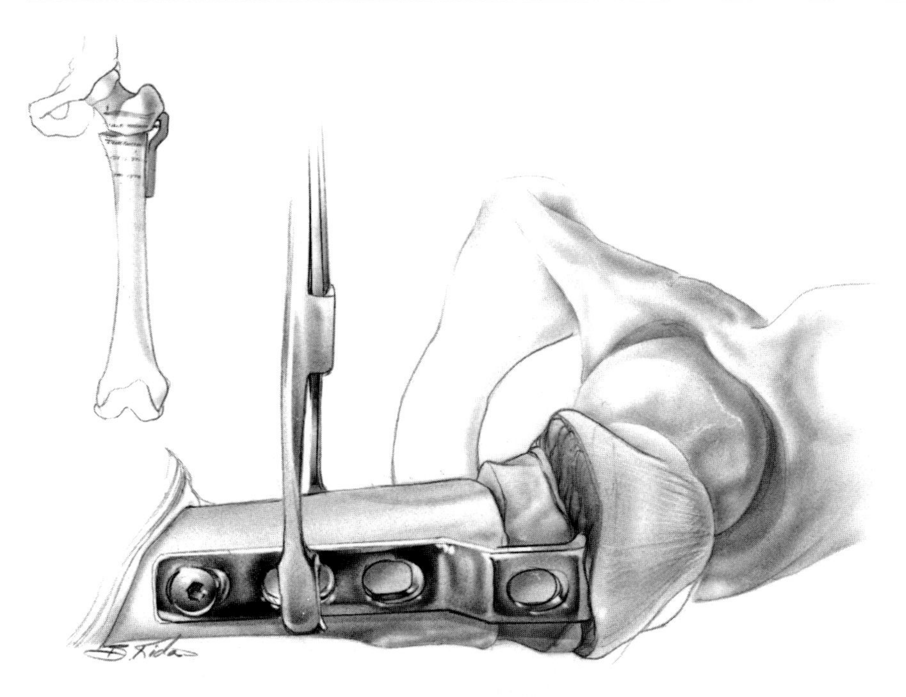

Figure 3–29

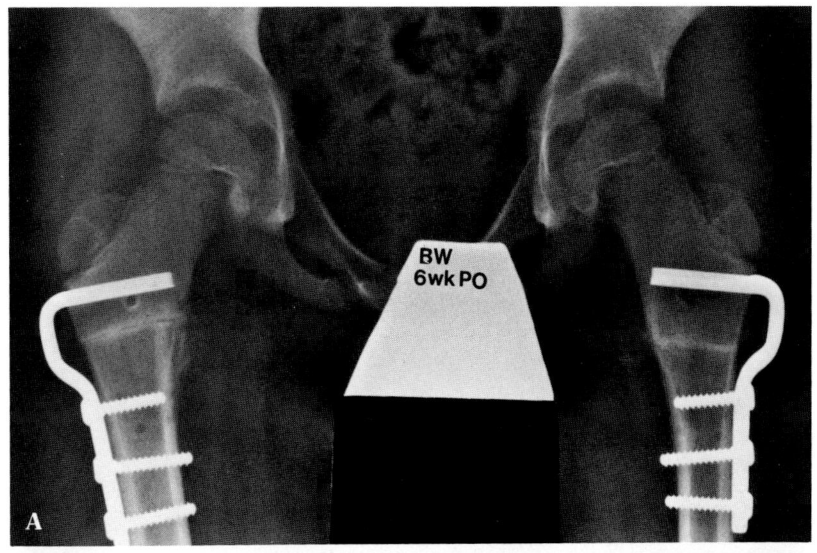

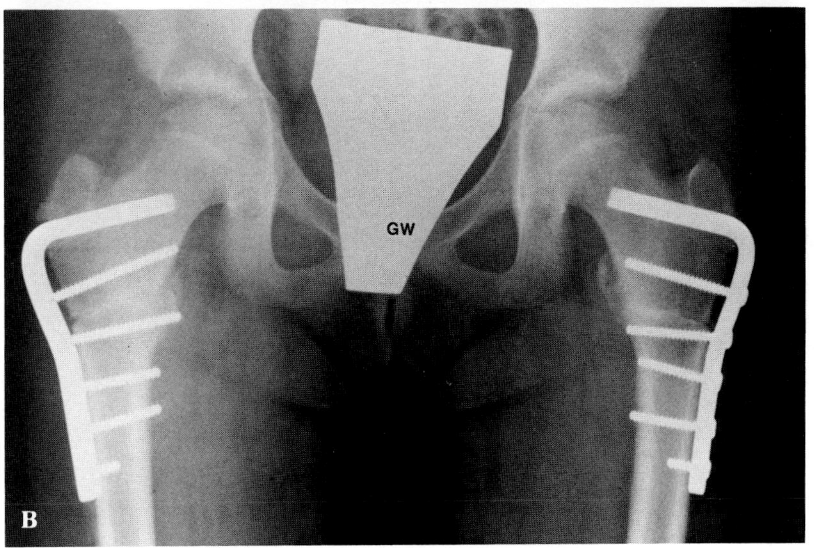

Figure 3–30

3.5 Southwick's Intertrochanteric Osteotomy

Although Southwick[1] originally described this biplane osteotomy as a means of primary treatment for chronic slips greater than 30 degrees, it is most often used today to correct residual deformity resulting from SCFE after in situ fixation.[2] The osteotomy is designed to create valgus and flexion, to which is added internal rotation of the distal fragment.

Chondrolysis has been described as a complication following this osteotomy.[2] In addition, it has gained a reputation as an osteotomy that is difficult to perform both from the aspect of the osteotomy itself and the method of fixation. A more important limitation of this and other osteotomies designed to correct severe deformity resulting from SCFE is the fact that they usually cannot produce enough change to correct the deformity completely. This does not negate the fact, however, that they can produce a considerable improvement in the range of motion.

The author has made three modifications in his use of the operation as originally described by Southwick. First, rather than removing a wedge of bone that spans one half of the width of the femoral shaft, the author fashions the wedge to include the entire diameter of the bone. This results in some shortening that Southwick attempted to avoid. In closing the osteotomy, however, some lengthening of the leg is achieved. Because of the adaptive shortening of the muscles and other tissues about the hip, this results in considerable pressure in the joint unless some shortening is achieved. If the osteotomy is difficult to close, additional bone is removed to reduce the pressure in the hip joint. Second, only the maximum wedge is removed. This avoids difficulty in complex estimates of the correct amount of bone to remove and is valid because this osteotomy is only done for severe slips. Third, rigid internal fixation with an angled plate is used.

Figure 3–31. The intertrochanteric area of the proximal femur is exposed as described for a varus intertrochanteric osteotomy. Care must be taken to expose the lesser trochanter adequately because release of the iliopsoas tendon is a part of this procedure.

Marks outlining the desired wedges are scored on the femoral shaft using an osteotome or saw. First, a vertical line is scored in the femoral shaft separating the anterior from the lateral femoral shaft (**a**).

Next, the base of the wedge is marked. It is the same on the lateral and anterior femoral surface and corresponds to a line perpendicular to the femoral shaft just cephalad to the lesser trochanter (**b**). (This is the same as the definitive osteotomy line [**b**] used in planning an intertrochanteric osteotomy.)

It now remains to determine the wedge that will be removed anteriorly to produce flexion and the wedge that will be removed laterally to produce valgus. The maximum angle of the Southwick templates is 45 degrees anteriorly (**c**) and 60 degrees laterally (**d**). This represents the maximum wedges that can be removed. The author prefers to use the angle templates from the Synthes osteotomy set to mark these wedges. They are marked to describe a wedge that will include the entire diameter of the femoral shaft.

Figure 3–32. The iliopsoas tendon will have to be released in most cases to reduce the tension on the osteotomy and lessen the pressure in the hip joint. This is done in a semiblind fashion. A Bennett retractor placed at the site of the lesser trochanter is twisted to push the soft tissues away. The iliopsoas tendon is now easily palpated and can be sectioned by using a #12 Bard-Parker knife blade.

Figure 3–33. Before the osteotomy is made, it is necessary to gain control of the proximal fragment. A large, smooth pin is drilled into the superior aspect of the greater trochanter aiming posteriorly. This gives good fixation and keeps this pin out of the path of the seating chisel.

The first cut is through the base of the osteotomy (**b**). This cut should be made to the medial cortex, which is best left intact until the other cut is made.

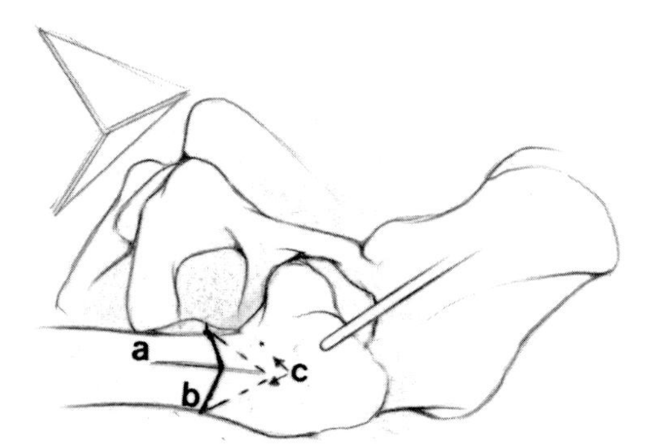

Figure 3–31

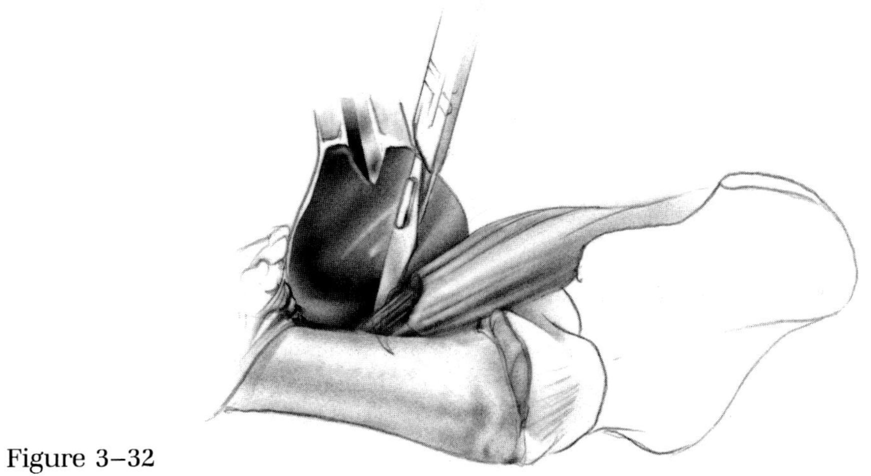

Figure 3–32

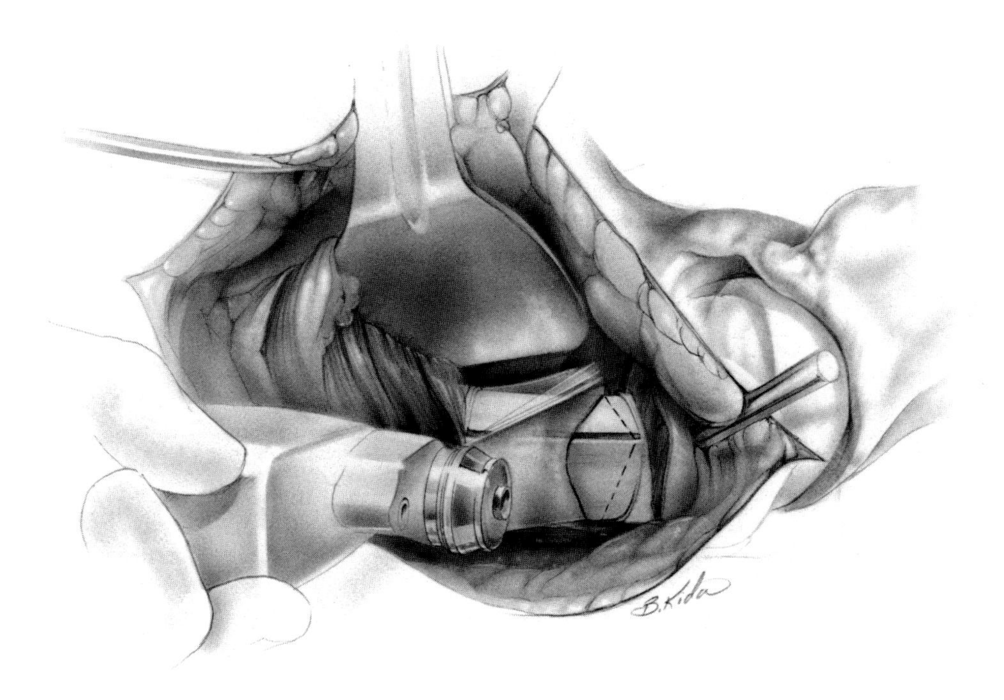

Figure 3–33

Figure 3–34. Confusion often arises in attempting to remove two separate wedges, one lateral and one medial. Rather, the next cut should remove one wedge—both the medial and lateral wedge as one piece. This is accomplished by starting the saw on the line separating the anterior and lateral aspects of the femoral shaft (see ***Figure 3–31a***). It is angled in such a way as to include both wedges, aiming toward the first cut at the medial cortex.

Figure 3–35. With the wedge of bone removed, the osteotomy is completed through the medial cortex and is ready to be closed. This is best accomplished by a combination of maneuvers. First, the support of the fracture table that holds the leg is both raised to produce flexion and abducted to produce valgus. The pin in the greater trochanter is used at the same time to pull the proximal fragment down, thus closing the osteotomy. Now the leg can be internally rotated the desired amount. This will usually not exceed 30 degrees and can be accurately noted by placing two pins on either side of the osteotomy as described for rotational intertrochanteric osteotomy.

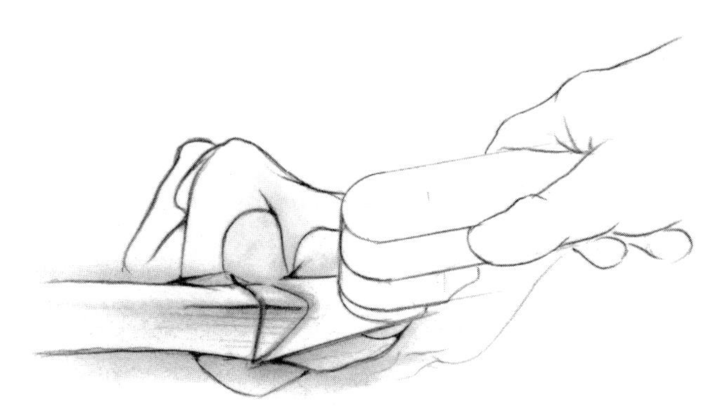

Figure 3–34

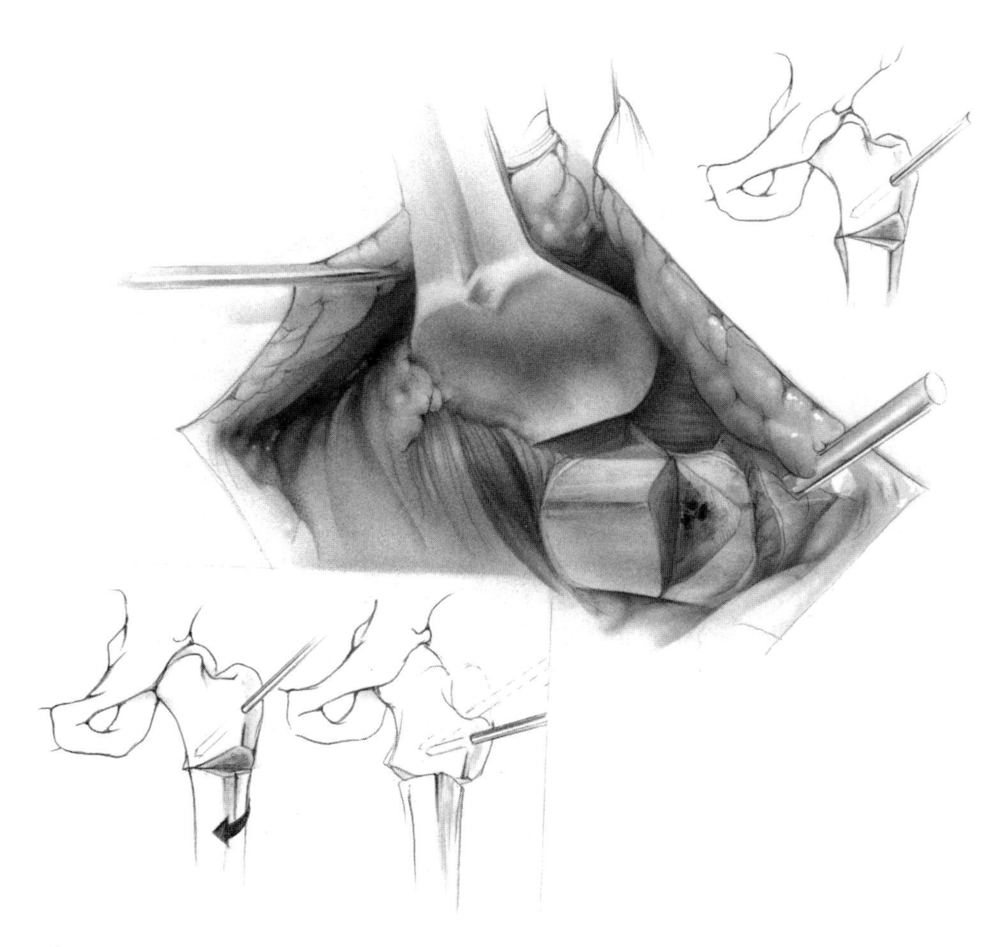

Figure 3–35

Figure 3–36. With the osteotomy held closed by an assistant using the heavy pin, the steps used to insert the blade plate as described in the technique of varus intertrochanteric osteotomy are performed. The angled plate used depends on the configuration of the bone at the completion of the osteotomy. The author has used both the 90-degree angled plate and the 120-degree repositioning plate.

For those with considerable experience in the use of the blade plates, there is an alternate method of inserting the blade and reducing the osteotomy. The 90-degree blade plate is designed so that the blade is inserted into the proximal fragment 1 to 1.5 cm proximal to the osteotomy cut, and the blade is kept parallel to the plane of the osteotomy cut in the proximal fragment. Thus, if the blade is inserted into the proximal fragment starting 1 to 1.5 cm proximal to the osteotomy and the flat surface of the blade is kept parallel to the plane of the osteotomy cut in the proximal fragment, when the osteotomy is closed, the plate will lie in correct apposition to the lateral aspect of the distal fragment, and the osteotomy will be closed.

At least four screws should attach the plate to the femoral shaft to provide sufficient fixation to avoid the need for a cast. The wound is closed and drained as for other intertrochanteric osteotomies.

Figure 3–37. ED is a 13-year-old boy with bilateral SCFE. He was initially treated with in situ fixation using a single cannulated screw (***Figure 3–37A***). After 18 months he still had −25 degrees of internal rotation in each hip, and flexion was limited to 60 degrees bilaterally. He was treated with bilateral Southwick osteotomies done 3 months apart at the patient's request to permit continued ambulation. The osteotomies were fixed with 90-degree angled blade plates (***Figure 3–37B***). This permitted early weight bearing and resulted in prompt healing of the osteotomies.

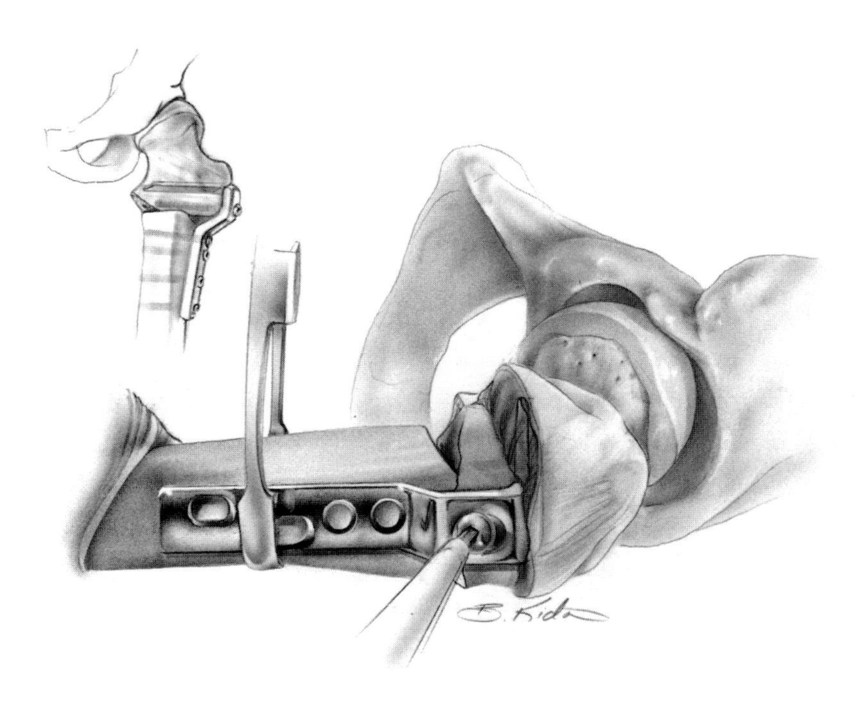

Figure 3–36

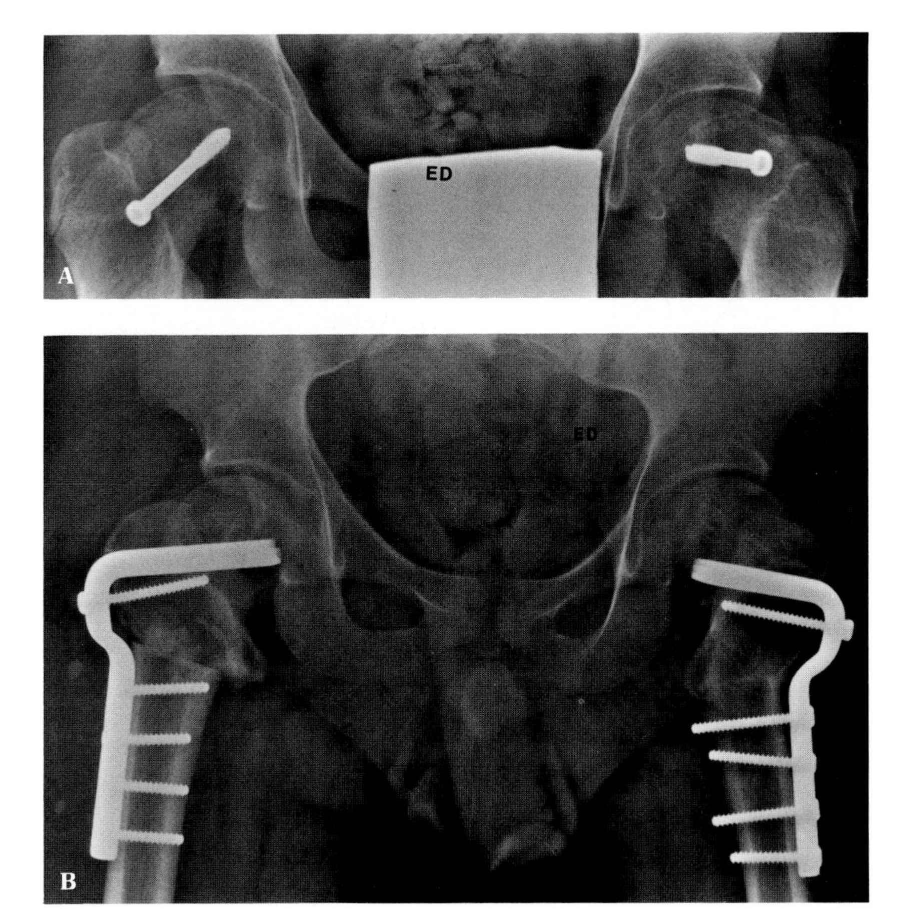

Figure 3–37

POSTOPERATIVE CARE

It is usually both undesirable and unnecessary to use a cast following a Southwick osteotomy that is adequately fixed. If there are questions about the patient's ability to comply with a partial weight-bearing crutch gait, bed rest and wheelchair may be used for the first 6 weeks. Full weight bearing is permitted at the first signs of radiographic healing, usually 6 to 8 weeks. Range-of-motion exercises are started from the first postoperative day and progress to muscle strengthening exercises as healing nears completion.

REFERENCES

1. Southwick WO. Osteotomy through the lesser trochanter for slipped capital femoral epiphysis. J Bone Joint Surg 1967;49A:807.
2. Morrissy RT. Slipped capital femoral epiphysis. In: Morrissy RT, ed. Lovell and Winter's pediatric orthopaedics. Philadelphia: JB Lippincott, 1989:897–900.

3.6 Transfer of Greater Trochanter

Whenever the growth of the proximal femoral physis is disrupted and that of the greater trochanter is not, an imbalance of the abductor musculature will result. This most often occurs as a result of Perthes's disease or avascular necrosis following treatment of congenital dislocation of the hip. The imbalance occurs because of the shortened resting length of the muscle as the insertion approaches the origin altering Blix's curve. It is important to recognize that the effectiveness of the abductor musculature is not only dependent on the height of the greater trochanter relative to the femoral head but also the distance of the greater trochanter from the center of the femoral head, which is the lever arm through which the force works.

Under normal circumstances the tip of the greater trochanter lies on a horizontal line connecting the center of the femoral heads and lateral to it by a distance that is equal to two to two-and-one-half times the radius of the femoral head.[1] Both of these relationships are important to the surgeon who is planning a transfer of the greater trochanter.

The indication for the operation should be based on clinical symptoms and findings in preference to the radiographic findings. A gluteus medius limp, especially after walking or standing, that is unacceptable to the patient is the usual indication. This situation will often be associated with a deformity of the femoral neck or acetabulum. It is usually possible and preferable to correct all of these abnormalities at the same operation. It is not advisable to operate on the radiographic findings of relative trochanteric overgrowth in the absence of clinical symptoms or findings. Despite the fact that this operation is not uncommon, there have been few reports in the English literature on the results of transfer of the greater trochanter to correct the clinical problem of a gluteus medius limp.[2,3]

Epiphysiodesis of the greater trochanter has been advocated as a method of preventing relative overgrowth of the greater trochanter in young patients, generally under 8 years of age.[4] This often seems to destroy the important lateral growth of the greater trochanter, however, and thus neglects one of the important biomechanical parameters of abductor function. Therefore, the author's preference is to wait until approximately 10 years of age when the trochanter is a sizable piece of bone whose transfer will result in lateral displacement.

Figure 3–38. As the patient is usually older when this procedure is performed, it is easier to operate with the patient on a fracture table. This permits good radiographic control and frees the surgeon from struggling with a large leg. The image intensifier should be positioned on the opposite side of the operating table for an unobstructed anteroposterior view of the femoral head and greater trochanteric region. In addition, the leg should be internally rotated so that the trochanter is directly lateral (***Figure 3–37A***) rather than behind the femoral shaft (***Figure 3–37B***). With the greater trochanter now in profile the epiphyseal plate (if present) should be clearly seen as a single straight line. This will make it easy to detach the entire greater trochanter through the epiphyseal plate with the guidance of the image intensifier.

A straight lateral incision is used extending from the tip of the greater trochanter distally for a distance that will allow sufficient exposure for the new location of the greater trochanter. The exposure is the same as for an intertrochanteric femoral osteotomy including elevation of the vastus lateralis from the lateral femoral shaft.

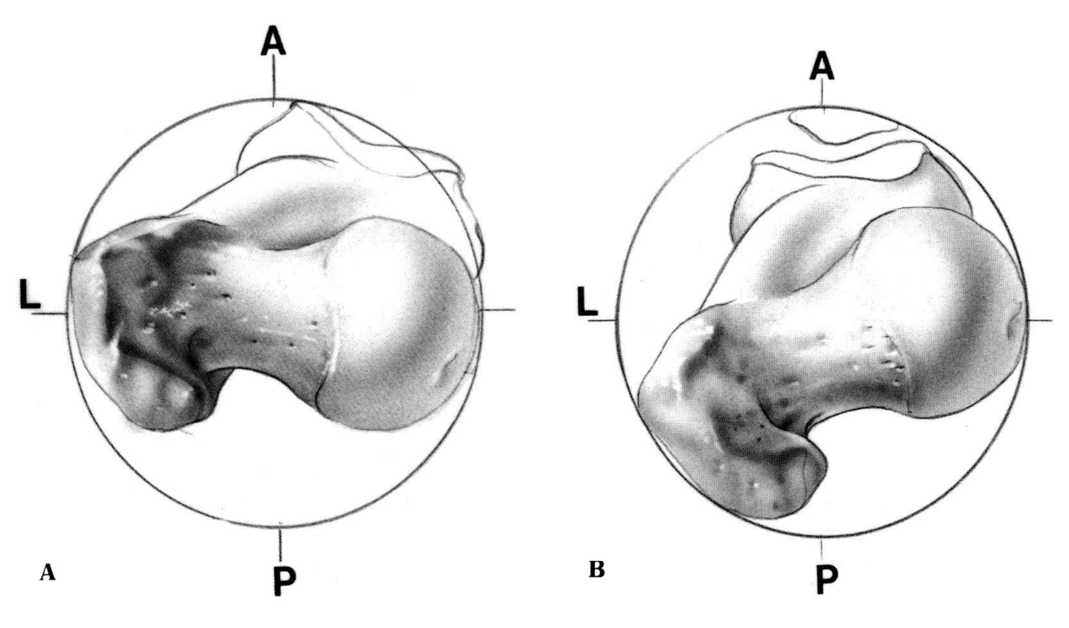

Figure 3–38

Figure 3–39. The anterior edge of the abductor muscles is identified and freed by blunt dissection. If the surgeon desires, a blunt elevator (*eg*, a Cushing or Crego elevator) can be passed between the abductor muscles and the capsule of the hip joint (***Figure 3–39A***). To accomplish this the elevator is passed beneath the abductor muscles, staying in close contact with the capsule over the femoral neck and aiming toward the trochanteric fossa. This step is not necessary if image intensification is available but is very useful if it is not. The posterior border of the abductor muscles can be identified by blunt dissection.

A Kirschner wire is now drilled into the greater trochanter to serve as a guide for the osteotomy (***Figure 3–39B***). In most circumstances this wire will lie along a line extending from the femoral neck. It can be placed under image intensifier control. Because of the location of the critical anastomosis of the ascending medial and lateral femoral circumflex arteries at the base of the femoral neck it is important to avoid drilling this wire completely through the bone (***Figure 3–39A***). It is important that as much bone as possible be included in the trochanteric fragment since lateral displacement is an important component of the transfer.

Figure 3–40. A retractor is placed posteriorly to protect the tissues while the elevator under the abductor muscles or another retractor protects the tissues anteriorly. An oscillating saw or an osteotome is used to create the osteotomy. However it is best if the saw does not penetrate the cortex to avoid damaging the vessels. An osteotome is used to crack through the remaining cortex, creating a "green stick" type of fracture. The greater trochanter can be elevated and pulled cephalad by grasping it with a large bone-holding forceps.

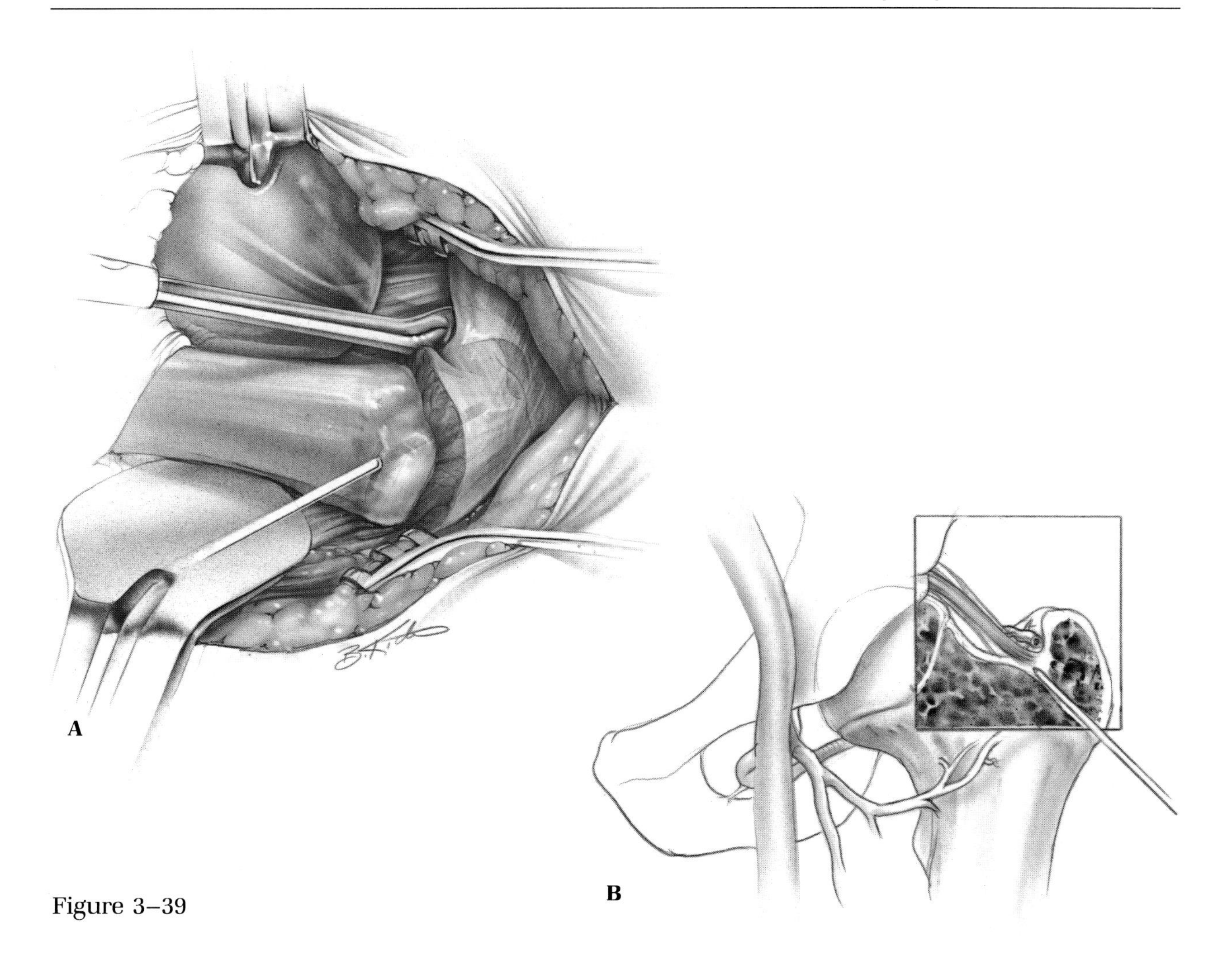

Figure 3–39

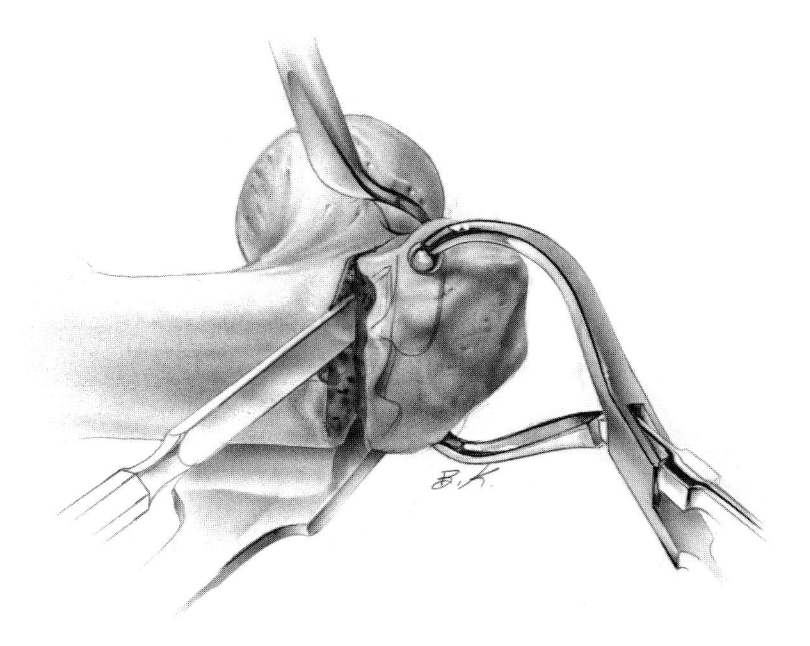

Figure 3–40

Figure 3–41. At first the trochanter will seem to be rigidly tethered with no sense of stretch when it is pulled. This is because of the fibrous connections between the muscle and the hip capsule. These fibrous connections and adhesions will have to be carefully released. This can be achieved with a combination of sharp and blunt dissection with care to avoid cutting in to the muscle or damaging the retinacular vessels. When there is a feeling of elasticity as the trochanter is pulled, the release is complete.

Figure 3–42. After roughening the cortex of the area to which the trochanter is to be transferred and contouring the surface of the fragment to provide good contact with the femur, the leg is abducted. The trochanteric fragment is then placed in the desired area and secured with two Kirschner wires. The use of a large bone hook to pull the greater trochanter distally avoids the complication of splitting the bone when a penetrating bone-holding clamp is used to grasp the bone. At this point the location of the trochanter can be verified with the image intensifier. Ideally the tip of the trochanter should lie on a horizontal line connecting the center of the femoral heads and be about two to two-and-one-half times the radius of the femoral head lateral to the center of the femoral head.

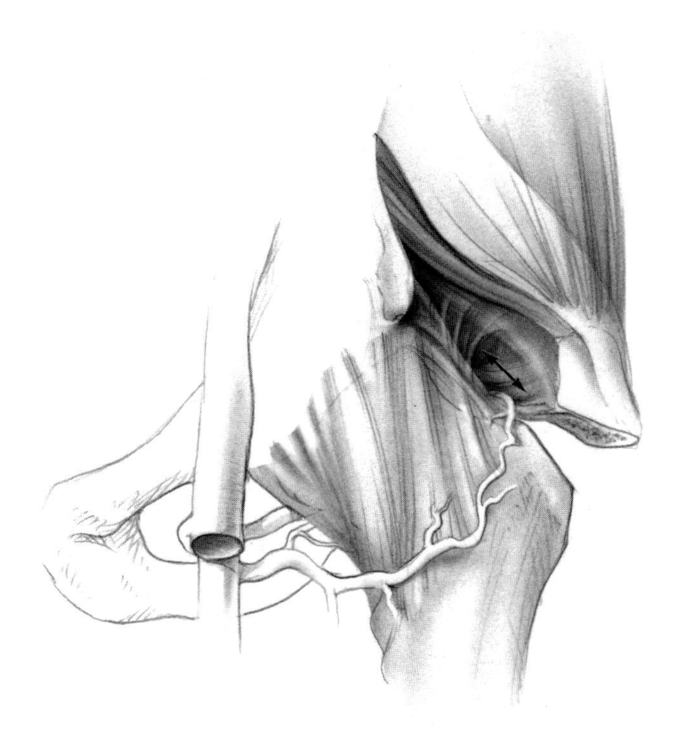

Figure 3–41

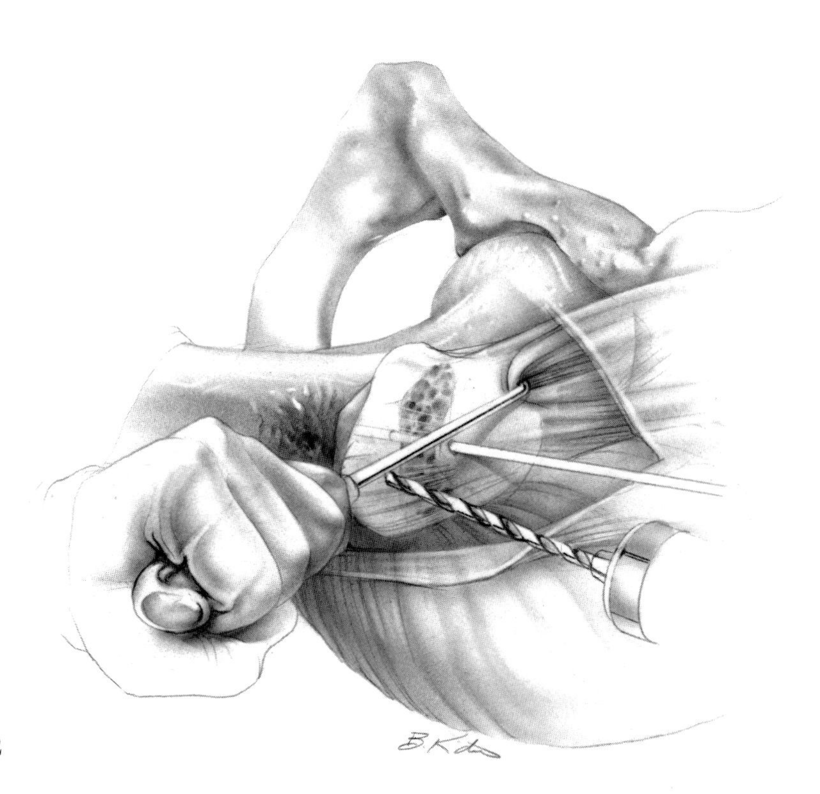

Figure 3–42

Figure 3–43. The trochanter is now fixed with two strong screws with washers. These screws should be directed distally and medially, and should penetrate the medial cortex. If the surgeon is unsure of the fixation, a tension band can also be used. The wound is closed in a routine manner over a drain.

Figure 3–44. Radiograph of a patient with a severe SCFE who underwent a Southwick osteotomy to correct the residual deformity (***Figure 3–44A***). This radiograph 6 months after the Southwick osteotomy demonstrates what turned out to be a delayed union with some loss of correction. This does not account for the entire problem with the trochanter, however: The varus component of the deformity was so severe that the largest wedge possible could not provide complete correction. One year after Southwick osteotomy, the bone had healed and the patient was very satisfied with his range of motion. He retained the abductor lurch during gait, however, which he had before the Southwick.

Three months following transfer of the greater trochanter (***Figure 3–44B***), the patient's abductor lurch was almost completely eliminated. Note that although the tip of the greater trochanter does not lie at the ideal level in relation to the femoral head, it has been lateralized to a significant degree.

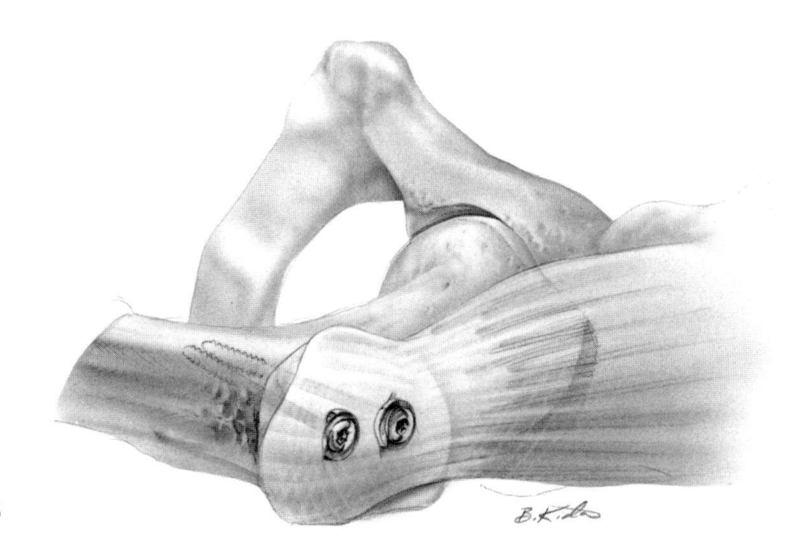

Figure 3–43

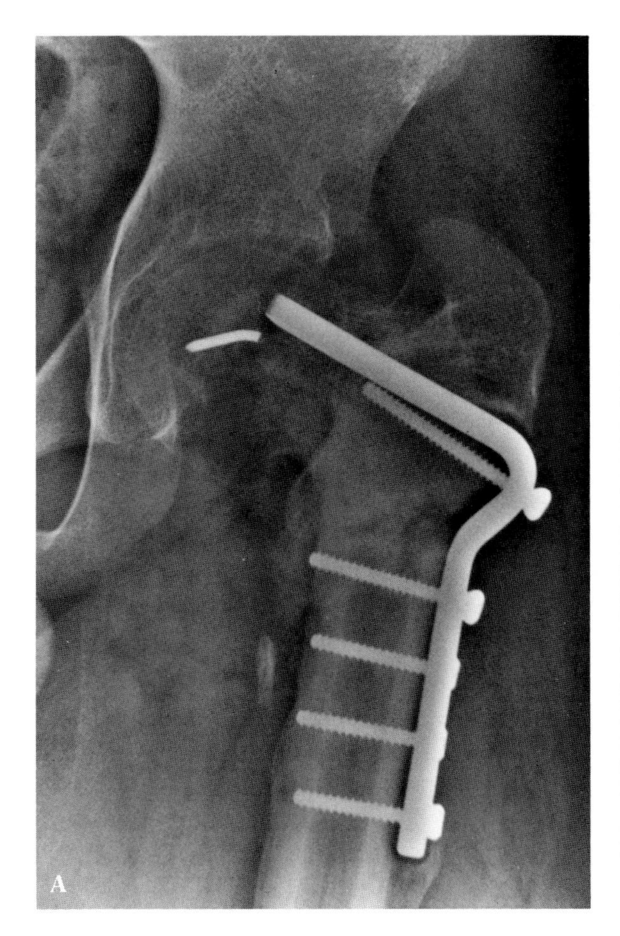

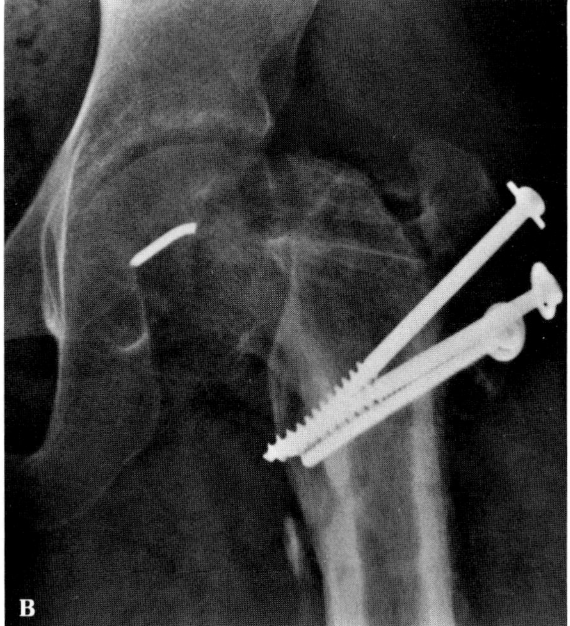

Figure 3–44

POSTOPERATIVE CARE

The patient is placed in traction with the leg slightly flexed and in abduction. Physical therapy begins passive and active-assisted motion the morning after surgery. By the second postoperative day the patient is usually ready to begin ambulation with a three-point partial weight-bearing crutch gait. The abduction contracture will gradually disappear. When healing of the fragment is confirmed radiographically, the patient is started on exercises to strengthen the abductor and extensor muscles around the hip. It is not unusual for it to take 6 months for the patient to recover full strength in the abductor muscles and for the lurching gait to disappear.

REFERENCES

1. Wagner H. Femoral osteotomies for congenital hip dislocation. In: Weil UH, ed. Progress in orthopaedic surgery, vol. 2. Acetabular dysplasia and skeletal dysplasia in childhood. Heidelberg: Springer, 1978:99–102.
2. Kelikian AS, Tachdjian MO, Askew MJ, Jasty M. Greater trochanteric advancement of the proximal femur: a clinical and biomechanical study. In: Hungerford DS, ed. The hip: proceedings of the 11th open scientific meeting of The Hip Society. St. Louis, CV Mosby, 1987:77–105.
3. Tauber C, Ganel A, Horoszowski H, Farine I. Distal transfer of the greater trocanter in coxa vara. Acta Orthop Scand 1980;51:611.
4. Langenskiold A, Salenius P. Epiphysiodesis of the greater trochanter. Acta Orthop Scand 1967;38:199.

3.7
Closed Intramedullary Femoral Shortening

Despite current trends, shortening is often preferable to lengthening in the femur as a means of achieving leg-length equalization for the patient at or near skeletal maturity. Closed intramedullary shortening of the femur is preferable to open techniques because morbidity is less and immediate weight bearing possible. Many surgeons are now familiar with the technique of closed intramedullary rodding for fixation of femur fractures, making this technique a viable option for an increasing number of surgeons who wish to learn it. In the hands of a surgeon skilled in the use of closed intramedullary shortening, this technique can also be applied to rotational femoral osteotomies and the correction of some angular deformities.

The key to the procedure is the intramedullary bone saw. This was initially developed by Kuntscher in 1962 and greatly improved by Robert Winquist working with the Boeing Company in 1973.[1] This saw allows a segment of bone to be cut from the diaphysis of the femur using the usual incision in the buttocks that is used for closed femoral rodding.

The procedure may be indicated in any patient at or near skeletal maturity who has a leg-length discrepancy of 6 cm or less that requires equalization. Shortening of greater than 6 cm is not advised because of the difficulty in quadriceps rehabilitation with greater shortening. A more detailed description of the preoperative clinical assessment and indications is given by Winquist[2] and Blair et al.[3] Winquist has also written more recently about the details of the shortening procedure as well as the use of this technique in rotational and angular corrective osteotomies of the femur.[4]

Figure 3–45. An anteroposterior and lateral radiograph of the entire femur is necessary for preoperative planning. Measurements should be made with a translucent ossimeter (Biomet, Warsaw, IN), which accounts for the magnification on the radiograph.

On the anteroposterior view, the narrowest intramedullary diameter should be identified. In the case illustrated, it is 9 mm. The segment of bone to be removed is marked on the radiograph, an equal portion (2 cm in this case) being taken from each side of the narrowest point. The width of the intramedullary canal and the outside diameter of the cortex is now measured 2.5 cm proximal and distal to these proposed osteotomy sites. It is desirable that a rod of sufficient width be used that provides secure fixation in this 2.5-cm section proximal and distal to the osteotomy. The largest diameter is proximal and measures 13 cm. It can also be noted that the cortex is quite thick in this region. Therefore, a 14- or 15-mm rod will be necessary for secure fixation. If it is determined that this area will be too wide for the widest available rod, an interlocking rod should be used to achieve rotational stability.

On the lateral view note should be taken of any unusual bow because this will cause eccentric reaming of the femur. The thickness of the linea aspera should be measured. This will be the thickest part of the femur, and this measurement will help to determine how much reaming is necessary to allow passage of a saw large enough to cut through the linea aspera.

Finally, the length of the rod is determined. The distance from the tip of the greater trochanter to the epiphyseal scar of the distal femur is measured. From this the amount to be shortened is subtracted. An additional 2 cm can be subtracted because a slightly shorter nail will lessen the tendency to distract the osteotomy site and will not result in substantial loss of fixation.

Figure 3–46. The intramedullary bone saw set is required equipment in addition to all of the equipment necessary for closed intramedullary femoral rodding.

The saw consists of two shafts: an inner one with a saw blade on the end and an outer one with a bushing set eccentrically on it just proximal to the saw blade. This bushing fits tightly inside the medullary canal. The size of the bushing on the saw defines the size of the saw, which ranges from 12 to 17 mm. In reality the size of the bushing is 0.5 mm smaller than the stated size—thus, it will fit into a canal reamed to the stated size. On the shaft opposite the saw blade is a T handle, an indexing scale marked 1 through 20, and a spring loaded index scale locking nut. This T handle rotates the saw blade out from behind the bushing. There is a measuring device on a threaded portion of the outer shaft. It consists of a trochanteric rest distally and a locking nut proximally. The use of this part of the saw to measure the amount of bone to be removed will be illustrated and described in ***Figure 3–53***.

The intramedullary chisel is a sharp, thick hook on the end of a strong rod. This is hooked on the distal end of the piece of bone to be split and driven out of the bone with the slotted hammer. Because the piece of bone to be split is a rigid ring, splitting one side of it will result in the other side of it splitting (see ***Figure 3–55***).

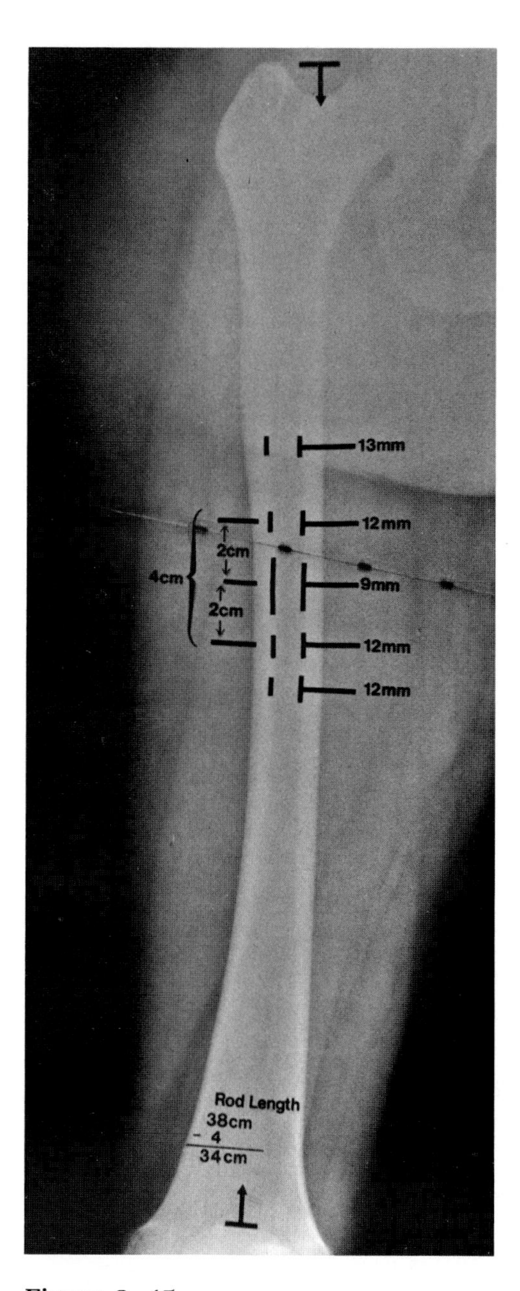

Figure 3–45

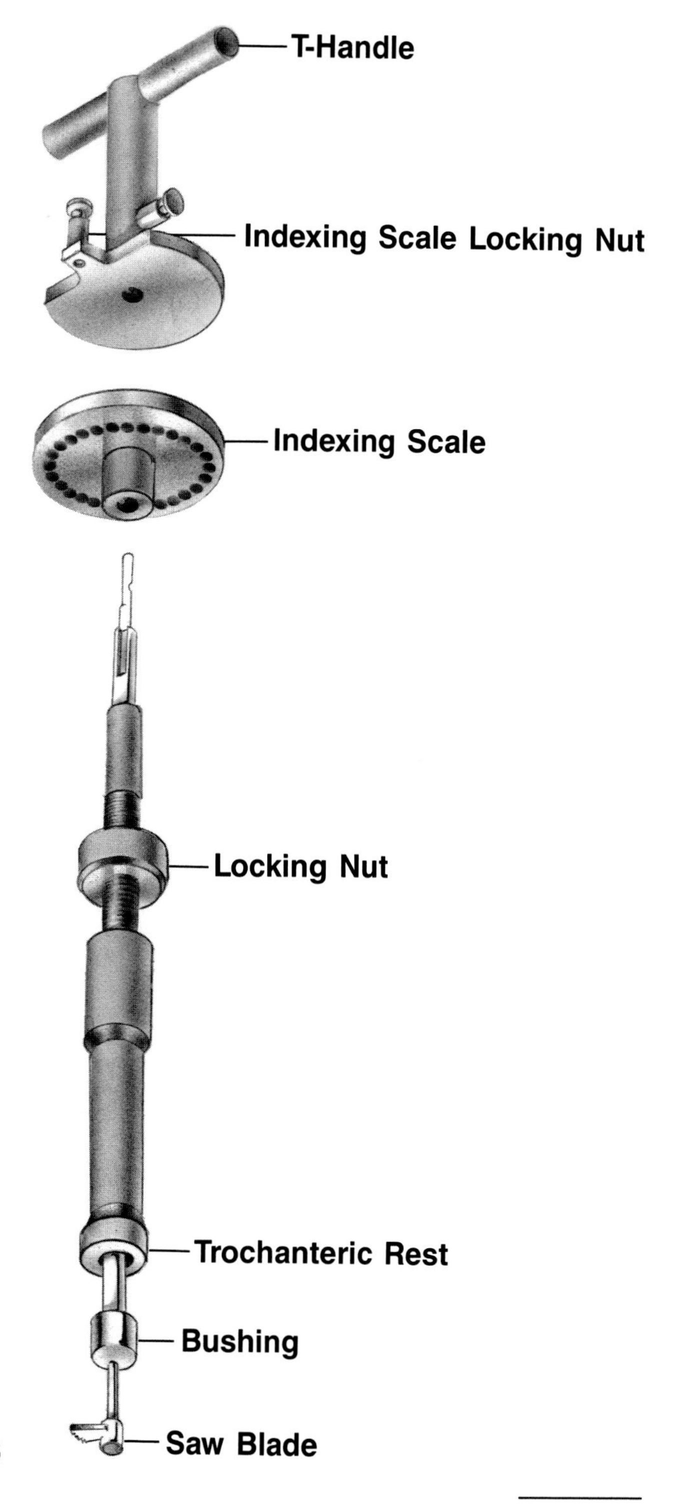

Figure 3–46

Figure 3–47. The operation begins as for any closed intramedullary rodding of the femur. The patient is placed on a suitable fracture table in either the supine or lateral position as the surgeon prefers. The gluteal area and leg down to and slightly below the osteotomy site is prepared. The reason for preparing the limb down to the osteotomy site is in case of the need to insert a percutaneous osteotome as will be described later. A transparent plastic barrier drape is ideal for draping the sterile field. The image intensifier is checked in both the anterior and lateral plane to be certain that an unobstructed view of the entire femur can be seen.

A 4-cm incision is made on the buttocks beginning 1 cm proximal to the tip of the greater trochanter and in line with the femoral shaft. This is deepened through the subcutaneous fat to expose the fascia of the gluteus muscles. The fascia is split sharply in the direction of the muscle fibers, and the muscle fibers are split bluntly exposing the tip of the greater trochanter and allowing palpation of the piriformis fossa.

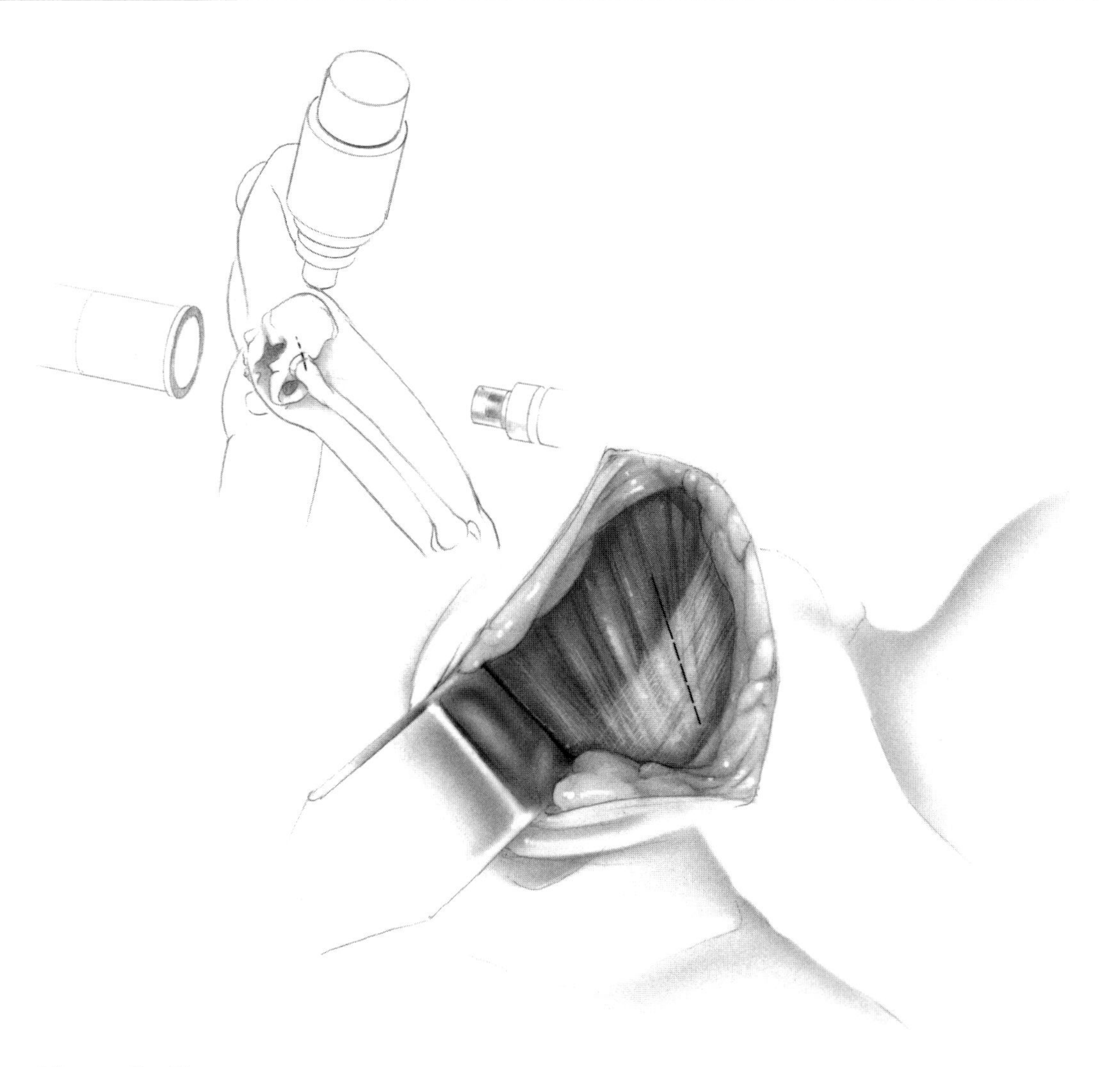

Figure 3–47

Figure 3–48. The T-handled awl is used to start the hole for reaming. It is of critical importance that this be in the correct place, just medial to the tip of the greater trochanter and slightly anterior to the piriformis fossa. This should be checked with the image intensifier in both the anterior-posterior and lateral plane.

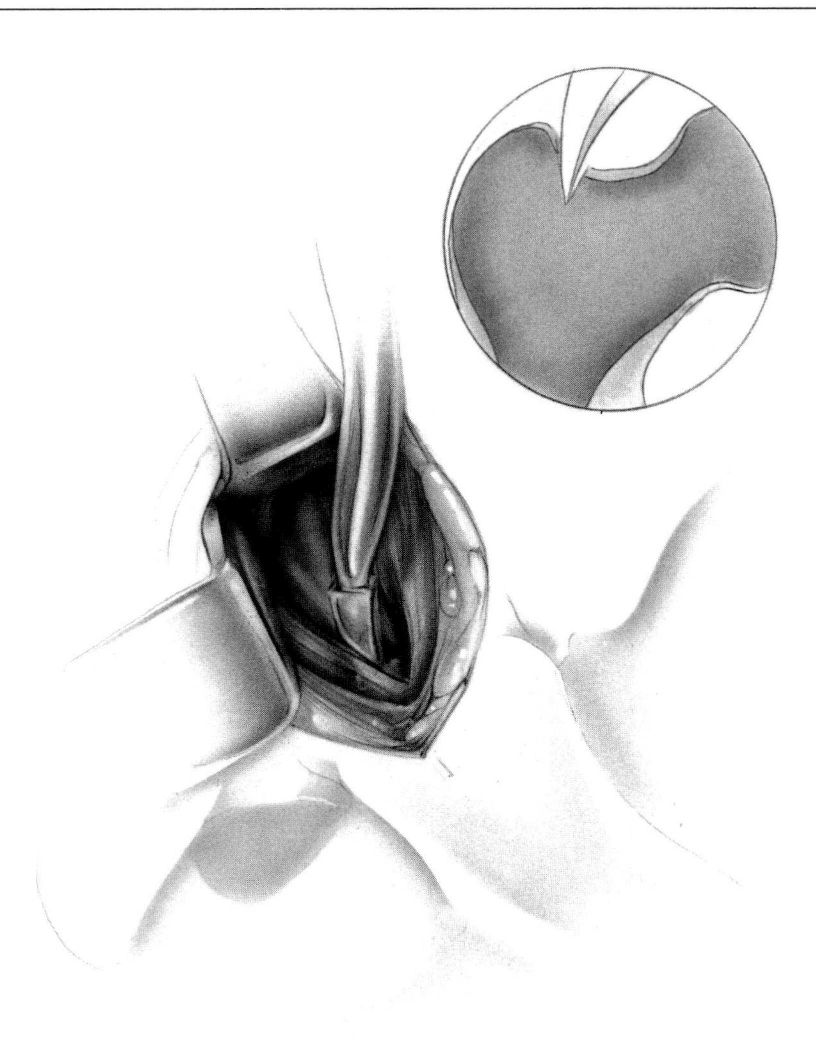

Figure 3–48

Figure 3–49. After this hole has been made, the bulb tip guide is passed to the distal end of the femur and reaming is started with the 8-mm reamer. Reaming can be continued in 1-mm increments until cortical bone is encountered, and then it progresses in 0.5-mm increments until the desired size reamer is reached. Reaming should be monitored on the lateral view because the anterior cortex will be thinned the most, and excessive thinning of this cortex should be avoided.

Reaming will deposit a large amount of bone distally within the medullary space, and this will interfere with the final few centimeters of rod passage causing distraction at the osteotomy site. This problem can be lessened by passing a 12.5-mm end-cutting reamer down the canal as the final reamer. This will help to remove the bone debris. To make passage of the saw easier, the proximal 3-cm of the femur can be over-reamed an additional 0.5 mm.

Figure 3–50. The saw is now advanced down the medullary canal. The distal cut is made first. The measuring device is set to allow the saw to pass down the shaft to the distance that was determined on the preoperative radiographs. This can be checked on the image intensifier; however, this will not be as precise. It is of critical importance that the trochanteric rest be held firmly against the tip of the greater trochanter at all times. Not only is this the reference point for all measurements, but it also ensures that the saw remains in the same cut in the bone.

To begin the osteotomy, the index scale locking nut is pulled back, and the indexing scale advanced one hole past the 0 mark. The T handle is then used to turn the saw through one or two complete revolutions. The osteotomy proceeds by advancing the indexing scale one hole at a time. Each time after it is advanced, the saw is turned 360 degrees, cutting a small thickness of the bone. Each time the indexing scale is advanced, the saw will protrude slightly more. When the saw has been advanced to 20 on the indexing device, it has reached its maximum penetration. The indexing device is now returned to 0, and the saw is withdrawn.

Occasionally, after the anterior cortex has been cut through, the saw will catch when it is rotated. Be certain that the measuring device is still firmly held against the tip of the trochanter. If this fails to correct the problem, retract the saw three or four stops and then begin to advance it one stop at a time. Care should be used because it is possible to break the saw.

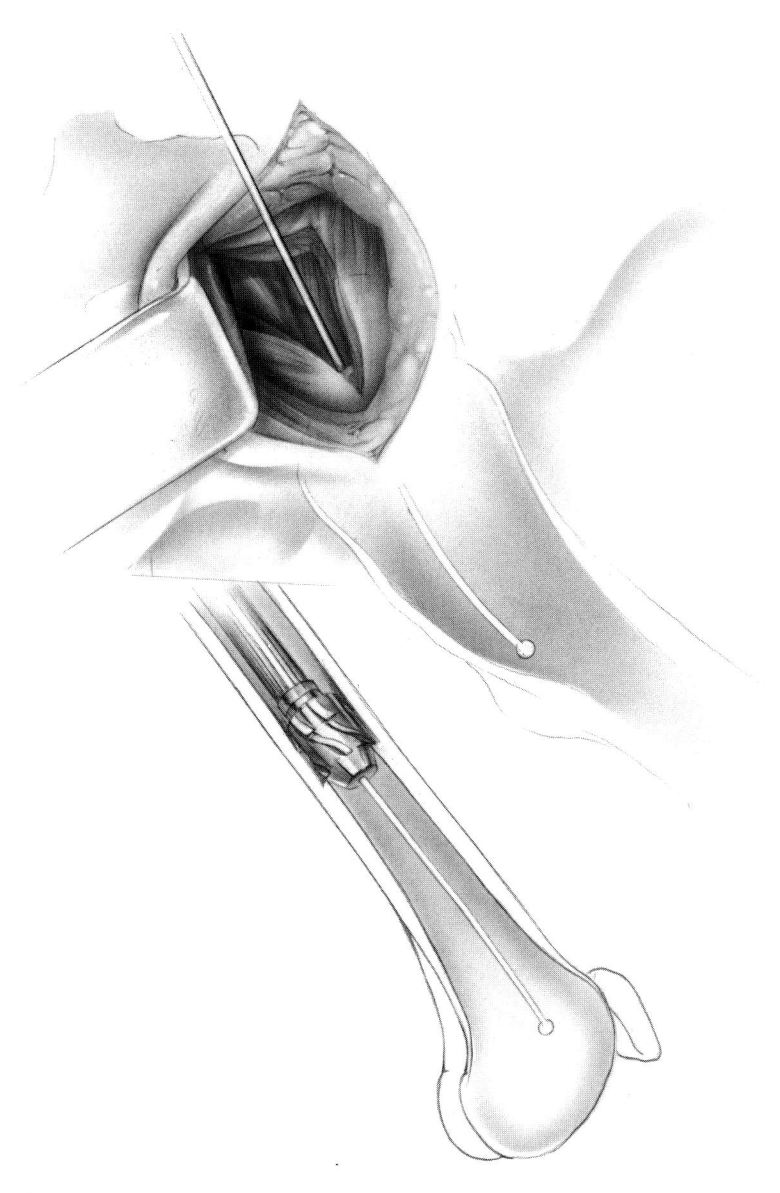

Figure 3–49

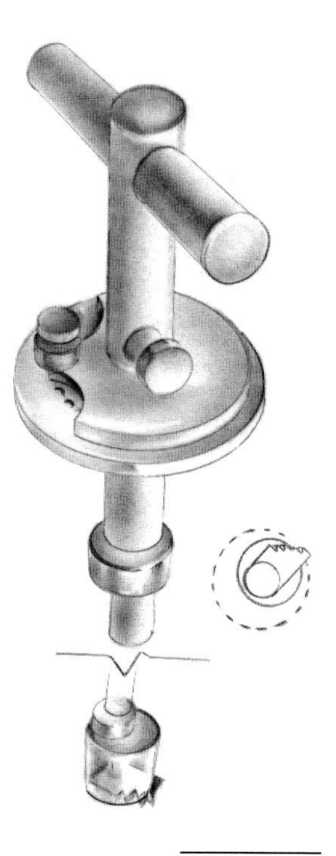

Figure 3–50

Figure 3–51. At this point osteoclasis of the femur is accomplished. This is a critical step in the operation. It is important that the periosteum be completely torn and stripped from the segment of bone that is to be removed. If this is not accomplished, it may not be possible to push the fragments of bone out of the way to allow shortening of the femur.

Osteoclasis is performed by the unscrubbed surgeon who is probably the most important individual in this operation. He removes the foot from traction, and with the knee in extension, bends the femur into varus to complete the osteotomy. Next, the two fragments of the femoral shaft are reduced, and the knee is flexed to 90 degrees to relax the sciatic nerve. Now the distal fragment is hyperextended at the osteotomy site to tear the linea aspera. The distal fragment is then bent into 60 to 70 degrees of valgus and then into the same amount of varus. With the osteotomy site held in valgus and then varus, the unscrubbed surgeon pushes the distal fragment cephalad to strip the periosteum from the fragment that will later be split and pushed to the side. Complete displacement and overlapping of the femoral fragments should be verified on the image intensifier. During this procedure the intramedullary saw should not be used to stabilize the proximal fragment as it may bend or break. If stabilization is necessary, a small intramedullary rod is passed down the canal to the site of the osteotomy.

Figure 3–52. In some circumstances the femur may not break. This is usually because the saw has failed to cut through the linea aspera. There are two ways to deal with this problem. The canal can be reamed larger, and a larger saw inserted. If this is not possible, the osteotomy can be completed by inserting a $\frac{1}{4}$-in osteotome through a stab wound in the lateral thigh over the osteotomy site. The osteotome is passed into the osteotomy site under image-intensifier guidance. The osteotome is then maneuvered posteriorly toward the linea aspera. With a firm grasp on the osteotome and the hand firmly against the thigh, the osteotome is struck sharply with a mallet to complete the osteotomy.

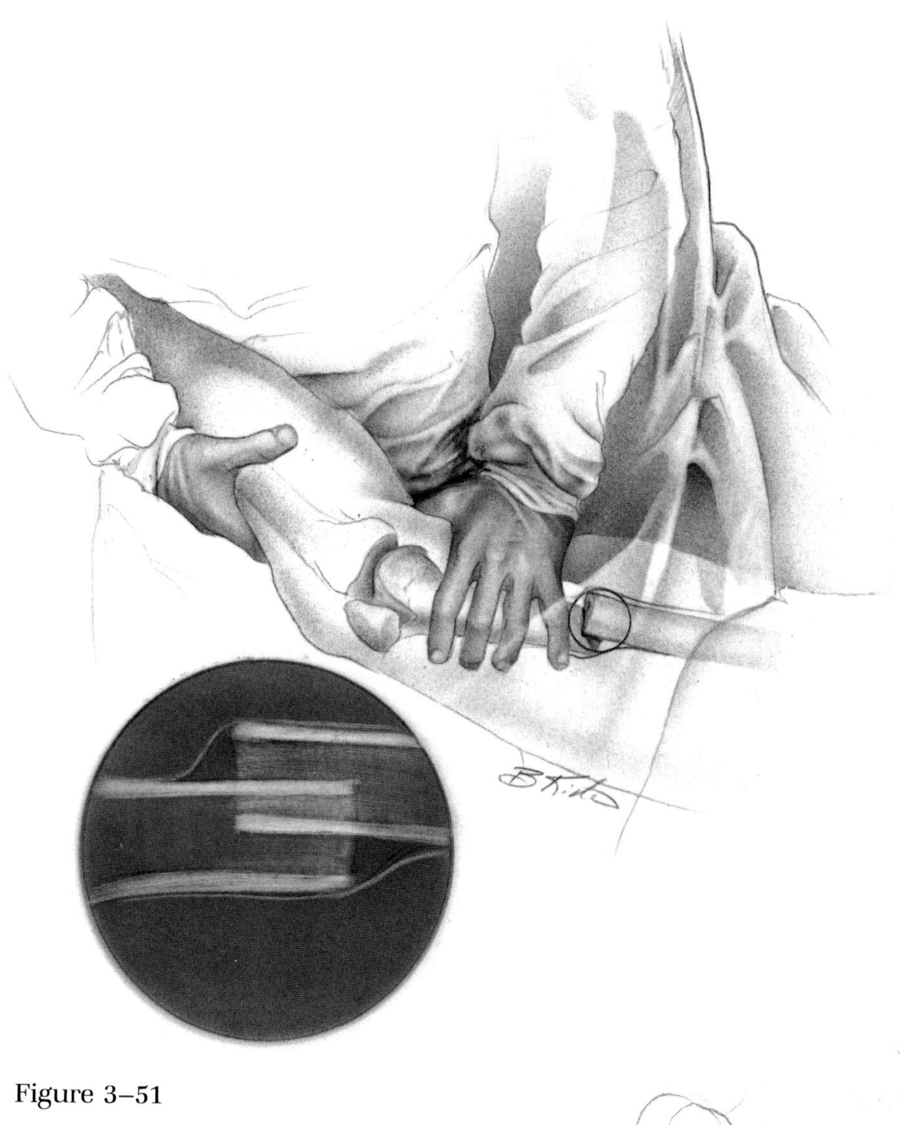

Figure 3–51

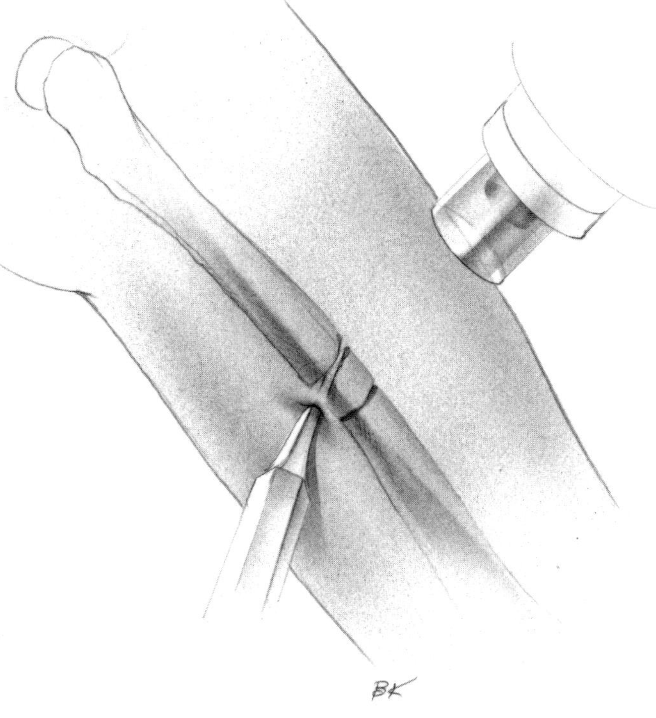

Figure 3–52

Figure 3–53. Adjustment is now made to the measuring device so that when the saw is pushed back down the medullary canal, the next cut will define the correct length of bone to be cut. To make this adjustment, the locking nut is held firmly in place while the portion that rests on the trochanter is advanced down the shaft toward the saw blade. When the desired amount of shortening is measured between the trochanteric portion and the locking nut, the locking nut is tightened down on the trochanteric rest to prevent its moving. This will result in a segment of bone of the correct length being cut.

Figure 3–54. The saw is now pushed down the shaft until the trochanteric rest sits firmly against the tip of the trochanter, and the entire procedure of cutting the bone is repeated at the proximal osteotomy site. It is now necessary to complete this osteotomy. This can usually be done by using the distal fragment of the femoral shaft as a lever to break this intercalary piece of bone off of the proximal fragment. If this is not possible, either of the two methods used to complete the first osteotomy can be used.

Figure 3–55. The intercalary fragment of femoral shaft created by the two osteotomies must now be split and moved out of the way to allow the femur to shorten. If the entire piece of bone or one large piece of bone is displaced, it may create a symptomatic enlargement that interferes with muscle movement.

The intramedullary chisel is inserted through the proximal and intercalary fragments, and the hook is directed posterolateral to catch on a thick part of the intercalary fragment. It is usually not possible to split the linea aspera, and if the thin anterior cortex is split, one large and one small fragment will result. With the hook in the proper location, the slotted hammer is used to drive the hook out of the canal. The image intensifier is used to verify that the intercalary fragment is split and to avoid splitting the proximal femoral shaft.

After the fragment is split, the hook is used to displace the pieces to each side. Additional manipulation of the fragments can be accomplished by pushing on them with the distal fragment of the femoral shaft as it is brought into apposition with the proximal fragment. It must be possible to displace the split fragments and bring the distal and proximal shaft into apposition.

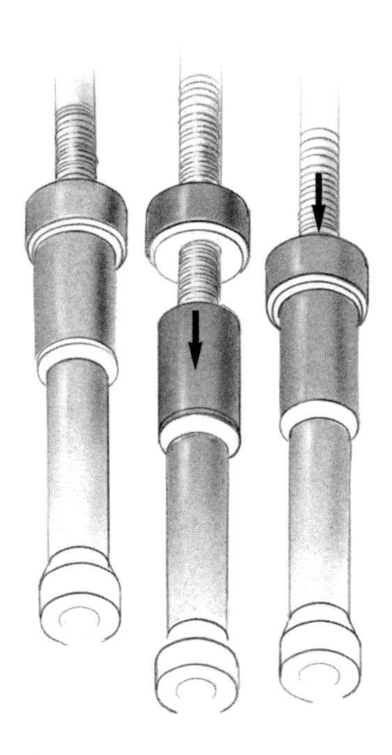

Figure 3–53

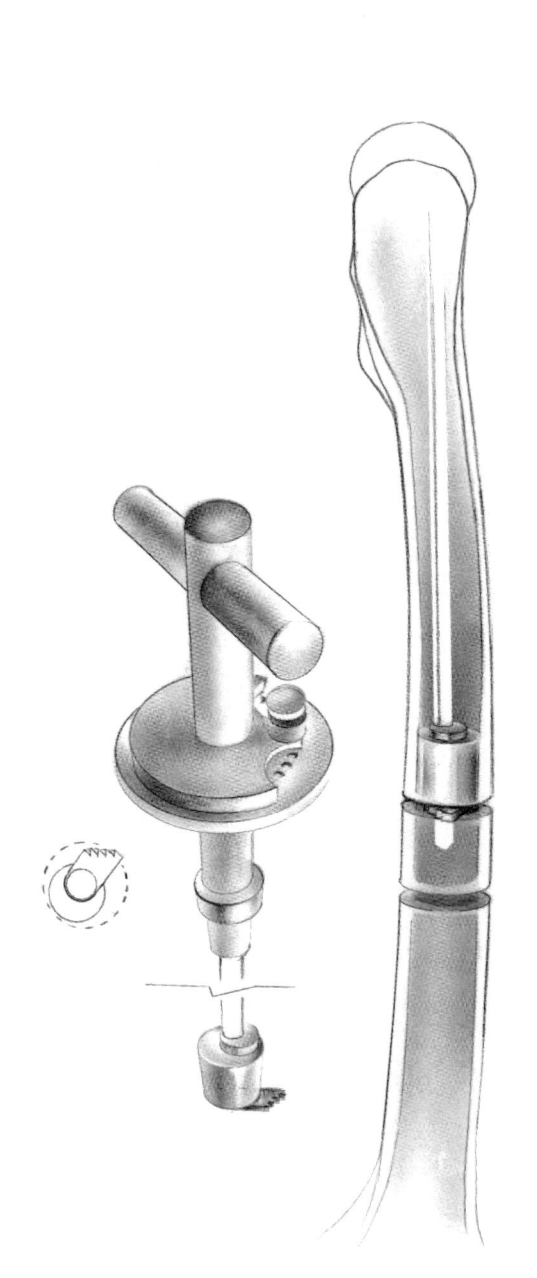

Figure 3–54

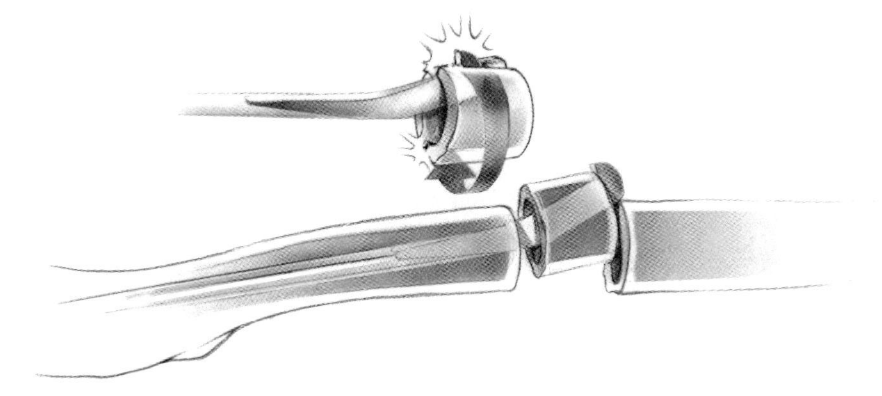

Figure 3–55

Figure 3–56. With the two fragments now in apposition, the distal one held by the unscrubbed surgeon, the correct size rod is driven down the canal. During this part of the operation it is important for the unscrubbed surgeon to maintain the correct rotation of the distal fragment and at the same time push cephalad on the bent knee to keep the osteotomy site from distracting. It is especially important to monitor the rod passing the osteotomy site on both the anteroposterior and lateral views. Next, the distal end of the rod is monitored. Remember, a rod shorter than usual was selected to avoid the problem of overdistraction.

Maintaining the correct rotation is a difficult problem. This is especially true because the leg will be removed from traction during the procedure. Visually maintaining the alignment of the leg as it was before the osteotomy and placing the leg in 20 degrees of internal rotation as is recommended for intramedullary nailing of fractures is usually reliable. Because this is so important it requires the most experienced member of the operating team. If shortening of greater than 3.5 to 4 cm is done, Winquist (personal communication, 1990) now recommends the use of an interlocking rod to maintain the correct rotation. The use of an interlocking rod necessitates absolute accuracy in the rotation of the two fragments because no adjustment will be possible after completion of the operation. This can be accomplished by placing one pin proximal and one pin distal to the osteotomy sites before they are made. The proximal pin is placed as far anterior in the greater trochanter as possible so as not to interfere with the reaming and rod passage. The second pin is placed in the lateral femoral condyle below the epiphyseal scar parallel to the first pin. These two pins will provide a visual reference for rotational alignment.

Occasionally a small spike will result from the osteoclasis in the region of the linea aspera. If this does not occur at both osteotomy sites and form a mirror image on the proximal and distal fragment, it will hold the fragments apart. Attempts should be made to break this off, but if it is not too large it can be accepted.

After the nail is in satisfactory position, the wound is closed. A drain is not necessary and if used usually blocks off early because of the debris that drains from the medullary canal. The patient is moved to the stretcher and the rotation of both legs inspected to be sure that no serious rotational malalignment exists. If manipulation of the leg cannot correct a discrepancy in rotation, it may be necessary to redo the nailing. If there is poor rotational stability, this needs to be accounted for in the postoperative management.

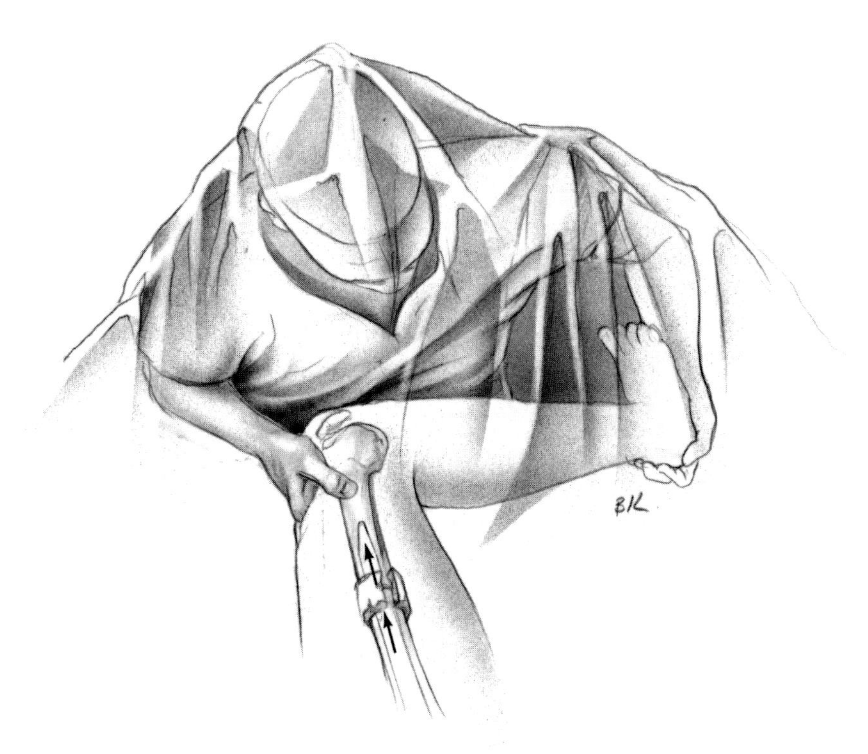

Figure 3–56

Figure 3–57. TL is a 14-year-old girl who 3 years previously sustained a closed fracture of the femur. She was treated with traction for 3 weeks followed by a spica cast for 3 months. Her final result was malunion with 4 cm of shortening (***Figure 3–57A***). Closed intramedullary shortening of the femur was chosen as the method to achieve leg-length equalization. The preoperative planning on the anteroposterior radiograph of the opposite leg is shown in ***Figure 3–45***.

Immediate postoperative radiograph is shown (***Figure 3–57B***). Note the excessive amount of bone medially that resulted from splitting the intercallary fragment in the wrong area. This was symptomatic to her for about 6 months when bending her knee past 60 degrees. Final result at 18 months following rod removal is seen (***Figure 3–57C***).

POSTOPERATIVE CARE

The patient should be placed in a derotation boot in the operating room to prevent external rotation of the leg if an interlocking nail was not used. This is maintained for 2 to 3 weeks while the patient is in bed. The hematocrit should be followed closely for several days because considerable bleeding into the thigh may occur.

Quadriceps exercises are started the day after surgery, and partial weight bearing is started within 24 to 48 hours. The patient is continued on crutches for 6 to 8 weeks. The rod can be removed at 1 year.

If there is no rotational stability or if pistoning of the bone is encountered, it is wise to apply a one-leg spica cast down to the knee when the swelling has decreased before discharge from the hospital. Within 3 to 4 weeks muscle tone and healing will provide sufficient stability to allow removal of the cast.

REFERENCES

1. Winquist RA, Hansen ST, Pearson RE. Closed intramedullary shortening of the femur. Clin Orthop 1978;136:54.
2. Winquist RA. Closed intramedullary osteotomies of the femur. Clin Orthop 1986;212:155.
3. Blair VP, Schoenecker PL, Sheridan JJ, Capelli AM. Closed shortening of the femur. J Bone Joint Surg 1989;71A:1440.
4. Winquist R. Intramedullary osteotomies. In: Browner BD, Edwards CC, eds. The science and practice of intramedullary nailing. Philadelphia: Lea & Febiger, 1987:349–363.

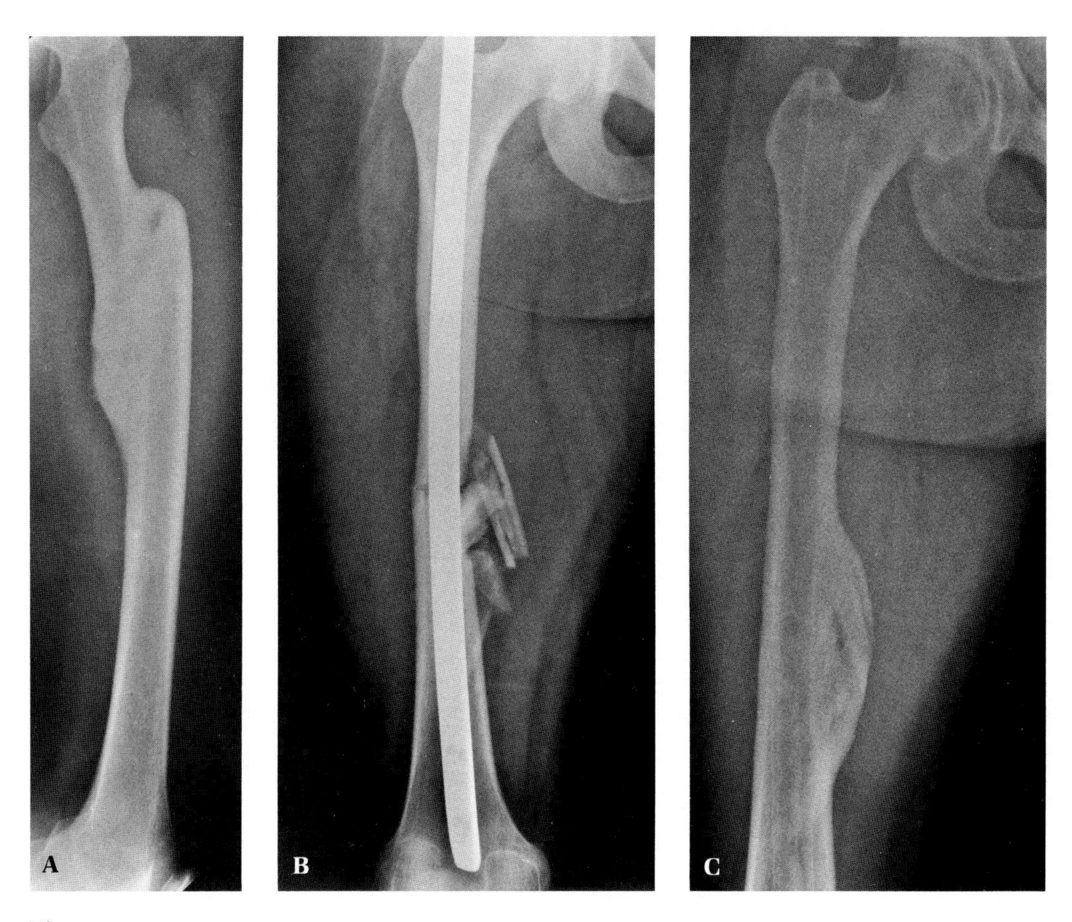

Figure 3–57

3.8 Wagner Technique of Femoral Lengthening for Congenitally Short Femur

The apparatus and principles for leg lengthening of Professor Heinz Wagner, introduced in the United States in the 1960s, made limb lengthening an accepted and routine procedure. The technique entails two distinct operative procedures: the actual lengthening and the osteosynthesis. Wagner[1] was especially careful to emphasize that function should not be sacrificed for length and that knee motion must be maintained during lengthening. Other series have emphasized the problems and complications that make attention to detail so important in what appears to be a relatively simple procedure.[2] The indications for leg lengthening are discussed by Moseley.[3]

One of the principles clearly stated by Wagner[1] is that all deformities should be corrected before the lengthening is begun. In addition, he emphasized that in congenital deformities, the soft tissues were abnormal, and resection of fascia and intermuscular septa was necessary. These principles are in contrast to those of the Ilizarov technique.

The Wagner device comes in two sizes. The smaller size is for use on the humerus but can also be used in small children. Both devices use two Schanz screws at each end to attach to the bone. One turn of the knob results in 1.5 mm of lengthening.

Figure 3–58. The case illustrated is of a lengthening for congenitally short femur. This incorporates an extensive soft-tissue release. If this lengthening were done for a post-traumatic deformity, the Schanz screws would be placed as discussed in the technique of femoral lengthening using the Orthofix device, and the osteotomy would be performed through a small incision between the two sets of Schanz screws.

The patient is positioned with a sand bag under the ipsilateral hip to tilt the lateral side of the femur up and with a large, soft roll under the knee to place the muscles about midway between flexion and extension before penetration with the Schanz screws (***Figure 3–58A***). Before lengthening of the congenitally short femur, the fascia lata must be lengthened and the lateral intermuscular septum excised. It is possible to do this at the same time the lengthening device is applied. This is accomplished through a long longitudinal incision from the greater trochanter proximally to the lateral condyle distally. The iliotibial band is identified. A longitudinal incision is made along its anterior border, and a second incision is then made along its posterior border (***Figure 3–58B***). A long oblique incision is then made in the iliotibial band, and it is elevated from the underlying muscle. (***Figure 3–58C***).

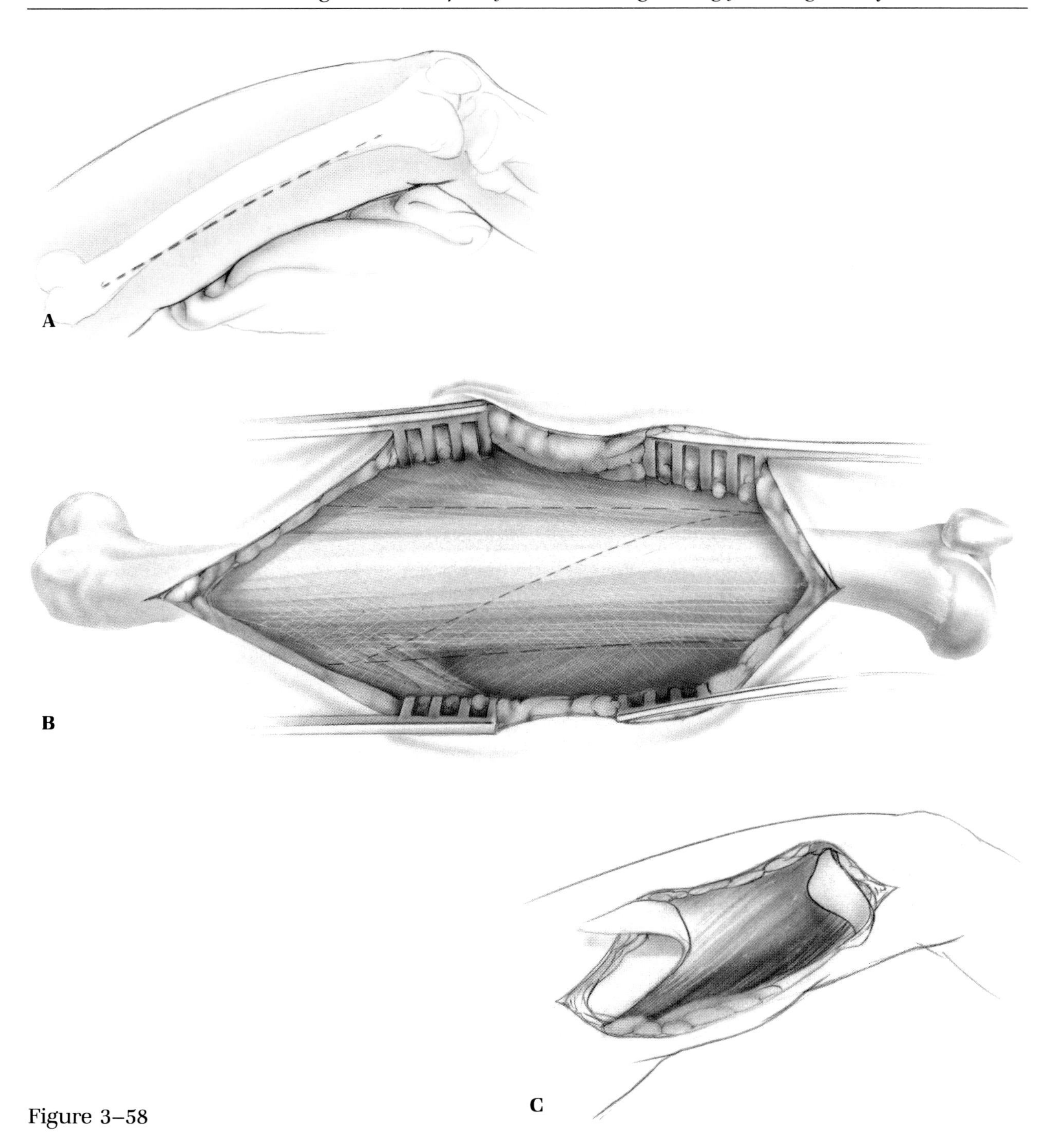

Figure 3–58

Figure 3–59. The vastus lateralis muscle is then elevated off of the lateral intermuscular septum, following this septum down to the bone. Likewise the biceps femoris muscle is elevated off of the posterior aspect of the septum down to the bone (***Figures 3–59A, B***). The lateral intermuscular septum is excised over the entire area of exposure. The fascia lata is now repaired but in a manner that lengthens it (***Figure 3–59C***).

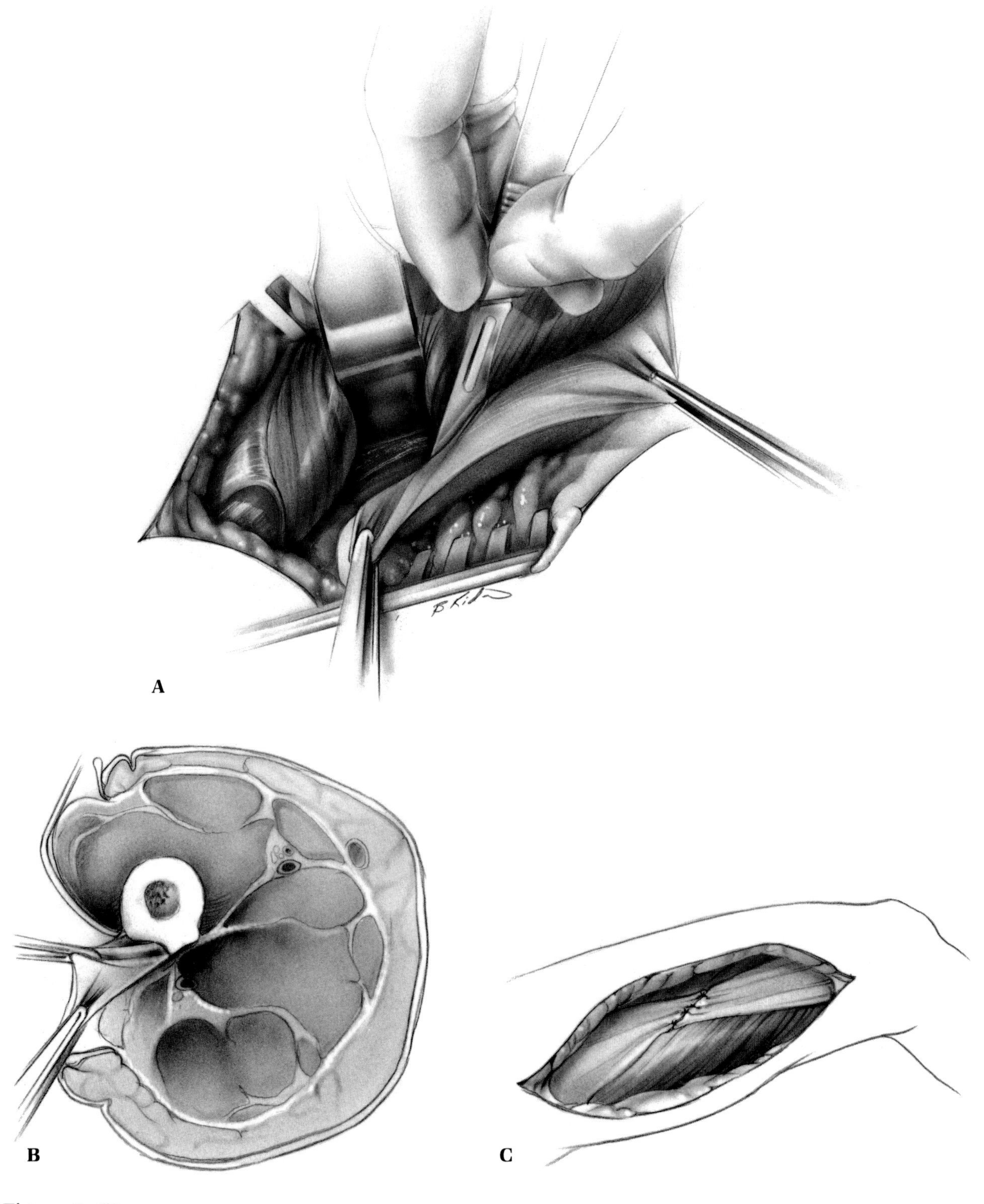

Figure 3–59

Figure 3–60. The center of the wound is approximated temporarily with interrupted sutures. The distal and proximal parts of the wound where the Schanz screws will be placed are left open.

The drill guide and template is used to position the proximal and then the distal screws. The proximal screw is placed at the level of the lesser trochanter and the distal screw in the supracondylar region. It is important that there be sufficient distance between the screws so that they will not interfere with placement of the plate during the osteosynthesis. Although the screw clamps will tilt about 20 degrees at each end to compensate for the proximal and distal sets of screws being in different planes, care should be taken to keep the two sets of screws closely aligned. In the femur the Schanz screws are selected so that at least 5 cm of the pin will project beyond the skin. This is necessary to allow enough distance between the skin and the lengthener for pin care (***Figure 3–60A***).

In the usual case of lengthening where this extensive dissection of soft tissue is not done, the technique of pin placement must follow the steps described in the discussion on Wagner lengthening of the tibia. In the usual femoral lengthening, one additional step is necessary for the distal pin insertion. Because the iliotibial band will move posterior when the knee is flexed, a second incision should be made in the iliotibial band extending anteriorly from the transverse incision (***Figure 3–60B***).

The Schanz screws should never be inserted with a power drill but rather by hand using the T-handled chuck. Because of the design of the Schanz screw, its tip has both a smooth flat surface and a threaded surface. To engage the threads of the screw in the cortex in the axis of the bone and at the same time avoid excessive protrusion beyond the cortex, it is necessary to align the tip of the screw in the cortex correctly (***Figure 3–60C***). The correct position is illustrated by the top screw and incorrect alignment is illustrated by the bottom screw.

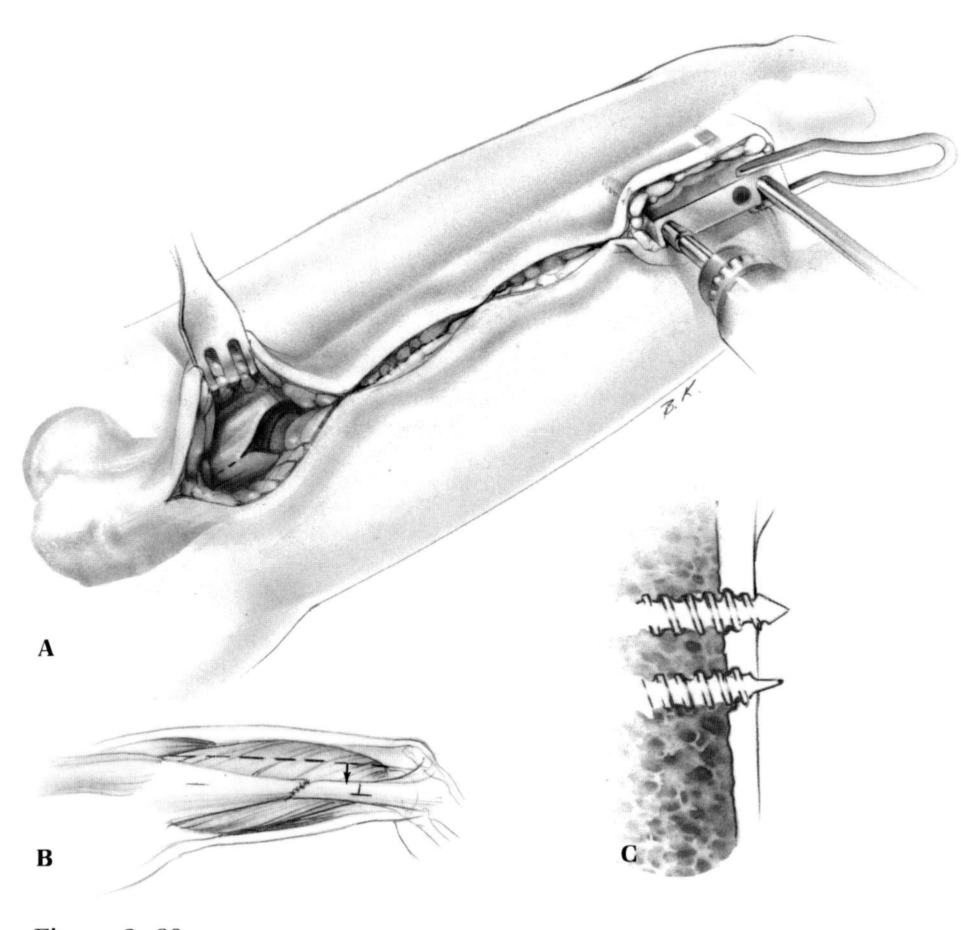

Figure 3–60

Figure 3–61. In the usual case of lengthening where an extensive soft-tissue release is not done, a separate incision is used after the screws are placed. This incision is posterolateral and midway between the screws. The approach to the femoral shaft is between the lateral intermuscular septum anteriorly and the biceps femoris posteriorly.

In the case illustrated here, the temporary sutures are removed from the middle section, and the diaphysis midway between the proximal and distal screws is exposed by elevating the vastus lateralis muscle and then the periosteum (***Figure 3–61A***). Although the original technique described transecting the periosteum circumferentially and cutting the bone with a power saw, the author has observed and adopted a different technique while visiting Professor Wagner in 1985. The bone is drilled through the cortex where accessible using a drill stop, and the drill holes are connected with an osteotome (***Figure 3–61B***). The lengthening device is attached to the Schanz screws keeping it parallel with the femur. It is placed under slight distraction so that completion of the osteotomy will be signaled by separation of the bone. The part of the cortex that is not possible to drill is now divided by using a Gigli saw thus completing the osteotomy (***Figure 3–61C***).

In a case such as congenitally short femur, the surgeon may anticipate that the leg will develop a varus deformity during lengthening. To obviate this complication, the leg should be aligned in slight valgus before the patient is awake. This is accomplished by placing a screwdriver in each of the remaining holes in the clamps. The nut holding the distal clamp is loosened by an assistant while the surgeon manipulates the screwdrivers to create about 10 to 15 degrees of valgus. The clamp is then tightened.

Figure 3–62. Note that the lengthener is applied with the knob toward the patient and the screw clamps anterior. The wound is carefully closed over a drain using interrupted sutures for the deep tissues and a continuous subcuticular suture for the skin. The skin is also closed around the pins. The author has experienced no problems with the pin tracks or the wound when using this technique. Before waking the patient, the knee is flexed past 90 degrees to further loosen the tissue around the pins.

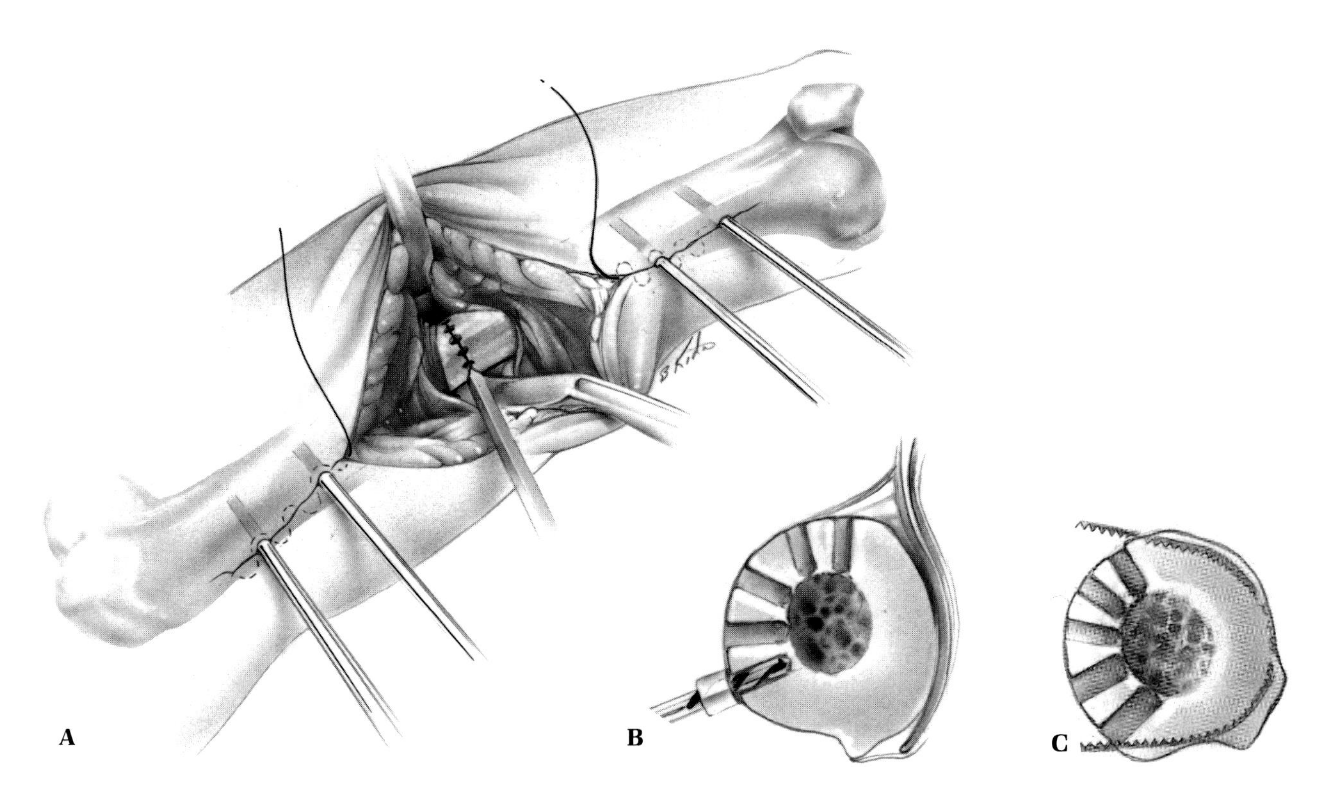

Figure 3–61

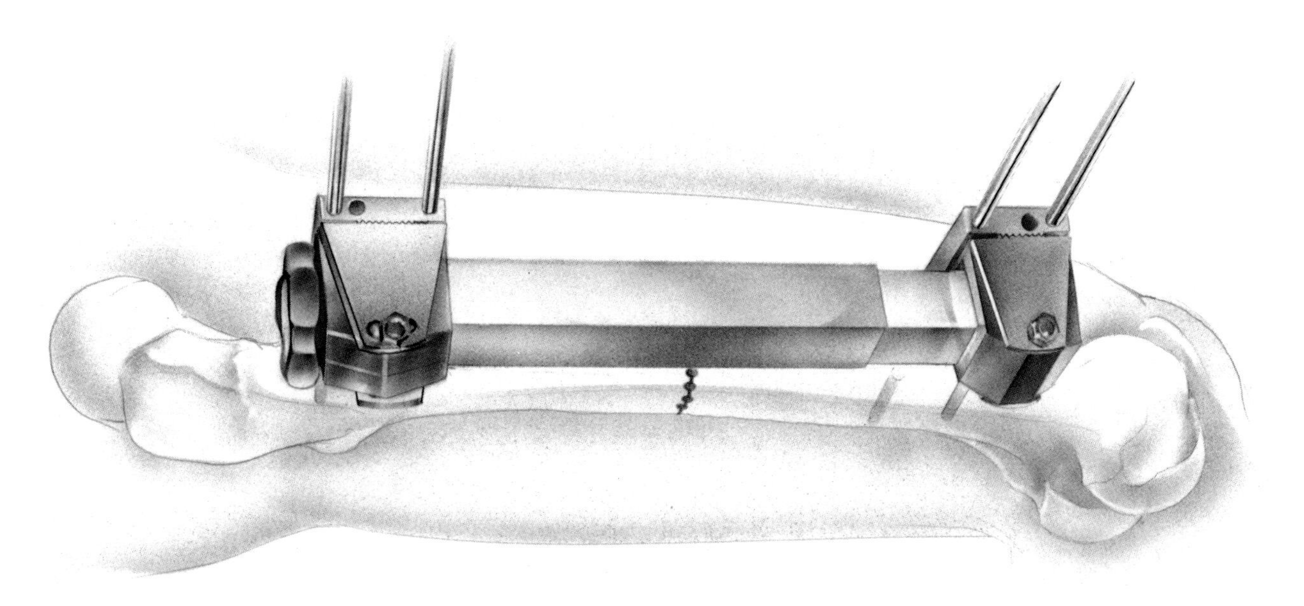

Figure 3–62

LENGTHENING

Physical therapy is started the day following surgery. It consists of active-assisted side-lying flexion and extension as well as sitting with the knee flexed. It is much easier to begin this on the first postoperative day than at 3 or 4 days after surgery. By the second or third postoperative day the patient should be ambulatory with a three-point partial weight-bearing crutch gait, which was taught preoperatively.

The leg is lengthened 1.5 mm per day by turning the knob one-quarter turn four times each day. Lengthening begins on the first postoperative day. The following parameters must be closely monitored during the lengthening: knee motion, knee subluxation, hip motion, hip subluxation, and pin sites.

Wagner has emphasized that active knee motion should be maintained between −15 degrees of full extension and 60 degrees of flexion. If the patient cannot achieve this, lengthening is stopped until motion is regained.

Subluxation of the knee is a particular problem in those with congenital limb shortening as they have tight soft tissue, deficient ligaments within the knee, and often a deficient lateral femoral condyle. In addition, subtle degrees of acetabular dysplasia often exist, and subluxation of the hip can be a rather "silent" occurrence. If motion becomes restricted, appropriate muscle release may be needed during the course of lengthening. If soft-tissue contractures are released before the lengthening, however, this is usually not a problem.

It is usually wise to monitor the progress of the lengthening every other week. A scanogram is obtained periodically to assess the true amount of length that is obtained. The marks on the lengthener should not be relied on. A lateral radiograph of the knee and an anteroposterior radiograph of the hip can be used to monitor subluxation and are definitely indicated if there is any significant loss of motion. As mentioned there is a tendency for the leg to angulate into varus. This is usually not a problem if accounted for by aligning the leg in slight valgus at the time of the initial osteotomy. Likewise, small amounts of varus can be corrected at the time of plate application. In the author's experience one of the proximal pins is almost always loose at the completion of lengthening, and this allows for movement of the fragments despite the fact that the fixator is still in place.

As the leg is lengthened, the pins will place pressure on the soft tissues. It is imperative that this be released when it occurs, or necrosis and subsequent infection will result. The author's preferred method of pin care is cleaning with hydrogen peroxide twice a day. In the femur with the large amount of soft tissue that is constantly moving around the pins, there will usually be some serous drainage requiring a dressing to keep the clothes clean.

When the correct amount of length has been achieved, lengthening is stopped. It is often desirable to wait a few weeks before the second operation for osteosynthesis to allow the pin tracks to heal.

Figure 3–63. For the osteosynthesis, the patient is placed in the prone position. The leg should be draped free, and the lengthening device must be isolated from the field while the posterior iliac crest is included. This is accomplished by wrapping the lengthening device in a sterile towel and enclosing the entire device and screw sites in a sterile adhesive plastic drape (***Figure 3–63A***).

The incision is posterolateral centered between the screws and over the interval between the vastus lateralis and the biceps femoris muscles. In the case illustrated this is the central part of the initial incision. In a lengthening for post-traumatic shortening or other noncongenital etiology, it will be the same incision used for the initial osteotomy, but extended both proximally and distally. If the lateral intermuscular septum has not been excised, the approach is between this septum anteriorly and the biceps femoris muscle posteriorly (***Figure 3–63B***). The posterior aspect of the femur is exposed for an adequate distance above and below the area of lengthening, but the screws should not be seen.

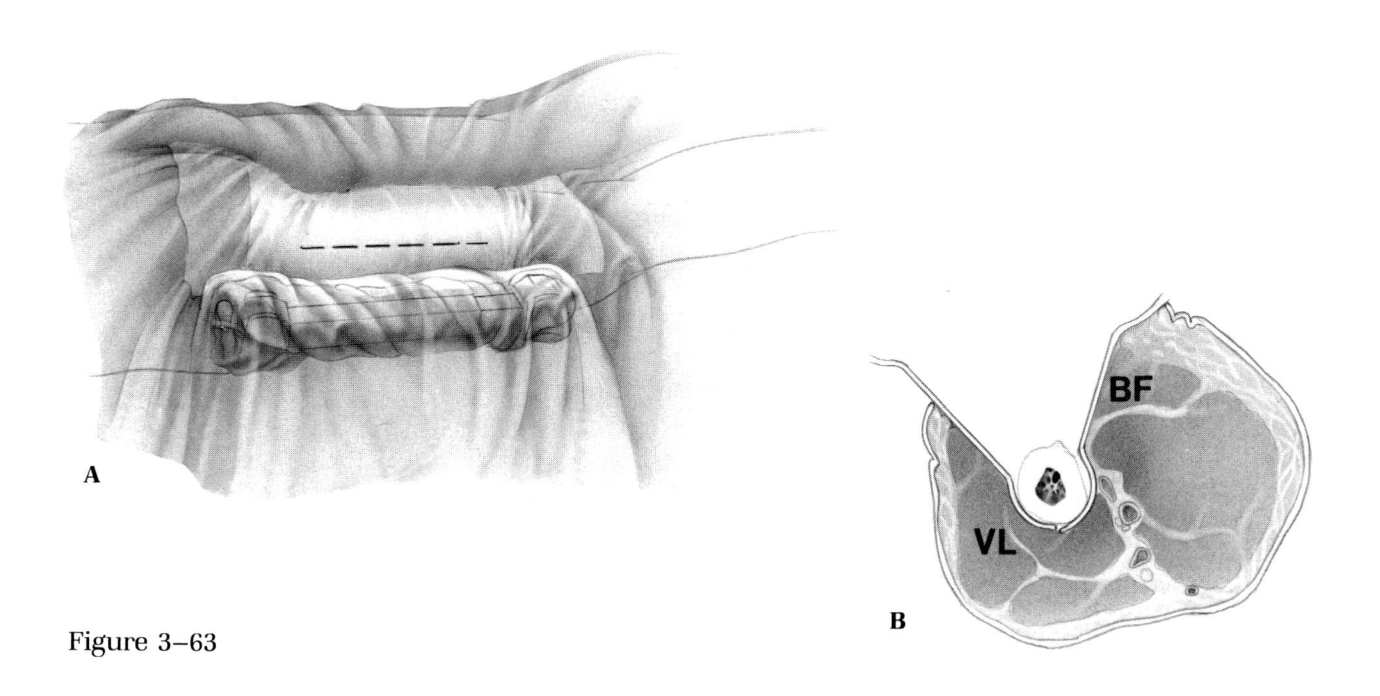

Figure 3–63

Figure 3–64. A special plate has been developed for osteosynthesis of a lengthened bone. It has five staggered holes at each end and is solid in the middle section. It is applied to the posterior, not the lateral, surface of the femur. In this way the entire width of the plate rather than the thickness of the plate resists the predominant tendency for lateral bowing. The plate should also be contoured with a slight anterior bow to conform to the natural anterior bow of the femur.

The gap between the bone ends will usually be filled with a fibrocartilaginous tissue. This will have to be removed with a curette to provide space for the bone graft. The surgeon may be tempted to believe that this will mature into bone. Having come this far, however, there is little reason not to fill the gap with fresh autogenous bone. After the bone graft is placed, the plate is secured to the bone. The wound is closed over suction drains. After the drapes are removed, the lengthening device and the screws are removed.

Figure 3–65. KM is a 12-year-old girl with a congenitally short femur and a projected discrepancy of 7 cm. She underwent lengthening as described. Three weeks after completion of 6 cm of lengthening (***Figure 3–65A***), she shows some early callus. This will not result in sufficient healing. In addition, she demonstrates the problem of varus deformity. At the time of initial lengthening, the fragments were not aligned in sufficient valgus. Radiographs after the osteosynthesis (***Figure 3–65B***) demonstrate correction of the varus even though the plate was not placed as far posteriorly as desirable. By 7 months (***Figure 3–65C***) considerable healing has occurred, but there is no development of a cortex apparent. At this time the Wagner plate was exchanged for a standard plate in which every other hole of the plate was used for fixation (***Figure 3–65D***).

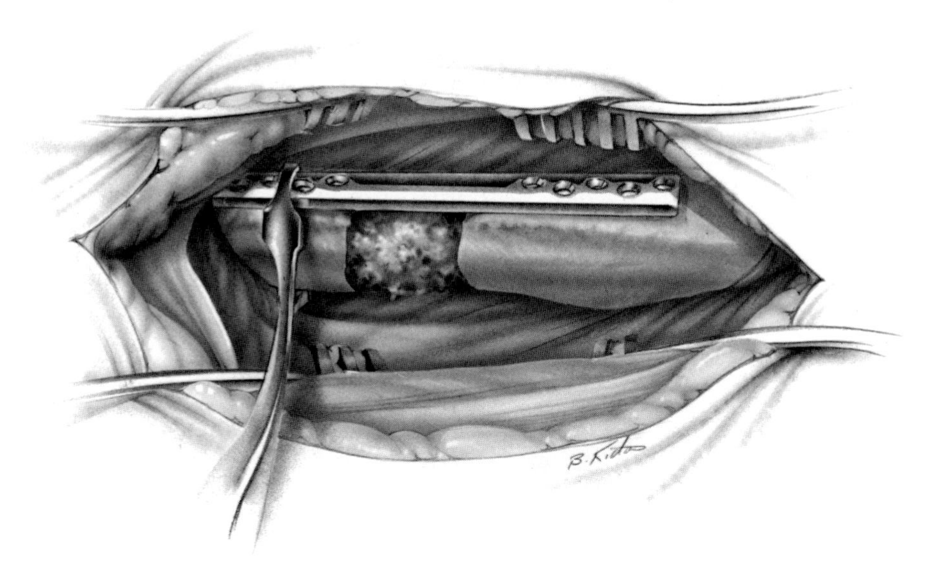

Figure 3–64

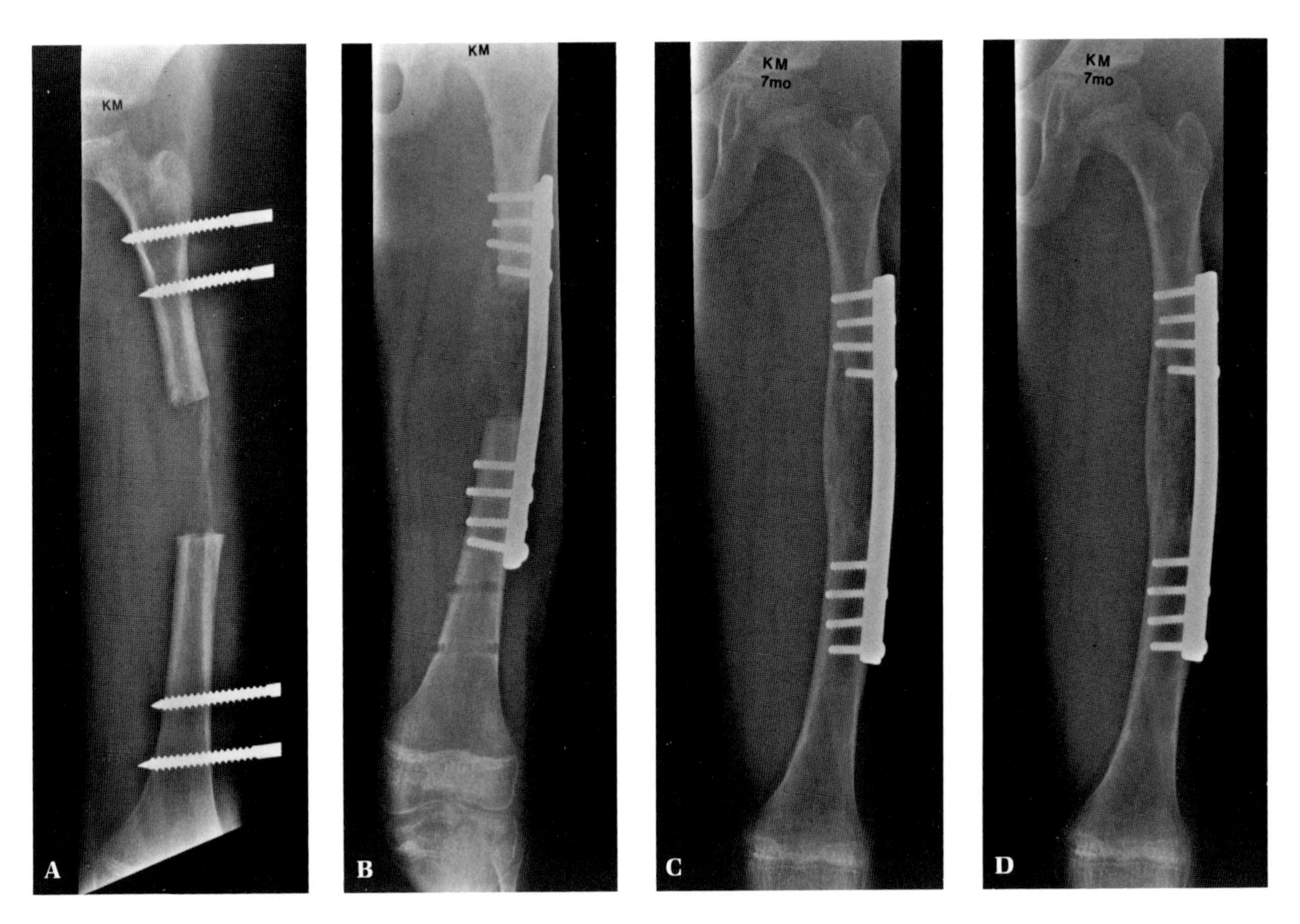

Figure 3–65

POSTOPERATIVE CARE

The drains are removed when the drainage is minimal, usually 24 hours after surgery. The patient is started on a three-point partial weight bearing crutch gait the day after surgery. The amount of weight bearing can be increased as consolidation of the bone is seen on the radiographs. Range-of-motion exercises for the knee are continued to regain the motion that was lost, and strengthening exercises for the knee and hip muscles are added as the acute pain subsides.

Because the Wagner osteosynthesis plate is so rigid it tends to stress shield the bone. If continuity of the bone is observed, but canalization and development of the cortex are not seen by 6 to 9 months, it may be necessary to exchange the special Wagner plate for a plate with less rigidity (*eg,* a tibial plate or semitubular plate). This is necessary both to prevent a stress fracture at the end of the plate and to allow increased stress in the bone. This plate is in turn removed when a good cortex has developed.

REFERENCES

1. Wagner H. Operative lengthening of the femur. Clin Orthop 1978;136:126.
2. Hood RW, Riseborough EJ. Lengthening of the lower extremity by the Wagner method. J Bone Joint Surg 1981;63A:1122.
3. Moseley CF. Leg-length discrepancy. In: Morrissy RT, ed. Lovell and Winter's pediatric orthopaedics, 3rd ed. Philadelphia: JB Lippincott, 1989:799.

3.9 Orthofix Technique of Femoral Lengthening

As with most lengthening devices, the name of the device also describes or is associated with unique biologic principles. The Orthofix lengthener was developed by De Bastiani and his colleagues[1] to be used with the principle of callotasis. It has certain advantages and disadvantages. In comparison with the Ilizarov apparatus, it is much better tolerated by the patients and much simpler for the surgeon. The template for insertion of the screws makes their precise alignment easier than with the Wagner device, and the lengthener permits up to three screws to be used at each end of the osteotomy, which helps in avoiding angulation during lengthening. Unlike the Wagner device, angular adjustment is possible without loosening the hold on the pins if the dynamic axial fixator is used in place of the lengtheners. The amount of angular correction, however, which is achieved acutely is limited for practical purposes to about 20 degrees, and rotational correction must be achieved at the time of the osteotomy and attachment of the lengthener. In the author's opinion this represents the best device today for most femoral lengthenings that do not require large angular or rotational corrections.

Figure 3–66. Like the Wagner apparatus, both the limb lengthener (***Figure 3–66A***) and the dynamic axial fixator (***Figure 3–66B***) are unilateral frames that use half-pins for fixation. The limb lengthener is a rigid telescoping device that does not allow for adjustment—thus, the need for a template to ensure precise placement of the screws. The dynamic axial fixator, however, allows for 34 degrees of adjustment at either end through a "ball and socket" joint. If this device is used for lengthening, the ball joints should be secured with methylmethacrylate after the adjustments are made to prevent any unintended motion.

Figure 3–67. Regardless of which device is used, the screws are inserted with the aid of a template, drill guide, and screw guide. This ensures precise alignment of the screws, which eliminates any tension on the screws and minimizes osteolysis around the screws. Different templates are available for the different size fixators and lengtheners.

Figure 3–68. The Orthofix screws differ from the Schanz screws used on the Wagner device in the thread design and the fact that they are tapered, becoming thicker toward the base. This is said to give them a securer fit in the bone. The standard cortical screw (***Figure 3–68A***) tapers from 6 mm at the base of the thread to 5 mm at the tip (6/5 mm). Smaller screws of 4.5/3.5 mm are also available (to be used in bones with a diaphyseal diameter <15 mm) as are 6/5-mm cancellous screws (***Figure 3–68B***). For leg lengthening these screws are now available with a cutting edge (***Figure 3–68C***) to minimize the tissue trauma at the leading edge of the pin during lengthening.

Figure 3–69. The patient is positioned in the supine position on a translucent operating table with an image intensifier opposite the surgeon. After the entire leg is prepared, a large soft roll is placed under the knee to flex the hip and knee. As the leg tends to fall into external rotation, it is also helpful to place a large roll under the buttocks.

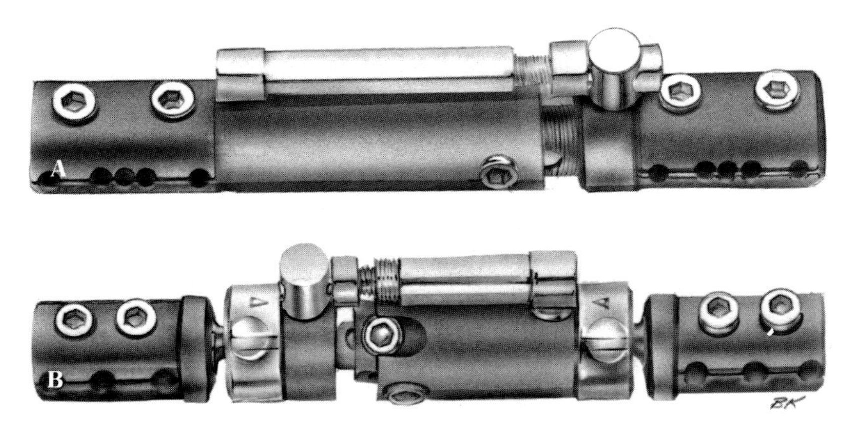

Figure 3–66

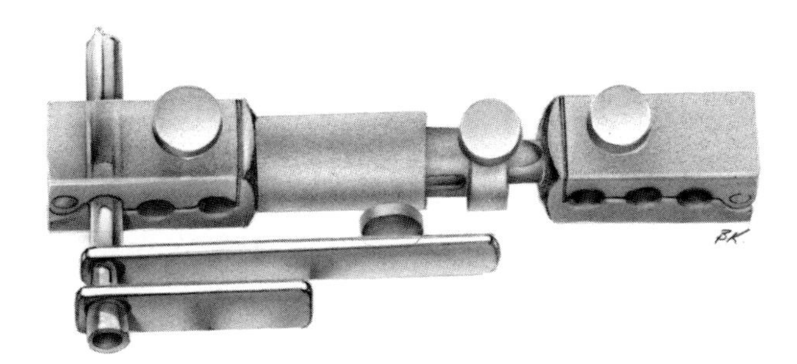

Figure 3–67

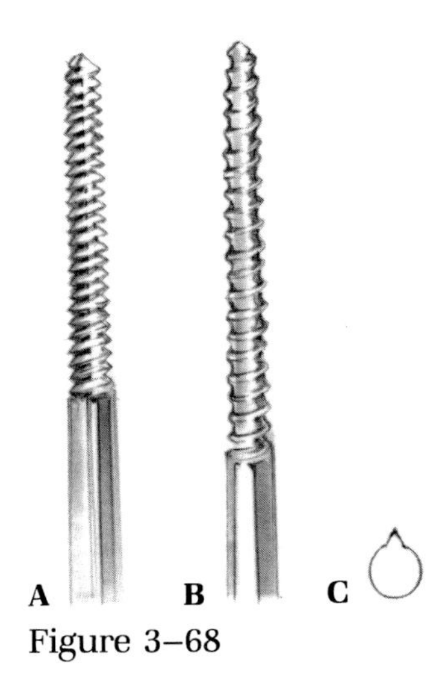

Figure 3–68

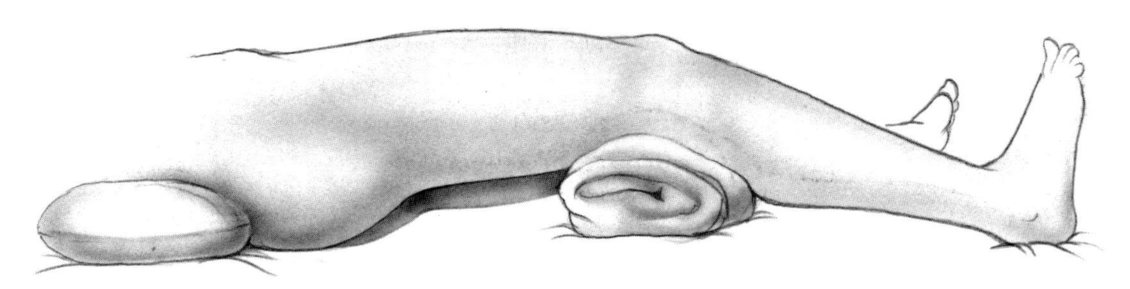

Figure 3–69

Figure 3–70. The most proximal screw is placed first. It should be placed just proximal to the lesser trochanter. Although it is possible to place this even higher in the femoral neck region to keep the osteotomy more proximal, this is not really necessary. After identifying the correct area by means of the image intensifier and a small Kirschner wire held over the thigh, a stab wound is made through the skin and fascia lata. This wound is then spread widely down to the bone with a large hemostat or scissors. The tendency is not to cut and spread as deeply or as widely as necessary. To prevent necrosis and subsequent infection, this wound should be large enough so that the screw does not put any pressure on the skin, muscle, or fascia.

Figure 3–71. A screw guide of appropriate length with the trochar inserted through it is passed down to the bone, and the center of the bone is found. The trochar is struck with a mallet to start the hole for the drill. The trochar is then removed, and the screw guide is struck with the mallet to drive its teeth into the bone and secure it.

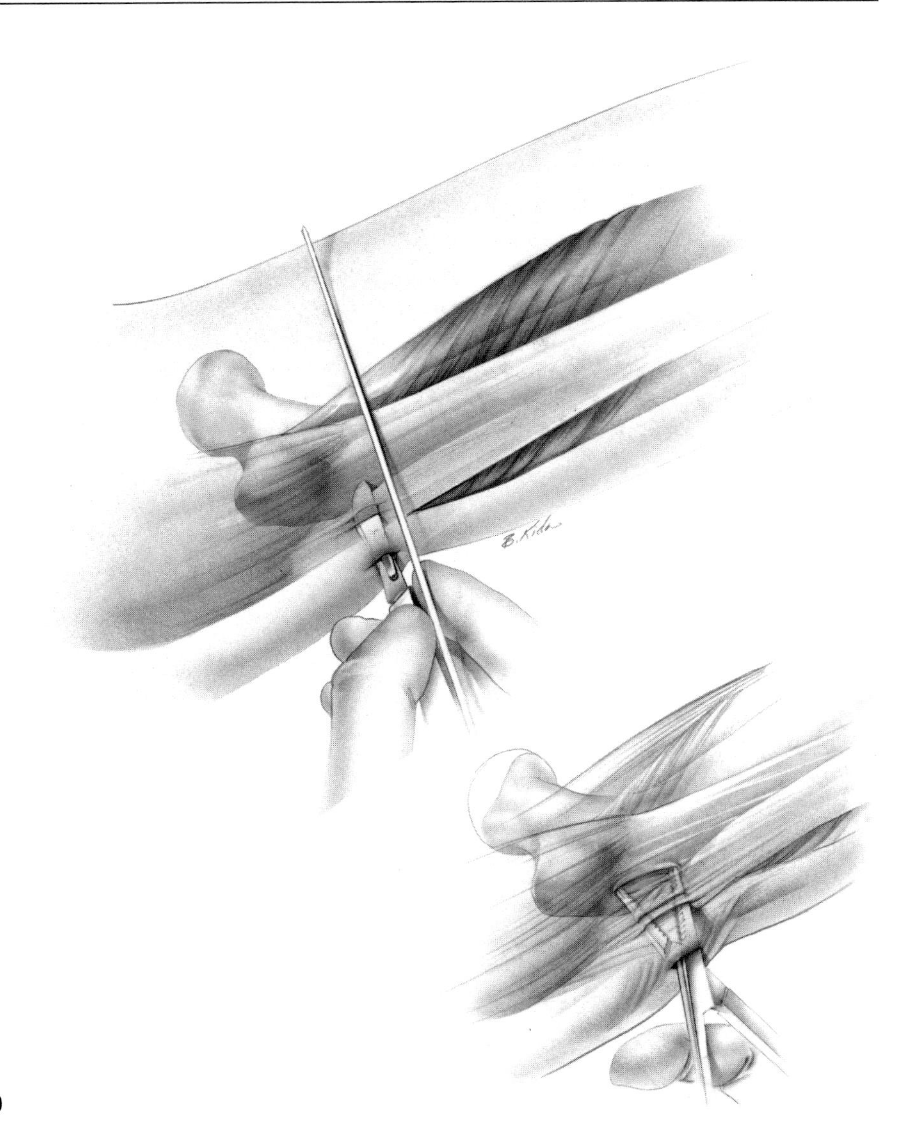

Figure 3–70

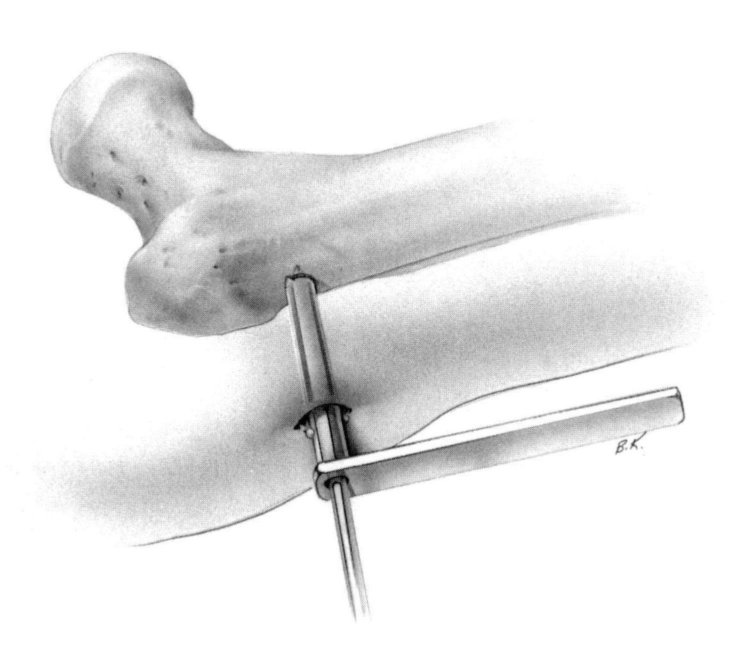

Figure 3–71

Figure 3–72. The drill guide of appropriate diameter and length is now passed through the screw guide. This will align the drill precisely within the screw guide. For the use of the 6/5-mm cortical screws, a 4.8-mm drill is used to make a hole through both cortices. A drill stop can be used to avoid over-penetration of the far cortex. First, the lateral cortex is penetrated, and the drill is advanced until the opposite cortex is encountered. Then the drill stop is adjusted to allow the drill to advance another 5 mm and penetrate the other cortex.

Figure 3–73. The drill and the drill guide are now removed and the proper length of screw is inserted using the T wrench. Although a cancellous screw can be used in this most proximal location, it is more flexible than the cortical screw and does not seem to offer any better purchase than a cortical screw that penetrates both cortices. Therefore, it is preferable to use a cortical screw here for its increased rigidity. After the far cortex is engaged, six to eight half-turns will usually result in two threads projecting through the opposite cortex, which is what is desired. There will be less resistance encountered with these screws than the surgeon is accustomed to, however. In addition, caution must be used not to advance these screws too far, because backing the screw out will result in loosening. Use of the image intensifier is helpful at this point. The screw guide is left in place because the holes of the template are designed to fit tightly around this guide.

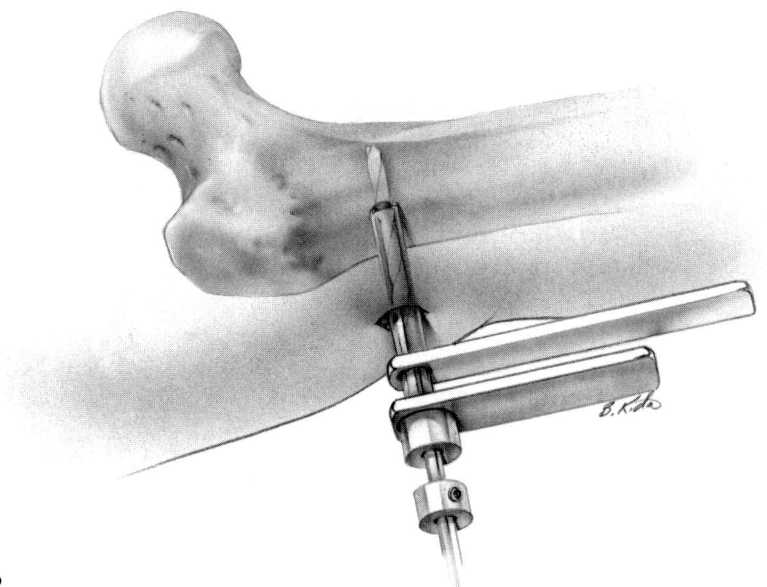

Figure 3–72

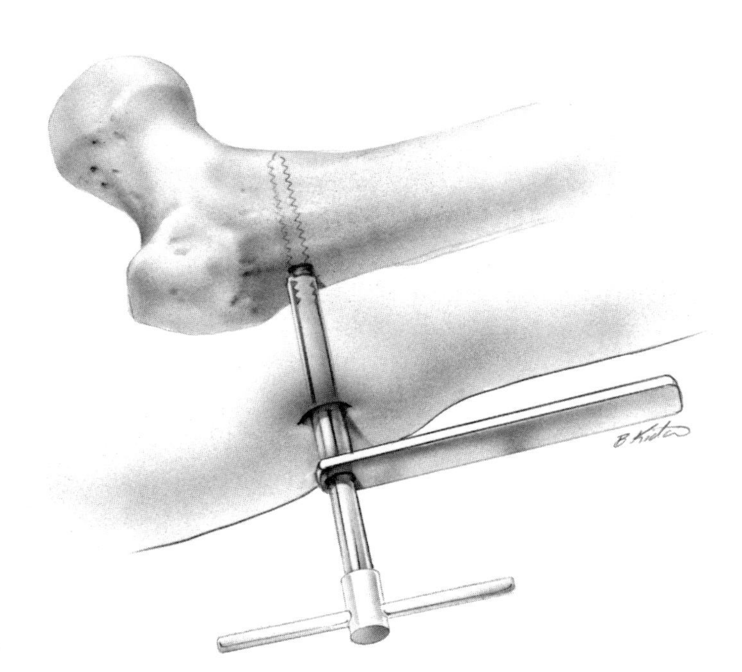

Figure 3–73

Figure 3–74. The proper size template for the limb lengthener being used is selected. For a 10-cm lengthener the standard template is fully extended, and for the 5-cm lengthener it is fully collapsed. The most proximal slot on the template is secured to the screw guide over the screw that was just placed. The template is now aligned with the femoral shaft, and the site for the most distal screw is marked. This is accurately done by passing a small knife blade on a long, thin handle through the slot in the template to initiate the stab wound in the skin. The most distal screw in the femur should be the second screw placed to ensure correct lateral alignment in the coronal plane.

Figure 3–75. All of the other screws are now placed as previously described. First, the screw guide is passed through the template and then the drill guide through the screw guide. After each screw is placed, the screw guide is left in place to provide a tight fit with the template and maintain precise alignment. In larger children, adolescents, and adults, three screws should be used at each end. In smaller children or for short lengthenings, two screws at each end may be sufficient.

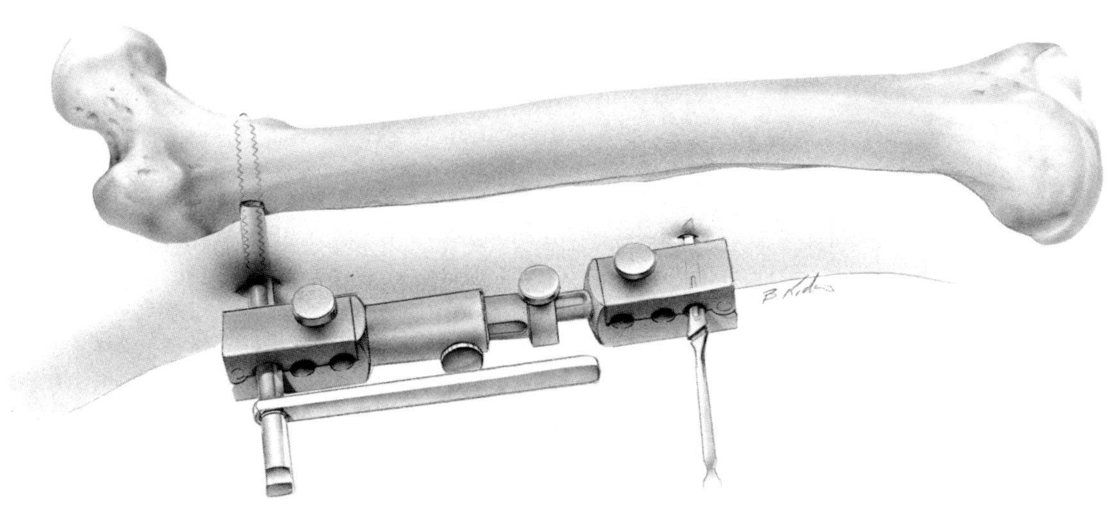

Figure 3–74

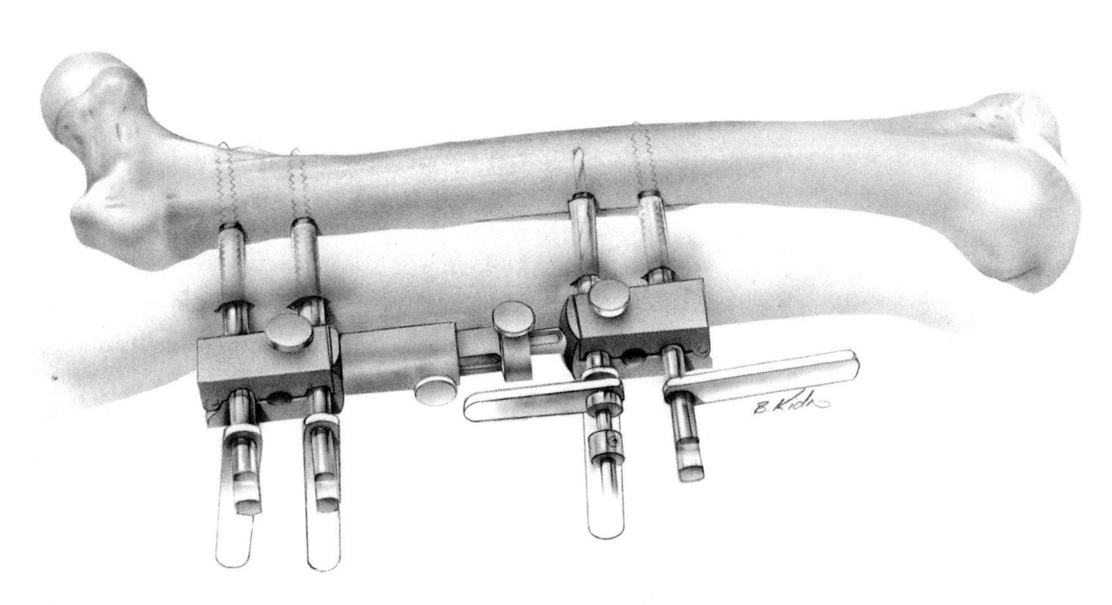

Figure 3–75

Figure 3–76. After all of the screws are placed, the template is removed, and the osteotomy is performed. It should be about 1 cm below the most distal of the proximal pins. This is accomplished through a small 4-cm incision placed on the anterolateral aspect of the thigh over the interval between the rectus and vastus lateralis muscles.

A longitudinal incision is made in the periosteum, and it is elevated circumferentially. Multiple drill holes are made in the bone. Although importance was initially attached to maintaining the intramedullary circulation, there has been no difference noted in bone healing when the posterior cortex is drilled by passing from the anterior cortex through the medullary canal with the drill. This greatly simplifies (and demystifies) the osteotomy and avoids the complication of a fracture propagating from the osteotomy into the nearest screw hole, which can occur when the posterior cortex is divided with an osteotome without drilling. To avoid excessive penetration of the posterior cortex, and particularly the posterior medial cortex where the deep femoral artery runs close to the bone, the drill stop can be used as described before. After multiple drill holes are made, they are connected with an osteotome. A power saw should not be used to make the osteotomy.

To be certain that the osteotomy is completed, the proximal and distal pins are grasped and rotated while observing the osteotomy. (An alternative method is to attach the lengthener to the pins, place the lengthener under slight distraction, perform the osteotomy, and verify the completeness of the osteotomy with the image intensifier.)

The osteotomy is now complete. The periosteum is approximated, and the wound is closed. Some surgeons think that the hematoma may actually aid in the callus formation and prefer not to use a drain.

Figure 3–77. The lengthener is now attached to the screws. The body of the lengthener or fixator (as illustrated here) should lie parallel to the diaphysis of the femur. In placing the fixator, it is important that the nut that locks the telescoping body (body-locking nut) faces outward, that the nuts tightening the clamp on the screws face up, and the distraction-compression bar faces up with the socket for the wrench toward the patient's head. If the dynamic axial fixator is used as illustrated here, the arrow on the cam should face up.

Once in place and tightened, the telescoping body is compressed with the distraction-compression bar and locked securely with the body-locking nut. The distraction-compression bar is now distracted until it is tight. This will keep it from falling out and will take up any slack in the bar, ensuring that the first turns on the bar begin to distract the bone.

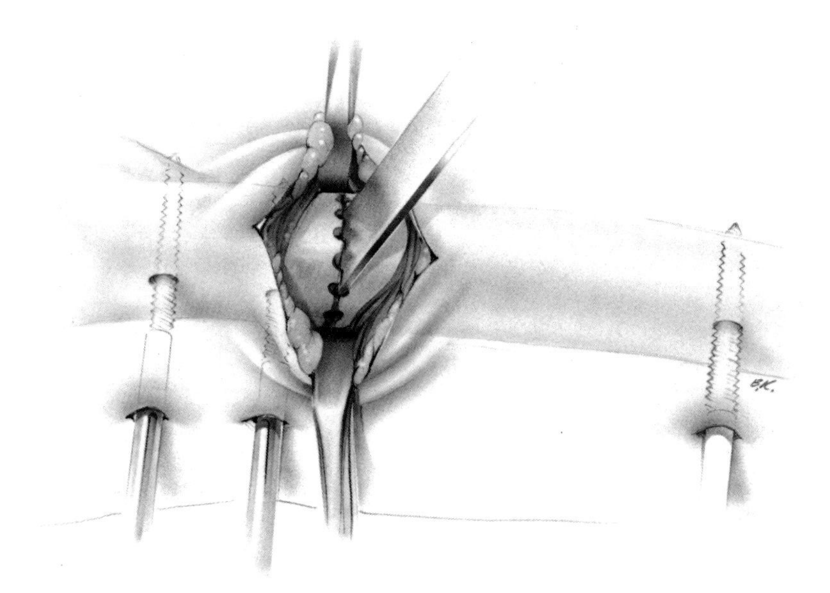

Figure 3–76

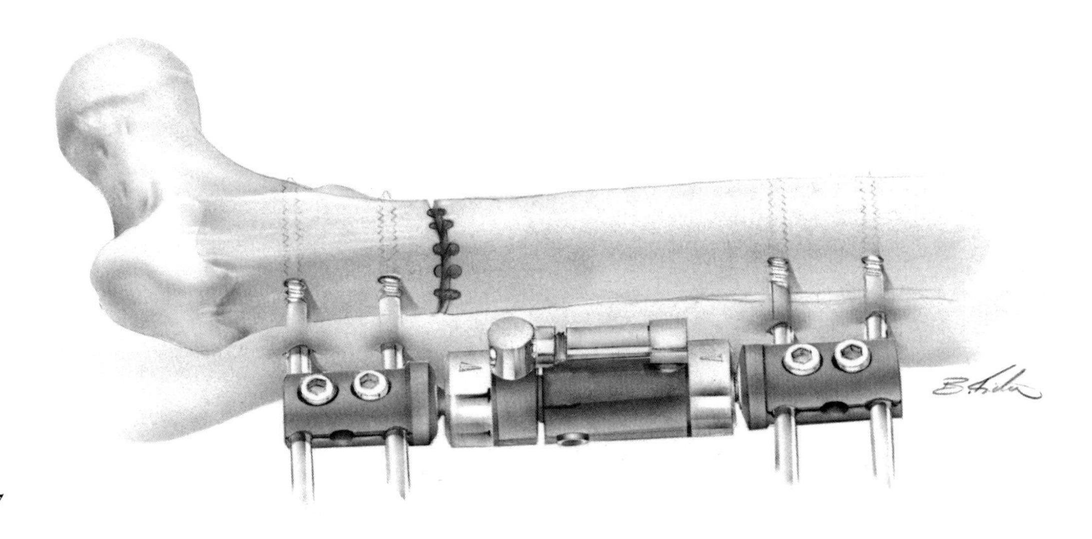

Figure 3–77

Figure 3–78. CQ is a 9-year-old girl with a congenitally short femur. At the time of lengthening her discrepancy was 6.7 cm with a projected discrepancy of 8 cm. Progression of the lengthening is shown in ***Figures 3–78A–C,*** at which time lengthening was discontinued. At this time she has gained 7 cm or 23% of the length of the femur. Maturation of the regenerated bone is seen in ***Figure 3–78D*** 9 months after lengthening was begun. (Courtesy of Charles T. Price, MD.)

POSTOPERATIVE CARE

On the first day after the surgery the patient is started on range-of-motion exercises for the hip and knee, and is ambulated with a three-point partial weight-bearing crutch gait. The osteotomy is quite stable, and the patient may bear as much weight as is comfortable. The first few days go much smoother and are more pleasant for the patient if continuous caudal analgesia is administered.

Pin care begins on the second postoperative day. The philosophy and methods of pin care vary so widely and involve such rigidly held beliefs that it is difficult to make any recommendations. That notwithstanding, the author's preference is to clean the skin and the pins daily with hydrogen peroxide only, avoiding any ointments or disinfectants that tend to form a build-up around the pins. The principle is to keep the local environment clean so the tissues remain healthy.

Distraction should begin when there is radiographic evidence of callus formation. In children this will be in 10 to 14 days, whereas in older adolescents and adults it may take longer. To begin lengthening, the body-locking nut is loosened. The patient distracts the leg 1 mm a day by four one-quarter turns of the distraction-compression bar each day.

It is important to monitor the distraction of the callus. An anteroposterior radiograph of the osteotomy site is taken at 1 week and then every 2 to 4 weeks as deemed necessary. It is important to maintain continuity of the callus. If a break in the callus is noted, distraction should be stopped and compression started at 1 mm a day. When radiographs demonstrate continuity of the callus, distraction is resumed. It is also necessary to be cautious of premature consolidation, a more unusual problem. If this appears to occur, distraction can be increased to 1.5 mm per day. When the desired lengthening is achieved, the body-locking nut is tightened. Now begins a period of consolidation. In general, this will last approximately one half of the time of distraction.

When the callus shows good consolidation, the body-locking nut is loosened, and the period of dynamic loading is begun.

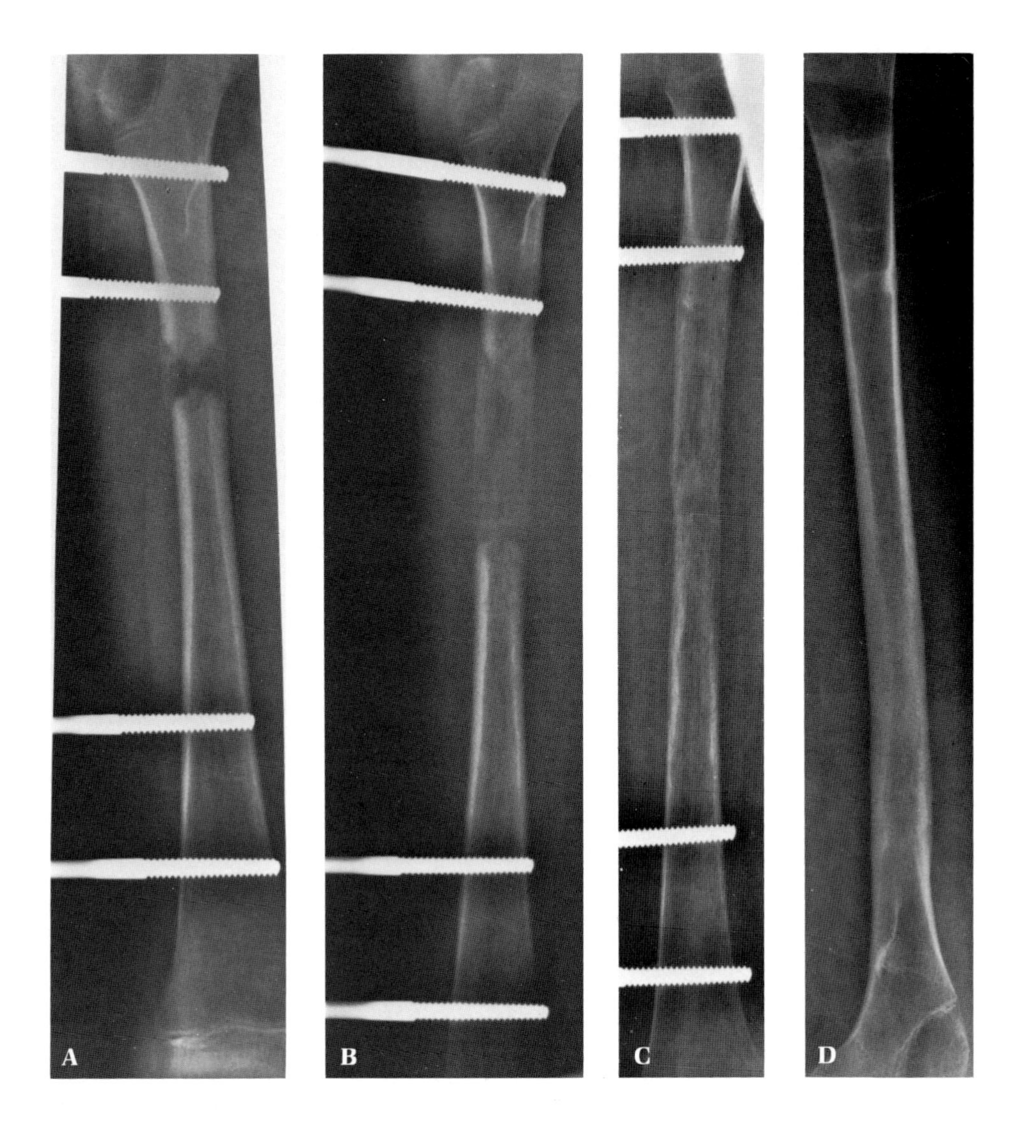

Figure 3–78

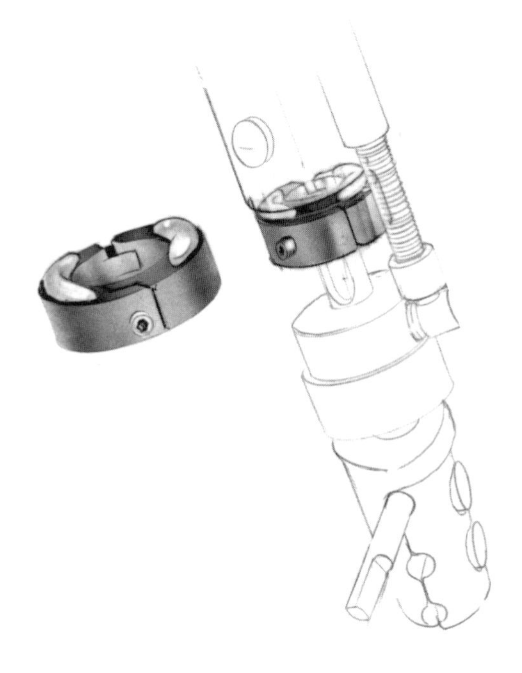

Figure 3–79

This can begin sooner and be safer if the dynamic locking collar is used. This ring locks rigidly to the telescoping bar (***Figure 3–79***). It is placed directly against the distracted body with the silicone rubber bumpers facing the body. This permits the device to collapse a few millimeters placing stress on the bone, but prevents any more collapse of the callus than that. This period of consolidation will also usually last about one half of the time of distraction. During this time the patient is encouraged to bear increasing weight. When cortical bone formation is observed, the device is ready for removal.

With the patient awake and the device still in place, the limb is stressed, particularly in compression. If this caused discomfort, the device should be left in place. If there is no discomfort, the device is removed, and angular and rotational stress is applied to the leg. If this demonstrates good stability without discomfort, the patient can be allowed protected weight bearing. It is wise to have the patient walk for several hours to a few days with the pins still in place in case there are signs of inadequate consolidation. If that occurs, the device can be reapplied.

The time to healing is expressed in the "healing index," which is the number of days of total treatment required to obtain 1 cm of lengthening. It is calculated by dividing the total treatment days by the number of centimeters of lengthening. According to De Bastiani et al,[1] the healing index is 36 days per centimeter for the femur.

REFERENCE

1. De Bastiani G, Aldegheri R, Renzi-Brivio L, Trivella G. Limb lengthening by callus distraction (callotasis). J Pediatr Orthop 1987;7:129.

3.10
Ilizarov Technique of Femoral Lengthening

The Ilizarov apparatus is a complex circular frame that is connected to the bone by wires that transfix the bone in multiple planes. There are many components that can be used in constructing a frame; although there is considerable latitude in the details, there should be no variation from the principles. Because of the complex nature of this apparatus and its varied applications, it is beyond the scope of this book to do more than describe its principles by illustrating a case of simple femoral lengthening. The details of erecting a frame and attaching the wires to the frame are described in more detail in the Ilizarov lengthening of the tibia.

As with any device, there are potential advantages and disadvantages to the use of the Ilizarov device in lengthenings of the femur. The biggest advantage that the Ilizarov device has over other methods of lengthening is its ability to correct angular and rotational deformities at the same time. The trade-off for the bulky frame proximally that interferes with daily functions is the fact the proximal pin fixation can be obtained in more than two planes at right angles to one another as opposed to the unilateral frames. This means secure fixation of the bone fragments and thus less deformity during lengthening.

Figure 3–80. For general guidelines in assembling the frames and a description of the various parts of the frame, see the discussion on Ilizarov lengthening of the tibia.

As much as possible the assembly of the frame should occur before the surgery. Exactly how the frame is constructed depends in large measure on the size of the patient. The proximal part of the frame can be made with two arches (90 or 120 degrees, small or large), or in the case of a small child one arch and a "dropped pin" that is attached to a multiple pin fixation clamp. This provides two levels of fixation of the proximal fragment in the horizontal or transverse plane. To achieve fixation in the coronal and sagittal plane, additional pins will transfix the bone in these various planes and attach to the frame.

The distal frame consists of two complete rings joined in the usual manner by connectors. Again, the principle is to achieve fixation of the distal fragment in two different horizontal planes. The distal ring will support two transfixion wires, and the proximal ring will support one or two transfixion wires depending on the need for stability. If the child is too small to permit the use of two rings, a "dropped wire" can be used. If there is fear that the distal ring will block knee flexion, a five-eighths ring can be used as the distal ring.

Between the 120-degree arch and the distal rings is a "dead ring." This ring is not attached to the bone. The proximal frame is connected to the dead ring by two oblique supports and two rigid rods. The dead ring will be connected to the more proximal of the distal rings with lengtheners or hinges that will be used to lengthen or correct the angular deformity. When initially constructed, the frame will conform to the deformity. This concept of the dead ring greatly simplifies the construction of the frame when it is used for angular correction.

The part of the apparatus that is preassembled—usually at least the distal rings and the dead ring—is first attached to the femur by the most distal transverse wire (see ***Figure 3–82a***). With the apparatus now attached to the bone through this wire, the frame can be adjusted to permit sufficient space between the rings and the skin, and the remainder of the frame can be assembled to fit the proximal thigh.

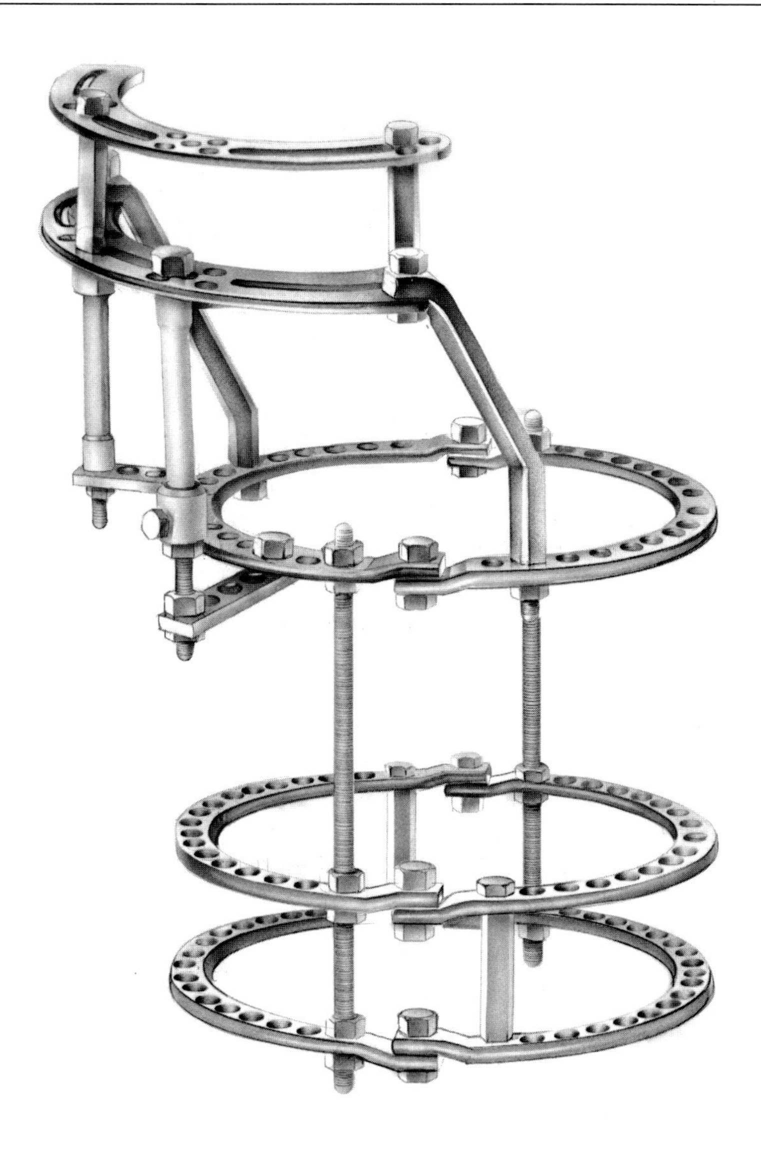

Figure 3–80

Figure 3–81. With the assembly of the frame completed and adjusted, the proximal half-pins are placed as illustrated. These can be either 4- or 5-mm pins depending on the size of the patient. The first pin placed is the lateral pin, which is placed directly distal to the greater trochanter (**b**) (***Figure 3–81A***). It is important that this pin be perpendicular to the mechanical axis (**m**) of the femur, which passes from the center of the femoral head through the center of the knee to the center of the ankle, not the anatomic axis (**a**) (***Figure 3–81B***). This half-pin is then attached to the ring, and the frame is further adjusted on the thigh. The apparatus is now fixed in position. Next, the anterior pin (**c**) is placed at 90 degrees to the lateral pin and is attached to the proximal arch. The third pin (**d**) is placed at a 45-degree angle to these two pins and attached to the lower arch (***Figure 3–81A***). In a large patient a fourth pin can be placed and attached to the lower arch.

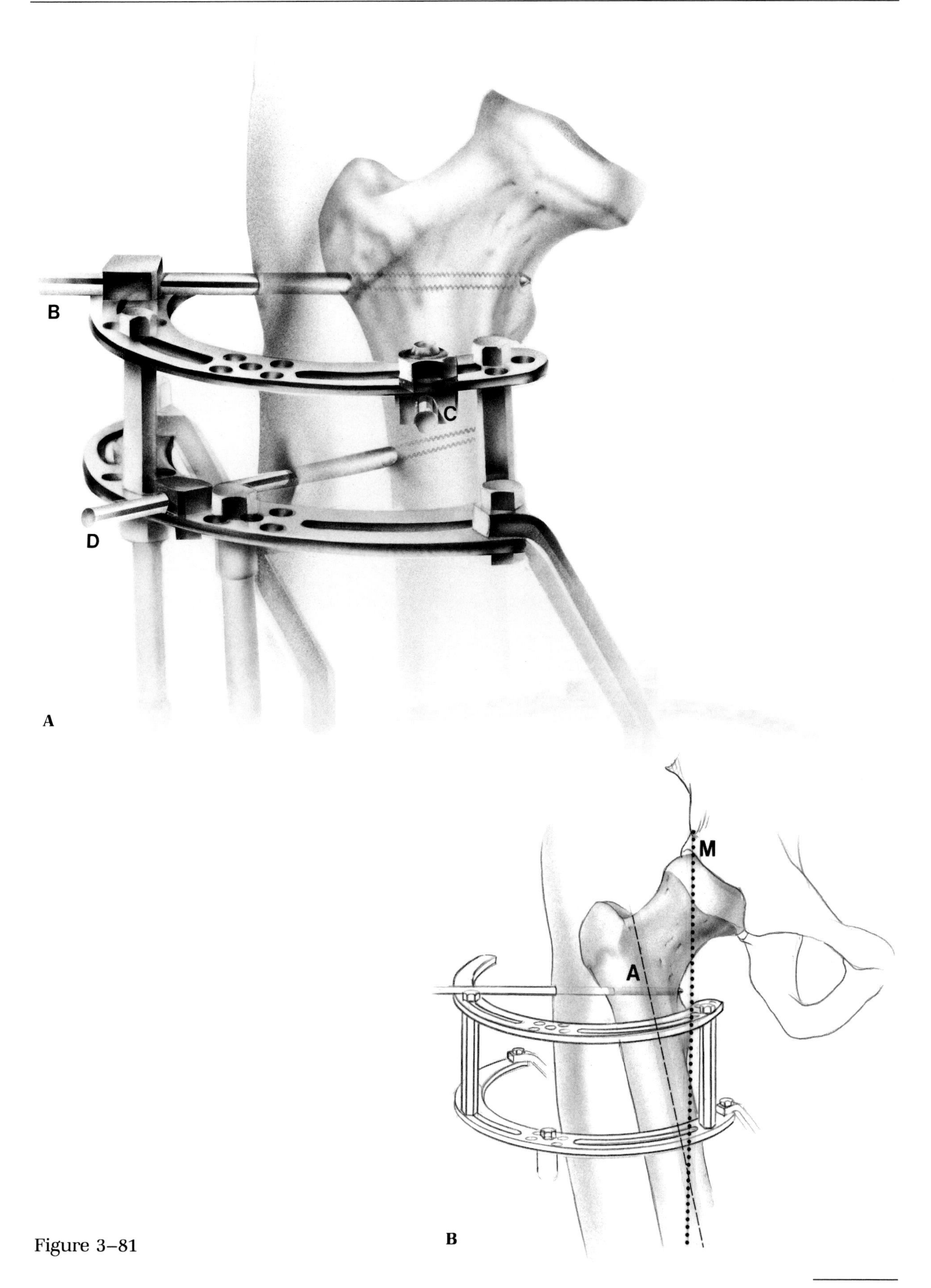

Figure 3–81

Figure 3–82. The distal wires are inserted in the following manner. The transverse pin on the distal ring was the first pin inserted (**a**). This pin should have an "olive" laterally. This first transverse pin should be placed parallel to the axis of the knee joint. The knee should be flexed when this pin is inserted to avoid fixing the quadriceps muscle in an extended position thus blocking flexion.

A second transverse wire with an "olive" medially is attached to the more proximal ring (**e**). Two additional pins will be needed. One of these should begin anterolateral (**f**) and another anteromedial (**g**) so that they tend to be at 90 degrees to each other. When the wire is passing through the quadriceps the knee should be flexed, and when the wire is exiting posterior and passing through the hamstring muscles, the knee should be extended.

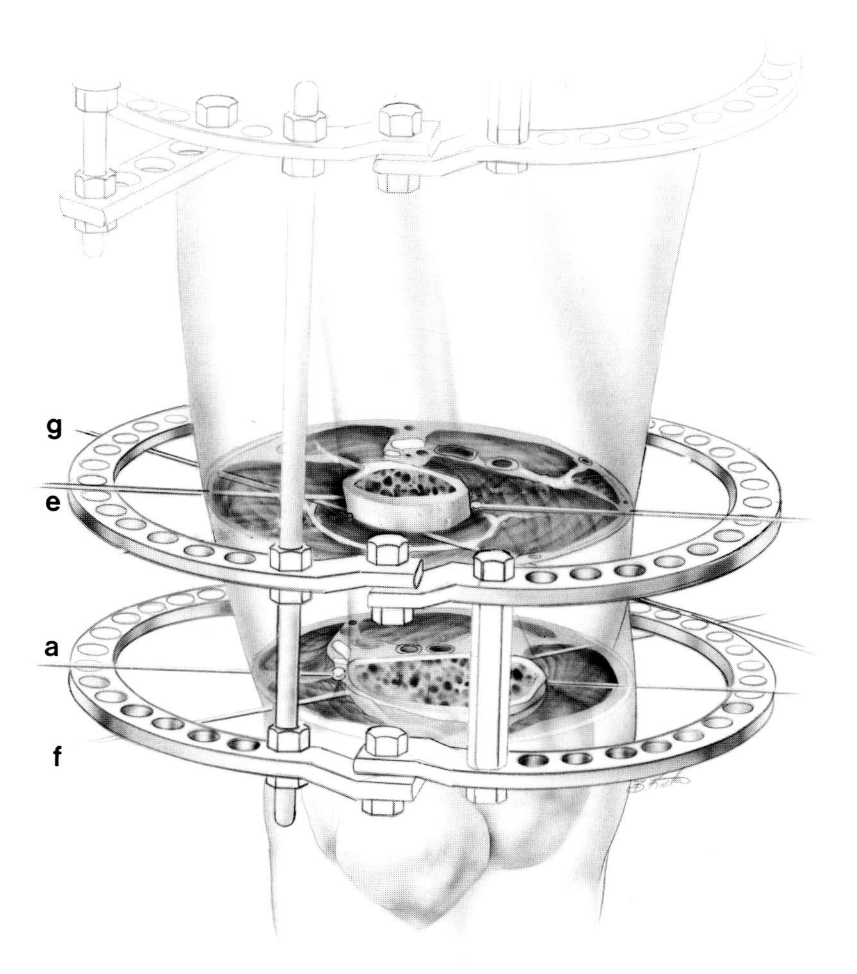

Figure 3–82

Figure 3–83. With the frame now attached to the leg, the connectors between the distal rings and the dead ring are removed in preparation for the osteotomy. The principles of the osteotomy and the technical aspects of its performance are described in the procedure for tibial lengthening with the Ilizarov technique. The osteotomy is performed in the distal femur approximately 1 cm proximal to the most proximal of the distal pins. This can be done through a lateral incision.

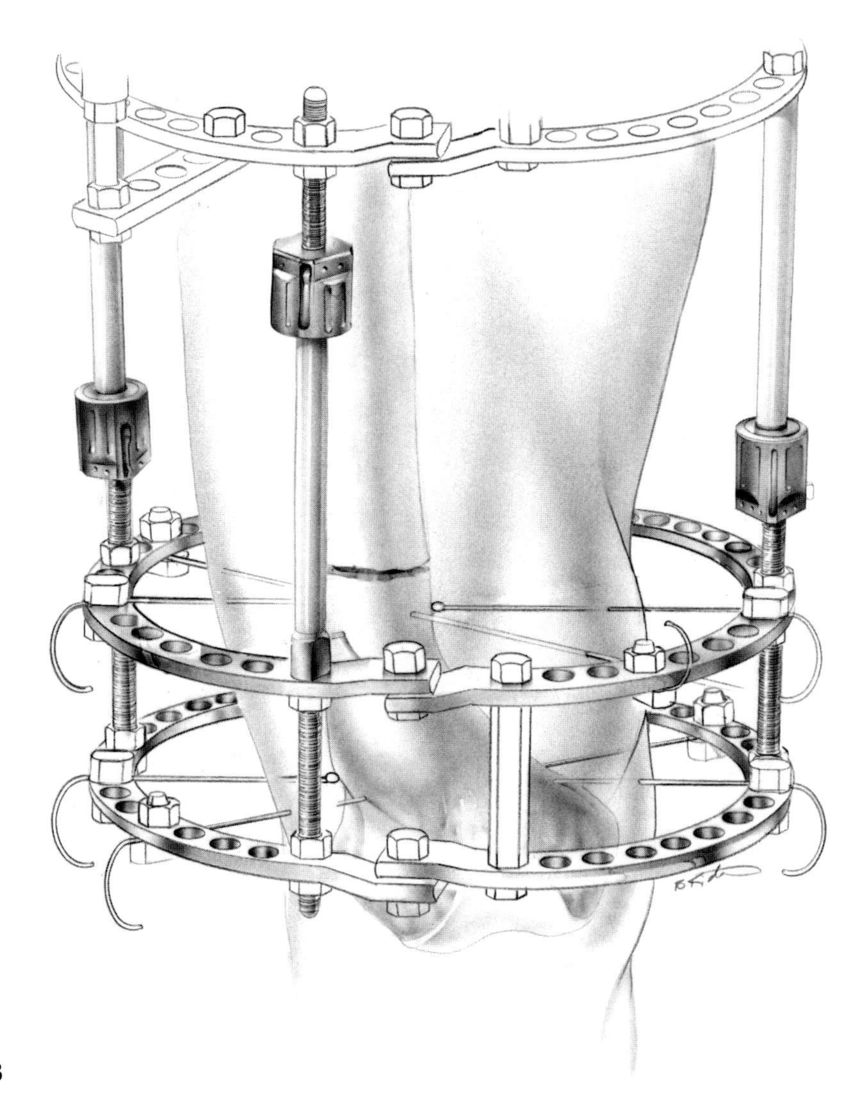

Figure 3–83

Figure 3–84. BH is a 6.5-year-old girl who sustained destruction of the distal femoral epiphysis secondary to sepsis as an infant. She has undergone several previous osteotomies, and her projected leg-length discrepancy is 15 cm (***Figure 3–84A***). The plan is to gain as much length as possible now, recognizing that further lengthening will be necessary in the future. It is anticipated that the translational deformity will be corrected during a future lengthening. Notice that despite the poor mechanical axis of the femur, her knee joint is parallel to the floor throughout the lengthening.

The progression of the callus distraction is illustrated at 4, 10, and 15 weeks (***Figures 3–84B–D***).

The result is seen at 6 months after removal of the apparatus (***Figure 3–84E***). (Courtesy of Peter Armstrong, MD.)

POSTOPERATIVE CARE

The lengthening begins between 3 and 10 days after the application of the device and osteotomy of the bone. In most children lengthening is started at 5 days. Lengthening is done at the rate of 1 mm per day in four stages. If the lengtheners are used, the patient's task is simplified because each click equals 0.25 mm. If threaded rods are used, the patient will have to adjust all of the nuts on all of the rods four times per day. During this period of lengthening weight bearing is encouraged, and physical therapy to maintain joint motion is done several times per day.

The lengthening is monitored radiographically to be certain that continuity of the callus is maintained. It should be remembered that 1 mm per day is a guide and that circumstances (*eg,* disruption of the callus or premature consolidation) call for either an increase or decrease in the rate of lengthening.

The apparatus should not be removed until cortical bone is present in the distraction callus. As the structure of the frame provides enough flexibility for mechanical loading of the bone, this cortex should develop without loosening the distraction such as is done during the period of consolidation in the Orthofix technique. Nevertheless, fracture is a problem as with all leg lengthenings, and the patient should be protected with a brace, crutches, or both as the circumstances dictate.

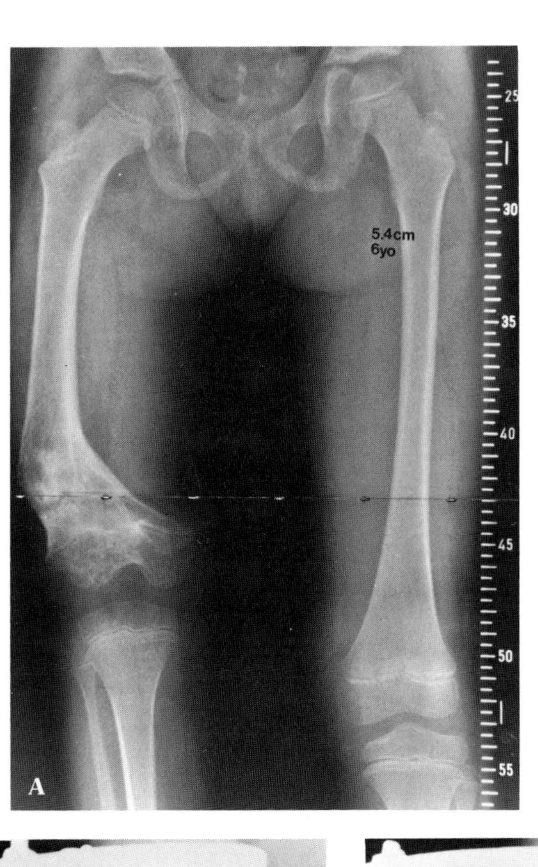

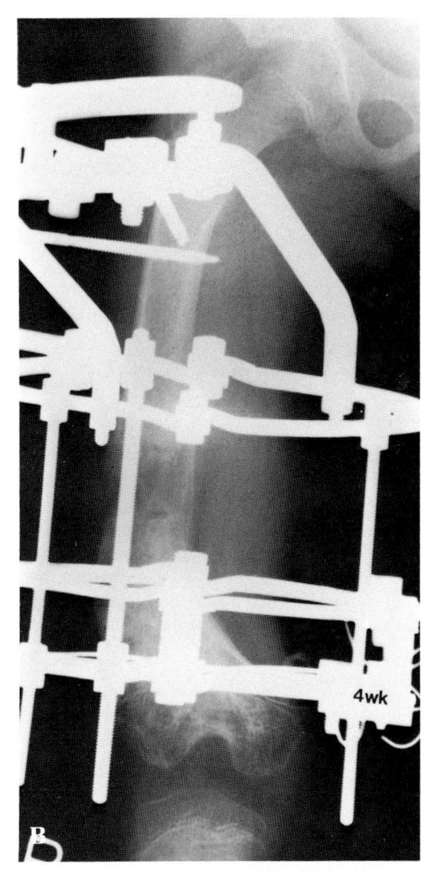

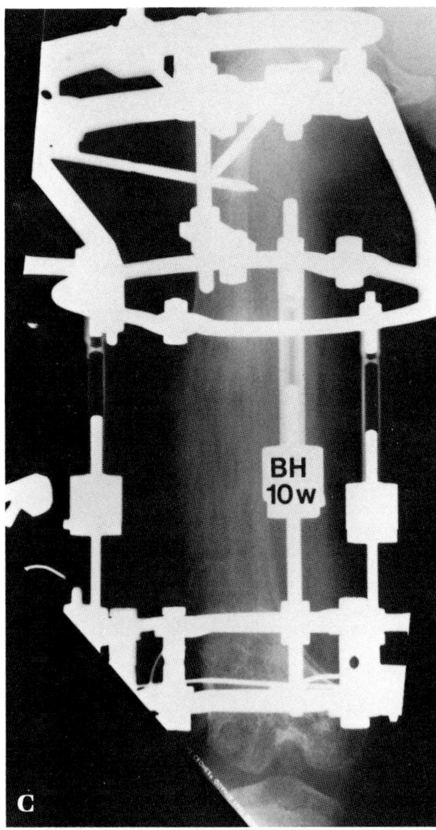

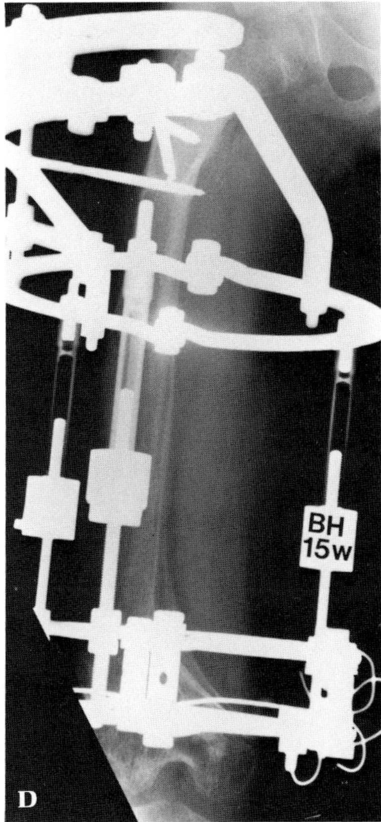

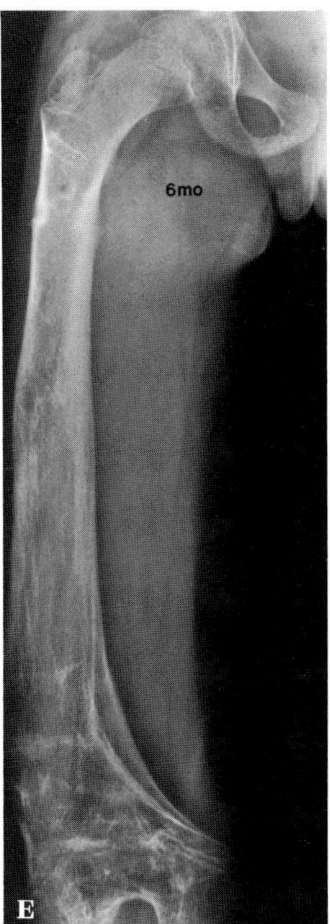

Figure 3–84

3.11 Distal Angular Femoral Osteotomy

There are many deformities in children that result in a growth disturbance of the distal femur. Among the commonest are infection, injury, and systemic growth disturbances (*eg,* rickets). In many cases, especially those that destroy a segment of the growth plate, varus or valgus may be combined with anterior or posterior angulation affecting predominantly one condyle. These combined deformities will create a plane of motion at the knee that is not in the mechanical or anatomic axis of the limb, and they require careful preoperative planning to correct each component of the deformity.

There is a particular risk in correcting valgus deformity, especially when severe and of long duration or when contemplating an opening wedge osteotomy. That risk is damage to the peroneal nerve. When this risk is foreseen, releasing the peroneal nerve distally past the fibular head is advisable.

Fixation around the knee (*ie,* the distal femur or proximal tibia) is often difficult in children because of the open growth plates. Crossed smooth Steinman pins have been used but have the dual disadvantage of being less rigid than desirable, necessitating a cast, and of risking infection if the pins are left outside of the skin. Rigid internal fixation with blade plates can be done in the usual manner if the growth plate is closed but if it is open, the blade must be inserted above the growth plate and the side plate recontoured. Often in smaller children the smaller right-angled blade plates can be used. Very careful preoperative planning, considering the location of the osteotomy and the type of plate, its length, and its off-set is required. A third alternative is the use of external fixation.

The osteotomy is generally performed and fixed from the lateral approach, although a severe valgus deformity can be corrected from a medial approach. It should be recognized that when a valgus deformity is corrected from a lateral approach the blade plate will be used as a buttress plate. If an opening osteotomy is used in this region, it is usually not necessary to add bone graft. Curretting bone from the metaphysis into the defect will usually result in prompt healing.

Limb length is also a consideration in angular deformities of the distal femur and should be accounted for in the preoperative planning. In addition to the projected discrepancy at the end of growth secondary to growth plate damage, there will be two factors regarding the limb length that should be considered in the planning. These factors are discussed in relation to tibial osteotomies by Canale and Harper.[1]

Figure 3–85. The first factor to consider in length is that any angular deformity will produce a functional shortening of the limb and correction of this angulation will produce a gain in length. The amount of length that can be gained (independent of the type of osteotomy performed) is dependent on the length of the limb below the osteotomy site and the degree of angulation. The amount of length to be gained can be derived from analysis of the geometry as shown.[1] It can more easily be estimated by drawing templates of the correction. If the deformity was created by a malunion and not a disturbance of growth, there is little value in this calculation because correction of the angulation will restore normal length. The calculation of this factor is of importance when correction is planned of a large angular deformity caused by a disturbance in the overall longitudinal growth of the limb.

Figure 3–86. The second factor to consider in the planning of the osteotomy is how much length will be gained or lost by an opening or closing wedge. Geometric analysis shows that the amount of length gained or lost is equal to the height at the center of the wedge.[1] Thus, this can be calculated either geometrically or from templates before surgery and measured directly at the time of surgery. Small corrections of length in the range of 1 to 2 cm are usually possible, but the surgeon should not expect to gain larger corrections by the method of the osteotomy alone.

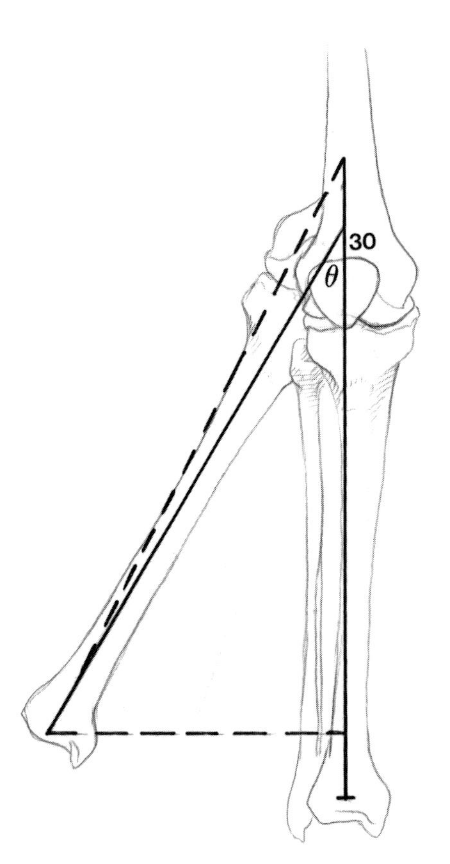

Figure 3–85

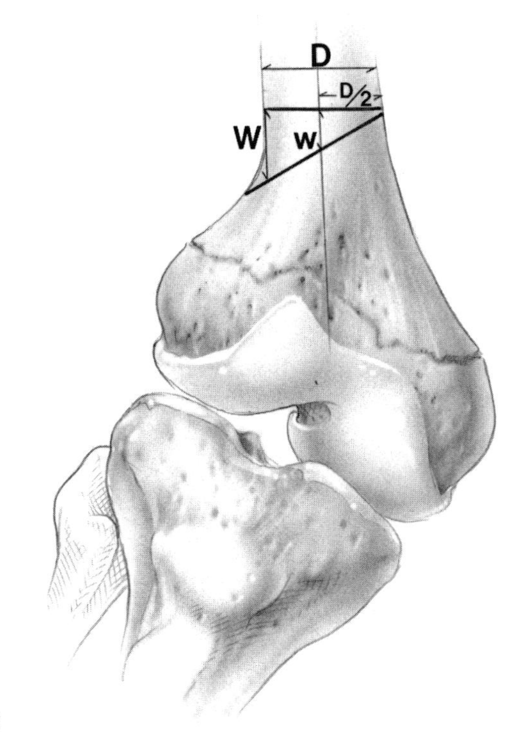

Figure 3–86

Figure 3–87. The patient is positioned supine on a translucent table. A sand bag is placed under the hip to compensate for the tendency of the leg to rotate externally and a soft roll placed under the knee to relax the muscles. The leg is draped free so that it can be moved. A sterile tourniquet can be used around the proximal thigh except in small children. The incision extends from the level of the knee joint proximal along a line that connects the midportion of the lateral femoral condyle and the greater trochanter.

Figure 3–88. The iliotibial band is identified after the subcutaneous tissue is divided. A divergence of the fibers distally can be identified: the fibers to the patellar retinaculum going anteriorly and the insertion of the iliotibial band into Gerdes tubercle continuing distal. The iliotibial band is divided starting in this interval.

Figure 3–89. The posterior edge of the vastus lateralis muscle is identified in the distal part of the exposure and is elevated anteriorly. After a short distance the vastus lateralis will be attached to the intermuscular septum from which it must be freed. This is done with a periosteal elevator. The muscle can be followed back to its insertion into the femur, from which it must also be freed. This would be a simple matter were it not for the superior geniculate artery crossing over the flare of the lateral femoral condyle and the perforating branches supplying the vastus lateralis muscle that come through the intermuscular septum close to the bone to enter the muscle. As the bone is approached, these vessels can usually be identified and cauterized if care is taken in the dissection.

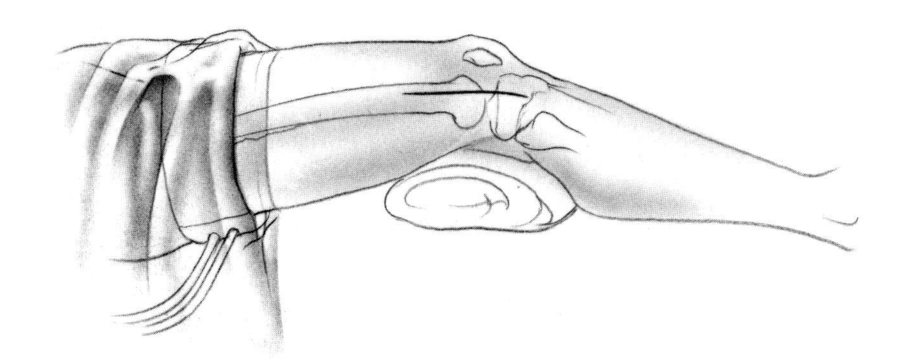

Figure 3–87

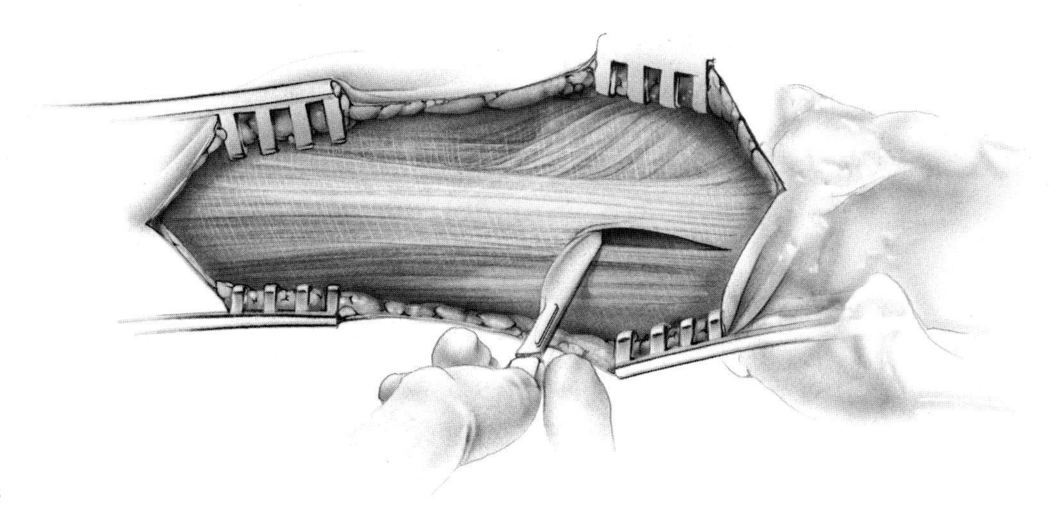

Figure 3–88

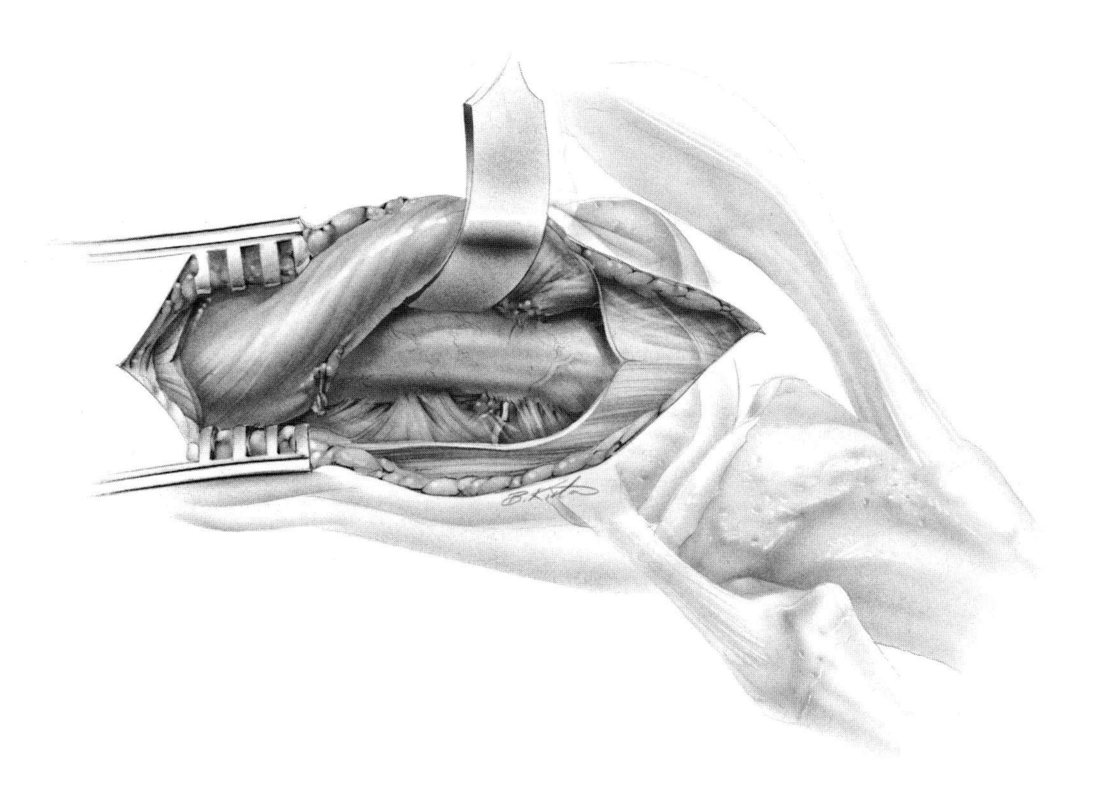

Figure 3–89

Figure 3–90. Because there will be a deformity the condylar guide cannot be used as it is for fracture fixation. The correction of the deformity, however, is dependent on the blade being placed in the distal fragment in exactly the correct position. This is usually parallel to the joint line. It is therefore best to identify the joint line by inserting a small, smooth Kirschner wire through the knee joint passing over both femoral condyles (**a**). This is easiest to do with the knee flexed 90 degrees. This wire will guide the insertion of the seating chisel in the frontal plane.

It is now necessary to determine the correct location and direction for the insertion of the seating chisel in the sagittal plane. A second smooth Kirschner wire can be passed over the anterior surface of the femoral condyles through the patellofemoral joint to determine the inclination (**b**). The correct starting point will be 1.5 cm proximal to the joint line and in line with the middle of the femoral shaft. Now a third Kirschner wire parallel to the joint line and at the proper inclination can be drilled into the femoral condyle 1 cm proximal to the joint, its location confirmed on the image intensifier, and then used as the guide for the seating chisel (**c**). The other two wires (**a, b**) can now be removed.

Figure 3–91. It is necessary to make an opening in the cortex before inserting the chisel so that its direction can be controlled. This can be done with a small osteotome or by making three holes with the 4.5-mm drill and drill jig, which can be connected with a small rongeur.

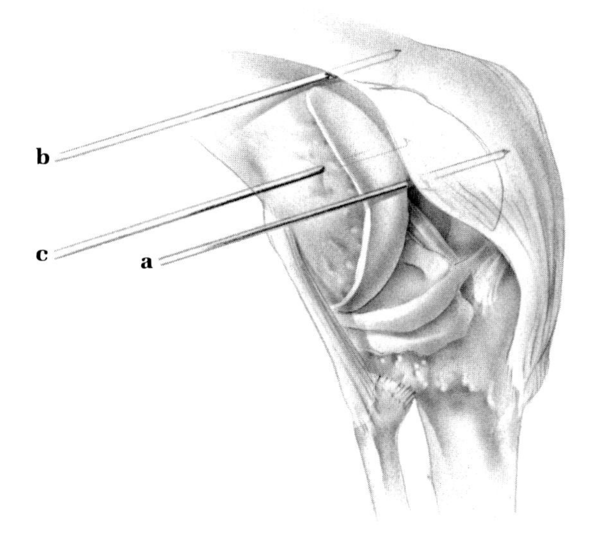

Figure 3–90

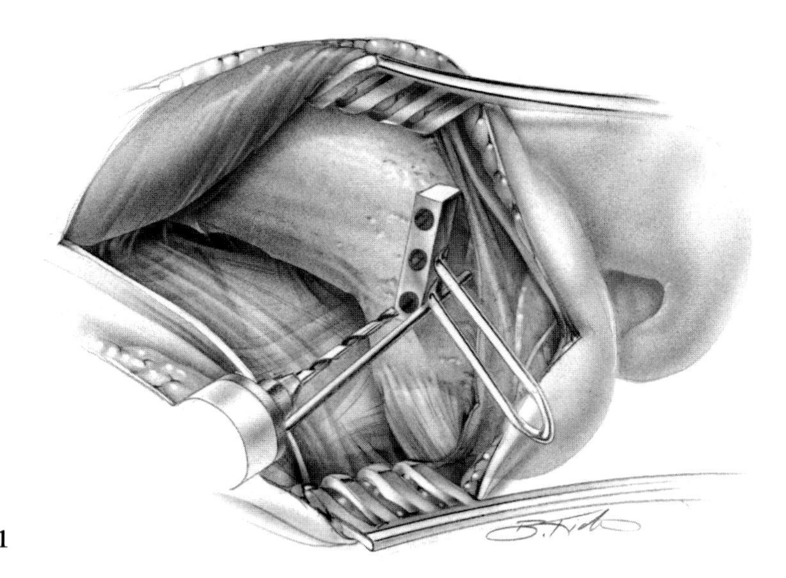

Figure 3–91

Figure 3–92. The seating chisel is now driven into the femoral condyles. It is helpful to use the seating chisel guide and the slotted hammer to maintain the proper rotation of the blade during insertion. If this is not done the plate will not contact the shaft of the femur.

Figure 3–93. If a valgus deformity is being corrected by an opening-wedge osteotomy to gain length, no further calculations need to be made. A simple transverse osteotomy is made in the supracondylar region. When the side plate is brought in contact with the femoral shaft, the alignment of the distal femur should be brought to normal.

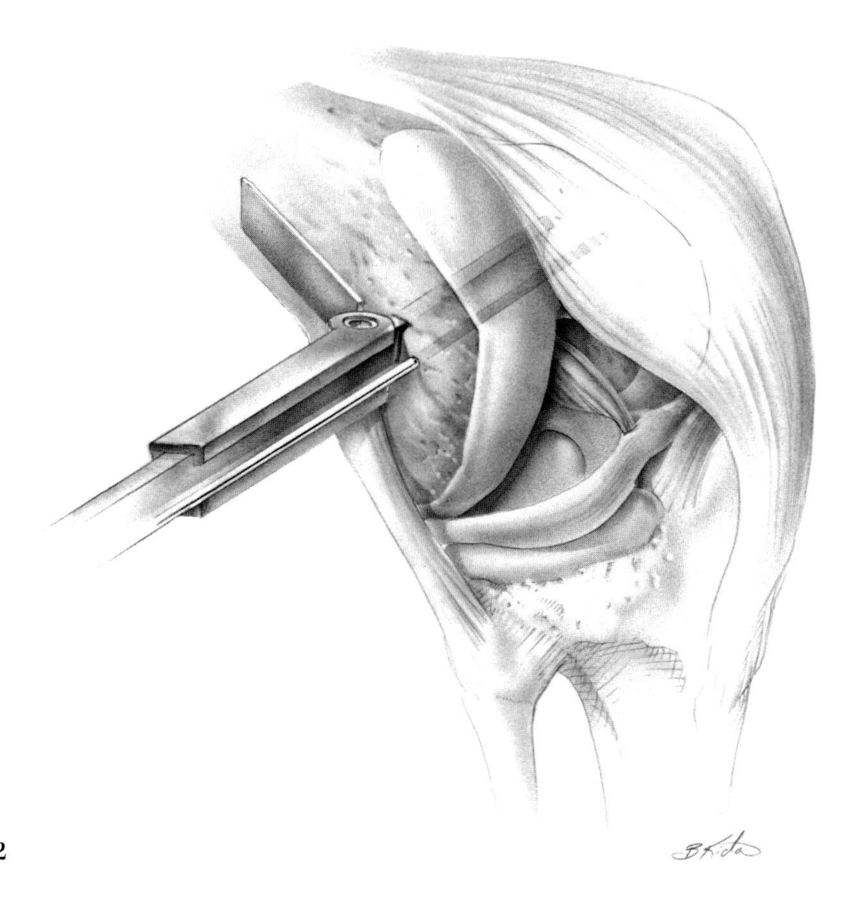

Figure 3–92

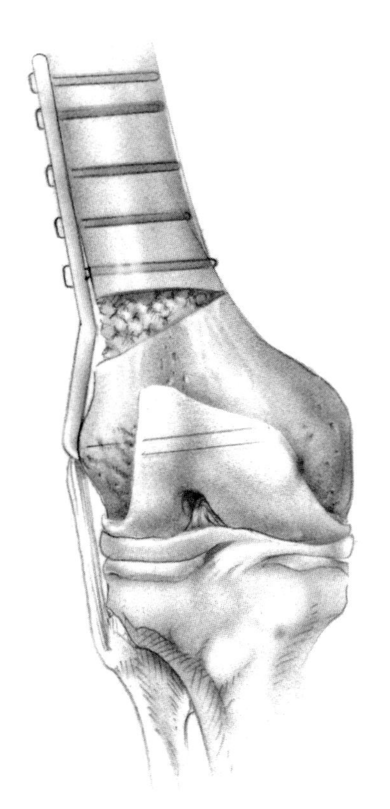

Figure 3–93

Figure 3–94. When a varus deformity is being corrected by a closing-wedge osteotomy, the size of the wedge needs to be determined. This should be done preoperatively, but may be confirmed by noting the angle formed by the seating chisel and the bottom of the condylar guide. A transverse osteotomy is made in the supracondylar region and then the appropriate-sized wedge is removed from the lateral one half of the proximal fragment if varus is being corrected or from the medial one half if valgus is being corrected without the need for additional length.

Figure 3–95. The two distal holes in the condylar plate are for the use of cancellous screws to provide for additional fixation of the distal fragment. After they are secured, the plate is held to the femoral shaft with a clamp and secured with screws. It is advisable in this osteotomy to use the compression device to obtain compression rather than rely on the compression obtained through the dynamic compression of the plate and screws alone.

The wound is drained and closure started at the iliotibial band.

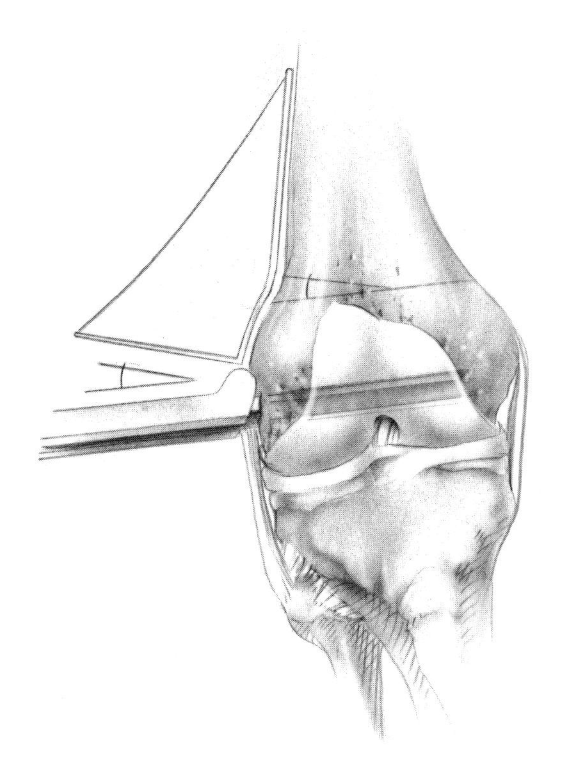

Figure 3–94

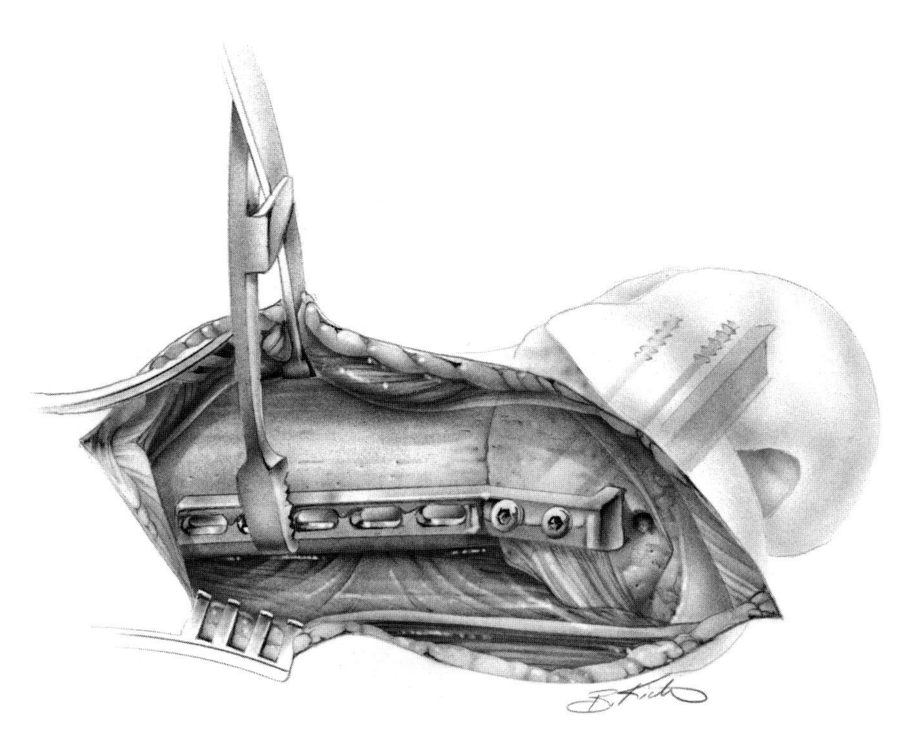

Figure 3–95

Figure 3–96. JT sustained a Salter II fracture of the distal femoral physis at 12 years of age with subsequent growth arrest of the lateral one half of the growth plate. When seen at 16 years of age, he had a significant valgus deformity and 4.5 cm of shortening of the femur as compared with the opposite side (***Figure 3–96A***). It was calculated that an opening-wedge osteotomy of the distal femur would produce 1.5-cm gain in length of the leg, leaving a 3-cm discrepancy. An opening-wedge osteotomy was performed using a condylar blade plate (***Figure 3–96B***). At the same operative session he also underwent a closed intramedullary shortening of the opposite femur to produce equalization of his limb lengths (***Figure 3–96C***). Today lengthening with angular correction using either the Ilizarov or Orthofix device would be another alternative to this treatment plan.

POSTOPERATIVE CARE

No immobilization is necessary postoperatively. The patient is started on active-assisted range-of-motion exercises the day after surgery and progressed to protected crutch weight bearing in a few days. As pain subsides, the patient begins active exercises to maintain quadriceps and hamstring strength. Healing of the osteotomy is monitored with radiographs and full weight bearing permitted when union is evident, usually within 6 to 8 weeks.

REFERENCE

1. Canale ST, Harper MC. Biotrigonometric analysis and practical applications of osteotomies of tibia in children. In: The American Academy of Orthopaedic Surgeons Instructional Course Lectures, vol XXX. St Louis; CV Mosby, 1981:85.

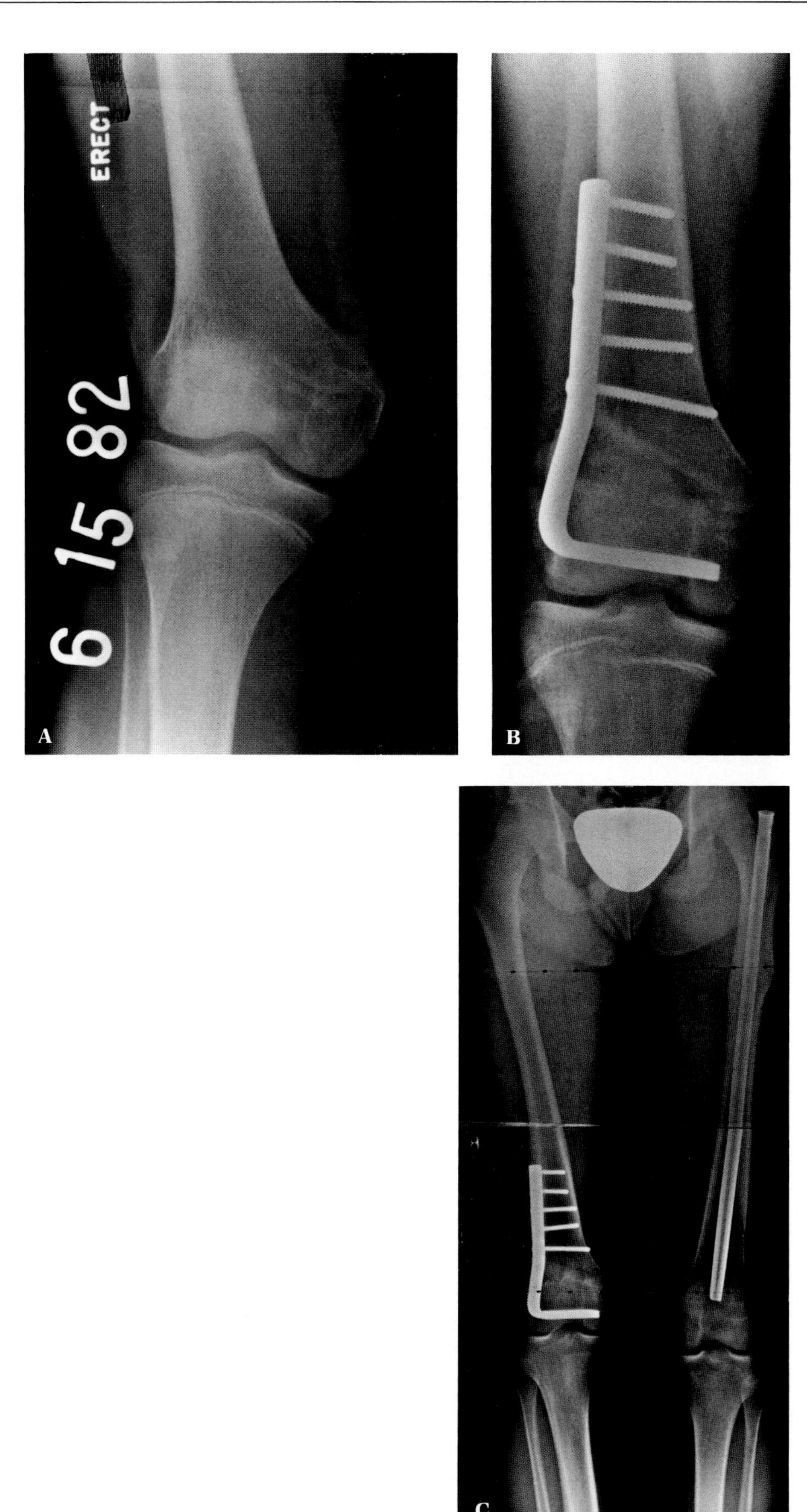

Figure 3–96

3.12
Distal Rotational Femoral Osteotomy Using External Fixation

Rotational malalignment in the femur can be corrected by osteotomy at any point in the bone. The rapid healing that occurs in the metaphyses, however, favors correction either in the intertrochanteric region or in the supracondylar region. Although many recommend that correction be done in the intertrochanteric region at any age, some prefer to perform the osteotomy in the supramalleolar region for children less than 9 years of age.[1,2] The indications for rotational osteotomy for excessive and persistent femoral anteversion have been given.[1–3] Because surgery is not indicated before 8 years of age and this technique is not recommended for children older than 9 years of age, it will find limited use for this indication.

The procedure was initially conceived on two principles: It does not matter where the rotational correction is achieved, and it is a smaller and simpler operation when done in the supracondylar region, leaving only a small scar and not requiring the removal of internal fixation. As originally performed, the procedure required no fixation other than a double-hip spica cast. After experiencing loss of position some surgeons began to place Steinmann pins into the bone and incorporate these into the cast. With the evolution of external fixation, it was logical that external fixation without a cast would be an additional option for treatment.

In addition to the potential loss of position if no fixation other than casting is used, medial overgrowth of the distal femur requiring reoperation has been reported.[4] The reason was not apparent but was likened to the valgus deformity that is seen after an incomplete proximal tibial fracture in a growing child.

Although the author has preferred to perform this correction in the intertrochanteric region, he has used a distal osteotomy in special circumstances (*eg*, a patient of the Jehova Witness faith). Considering all of the factors, it is the author's choice to use an external fixator when performing this osteotomy—trading the pin track scars for secure fixation. In choosing a fixator the Orthofix device would seem to be ideal. It permits rotational adjustments after it is applied, as well as dynamic loading of the osteotomy site to promote more rapid healing. With this approach the consideration of scars is not paramount, and the osteotomy can more easily be performed from the lateral approach. If the presence of the scars is paramount and the risks of valgus deformity and loss of position are balanced by this, a medial approach to the osteotomy and double-spica cast is the best approach.

Figure 3–97. The patient is positioned flat on a radiolucent table. A sterile bolster beneath the knee facilitates placing the pins but must be removed when checking the rotation.

The appropriate-sized Orthofix fixator and its template are chosen. The body of the template should be extended 2 to 3 cm. This is to allow for the shortening of the device that will occur as the bone is rotated, bringing the two sets of pins closer together. Just as important, having the device extended will permit dynamic loading of the osteotomy site to promote more rapid healing. The template is aligned with the femoral shaft, and the most proximal two pins are placed first as described for lengthening.

Figure 3–98. The most distal pins are placed next. Because the distal fragment will be rotated externally, however, these pins will not be placed in the same axis as the two proximal pins. Rather, they will be placed at an angle to the proximal two pins that approximates the degree of correction that is desired. These distal pins should not simply start at a different angle in the same longitudinal axis as the other two pins, but actually start on that surface of the bone that will come to lie in the axis of the proximal pins after the rotational correction is achieved (***Figure 3–98A***).

If these distal pins are placed straight through the skin, they will produce severe pressure and subsequent necrosis of the skin after they are rotated to produce the correction. To avoid this the skin of the distal thigh is rotated anteriorly and held there while these distal pins are inserted (***Figure 3–98B***). The ball joints of the template are rotated to permit the insertion of these pins in a different axis but parallel to the femur (***Figure 3–98C***). They are inserted in the manner previously described for the Orthofix device with one addition. Because these pins will rotate through the muscle and particularly the fascia lata, the incision in the fascia lata is "T'd" posteriorly, and the hemostat is spread in both a longitudinal and transverse direction.

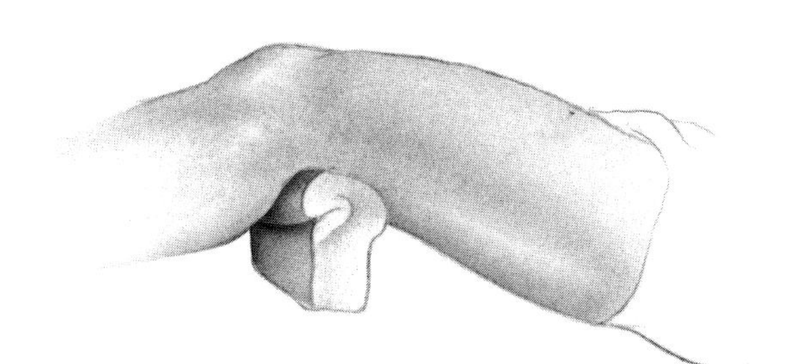

Figure 3–97

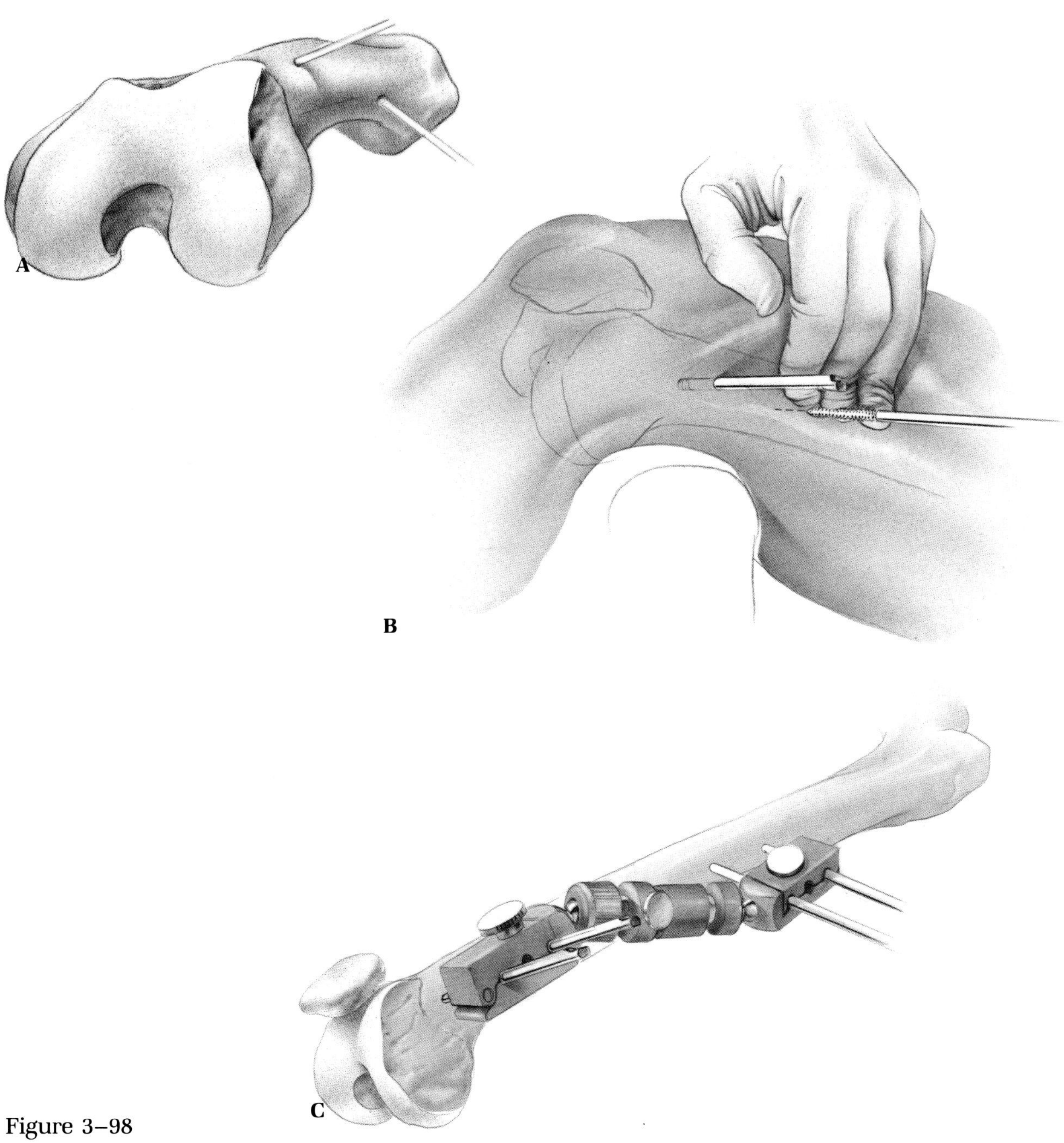

Figure 3–98

Figure 3–99. After the pins are inserted, the template is removed and a small incision is made posterolaterally, extending proximal for about 2 cm from the level of the most proximal of the distal two pins (***Figure 3–99A***).

The vastus lateralis is elevated off of the intermuscular septum and followed to the bone. A longitudinal incision is made in the periosteum, which is elevated circumferentially. Multiple drill holes are made in the bone, extending through the opposite cortex. The drill stop can be used to avoid overpenetration on the medial side. The osteotomy is completed with a small osteotome (***Figure 3–99B***). The pins are grasped and twisted to be certain that the osteotomy has been completed and that there is sufficient mobility between the two fragments. The wound is then closed over a drain.

Figure 3–100. The fixator is now applied to the pins, and the fracture reduction clamps are applied (only one clamp is shown for clarity). With the bolster removed and the leg flat on the table, the rotational correction is accomplished. The ball joints are locked with the torque wrench. The compressor-distractor is now applied and the osteotomy site compressed. The body-locking nut is tightened. The knee is flexed past 90 degrees to ensure that the pins are loose enough in the muscle to permit knee motion.

After the second leg is done, the drapes are removed, and the rotation of the two is compared. If any adjustments are necessary, they can be accomplished before the patient emerges from the anesthetic.

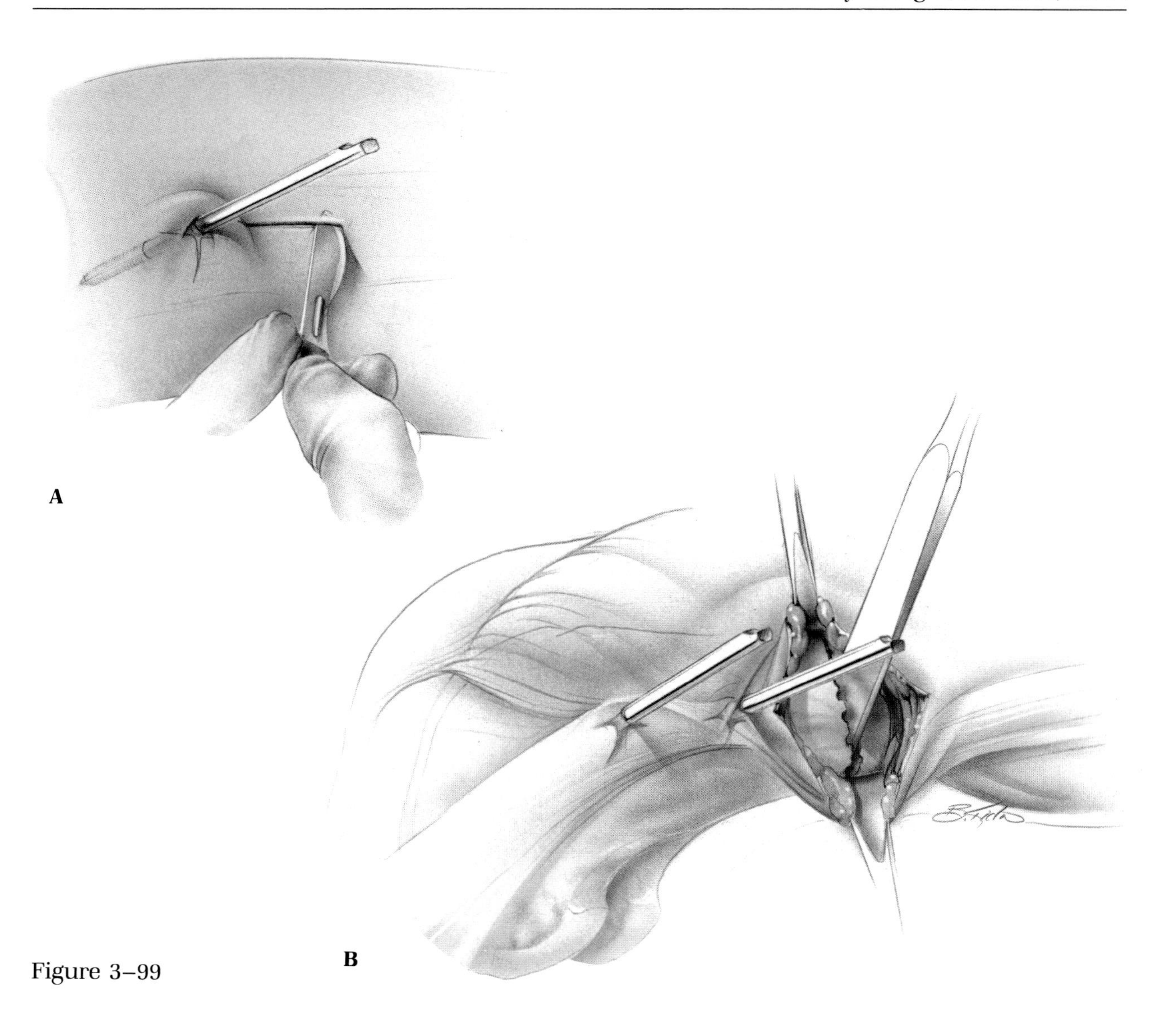

Figure 3–99

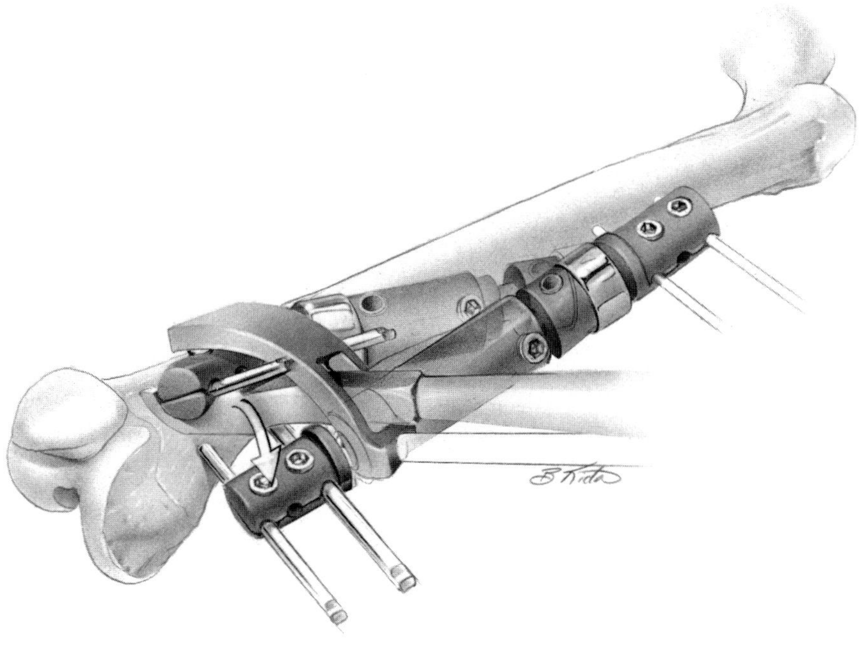

Figure 3–100

Figure 3–101. Immediate postoperative anteroposterior radiographs of an 11-year-old girl following a bilateral distal rotational femoral osteotomy (***Figure 3–101A***). The Synthes external fixator was used for fixation. The osteotomies were done higher than necessary but were healed sufficiently in 8 weeks to allow removal of the fixators. The lateral radiograph of the right femur (***Figure 3–101B***) demonstrates the displacement that occurs when the linea aspera is not stripped for a long distance: It acts as a tether at one point on the radius of the bone, causing one fragment to rotate out of the axis of the other fragment. This is illustrated in the technique of proximal rotational femoral osteotomy. The result at 8 weeks is shown (***Figure 3–101C***).

POSTOPERATIVE TREATMENT

The drains can usually be removed on the first postoperative day. Range-of-motion exercises are also started on the first postoperative day. By the second day the patient is out of bed and may progress to four-point crutch gait as tolerated. At 3 to 4 weeks the body-locking nut is loosened, and the compressor-distractor is removed. Healing should be sufficient to prevent distraction at the osteotomy site, and pain should be minimal so that dynamic compression of the osteotomy site can begin. When the osteotomy is healed, the fixator and the pins can be removed.

REFERENCES

1. Kumar SJ, MacEwen GD. Torsional abnormalities in children's lower extremities. Orthop Clin North Am 1982;13:629.
2. Kling TF, Hensinger RN. Angular and torsional deformities of the lower limbs in children. Clin Orthop 1983;176:136.
3. Staheli LT. The lower limb. In: Morrissy RT, ed. Lovell and Winter's pediatric orthopaedics, 3rd ed. Philadelphia: JB Lippincott, 1990:745.
4. Fonseca AS, Bassett GS. Valgus deformity following derotation osteotomy to correct medial femoral torsion. J Pediatr Orthop 1988;8:295.

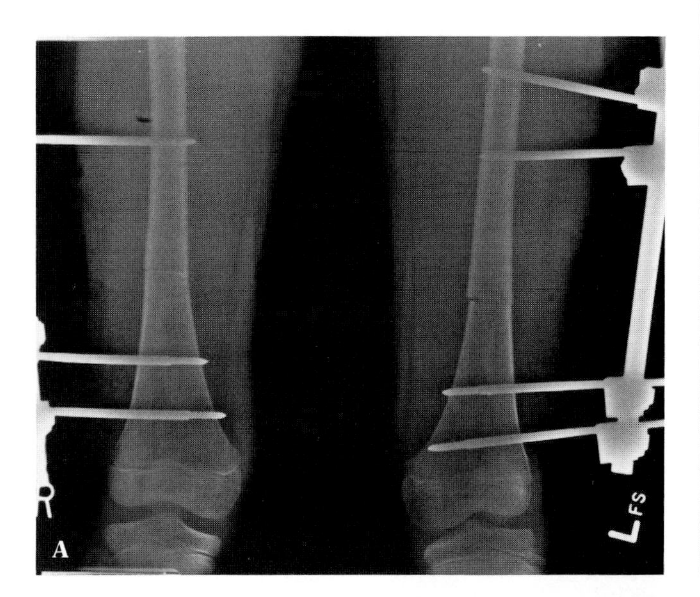

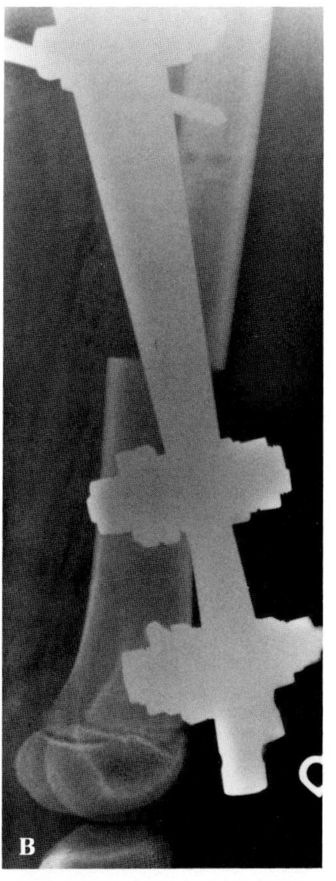

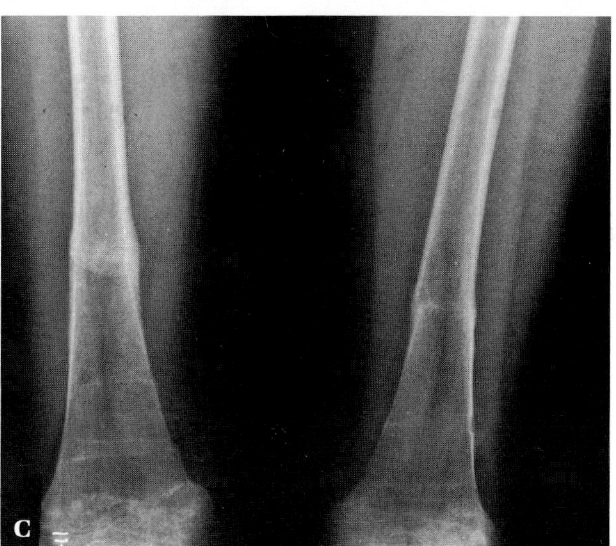

Figure 3–101

3.13 Distal Femoral Epiphysiodesis, Phemister Technique

Arrest of the physeal plate as originally proposed by Phemister remains the commonest and most practical method of correcting mild to moderate leg-length discrepancy in the growing child.[1] It is relatively easy to perform compared with other methods of leg-length equalization and has a decidedly lower morbidity than any other method. It may in fact be deceptively easy, for complications (*eg*, asymmetric arrest of growth) do occur.[2] The key to the success of epiphysiodesis lies in the preoperative planning to estimate correctly the timing of the surgery and the thoroughness of the destruction of the physeal plate.

Performance of this operation percutaneously has recently been described.[3] The author's experience with this percutaneous technique has led him to return to the open technique for the following reasons. The amount of bleeding through the large, open hole in the cortex with subsequent swelling and knee stiffness is much worse than with the open technique. Radiation is substituted for direct vision as a means of identifying the plate, and this can be a fairly large dose to the physician and the patient. Finally, experience with the percutaneous technique taught the author that the incision necessary to remove a block of bone and permit curettement of the plate under direct vision need not be much larger than the incision for the percutaneous technique and is not troublesome to the patient.

Figure 3–102. The patient is first positioned for surgery on the lateral side with a sand bag under the buttocks. When completed, the sand bag can easily be removed, allowing the patient to roll flat, facilitating the medial approach. A tourniquet is used. An incision about 3 cm in length is centered over the physeal plate. This incision is often made unnecessarily large with the result being an unsightly scar. It should be remembered that the exposure only needs to be large enough to excise the block of bone; the remainder of the surgery is done through the resulting hole in the bone. If the surgeon is not able to identify the region of the epiphyseal plate by the external anatomic landmarks, an image intensifier can be used.

Figure 3–103. The incision is deepened through the fascia lata and the posterior border of the vastus lateralis is identified, freed, and retracted anteriorly. This will expose the periosteum, which is incised, creating two flaps that are elevated with a periosteal elevator. These flaps can be cut in the periosteum with a coagulation current to cauterize the numerous vessels that cross this operative site. This will help to prevent excessive bleeding and swelling after the tourniquet is removed. The physeal plate is easily identified if exposed by elevating the periosteum. The exposure can be enhanced by also incising the periosteum directly over the plate at 90 degrees to the first incision, producing a cruciate incision. It is more difficult to secure a tight closure with this cruciate incision. It is important to recognize that it is not necessary to perform excessive periosteal stripping and expose large areas of the physeal plate. Only an area sufficiently large to permit removal of a block of bone no larger than $\frac{3}{4}$ to 1 inch square is necessary. This block of bone will create a bony bridge across the plate while the hole it makes will allow access for the destruction of most of the physeal plate.

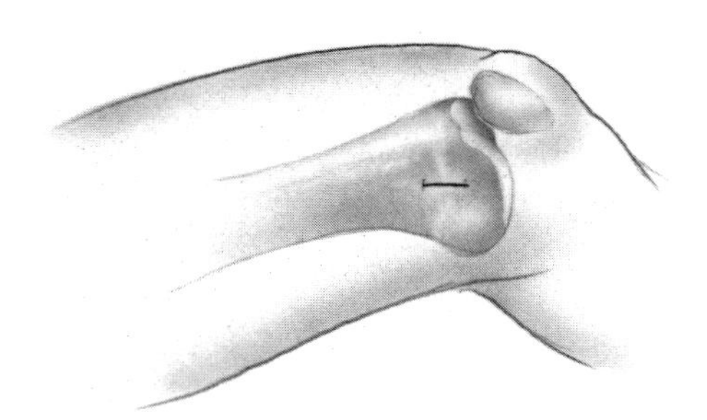

Figure 3–102

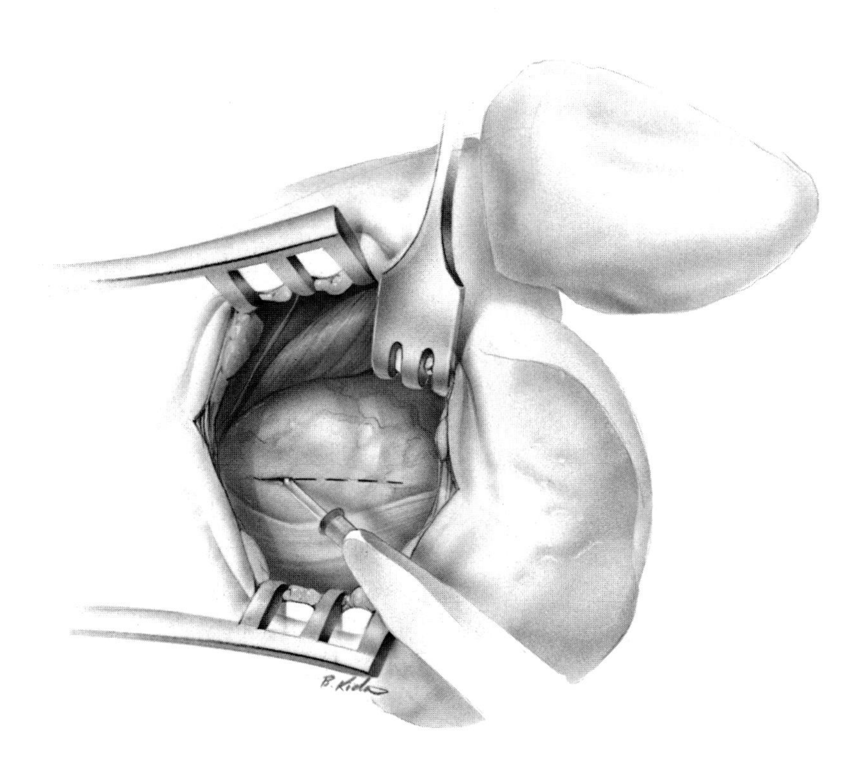

Figure 3–103

Figure 3–104. The next step is to remove a square or rectangular piece of bone, which includes the physeal plate. This can be accomplished with ordinary osteotomes or a mortising chisel as described by White and Stubbins[4] (***Figure 3–104A***). If osteotomes are used, $\frac{5}{8}$ to $\frac{3}{4}$ in is a good size. This block of bone should be removed to a depth of approximately 1 in or more if the size of the femur permits. This makes removal of the surrounding physeal plate easier. It is also important that this block of bone be kept intact so that when it is replaced, it will seal off the bleeding from the cancellous bone, a significant cause of postoperative swelling resulting in knee stiffness.

In removing the bone block, attention should be given to the anteroposterior radiograph of the distal femoral physis. If this is not done, it is easy to miss most of the physeal plate in the bone block as the plate undulates and is not straight across (***Figure 3–104B***).

Figure 3–105. After the bone block is removed, it is necessary to curette out a large portion of the remaining physeal plate (***Figure 3–105A***). This is not so easy as it first appears. The undulating physeal plate has a way of disappearing and proves quite resistant to quick and effortless removal. Techniques have been described using drills and other power tools but in the author's experience, the soft and resilient cartilage of the plate proves much more resistant to removal by these means than the surrounding cancellous bone.

The most reliable tool is a sharp curette, which is used to remove the physeal cartilage by rotating the curette into the plate (***Figure 3–105B***). Frequent irrigation and suctioning is necessary to visualize the plate. It is not necessary to destroy the most peripheral parts of the physeal plate; indeed, this would cause unnecessary instability and bleeding into the joint. When the surgeon judges the lateral half of the plate to be sufficiently destroyed, a moist sponge is placed in the wound, the sand bag removed, and the procedure is repeated on the medial side of the leg.

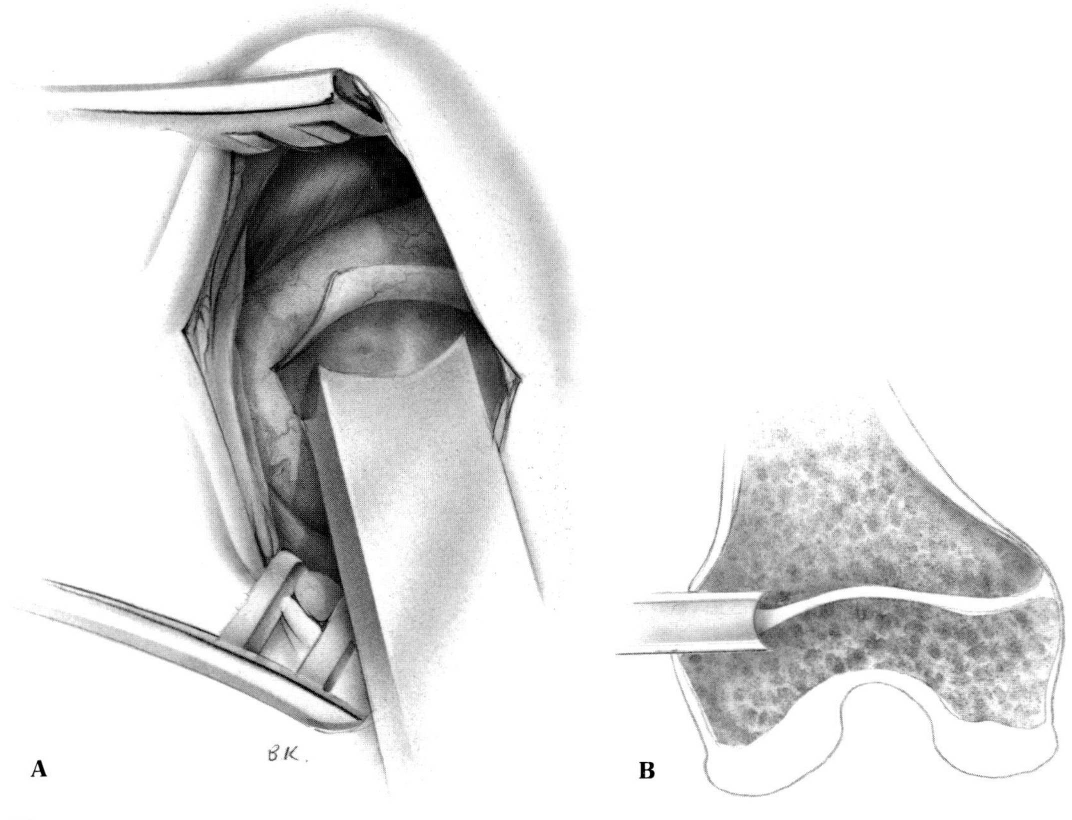

Figure 3–104

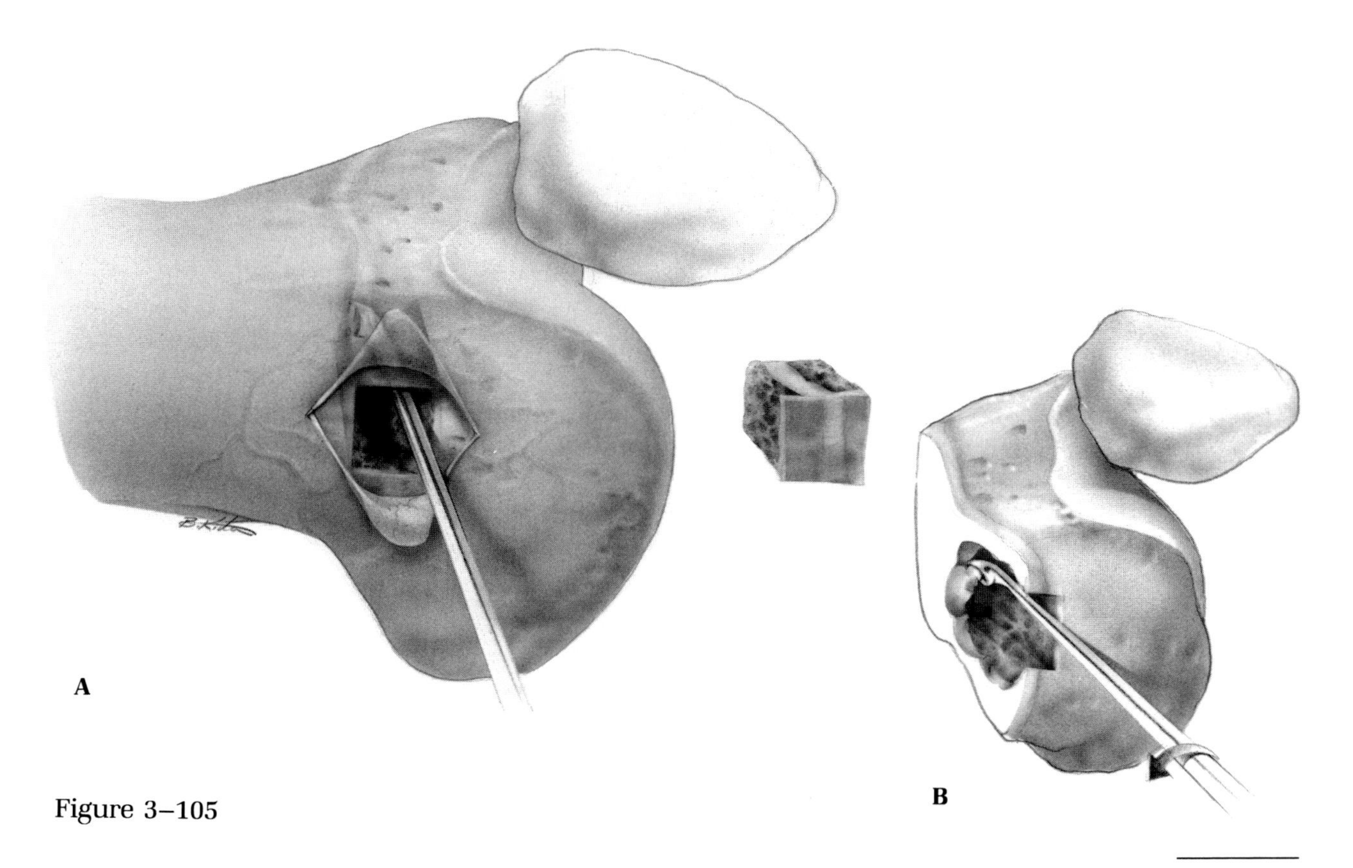

Figure 3–105

Figure 3–106. The incision on the medial side is identical to the lateral incision being about 3 cm in length and centered over the physeal plate. After the bone block is removed, curettement of the plate proceeds toward the opposite side until it joins the curetted area on the lateral side. This is advisable because it is easy to assume that more of the physeal plate has been removed than actually has been. After this, removal of the plate occurs in a centrifugal manner until the surgeon again judges that sufficient plate has been destroyed.

Figure 3–107. To complete the operation, the bone blocks are now reinserted into the area from which they were removed. In doing this, however, they are rotated: 90 degrees if a square block was removed, and 180 degrees if a rectangular block was removed. The periosteal flaps are closed as tightly as possible, and the remainder of the wound is closed. Drains do not seem effective in that they never drain more than a few milliliters of blood. If the surgeon is unsure of the completeness of the epiphysiodesis, an anteroposterior and lateral radiograph can be obtained before wound closure. Interpretation of this radiograph must be done, however, recognizing its limitations as a two-dimensional image in reflecting a three-dimensional problem—the depth of the curettement.

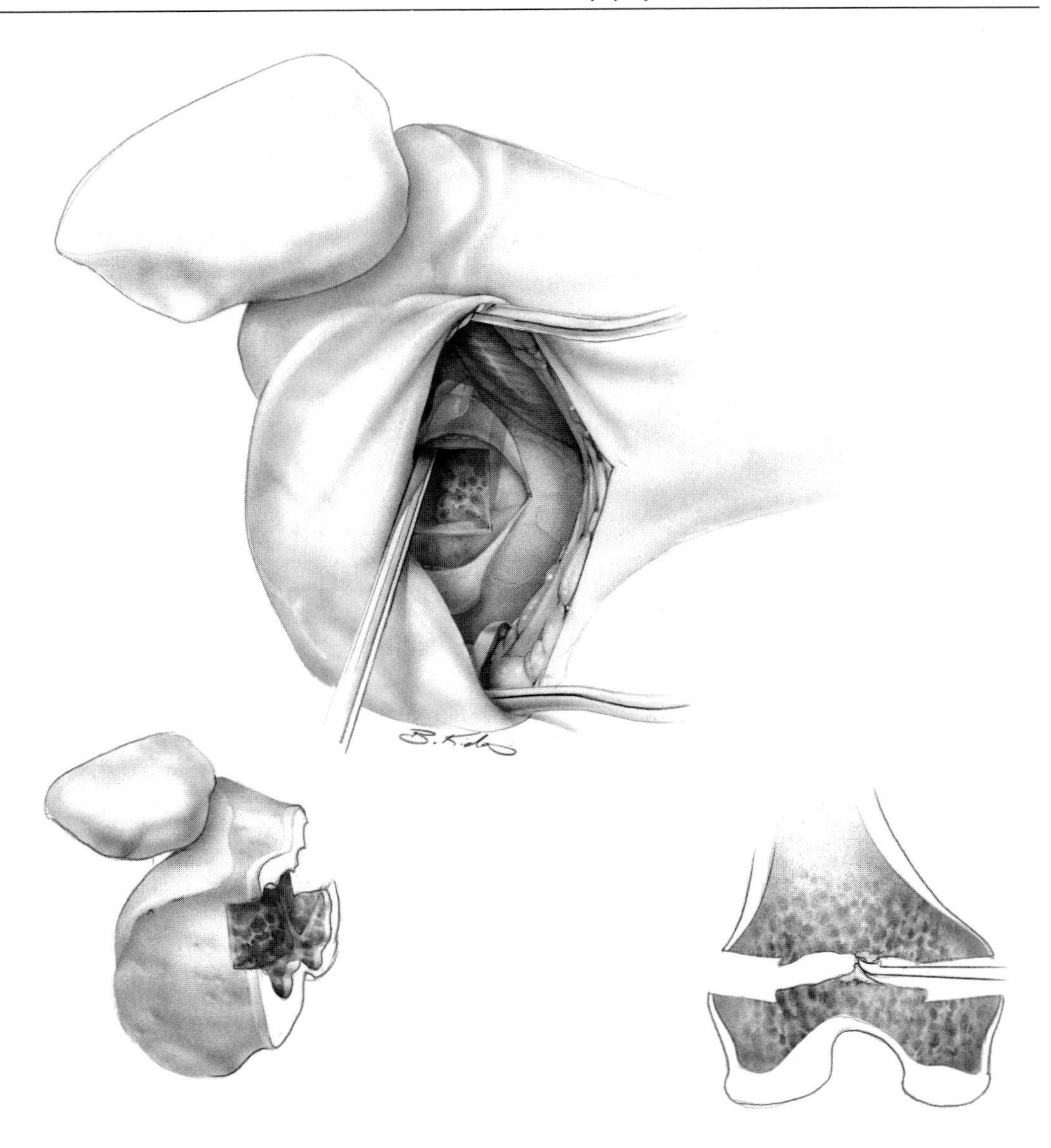

Figure 3–106

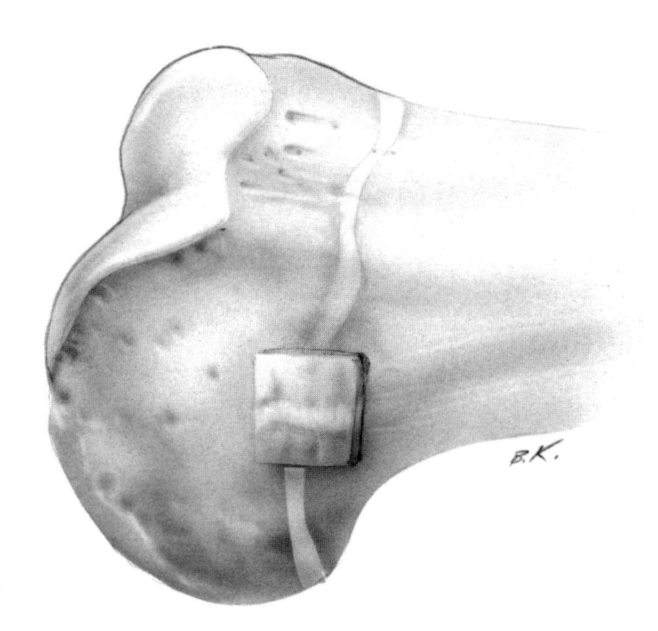

Figure 3–107

Figure 3–108. Radiographs taken immediately after surgery demonstrate adequate destruction of the physeal plate (***Figures 3–108A, B***). Two months later, radiographs (***Figures 3–108C, D***) confirm complete closure of the plate.

POSTOPERATIVE CARE

At the completion of surgery, the patient is placed in a velcro-fastening knee immobilizer. On the first postoperative day, a three-point partial weight-bearing crutch gait is begun along with quadriceps-setting exercises and active-assisted range of motion. The patient can usually be discharged by the second postoperative day. Physical therapy is continued at home with supervision as necessary. If the patient is reliable on crutches, the immobilizer can usually be discontinued by 4 to 6 weeks. Crutches are continued until radiographic evidence of bone union is seen. This is preferable to discontinuing the crutches and maintaining the immobilizer or a cast because it permits earlier rehabilitation of the knee.

Radiographs at 6 to 12 weeks should demonstrate the areas of bone fusion across the physeal plate. This should be assessed so that the potential of developing angular deformity from an inadequate area of fusion is not ignored. The patient should be examined clinically for leg-length discrepancy every 4 to 6 months to be certain correction is occurring and that the proper correction is obtained. Periodic scanograms for length or radiographs to assess the adequacy of plate closure may be necessary and depend on the clinical situation.

REFERENCES

1. Phemister DB. Operative arrestment of longitudinal bone growth in the treatment of deformities. J Bone Joint Surg 1933;15:1.
2. Green WT, Anderson M. Epiphyseal arrest for the correction of discrepancies in length of the lower extremities. J Bone Joint Surg 1957;39A:353.
3. Canale ST, Christian CA. Techniques for epiphysiodesis about the knee. Clin Orthop 1990;255:81.
4. White JW, Stubbins SG. Growth arrest for equalizing leg lengths. J Am Med Assoc 1944;126:1146.

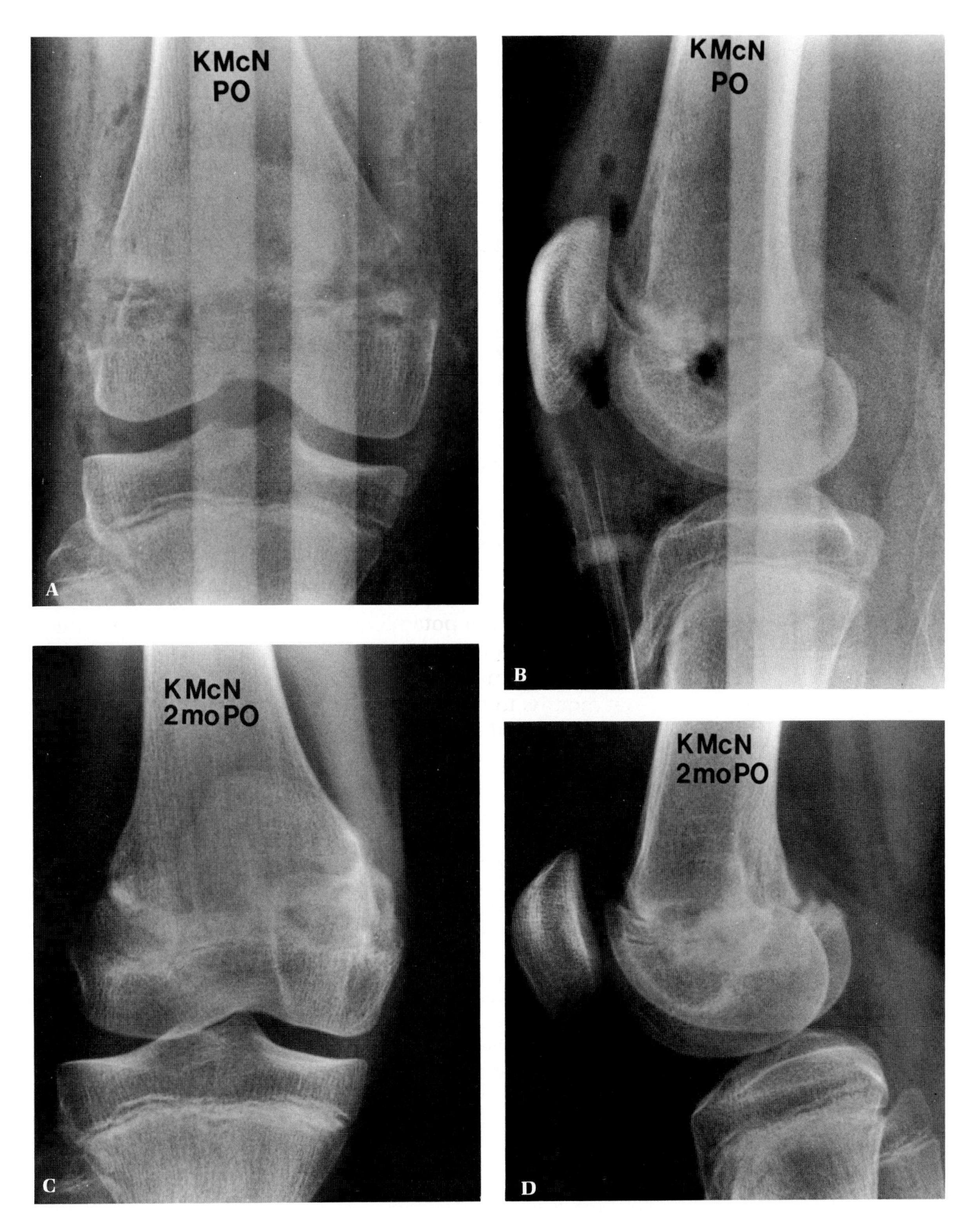

Figure 3–108

3.14 Distal Hamstring Lengthening and Posterior Capsulotomy

Knee flexion contracture is one of the commonest and most easily noticed of all the deformities in the patient with cerebral palsy. In addition, its correction is the most likely to produce worsening of the patient's functional abilities if the surgeon does not observe all of the prerequisites and indications. These are discussed by Rang[1] and Bleck.[2] The hamstring muscles are three: semimembranosus, semitendinosus, and biceps femoris. The gracillis muscle is often considered for lengthening during this operation, but care should be given to its inclusion because this is one of the muscles that initiates the swing phase of gait.[2]

The technique of fractional lengthening of the hamstring tendons was first described by Green and McDermott[3] in 1942 and is still the technique used by most surgeons today.

Figure 3–109. Distal hamstring lengthening can be performed in either the prone or supine position. Although it is a bit easier for the surgeon to have the patient in the prone position, this makes it impossible to perform any associated operations around the hip (*eg*, adductor release) and does not permit testing of the lengthening by straight leg raising. If the patient is prone, the incision can be a midline incision, which should extend from the popliteal crease proximally to the junction of the middle and lower one third of the thigh (***Figure 3–109A***). This length is necessary to allow exposure of both medial and lateral structures. An alternative is two incisions, one medial and one lateral, placed over the hamstring tendons (***Figures 3–109B, C***). These incisions can be used in either the prone or the supine position. The author's preference is to use a medial and lateral incision with the patient in the supine position. These incisions are placed slightly anterior to the tight hamstring tendons beginning just proximal to the knee joint and extending proximal for approximately 5 cm.

Posterior capsulotomy can be done through either of these incisions. If posterior capsulotomy is to be done through the two incisions, all of the structures posterior to the capsule are bluntly dissected free and retracted posteriorly, allowing the origins of the gastrocnemius muscle and the capsule to be divided. This approach, while seeming more difficult at first, is actually easier because dissection of the popliteal space is avoided.

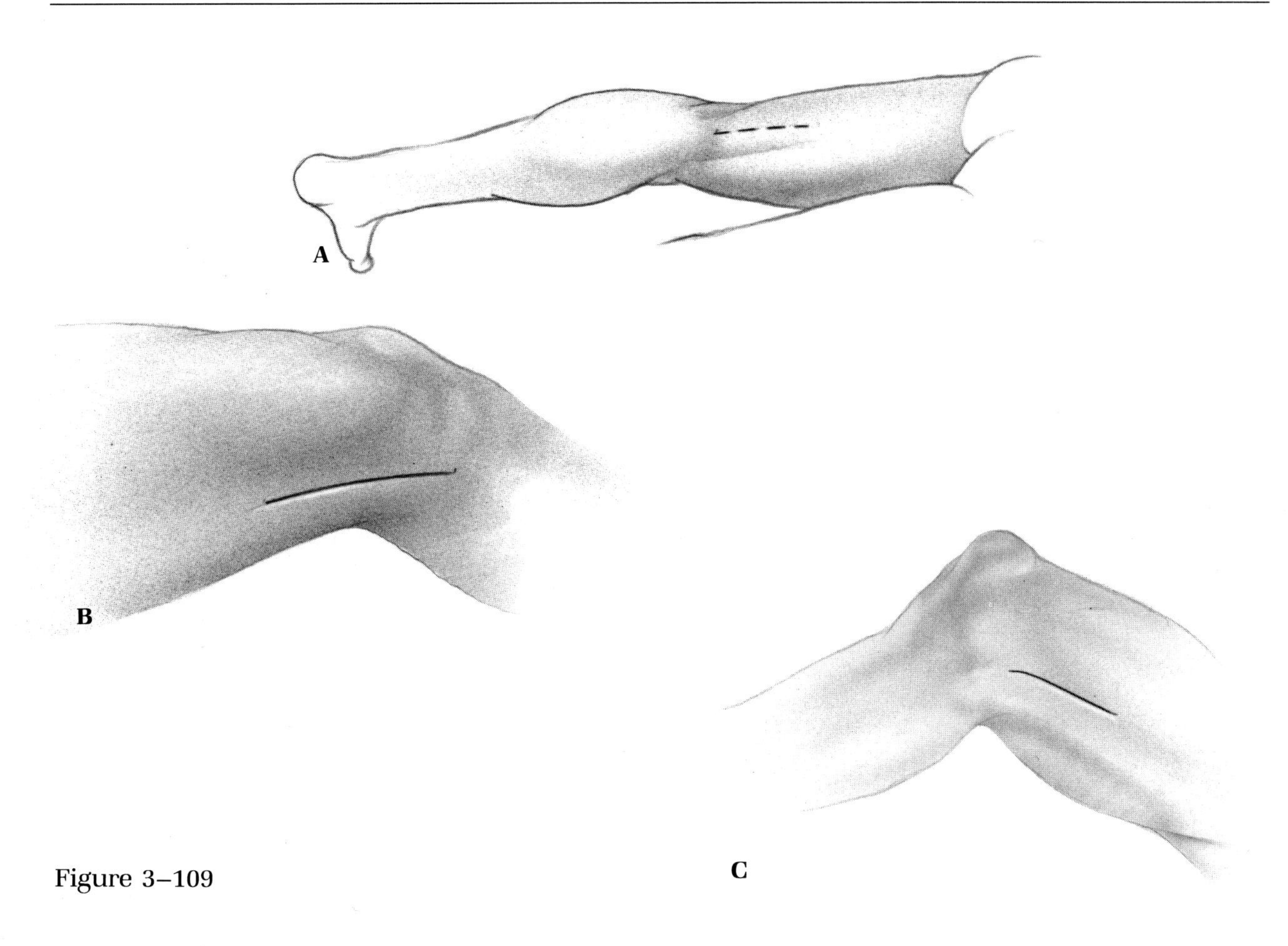

Figure 3–109

Figure 3–110. The leg is flexed at the hip and externally rotated. The medial incision is made between the palpable tendons of the gracillis anterior and the semitendinosus posterior. These two tendons usually stand out clearly with the knee extended and can be identified before the incision is made. If there is a question, abduction of the hip with the knee extended will identify the gracillis as it will become tight in adduction.

The arrangement of the tendons on the medial side of the knee is shown (***Figure 3–110A***). The sartorius muscle is the most superficial and anterior. It is not easily confused with the hamstring tendons. Deep and posterior to the sartorius muscle is the tendon of the gracillis muscle. It is a small round tendon at this location. A second small round tendon, that of the semitendeninosus muscle, can be identified posterior to the gracillis tendon. It is somewhat larger than the gracillis tendon. It is shown here sutured together after a "Z" lengthening. At this location it is crossing over the posterior aspects of the broad musculotendinous portion of the semimembranosus muscle, coming to lie lateral to it. The semimembranous muscle is not easily confused with any other because in this location it has a broad muscle belly that is transitioning into a thick tendinous aponeurosis.

After the subcutaneous fat is divided, the semitendinosus tendon is easily identified by palpation but is not so easily seen. This is because it is enclosed in a sheath. Cutting down on the tendon with a sharp knife will open this sheath (***Figure 3–110B***). A scissors is then used to expose a sufficient length of this tendon to perform a "Z" lengthening. This is often difficult in small children. Bleck[2] reports no noticeable difference between "Z" lengthening and release of this tendon. If the surgeon wishes to lengthen the gracillis, it is exposed in the same manner.

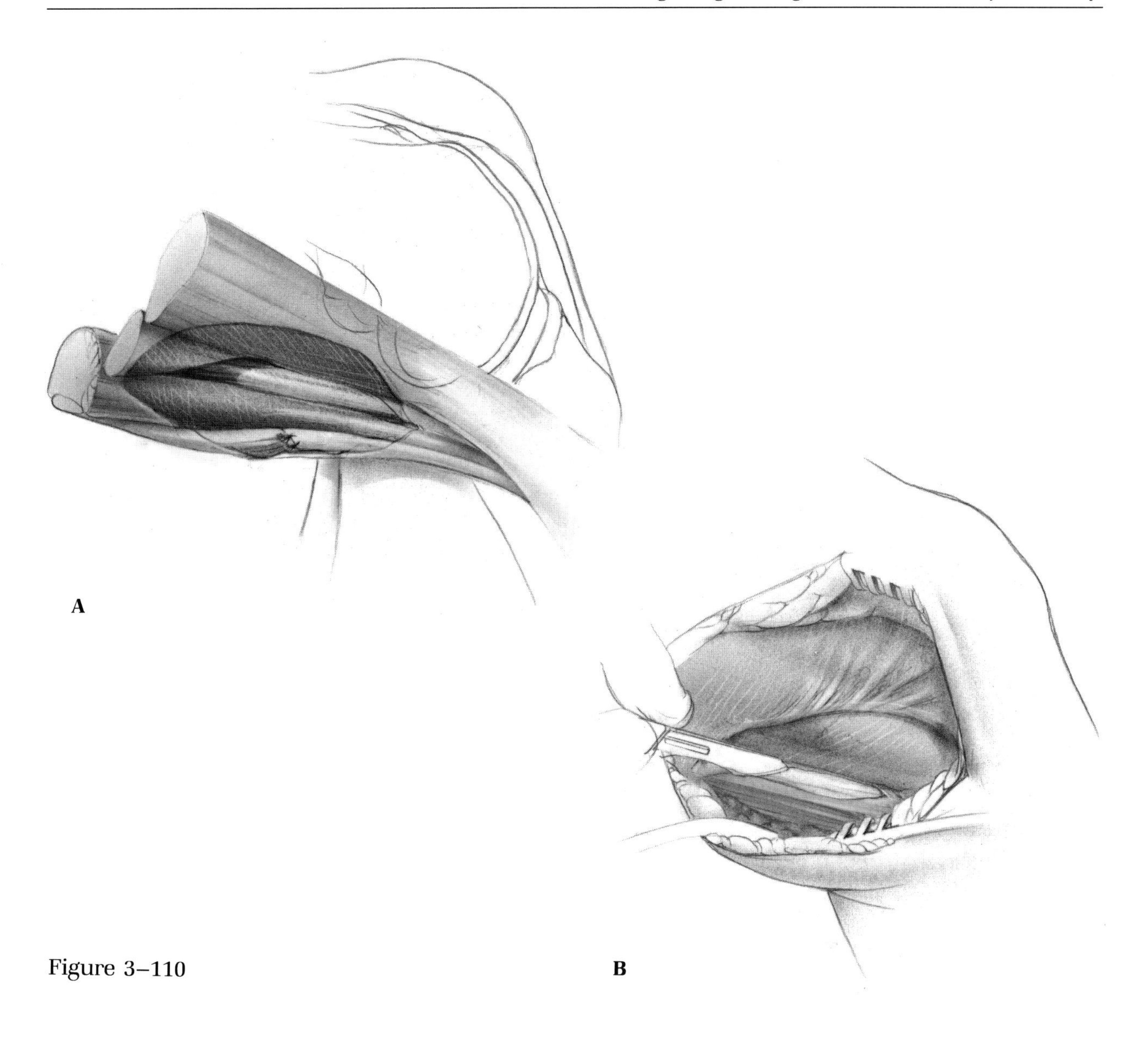

Figure 3–110

Figure 3–111. The semimembranosus is relatively easy to identify deep to the semitendinosus. As mentioned, it has a broad aponeurosis that is very thick, surrounds the muscle in the proximal part of the wound, and fans out into a more tendinous structure distally. This muscle and the biceps femoris do not lend themselves to a "Z" lengthening because of their thick and muscular insertions. They will be lengthened by division of their surrounding aponeurosis.

Once the muscle and its aponeurosis is identified, it should be exposed completely on all sides so that part of the aponeurosis is not missed and left intact. The aponeurosis is now incised with two or three chevron cuts. These should not extend into the muscle and must include all of the aponeurosis. Because the goal is to leave the muscle in continuity, these cuts should not be made too distal. Straight leg raising is now gently performed to stretch the muscle. The aponeurosis will be observed to spread apart. Great force should not be used for two reasons: The sciatic nerve is tight and may be injured, and the muscle should not be disrupted.

Figure 3–112. If posterior capsulotomy is to be performed, the medial side of the posterior capsule is now exposed and divided. Starting at the posteromedial corner of the femoral condyle, all of the soft tissues are reflected posteriorly off of the gastrocnemius muscle and the posterior aspect of the knee capsule. This will include the hamstring tendons and the neurovascular structures. This is accomplished by dissecting the tissue with a broad periosteal elevator. It will be necessary first to work anteriorly, exposing the capsule up to the medial collateral ligament. Then the dissection is carried posteriorly around the insertion of the medial head of the gastrocnemius muscle. Care is taken to stay close to the capsule between it and the fat that surrounds the structures in the popliteal space. The medial head of the gastrocnemius, which inserts on the posterior aspect of the femoral condyle, covers the posterior capsule. After dividing this medial head, it is reflected distal to expose the capsule. Opening of the capsule can wait until the lateral side has been exposed and the surgeon is certain that all of the vital structures are safely out of the way.

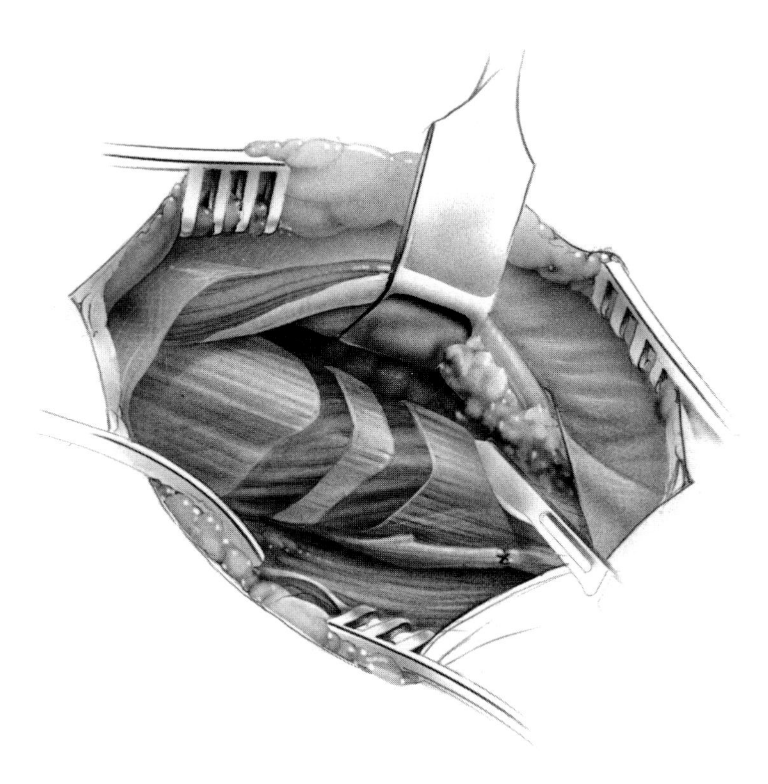

Figure 3–111

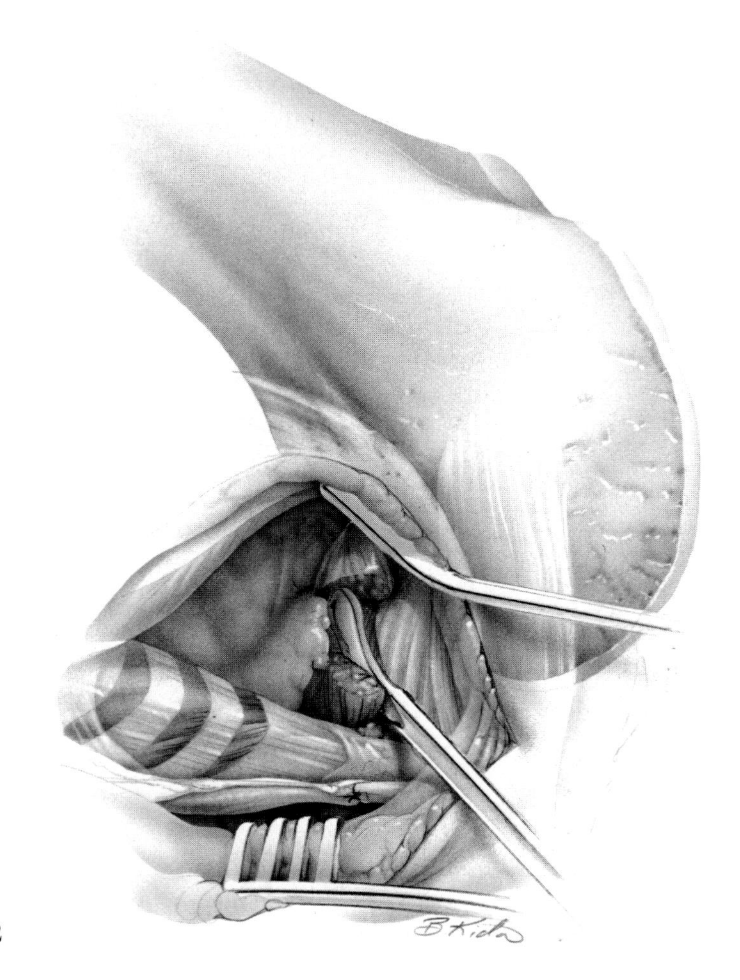

Figure 3–112

Figure 3–113. The hip is now internally rotated, and the lateral incision is made just anterior to the taut biceps femoris tendon. The aponeurosis of this tendon is exposed, and two or three chevron cuts are made in it just as was done for the semimembranosus.

Figure 3–114. The soft tissues are reflected off of the lateral head of the gastrocnemius and posterior aspect of the knee just as on the medial side (***Figure 3–114A***). This dissection should join that of the medial side, ensuring that all vital structures are retracted posteriorly. The gastrocnemius head is divided and reflected distal to expose the underlying capsule.

A moist 4 × 4 sponge is passed through the exposure and is used to retract the hamstrings and the neurovascular structures posteriorly (***Figure 3–114B***). The lateral capsule is incised and the joint identified. There is a tendency to make this incision too proximally. It should be started at the most prominent part of the femoral condyles or it will be difficult to divide the midportion of the capsule. Once the joint is identified, a curved Mayo scissors is used to divide the capsule as far medially as possible. The division should also be done going anteriorly, stopping just before reaching the lateral collateral ligament. The division of the capsule can now be completed through the medial incision, again extending as far anteriorly as the medial collateral ligament.

A closed suction drain is placed in the wound. The deep fascia, subcutaneous fascia, and skin are closed.

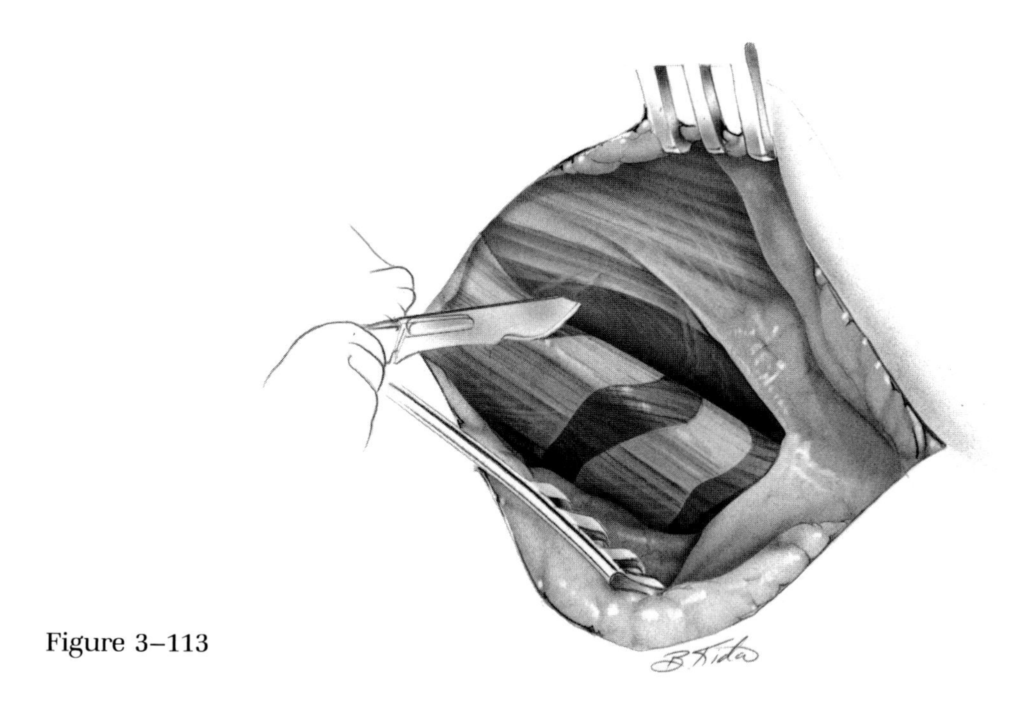

Figure 3–113

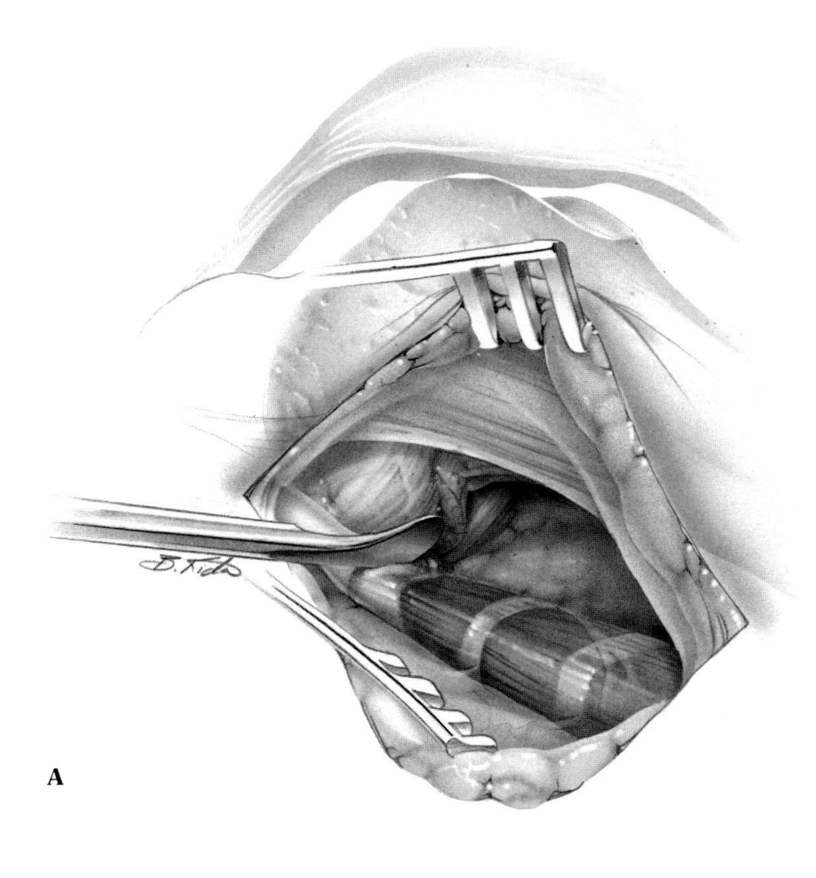

A

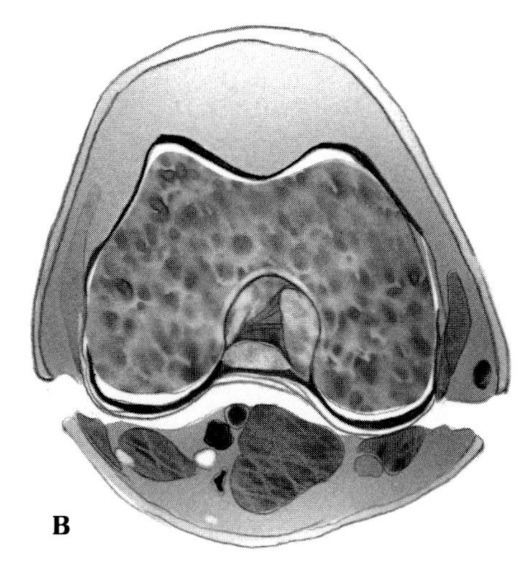

B

Figure 3–114

POSTOPERATIVE CARE

If posterior capsulotomy was necessary, it is unlikely that the knee will straighten completely without force. Therefore, to avoid stretching the sciatic nerve, the leg should be casted in the amount of extension that can be obtained without force. The cast should be applied and padded with the plan to wedge it into more extension during the postoperative period. Just before discharge at 3 to 4 days, the cast is wedged. This can be repeated at weekly intervals until correction is satisfactory. An alternate approach is to remove the anterior one half of the cast from a point above the patella distal. Stretching is then done several times a day. As further extension is gained, a new cast is applied, the anterior one half removed, and the entire process repeated until correction is achieved.

REFERENCES

1. Rang M. Cerebral palsy. In: Morrissy RT, ed. Lovell and Winter's pediatric orthopaedics, 3rd ed. Philadelphia: JB Lippincott, 1990:492.
2. Bleck EE. Orthopaedic management in cerebral palsy. Philadephia: JB Lippincott, 1987:344–355.
3. Green WT, McDermott LJ. Operative treatment of cerebral palsy of the spastic type. JAMA 1942;118:434.

CHAPTER FOUR
THE KNEE

4.1
Proximal Patellar Realignment (Insall Technique)

With subluxation or dislocation of the patella in childhood, the surgeon's options are limited by the open growth plate of the tibial tubercle, which prohibits operations that transfer the origin of the patellar tendon. For the growing child with recurrent subluxation or dislocation of the patella—whether owing to malalignment, trauma, or mild ligamentous laxity (*eg*, seen in Down's syndrome)—the proximal soft-tissue realignment described by Insall et al[1,2] provides a method of realigning the forces on the patella. To the author, this method seems preferable to detaching and then advancing the vastus medialis muscle. In cases in which advancement of the medialis muscle seems necessary, the muscle is usually so deficient that little is gained, and it is difficult to secure the muscle in place. The proximal realignment provides a secure repair with little tension on the suture lines and, thus, earlier rehabilitation.

In cases of congenital dislocation associated with defficiency of the lateral femoral condyle or muscle structure, however, this operation is usually not sufficient. This is also true for the child with Down's syndrome or other collagen disorders who have severe ligamentous laxity and poor tissue for repair. For such cases the author prefers to combine elements of this procedure with the semitendinosus tenodesis of the patella.[3]

Figure 4–1. The operation is performed with the patient supine and a bolster under the hip to avoid having to have an assistant hold the leg in internal rotation. The incision begins in the midline just below the junction of the middle and lower one third of the thigh, and extends distally across the center of the patella to the tibial tubercle. The incision must be long enough to expose the entire quadriceps tendon.

Figure 4–2. The flaps are reflected medially and laterally sufficiently to expose the medial and lateral border of the patella as well as the insertion of the vastus medialis and lateralis into the quadriceps tendon proximal to the patella. The first incision begins as far proximally as the quadriceps tendon and detaches the vastus medialis from this tendon, leaving just enough tendon on the muscle to hold sutures. As this incision is carried distally, it should be directed to cross the patella, dividing the medial one third from the lateral two thirds and then continuing down along the medial border of the patellar tendon. The quadriceps expansion overlying the medial one third of the patella is then elevated subperiosteally from the patella (***Figure 4–2A***). This will now allow the patella to be turned up laterally, exposing the joint. By dividing the fat pad, the undersurface of the patella and the joint can be inspected (***Figure 4–2B***).

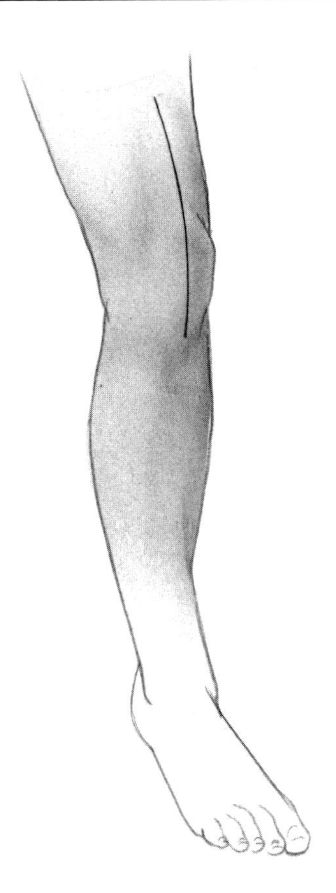

Figure 4–1

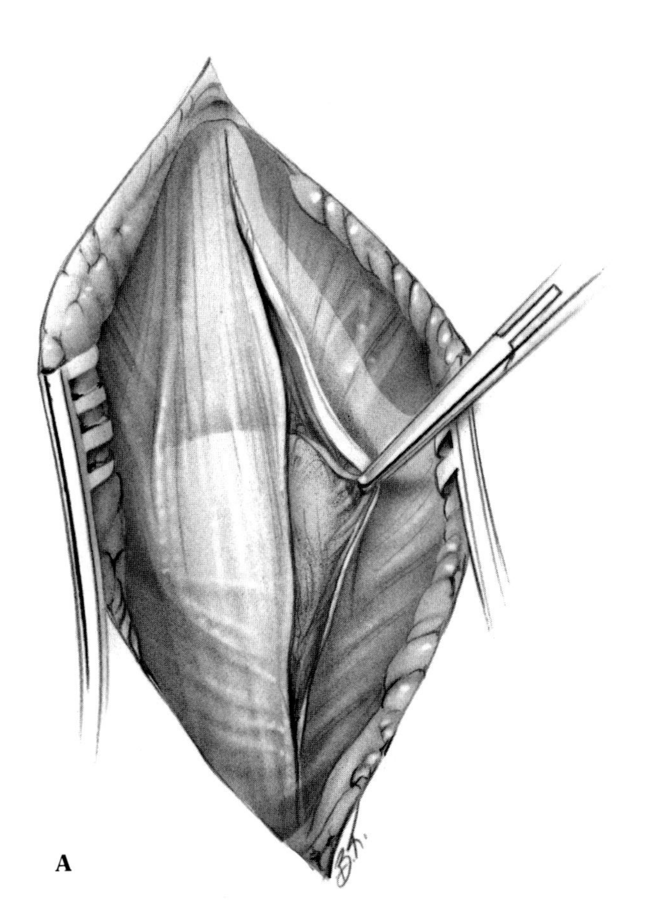

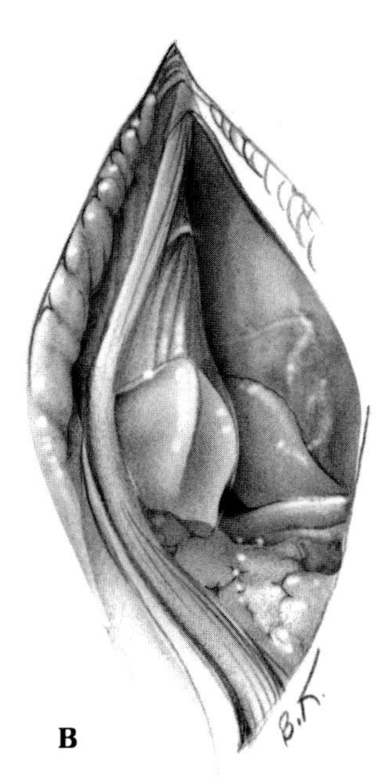

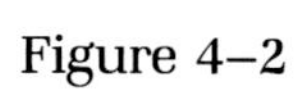

Figure 4–2

Figure 4–3. The next incision will divide the lateral patellar retinaculum and separate the vastus lateralis from the quadriceps tendon. This incision will begin in the quadriceps tendon proximally, opposite the medial incision. Detach the vastus lateralis, leaving a rim of tendon for suturing. As this incision approaches the patella it will skirt the lateral margin of the patella. The synovium should also be divided with care taken to identify and coagulate the vessels that will be encountered. If the surgeon desires, the tourniquet can be released at this point to control any bleeding and then reinflated before beginning the repair.

Figure 4–4. The repair is started proximally by bringing the cut edge of the vastus medialis and vastus lateralis together over the remaining portion of the quadriceps tendon, which is pushed deep to the repair. As the repair reaches the proximal pole of the patella, the patella will begin to rotate medially, elevating the lateral portion of the patella. It is not necessary nor possible to continue this repair across the entire patella, because the medial periosteal flap will not reach the lateral retinaculum. Rather, when the patella is rotated and displaced medially to a sufficient degree, the medial flap is sutured to the periosteum on the lateral two thirds of the patella without further effort to pull the patella medially. The knee can now be flexed to test the stability of the patella. The lateral incision is left open.

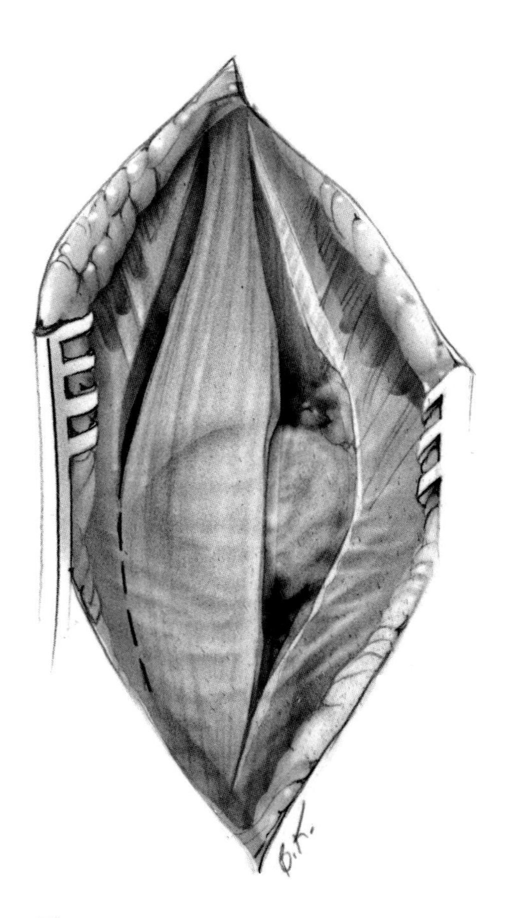

Figure 4–3

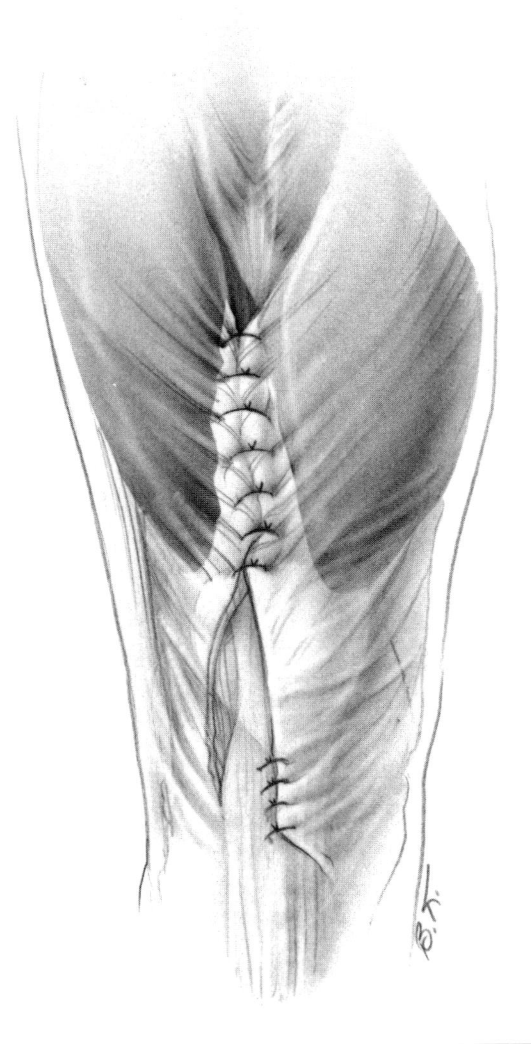

Figure 4–4

POSTOPERATIVE CARE

A compression bandage is applied about the knee for the first few days. This may be supplemented by a knee immobilizer for comfort, but this is not necessary to protect the repair. The patient can begin to ambulate with a three-point crutch gait as soon as possible, usually the second postoperative day. The pressure dressing can be removed in 3 days, and physical therapy begun with active-assisted flexion and extension. It is best to discontinue the knee immobilizer early and rely on crutches for support, because this will promote use of the knee. Children often come to rely on the immobilizer, which slows their progress. A full program of knee rehabilitation can be started at 3 weeks. The subsequent progress of the patient is very much dependent on the patient as well as the underlying condition; however, most children should be back to normal within 6 months.

REFERENCES

1. Insall J, Falvo KA, Wise DW. Chondromalacia patellae. J Bone Joint Surg 1976; 58A:1.
2. Insall J, Bullough PG, Burstein AH. Proximal "tube" realignment of the patella for chondromalacia patellae. Clin Orthop 1979; 144:63.
3. Baker RH, Carroll N, Dewar FP, Hall JE. The semitendinosus tenodesis for recurrent dislocation of the patella. J Bone Joint Surg 1972; 54B:103.

4.2 Semitendinosus Tenodesis of Patella for Recurrent Dislocation

The use of the semitendinosus tendon to realign the patella was first described by Galeazzi in 1922, and was first reported in the American literature in 1957.[1] Subsequent reports have been favorable.[2,3] This procedure addresses several problems that the orthopaedic surgeon often encounters in the child with recurrent dislocation of the patella: ligamentous laxity, deficient lateral condyle, deficient medial musculature, and open growth plates. In all of the various conditions in which recurrent dislocation of the patella is encountered (eg, Down's syndrome, congenital dislocating patella, etc), the semitendinosus tendon is usually normal. Thus, the author has found this to be an excellent solution to the unusual problem of recurrent dislocating patella in skeletally immature children, often combining it with a proximal realignment.

Figure 4–5. The patient is placed supine on the operating table, and the entire leg is draped free. A tourniquet is used. One incision is used. Although a medial parapatellar incision makes it slightly easier to reach the semitendinosus tendon, a long midline incision as described for proximal realignment is cosmetically better. The tendons on the medial side of the knee are illustrated (***Figure 4–5A***). Note the broad expanse of the sartorius, which is the most anterior. The gracillis tendon lies just behind the sartorius. The semitendinosus is the most posterior behind the knee and is the deepest or most posterior tendon inserting into the tibia. It is easily distinguished from the gracillis not only by the location of its insertion but also by the fact that it is a much larger tendon. The surgeon should not make the mistake of taking the gracillis tendon for the repair.

The medial skin flap is extensively elevated around the medial side of the knee. The dissection must be carried both posterior and proximal. Flexing the knee will aid in this dissection. The infrapatellar branch of the saphenous nerve will usually be noted emerging from the sartorius. Although a few of its sensory twigs may be divided, care should be taken with this nerve to avoid a large area of anesthesia (***Figure 4–5B***).

Figure 4–6. With the knee flexed, the skin flap is retracted with a long blade retractor, and blunt dissection is continued posterior and proximal (***Figure 4–6A***). At this point care should be taken to avoid injury to both the infrapatellar branch of the saphenous nerve or the saphenous nerve itself (**see *Figure 4–9***). The tendon can be palpated. As mentioned before, it is a larger structure than the gracillis tendon, which may be taken by mistake. It lies posterior to the sartorius and gracillis tendons in this location. Once the tendon is identified and exposed, it should be followed to its musculotendinous junction where it is divided.

Next the tendon should be followed to its insertion posterior to the sartorius and gracillis tendons, freeing all extraneous attachments with care to avoid cutting the saphenous nerve (***Figure 4–6B***). If the tendon is not completely freed to its insertion, it will not have the proper direction and will soon become loose as the fascia that tethered it becomes stretched.

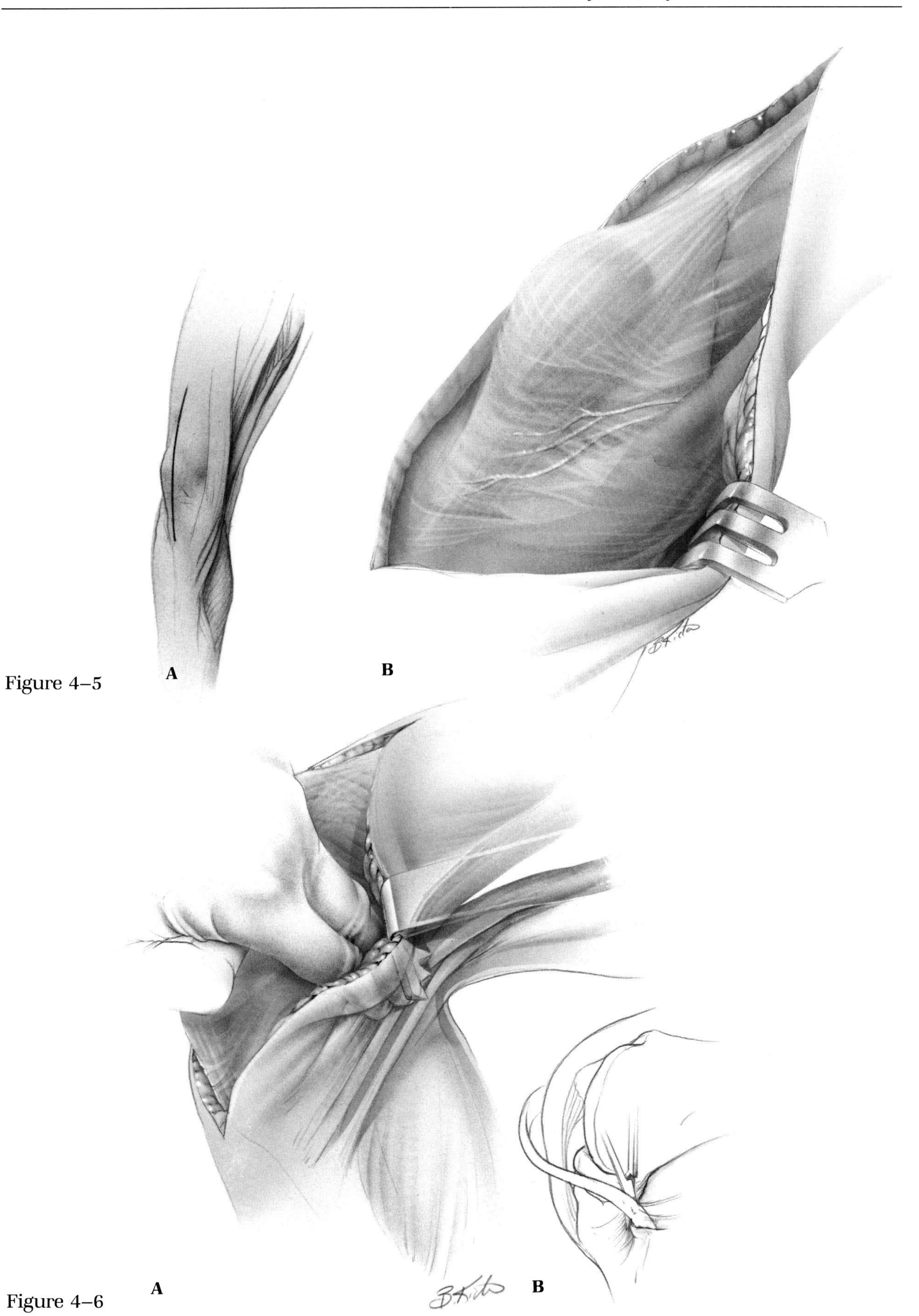

Figure 4–5

Figure 4–6

Figure 4–7. The lateral flap is now dissected to expose the lateral border of the patella. At the minimum a complete lateral release should be performed, including both capsule and synovium. At this point the decision can be made to do a more extensive realignment of the patella with advancement of the vastus medialis muscle or complete proximal realignment. If nothing more is to be done (as illustrated here for simplicity) a small incision should be made in the medial capsule at the distal end of the patella. This will allow palpation of the inferior surface of the patella for more accurate placement of the drill hole.

Figure 4–8. With the patella held in the desired position and the tendon pulled across the surface of the patella, the proper direction for the drill hole can be determined (***Figure 4–8A***).

Starting at the inferior medial edge of the patella, a hole of sufficient size to allow passage of the tendon is drilled, emerging at the superior lateral corner of the patella (***Figure 4–8B***). Care must be taken in directing the drill not to penetrate the articular surface.

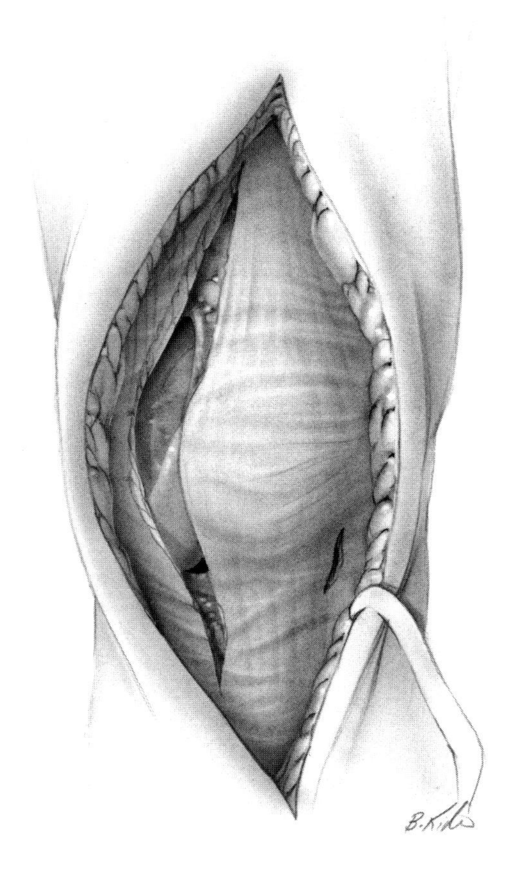

Figure 4–7

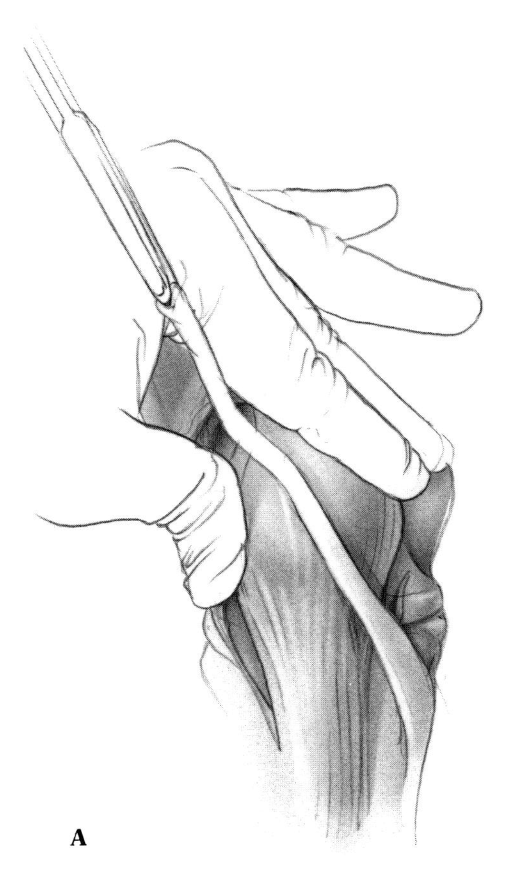

A

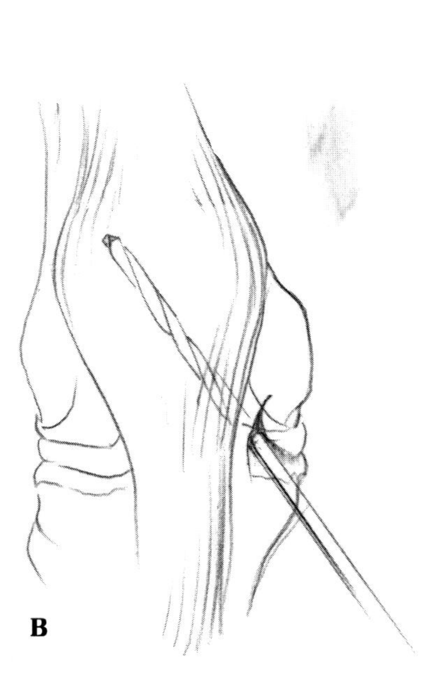

B

Figure 4–8

Figure 4–9. The tendon is drawn through the hole and pulled back on itself. Sufficient tension should be placed on the tendon to hold the patella in line with the intercondylar notch. This can be tested by flexing the knee while an assistant holds tension on the tendon. Tension should be sufficient to create a laxity of the patellar tendon.

Note the infrapatellar branch of the saphenous nerve that penetrates the sartorius muscle and branches over the medial capsule of the knee. The main branch of the saphenous nerve emerges from between the sartorius and gracillis tendons to continue down the leg. Care needs to be taken both during the dissection and the routing of the tendon to be certain that these nerves are neither cut nor kinked.

The operation is completed by suturing the semitendinosus tendon to the periosteum of the patella and if sufficient length is available, to itself.

Figure 4–10. To restore tension to the patellar tendon and effect some redirection in its line of pull, a Goldthwait procedure can be added.[4] This entails splitting the patellar tendon in one half, detaching the lateral one half, directing this one half under the medial one half of the tendon, and attaching it to the periosteum of the tibia under moderate tension.

At the completion of this step any muscle advancements or other steps to augment the realignment are completed, and the wound is closed over a suction drain.

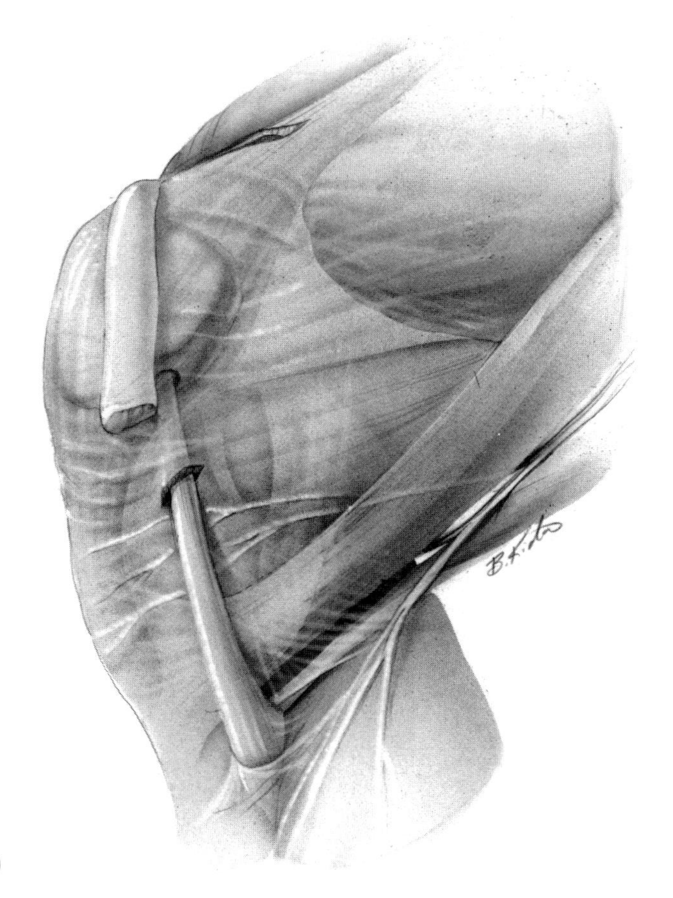

Figure 4–9

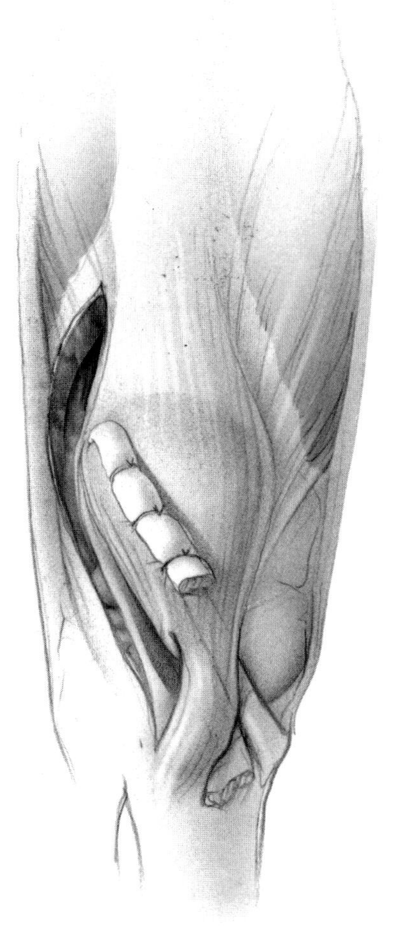

Figure 4–10

POSTOPERATIVE CARE

The knee is immobilized in extension for 6 weeks. The drain can usually be removed the day following surgery and the patient discharged on a three-point partial weight-bearing crutch gait within 3 days. Attempts to begin isometric quadriceps exercises can be started 1 to 2 weeks after surgery. Following the discontinuation of immobilization, a rehabilitation program for the knee is started.

REFERENCES

1. Dewar FP, Hall JE. Recurrent dislocation of the patella. J Bone Joint Surg 1957; 39B:798.
2. Baker RH, Carroll N, Dewar FP, Hall JE. The semitendinosus tenodesis for recurrent dislocation of the patella. J Bone Joint Surg 1972; 54B:103.
3. Hall JE, Micheli LJ, McNamara GB Jr. Semitendinosus tenodesis for recurrent subluxation or dislocation of the patella. Clin Orthop 1979; 144:31.
4. Goldthwait JE. Slipping or recurrent dislocation of the patella with the report of eleven cases. Boston Med Surg J 1904; 150:160.

4.3
Quadriceps Plasty and Reduction of Congenital Dislocation of Knee

Congenital dislocation of the knee is a rare disorder, especially if distinguished from congenital hyperextension. Curtiss and Fisher[1] distinguish three types of deformity: recurvatum, subluxation, and dislocation. An occasional hyperextended knee will resist manipulation and require surgical treatment. More often it is the subluxated knee and almost always the dislocated knee that will require surgery for reduction. The need will be apparent after a trial of manipulation and casting. It is debatable whether or not a trial of skeletal traction is desirable before an open reduction in view of the high incidence of epiphyseal injury and femoral fracture that is reported with its use.[2]

Descriptions of the pathology in the dislocated knee have been similar.[1,3,4] The axis of the tibia lies anterior to the axis of the femur. The quadriceps mechanism is shortened with poor development of the entire muscle. The suprapatellar pouch is obliterated and filled with dense fibrous tissue by which the quadriceps mechanism is bound to the anterior surface of the femur. In many cases the muscle fibers of the quadriceps including the medialis and the lateralis as well as the entire capsule are adherent to the femur. The anterior capsule is very short, and the collateral ligaments run anterior to the tibia and are shortened. The hamstring tendons are usually subluxated anterior as well, acting as extensors. In about one half of the cases the patella will be subluxated laterally, and the tibia will be in valgus and external rotation. The cruciate ligaments have been described as usually present,[1] usually absent,[4] and shortened.[5]

This is the pathology that must be corrected to allow the tibia to be reduced and flexed on the femur. Although there are consistent features, it appears that not all cases will demonstrate exactly the same pathology or the same severity. The basic steps that must be taken to effect a reduction are: Free the quadriceps and lateral retinaculum from the underlying femur; divide the anterior capsule and extensor retinaculum; and lengthen the quadriceps mechanism. Although it has been recommended that the absent anterior cruciate ligament be reconstructed[4] or, if stretched, advanced,[3] this author doubts that this can be achieved with the precision that we now recognize as necessary to be beneficial to the long-term stability of the knee.

Figure 4–11. The patient is positioned supine, and a midline longitudinal incision is made from the tibial tubercle to the midthigh. Sharp dissection is used to expose the quadriceps muscle, the patella, the patellar tendon, and the lateral retinaculum. The subluxated hamstring tendons and the collateral ligaments should also be identified but do not usually require extensive exposure.

Figure 4–12. The most striking feature of the anatomy is the appearance of the quadriceps muscle. The amount of muscle is small, and the medial and lateral fibers insert into the quadriceps tendon well above the patella. Before proceeding, the surgeon must decide how the quadriceps mechanism will be lengthened. This author prefers a "V" to a "Y" advancement.

To accomplish this, as much of the quadriceps tendon proximal to the patella as possible should be exposed. The medial and lateral fibers are detached from the tendon, leaving a small amount of tendinous tissue attached to the muscle for later repair. This incision is then carried distally on each side of the patella to divide the medial and lateral retinaculum as far as the collateral ligaments. If the tibia is in valgus and external rotation, it is important to divide the iliotibial band at this point.

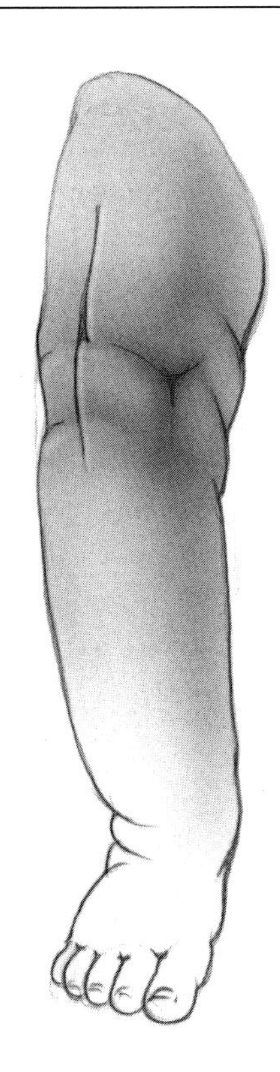

Figure 4–11

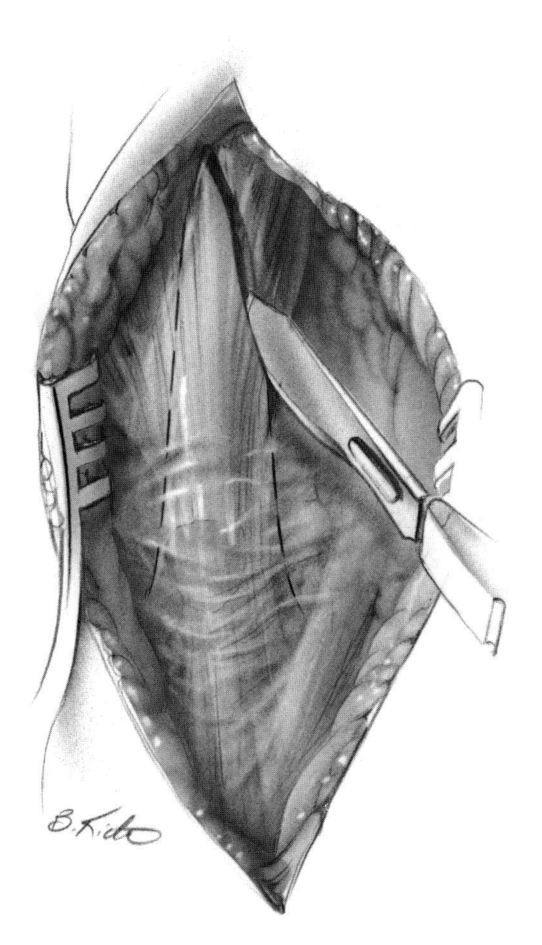

Figure 4–12

Figure 4–13. At this point the joint can be inspected. The menisci are usually present and normal. The pathology in the cruciate ligaments is variable. The most striking feature, however, is the adherence of the quadriceps muscle and lateral retinaculum to the femur. This will usually prevent complete reduction and flexion of the dislocated tibia at this point. Therefore, it will be necessary to dissect these tissues free, both to permit the tibia and the collateral ligaments to slide posteriorly and to allow sufficient mobilization of the quadriceps muscle for excursion and repair. To accomplish this the posterior border of the lateralis (*scissors*) and the medialis (*dotted line*) are sharply divided, and the flap of muscle created is dissected free of its underlying attachments to the femur. At the completion of this step there should be some elasticity noted when pulling on the muscle.

Figure 4–14. The knee can now be flexed and reduced. The amount of extension that permits redislocation should be noted. With the knee flexed about 45 degrees, the medialis and lateralis are reattached to the quadriceps tendon in their new position. It is at this point that the surgeon will appreciate the time spent to plan the lengthening of the quadriceps for there is seldom an excess of tendon for the repair. The retinaculum cannot be closed, and no attempt should be made to do so.

Drains are placed, the wound is closed, and the leg is immobilized in the degree of flexion that was chosen for repair of the quadriceps muscle. This should be in sufficient flexion so that there is no tendency for the tibia to subluxate anteriorly—usually 45 degrees.

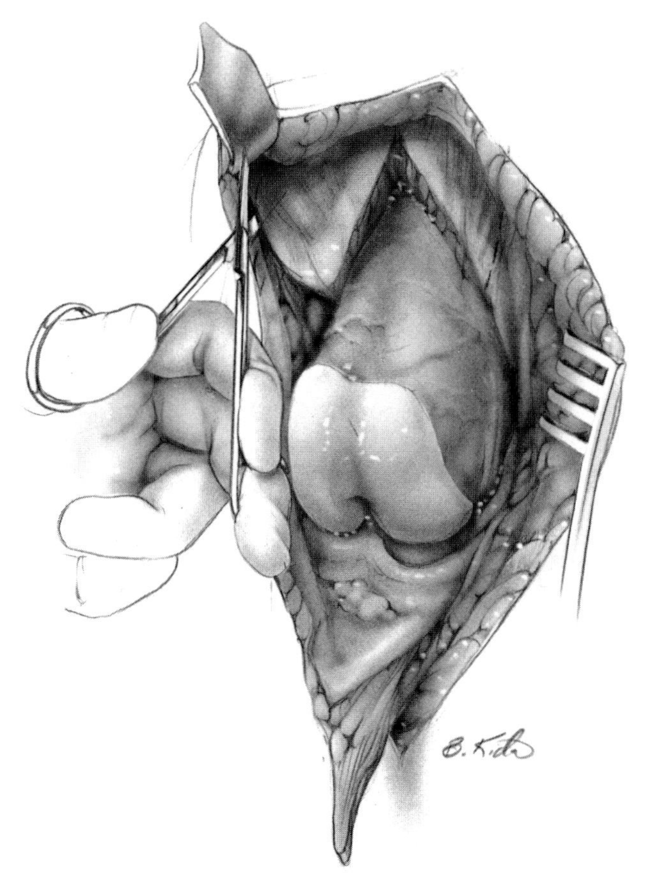

Figure 4–13

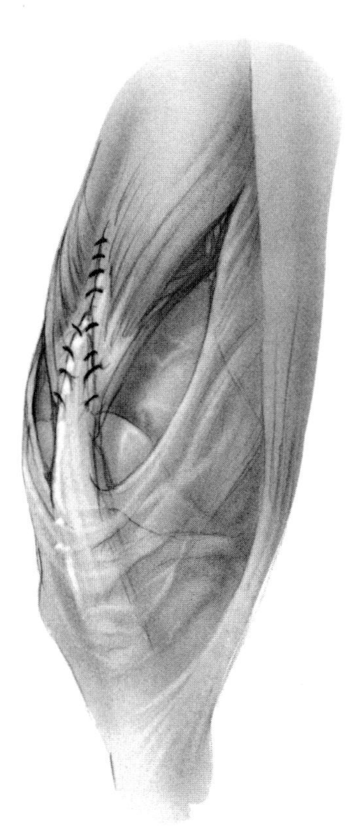

Figure 4–14

POSTOPERATIVE CARE

The knee is immobilized for 6 weeks. It may be advisable to obtain a lateral radiograph between 1 and 2 weeks to be certain that the knee has not redislocated. At 6 weeks the immobilization is discontinued, and the patient is allowed to kick free. The parents are taught techniques to stimulate quadriceps contraction, and gentle passive flexion and extension stretching is begun.

REFERENCES

1. Curtiss BH, Fisher RL. Congenital hyperextension with anterior subluxation of the knee. J Bone Joint Surg 1969; 51A:255.
2. Jacobsen K, Vopalecky F. Congenital dislocation of the knee. Acta Orthop Scand 1985; 56:1.
3. Niebauer JJ, King DE. Congenital dislocation of the knee. J Bone Joint Surg 1960; 42A:207.
4. Katz MP, Grogono BJS, Soper KC. The etiology and treatment of congenital dislocation of the knee. J Bone Joint Surg 1967; 49B:112.
5. Austwick DH, Dandy DJ. Early operation for congenital subluxation of the knee. J Pediatr Orthop 1983; 3:85.

CHAPTER FIVE
THE TIBIA

5.1
Dome Osteotomy of Proximal Tibia

Osteotomy of the proximal tibia in the growing child is always difficult. Although the deformity usually occurs at the physis, the osteotomy must be performed at some distance from the physis to avoid damaging further growth potential. At the same time, the need for internal fixation will cause the osteotomy to be performed even further from the site of deformity. All of the techniques of proximal tibial osteotomy in the growing child should aim for the same goals: be as close to the site of the deformity as possible, provide a large surface of bone for stability and rapid healing, provide fixation that will avoid loss of correction, and restore or preserve the normal mechanical axis of the leg.

A discussion of the following four operations describes various techniques for proximal tibial osteotomy in the growing child. Their virtues and drawbacks are discussed. All of them have been and can be used successfully.

The classic osteotomy of the proximal tibia is the "dome" osteotomy in which a semicircular cut is made in the bone, and the distal fragment is simply rotated into the correct position. There are several problems with this technique that have led this author to abandon it in favor of other techniques that answer these problems. Because this is still the most common technique used, however, it is described. The incision and dissection described for this osteotomy is the same for all others described here. This approach has the advantage of good exposure, good cosmesis, and only one incision is necessary for both the tibial and fibular osteotomy.

Problems with the dome osteotomy are the lack of inherent stability at the osteotomy site and the near impossibility of producing the perfect dome in a bone that is triangular in cross-section. Fixation of this osteotomy has traditionally been accomplished with crossed Steinmann pins (see discussion on proximal tibial osteotomy by transverse wedge). Crossed pins are difficult to insert through the thick tibial cortex at the desired oblique angle and may not produce the degree of rigidity that is necessary to resist the pull of the quadriceps on the proximal fragment. It is important to note, however, that none of these problems is insurmountable and that many of the goals for the ideal osteotomy are met: Length is not altered, and the cancellous surface is maximized for rapid healing.

Figure 5–1. Visual inspection of the alignment of the leg is of critical importance to the surgeon. For this reason, as much of the leg as possible should be clearly visible to the surgeon. If a tourniquet is applied to the thigh and the leg then prepared and draped, there will be very little of the thigh visible in the child. If loose-fitting stockinette is covering the leg, the exact alignment of the tibia will also be obscured. For this reason, it is the author's preference to prepare and drape the leg from groin to toes and then wrap the leg in an adhesive, translucent, flexible plastic drape (*eg*, Op Site). A sterile (gas autoclaved) tourniquet is then placed about the proximal thigh. This permits excellent visual inspection of the overall alignment of the leg.

The incision is oblique, beginning at the medial flare of the tibia and extending downward and lateral across the tibial tubercle. It is not necessary to extend the incision around the leg to provide access to the fibula.

Figure 5–2. The entire incision is deepened through the subcutaneous tissue to expose the investing fascia of the muscles of the anterior and lateral compartment as well as the periosteum of the medial face of the tibia. The fibula can be divided first. The subcutaneous tissue is elevated from the fascia of the anterior tibial, extensor digitorum longus, and the peroneus longus muscles. At this point the sharp lateral border of the fibula can be palpated. This approach takes the surgeon posterior to the peroneal nerve.

A long blade retractor (*eg*, an Army-Navy or small Myerding) is used to pull the skin and subcutaneous tissue away from the muscle while a small sharp rake retractor or small Myerding retractor is used to pull the peroneus longus anteriorly (***Figure 5–2A***). The fascial interval between the peroneus longus and the soleus muscle is easily identified, and opened with a knife. This plane can be followed to the fibula, whose periosteum is exposed for a short distance by elevating the muscle with a periosteal elevator (***Figure 5–2B***).

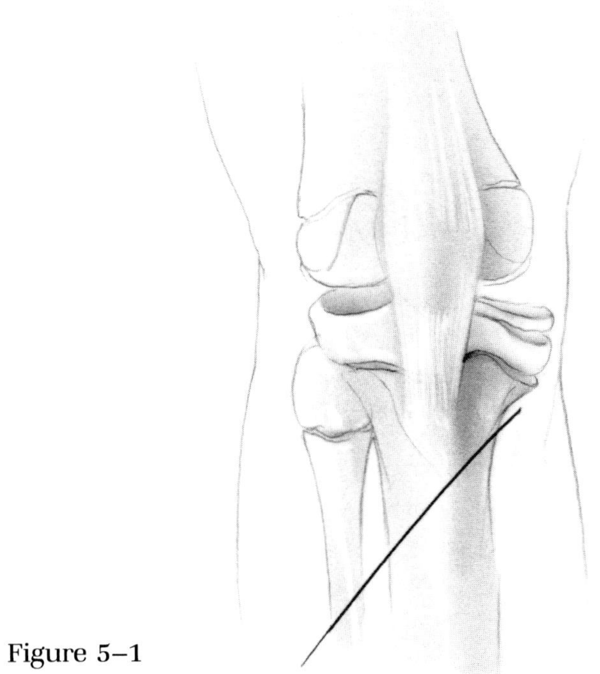

Figure 5–1

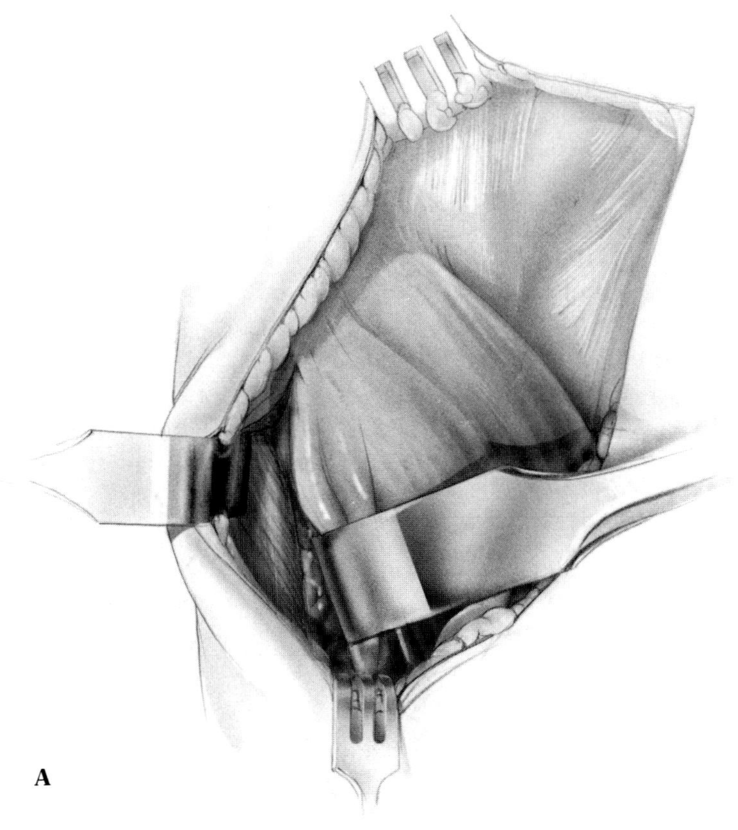

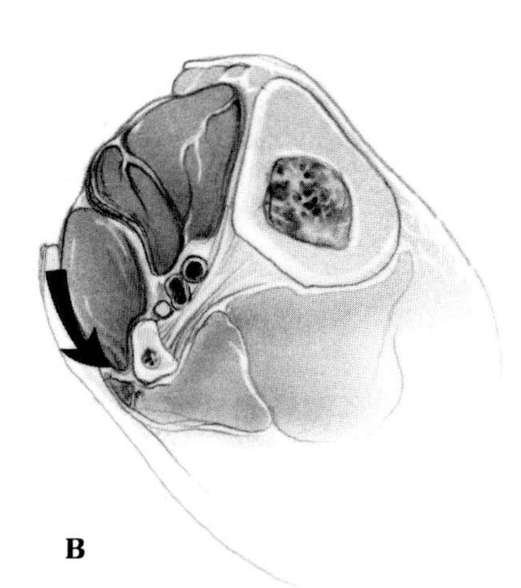

Figure 5–2

Figure 5–3. The periosteum is sharply incised, the fibula exposed subperiosteally, and two small Chandler or similar retractors are placed around the fibula. The bone can now be safely divided or a section removed. Care should be used in applying more retraction than necessary with the Chandler retractors to avoid traction injury to the peroneal nerve. No attempt is made to close this exposure; the muscles are simply allowed to fall back into place.

Figure 5–4. The exposure of the tibia is achieved by first incising the periosteum along the medial flare of the tibia, passing beneath the tibial tubercle, and continuing down the anterior crest of the tibia. The medial surface of the tibia is now exposed by subperiosteal dissection around to the posterior surface of the tibia.

To expose the lateral surface of the tibia, it is necessary to detach a variable portion of the origin of the anterior tibialis muscle and reflect this muscle off of the lateral face of the tibia. To accomplish this an incision is made along the lateral flare of the tibia joining the first incision below the tibial tubercle. In an effort to remain below the physeal plate, some of the muscle fibers may be cut, but this is of no concern. This muscle is now elevated subperiosteally, exposing the lateral surface of the tibia.

Some surgeons prefer to enter the anterior compartment to expose the lateral surface of the tibia. This is done by incising the fascia over the tibialis anterior muscle close to the tibial crest, retracting the muscle, and then incising the periosteum over the tibia just lateral to the crest. The incision of the fascia over the tibialis muscle is done as far distal as possible to accomplish a fasciotomy of the anterior compartment.

It is important here, as on the medial side, to carry the subperiosteal dissection around the posterior corner of the tibia. Sufficient detachment of the muscle origins from the lateral flare of the tibia should be done to permit this exposure. The use of a curved periosteal elevator (*eg*, the large Crego elevator) is also helpful in exposing the posterior surface of the tibia. During this exposure the knee should be flexed and any pressure on the back of the tibia relieved so that the neurovascular structures are permitted to fall away. At the completion of this dissection, it should be possible to pass retractors behind the entire tibia to assure protection of the soft tissues. This can usually be accomplished with a combination of different retractors (*eg*, a small malleable retractor, a Chandler retractor, a Blount knee retractor, etc).

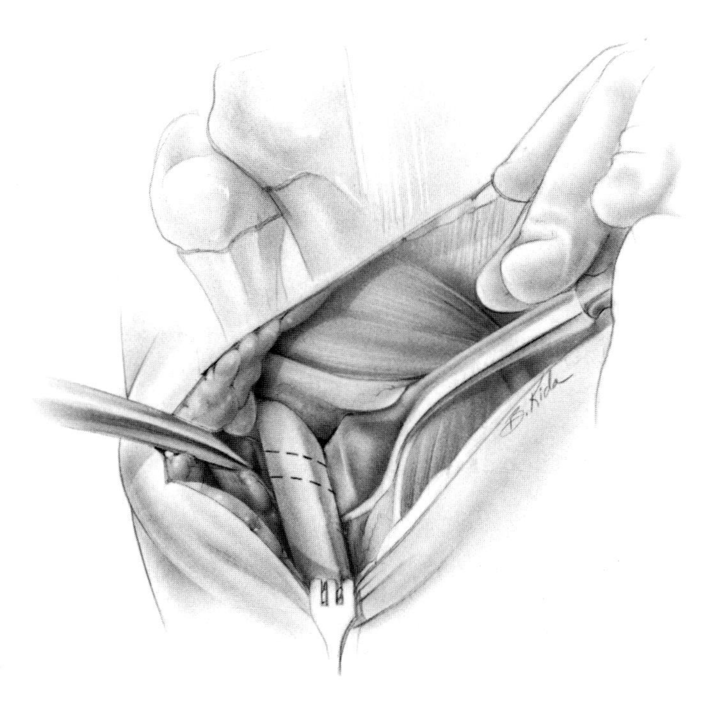

Figure 5–3

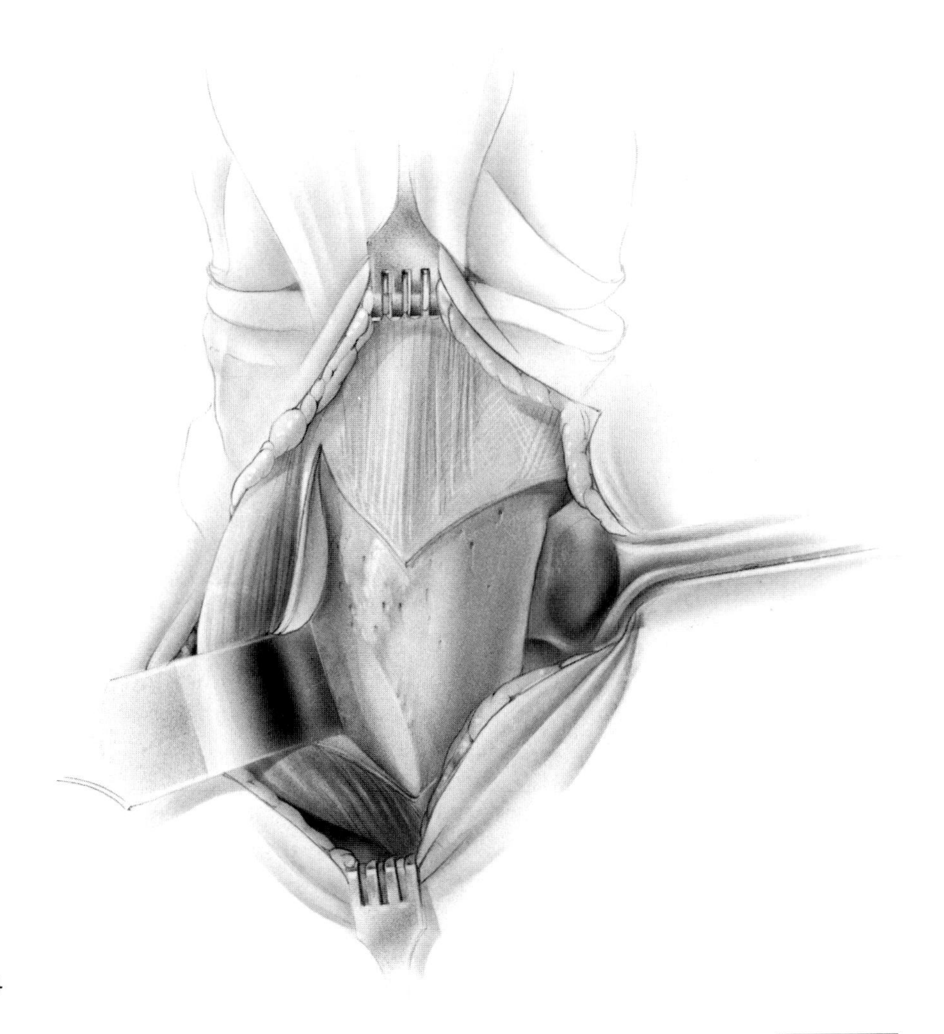

Figure 5–4

Figure 5–5. The dome to be cut in the tibia is outlined with multiple drill holes. The apex of the dome should be the first hole drilled and should lie about 1 cm beneath the tibial tubercle. It is easiest to drill the holes in the medial and lateral face of the tibia by keeping the drill perpendicular to the surface of the bone. To preserve the same contour in the posterior surface, however, the drill should then be passed in a straight anterior to posterior direction when drilling the holes in the posterior cortex.

Following this the holes are connected with an osteotome, first cutting the anterior cortex, then the medial and lateral cortex, and finally the posterior cortex. Again, care should be taken to be sure that retractors are protecting the soft tissues posteriorly.

Figure 5–6. The osteotomy is now manipulated into the correct position. It is possible to correct both varus and valgus, flexion and extension, and rotation. After all of the correction in the various planes is achieved, the osteotomy seldomly retains the characteristics of the perfect dome. Therefore, some adjustment is usually needed to the osteotomy surfaces to achieve good coaption and remove bony prominences. This is most easily accomplished with a rongeur. Much of the difficulty in achieving good coaption between the two surfaces is due to the fact that the bone is triangular in cross-section in the area of the osteotomy.

After the desired correction is achieved, two smooth or threaded Steinmann pins are passed across the osteotomy site; one from medial and one from lateral. It is important that the pins cross as far as possible above or below the osteotomy site, or in other words, are as far apart as possible when they cross the osteotomy. If the pins cross at the osteotomy site or are close together, there will be no rotational stability. If the pins cross the physeal plate they should be smooth. Whether the pins are left out through the skin or buried beneath the skin is the surgeon's choice, with the pros and cons being obvious.

The final position and fixation should be checked radiographically. The position is best checked with a long radiograph, but the fixation is best checked with an image intensifier while stressing the osteotomy site. It is important when verifying the degree of correction that the osteotomy not be held forcibly in position, because opening of the joint space could lead the surgeon to believe that more correction had been achieved than really had been (see discussion on oblique coronal osteotomy of the proximal tibia).

The wound is then closed by loosely approximating the periosteum and reattaching the muscle origin of the anterior tibialis muscle. It is neither possible nor desirable to close the periosteum completely. A suction drain is placed in the subcutaneous space and the remainder of the wound is closed. A long leg cast is applied with the position depending on the surgeon's preference. Usually the knee is flexed about 45 degrees. This position will aid in elevation in the postoperative period and permit non–weight-bearing during ambulation if done as a unilateral procedure. This position will make it impossible to check the alignment of the osteotomy in the postoperative period, however, and decreases the ability of the cast to immobilize the osteotomy site as compared with a straight leg cast. For these reasons the surgeon may prefer to cast the leg with the knee extended but risk the fact that the child will almost certainly bear weight on the leg.

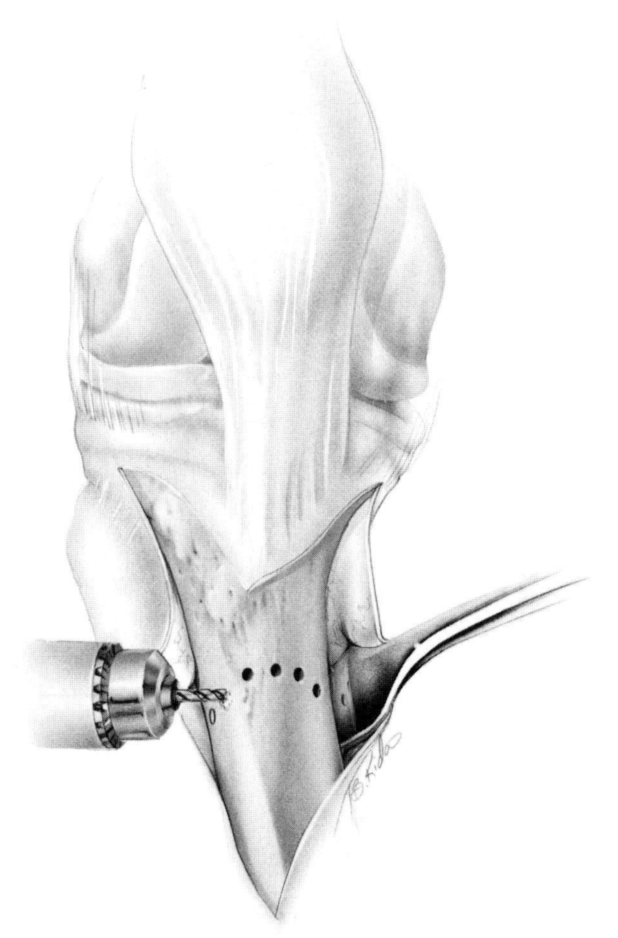

Figure 5–5

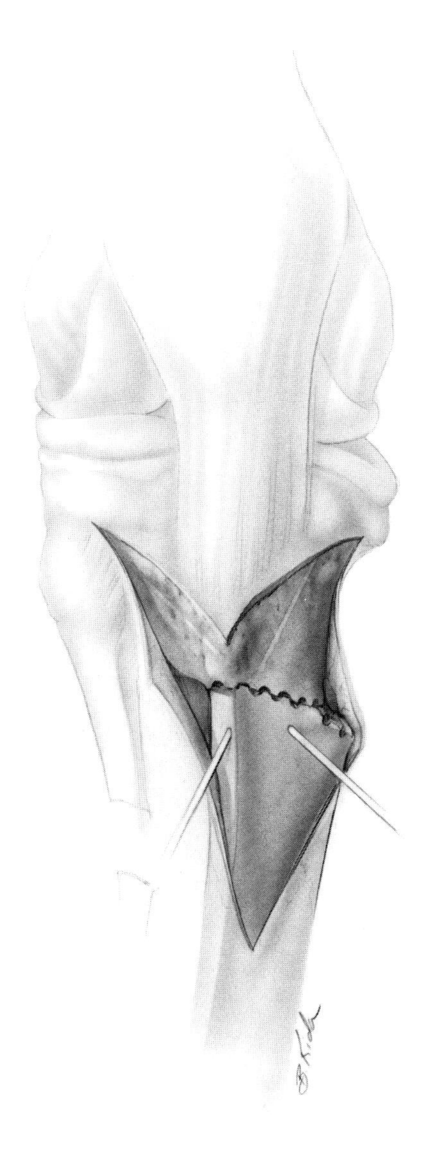

Figure 5–6

Figure 5–7. The problems with using two crossed Steinman pins for fixation are illustrated in these postoperative radiographs of a 13 + 8-year-old male with adolescent Blount's disease who underwent a closing transverse wedge osteotomy with crossed-pin fixation (***Figure 5–7A***). The anteroposterior radiograph demonstrates the anatomic difficulty of gaining secure fixation. If this osteotomy were done more proximally as it could have been, it would have been even more difficult to obtain fixation. If the pins are started distally, it can be very difficult to penetrate the thick tibial cortex at the necessary angle. The lateral radiograph (***Figure 5–7B***) illustrates the anterior angulation that results by the pull of the quadriceps tendon that is poorly resisted by the fixation.

Figure 5–8. An alternative to crossed-pins is the use of the T-buttress plate as illustrated in this 3 + 9-year-old child with Blount's disease (***Figure 5–8A***). The immediate postoperative radiograph shows the osteotomy done in the correct location just beneath the tibial tubercle (***Figure 5–8B***). Three months later the osteotomy is healed (***Figure 5–8C***). (Courtesy of Douglas H. Kehl, MD.)

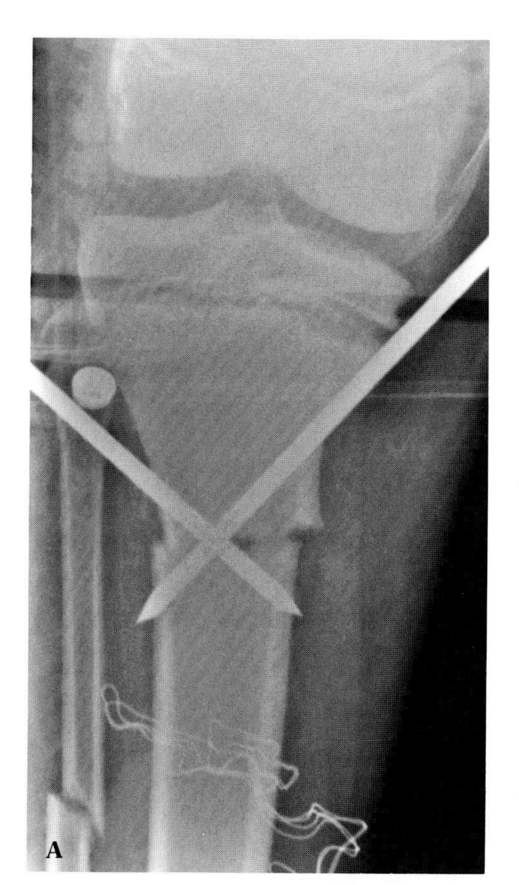

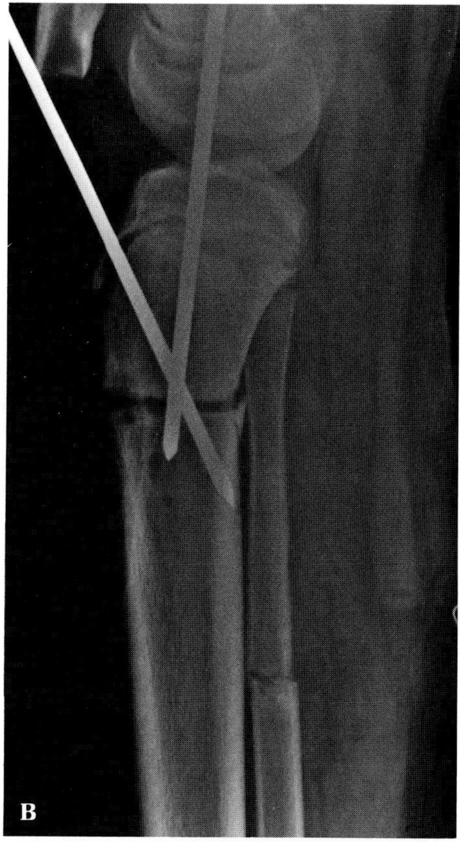

Figure 5–7

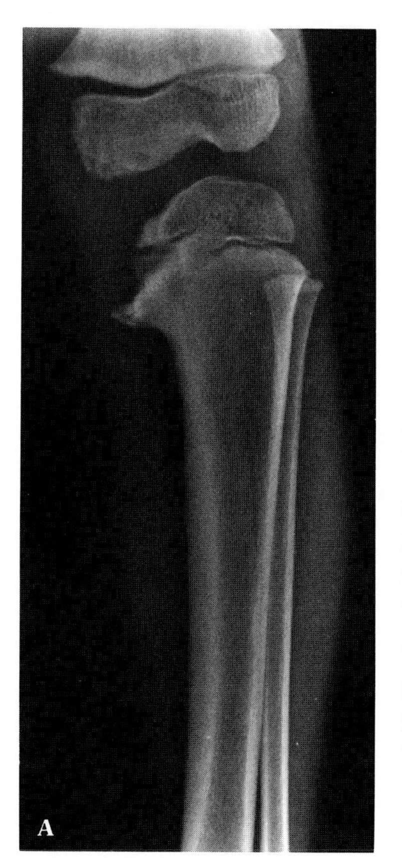

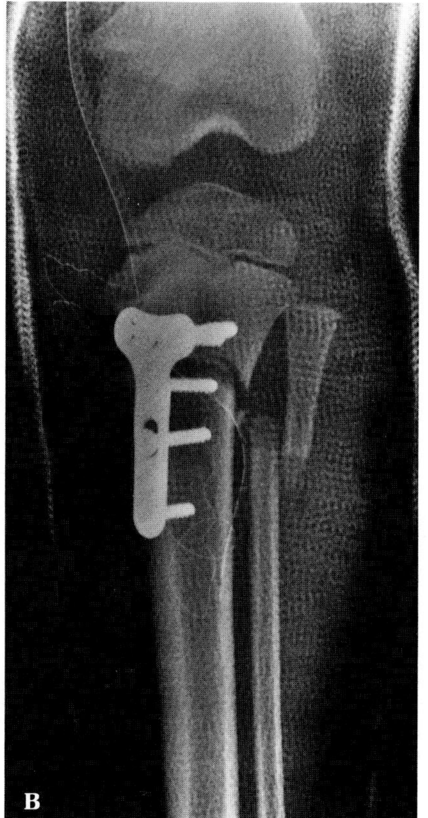

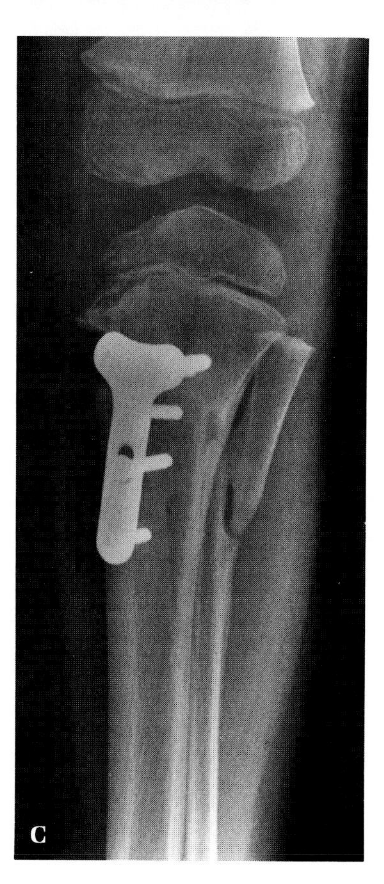

Figure 5–8

POSTOPERATIVE CARE

The drain is removed when the drainage has slowed. If the procedure is unilateral, the patient can be ambulated as soon as comfortable and depending on age. It is important that weight-bearing not be permitted. Therefore, if the patient is not to be trusted in this regard, it is best to obtain a rental wheel chair for a bed-to-chair program until the radiographs show sufficient healing to permit removal of the pins and weight-bearing. This will usually be between 6 and 8 weeks postoperatively, and depending on the degree of healing and the reliability of the patient. Application of a long leg cast with knee flexed 10 degrees can be used at any time the surgeon thinks that weight-bearing is either permissible or desirable.

5.2 Transverse Wedge Osteotomy of Proximal Tibia

Transverse wedge osteotomy is the second most popular technique for correcting angular deformity of the proximal tibia in the growing child after dome osteotomy. This is probably due to the surgeon's familiarity with this technique in adults. There are problems with this osteotomy in the growing child, however, that are not present in the adult. These do not necessarily make this a poor choice, but the surgeon should be aware of these differences.

Figure 5–9. In the child with open growth plates the osteotomy is performed below the tibial tubercle rather than above it. This region of the tibia tapers rapidly, resulting in a large change in the circumference of the bone over a very short distance. After removal of a wedge of bone, the circumference of the distal segment will be smaller than the circumference of the proximal segment. Thus, cortical apposition will not be possible at some point around the circumference of the bone. The result is that there will be a loss of intrinsic stability at the osteotomy site in the area where the cortex of the smaller distal segment is opposed to the cancellous area of the larger proximal segment. This can result in further displacement of the osteotomy as the cortical bone of the smaller fragment sinks into the cancellous bone of the larger fragment. This problem can be aggravated by the strong pull of the quadriceps muscle on the proximal fragment, which tends to angle the osteotomy anteriorly. These factors place an increased importance on the method or strength of the fixation. This is a greater problem in the older heavier child (*eg*, the patient with adolescent Blount's disease) in whom the fixation cannot provide sufficient stability and collapse at the osteotomy site can lead to secondary deformity (*eg*, anterior angulation or loss of correction). The ideal fixation for this osteotomy in the child does not exist. The T-buttress plate is one solution. Some surgeons are now using external fixation for these osteotomies.

Figure 5–10. Another potential disadvantage to the transverse wedge osteotomy is the displacement of the distal segment that can result if the closing of the wedge is not accompanied by displacement of the distal fragment. This is seldom a problem with a single osteotomy (***Figure 5–10A***), but with second and subsequent wedge osteotomies hinged on the medial cortex, as may be required in Blount's disease, this can result in significant displacement of the mechanical axis of the leg as the smaller distal segment shifts slightly medial to the knee joint with each osteotomy (***Figure 5–10B***). The solution to this problem is to combinemedial or lateral displacement depending on the osteotomy with the valgus or varus correction (***Figure 5–10C***).

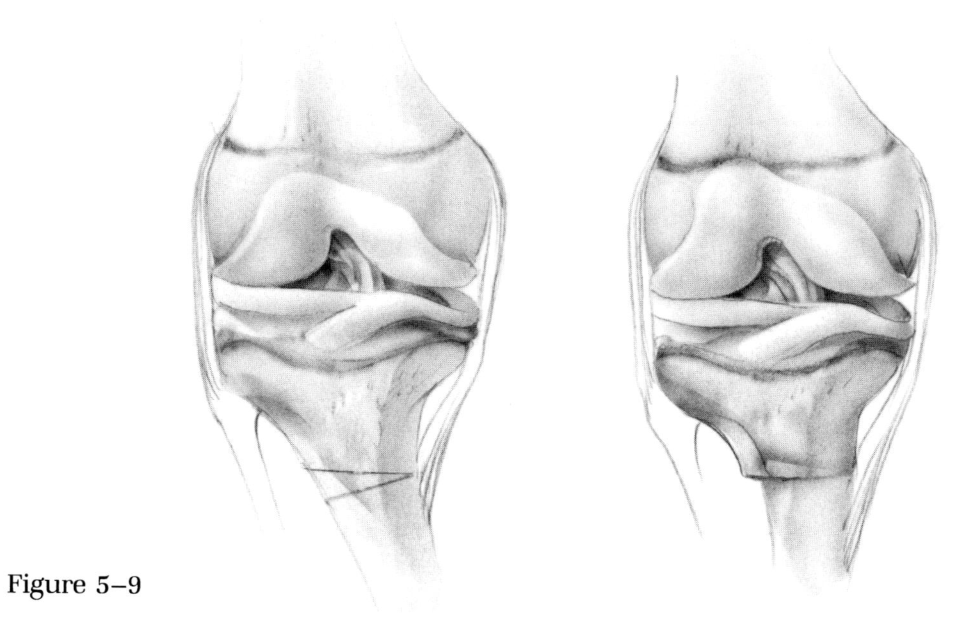

Figure 5–9

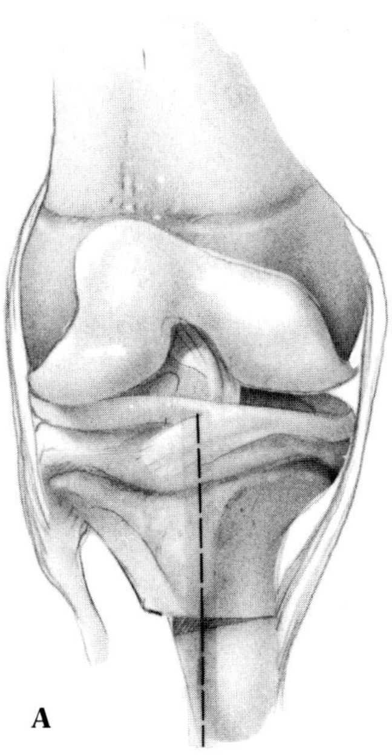

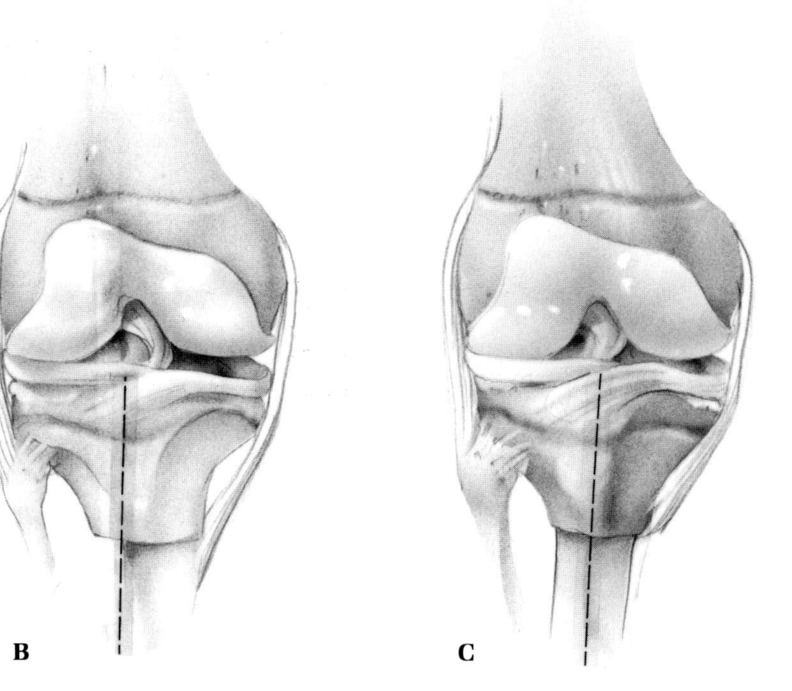

Figure 5–10

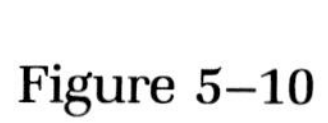

Figure 5–11. The final problem with the transverse wedge osteotomy is the calculation of the size of the wedge to be removed. Although this author cannot verify the accuracy of all of the calculations, an excellent discussion of the principles involved is provided by Canale and Harper.[1] According to the authors, the usual rule of one millimeter for every degree of correction is a reasonable approximation for tibias that are 5 to 6 cm in diameter. In smaller tibias, however, this rule will result in too large of a wedge being removed and overcorrection.

There are several methods to calculate accurately the width of the base of the wedge to be removed. The first is to draw the correction on a preoperative radiograph and measure the template for the necessary wedge. Care must be taken to account for the magnification factor of the radiograph, which can vary but is usually assumed to be about 20%.

A second method of preoperative planning is illustrated. This can be done either preoperatively on the radiographs (again with care to include the magnification factor) or at the time of operation to measure its diameter. First drill a wire through the bone at the proposed site of the osteotomy to determine the diameter of the bone. Then along with the desired angle of correction apply the following formula:

$$W \text{ (wedge)} = D \text{ (diameter)} \times \text{tangent of angle}$$

Canale and Marion state that the following formula gives a reasonable approximation of the preceding formula without the need to calculate the tangent:

$$W = D \times 0.02 \times \text{angle}$$

Figure 5–12. A final method to calculate the size of the wedge is done at the time of surgery and avoids mathematical calculations. The diameter of the bone at the proposed site of the osteotomy is measured by passing a guide through the bone. A nomogram with the desired angle of correction relating various diameters and various widths of wedges is drawn to scale with the desired angle of correction before surgery and brought to the operating room. Once the diameter of the bone is known, the size of the wedge can be measured directly from the nomogram.

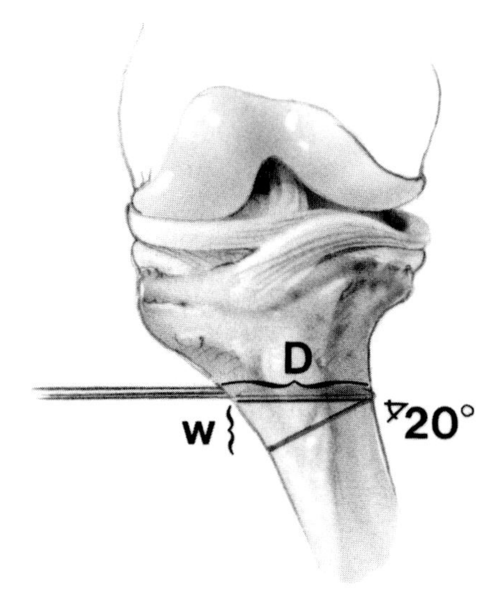

Figure 5–11

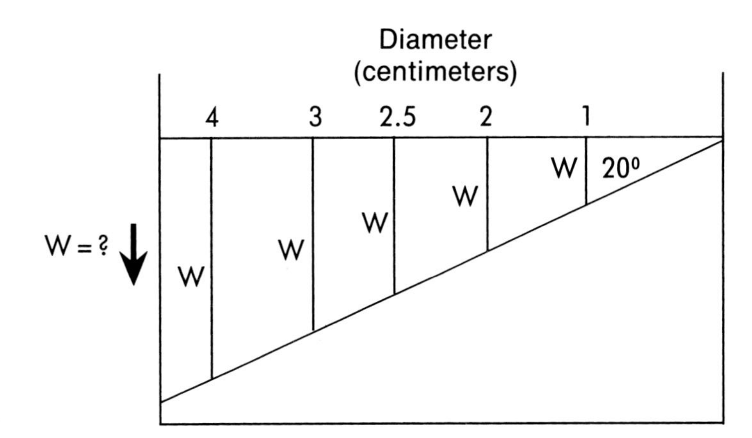

Figure 5–12

Figure 5–13. The incision, the exposure of the tibia, and the exposure and division of the fibula are the same as described for the dome osteotomy. In the case illustrated, a lateral wedge will be removed below the tibial tubercle for the correction of a varus deformity in a growing child. In this circumstance the lateral dissection will have to be thorough to allow the wedge to be removed and the T-buttress plate to be secured.

The first consideration is accurate placement of the wedge. The common mistake is to place the wedge too distally for fear of injury to the tibial tubercle. Often the surgeon is afraid to dissect sufficiently to identify the tubercle. For these reasons it is wise to verify the level of the proximal transverse cut by drilling a guide wire transversely through the tibia just proximal to the proposed site of the cut and visualizing this radiographically. This cut should be about 1 cm distal to the tibial tubercle. The base of the wedge can be measured, and the distal cut marked with an osteotome or a saw.

Figure 5–14. A power saw is used to remove the wedge of bone. Care should be taken to protect the soft tissues behind the tibia. If neither rotational correction nor displacement is needed, a small portion of the medial cortex can be left intact and fractured as the osteotomy is closed. Although this will result in slight medial displacement of the leg under the knee joint it will confer an increased stability to the osteotomy. If the correction is large, if this is a repeat osteotomy, or if it is desired to unweight the medial side of the knee, however, it may be desirable to displace the distal fragment laterally.

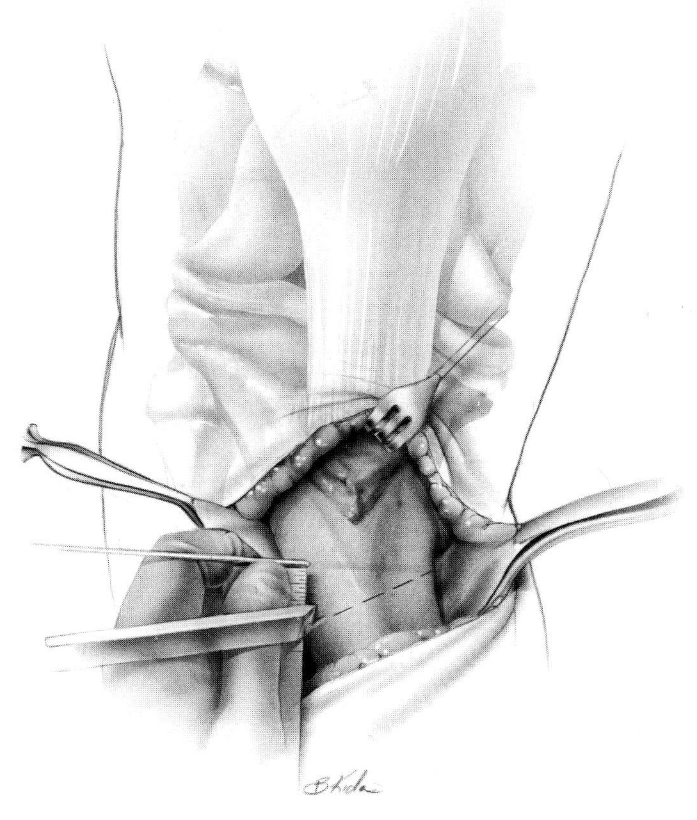

Figure 5–13

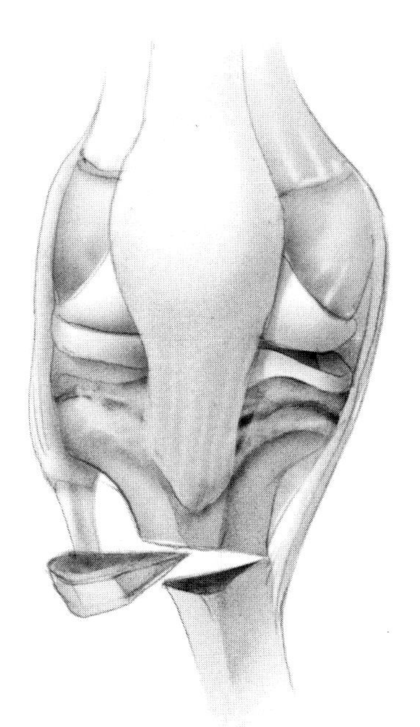

Figure 5–14

Figure 5–15. After removal of the wedge the osteotomy is closed. The leg should be visually inspected to be certain that the desired correction has been achieved. If any questions exist, the osteotomy should be fixed temporarily with a smooth Kirschner wire and a radiograph obtained. The osteotomy should not be held closed by manual force while this radiograph is obtained as this will force open the medial joint line, creating the impression of more correction than has actually been obtained at the osteotomy site (see discussion on oblique coronal osteotomy of proximal tibia).

When satisfactory correction has been obtained, a T-buttress plate is contoured to the lateral tibia and fixed in place. The proximal limb of the "T" will lie just beneath the physeal plate.

The periosteum is loosely approximated, a suction drain is placed superficial to the muscles and the periosteum, and the subcutaneous tissue and skin are closed. A long leg cast is applied with the knee bent 45 degrees.

Figure 5–16. Immediate postoperative lateral radiograph of a closing transverse wedge osteotomy for adolescent Blount's disease is shown (***Figure 5–16A***). Notice the overhang of the proximal fragment posteriorly. Eight weeks later (***Figure 5–16B***) there is anterior angulation and delayed healing with collapse and resorption posteriorly. This method of fixation is not ideal for the very large adolescent as it resists the pull of the quadriceps poorly and cortical apposition in all areas is not always achieved.

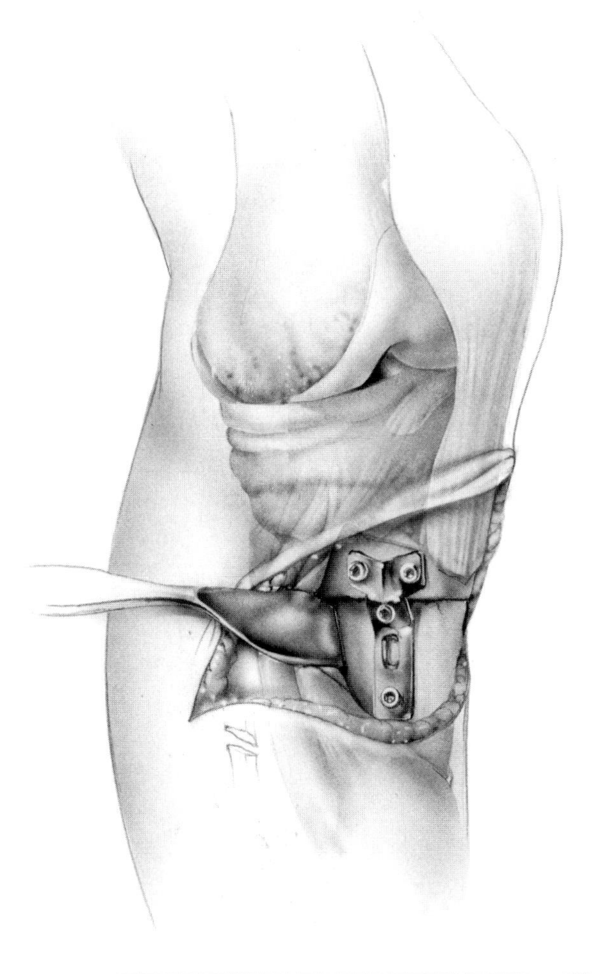

Figure 5–15

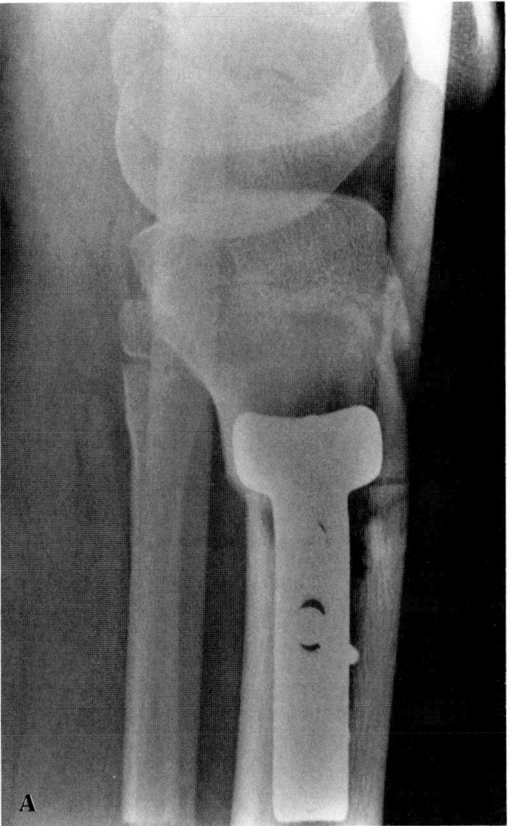

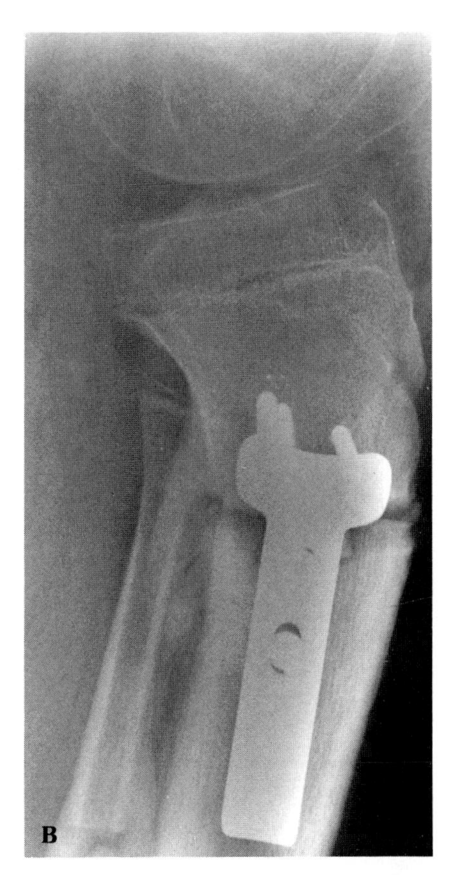

Figure 5–16

POSTOPERATIVE CARE

The fixation is not secure enough to permit weight-bearing. Therefore, the patient is kept non–weight-bearing for the first 6 weeks, at which time healing is usually sufficient to permit removal of the cast, resumption of weight-bearing, and rehabilitation of the knee. It is probably advisable to plan removal of the fixation.

REFERENCE

1. Canale TS, Harper MC. Biotrigonometric analysis and practical applications of osteotomies of tibia in children. In: Murray DG, ed. Instructional course lectures, vol XXX. The American Academy of Orthopaedic Surgeons. St Louis: CV Mosby, 1981:87.

5.3 Oblique Wedge Osteotomy of Proximal Tibia

An alternative to the classic transverse wedge osteotomy is the oblique wedge. The author ascribes this osteotomy to Professor Heinz Wagner (although he cannot reference this). There is a reference to this technique in adults that also describes a precise way in which to measure the wedge.[1]

The advantages of this type of wedge are the inherent stability, the rapid healing owing to the broad cancellous surface, and the fact that axial displacement of the tibia is minimized. Rotational correction is also possible with this osteotomy and is achieved by the shape of the wedge removed. The author favors this osteotomy for correction of deformity in the proximal tibia, especially in older children and adolescents.

Figure 5–17. The incision is the same as described for the dome osteotomy of the proximal tibia with the exception that it should be made slightly more oblique to give more distal exposure. If the osteotomy is being done to correct valgus, the dissection of the muscles and periosteum on the lateral side should be minimized as it is not needed and the intact lateral periosteum provides a good hinge for the osteotomy. The same is true for the dissection on the medial side if varus is being corrected. It may also be necessary to extend the incision in the periosteum more distal than with other osteotomies.

Figure 5–18. For correction of a varus deformity as illustrated here, the tibialis anterior muscle must be elevated subperiosteally to permit the lateral-based wedge to be removed. ***Figure 15–18A*** shows the extent of the incisions in the periosteum that are possible through this oblique skin incision. The periosteal elevation will extend more distally than with other proximal tibial osteotomies to permit the wedge to be oblique. Perhaps the most difficult part of the operation is to make the wedge oblique enough to realize its advantages. The perosteum should not be elevated in the proximal medial corner where the osteotomy will hinge.

A guide wire is then drilled from distal-lateral to proximal-medial. It should penetrate the medial cortex just beneath the physeal plate. This wire will mark the proximal cut of the wedge. If desired a second guide wire can be drilled into the bone to mark the distal cut (***Figure 5–18B***).

Figure 5–19. The exact width of the wedge can be calculated[1] or estimated. The author has found it rather easy to estimate the size of the wedge correctly: For some reason it seems much more intuitive than estimating the amount of a transverse wedge. If the surgeon miscalculates, more bone can be removed or a small piece of bone from a too-large wedge replaced. Because of the large cancellous surface, healing will not be impaired.

If only correction of varus or valgus is desired, the wedge of bone that is removed will be as wide anteriorly as posteriorly (***Figure 5–19A***). If correction of internal rotation is desired in addition to correction of the varus, however, the wedge of bone removed is cut wider anteriorly than posteriorly (***Figure 5–19B***). Thus, when the osteotomy is closed, the distal fragment will rotate laterally producing the desired correction.

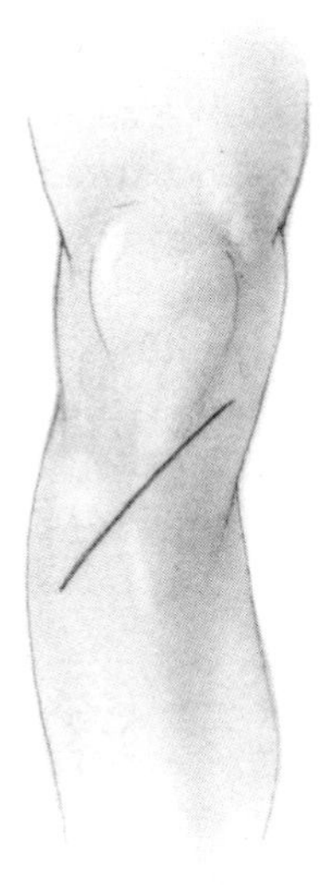

Figure 5–17

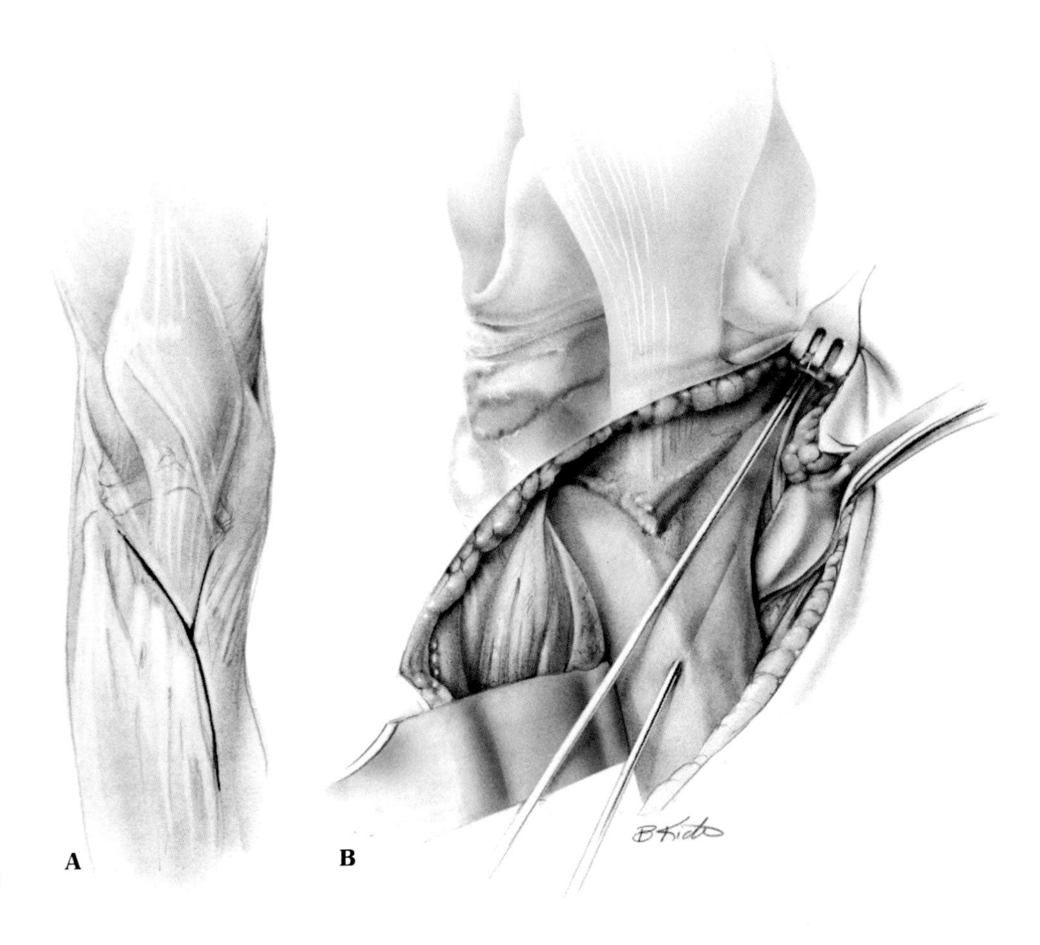

Figure 5–18

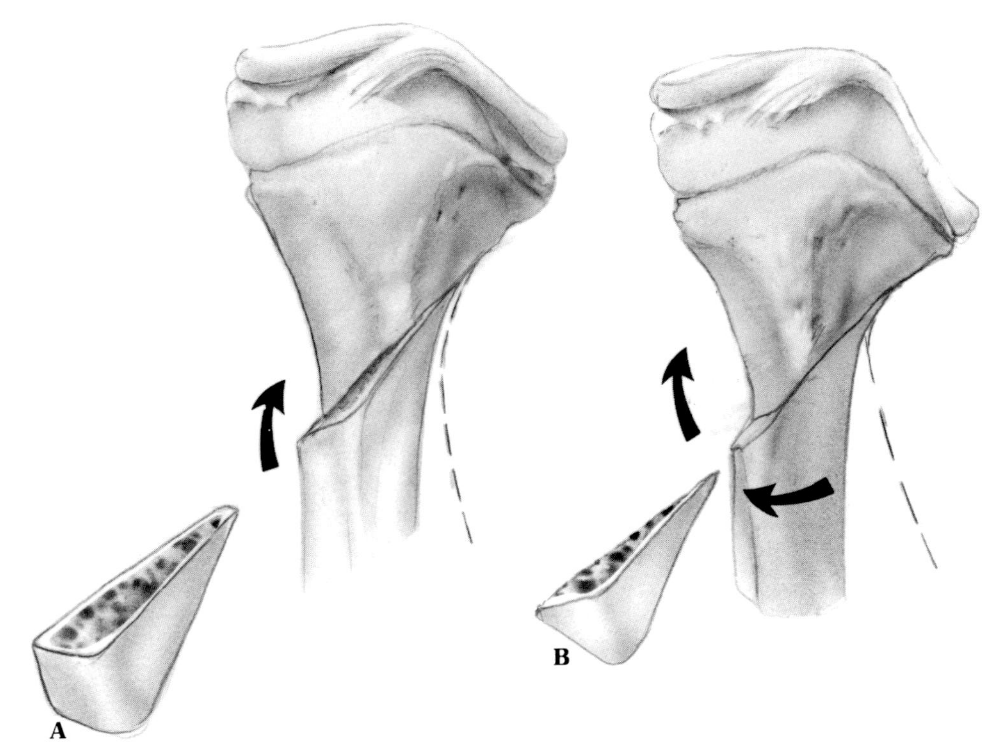

Figure 5–19

Figure 5–20. A power saw is used to remove the wedge. The posterior soft tissues are protected by a small, malleable retractor passed behind the osteotomy site from the lateral side. If only varus is to be corrected the wedge should be removed so as to leave a small, thin segment of the medial cortex intact that can be fractured as the osteotomy is closed. If internal rotation is also part of the correction, the bone should be completely divided; however, an effort should be made to leave the periosteum intact as this will make it easier to close and fix the osteotomy.

Figure 5–21. The osteotomy site is closed and fixed with two cortical screws that are inserted perpendicular to the plane of the osteotomy from the medial side. Because of the obliquity of the incision, it is often not possible to insert the distal screw in the proper direction through the incision. In such cases it is inserted through a small stab wound over the subcutaneous border of the tibia. Subsequent removal of the screws is actually easier if both are placed through stab wounds, because they can be difficult to palpate, but the small scars show exactly where they are.

The wound is now closed over a suction drain and a long leg cast applied. Because it is possible with this osteotomy to achieve a tight closure of the periosteum, the surgeon may wish to perform a fasciotomy of the anterior compartment at this time.

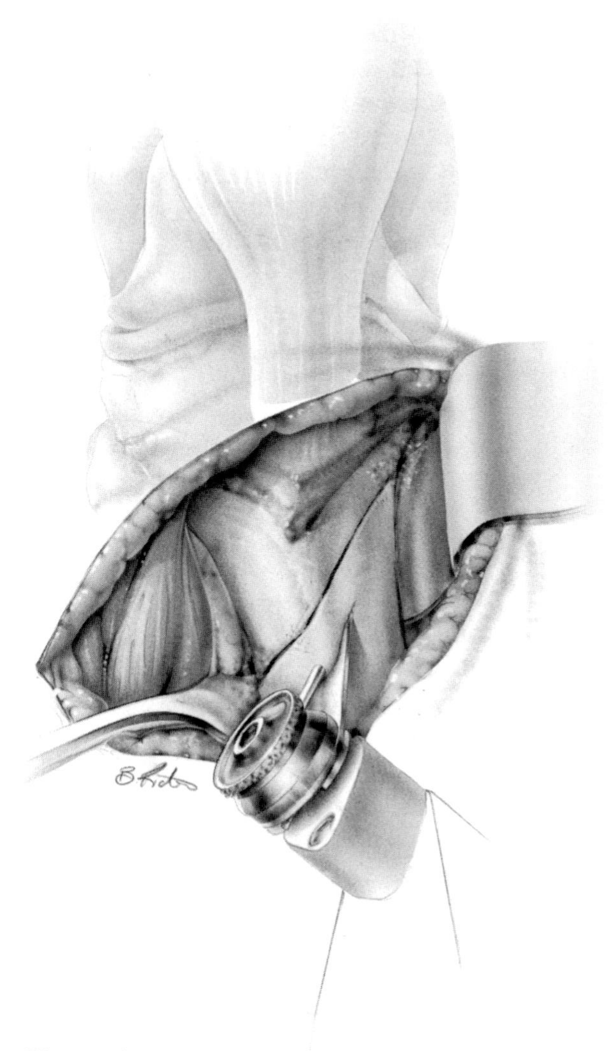

Figure 5–20

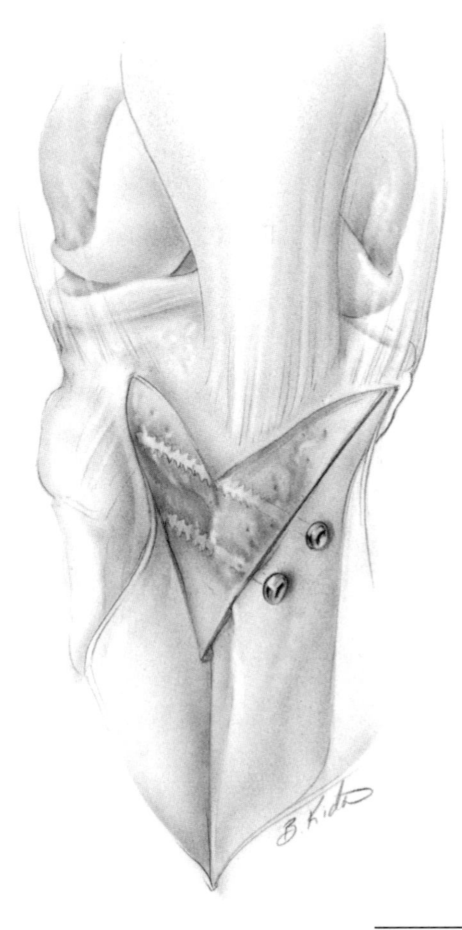

Figure 5–21

Figure 5–22. BM is a 12-year-old boy with idiopathic genu valgum. Correction of the deformity was done at the parents' request because of his appearance and the social problems it was causing him (***Figure 5–22A***). The osteotomies of the right (***Figure 5–22B***) and left leg (***Figure 5–22C***) were done differently and serve to emphasize several technical points. The right osteotomy is more oblique than the left, which is desirable but more distal. Placing the screws in an osteotomy done to correct valgus is more difficult than in an osteotomy to correct varus. In long-standing deformities of the legs there is deformity on the femoral as well as the tibial side of the joint. The optimum correction of the knee mechanics would require both a femoral and tibial osteotomy. ***Figures 5–22D, E*** show the patient at 6 weeks after the surgery, at which time the casts were removed and protected weight-bearing with a four-point crutch gait begun.

POSTOPERATIVE CARE

The drain can usually be removed on the first postoperative day. If the patient is old enough to ambulate reliably with a three-point partial weight-bearing crutch gait, that is started on the second postoperative day. Healing is usually sufficient in 6 weeks to permit removal of the cast, progression to full weight-bearing, and vigorous rehabilitation of the knee.

REFERENCE

1. Williams AT. Tibial realignment by oblique wedge osteotomy. Int Orthop 1986;10:171.

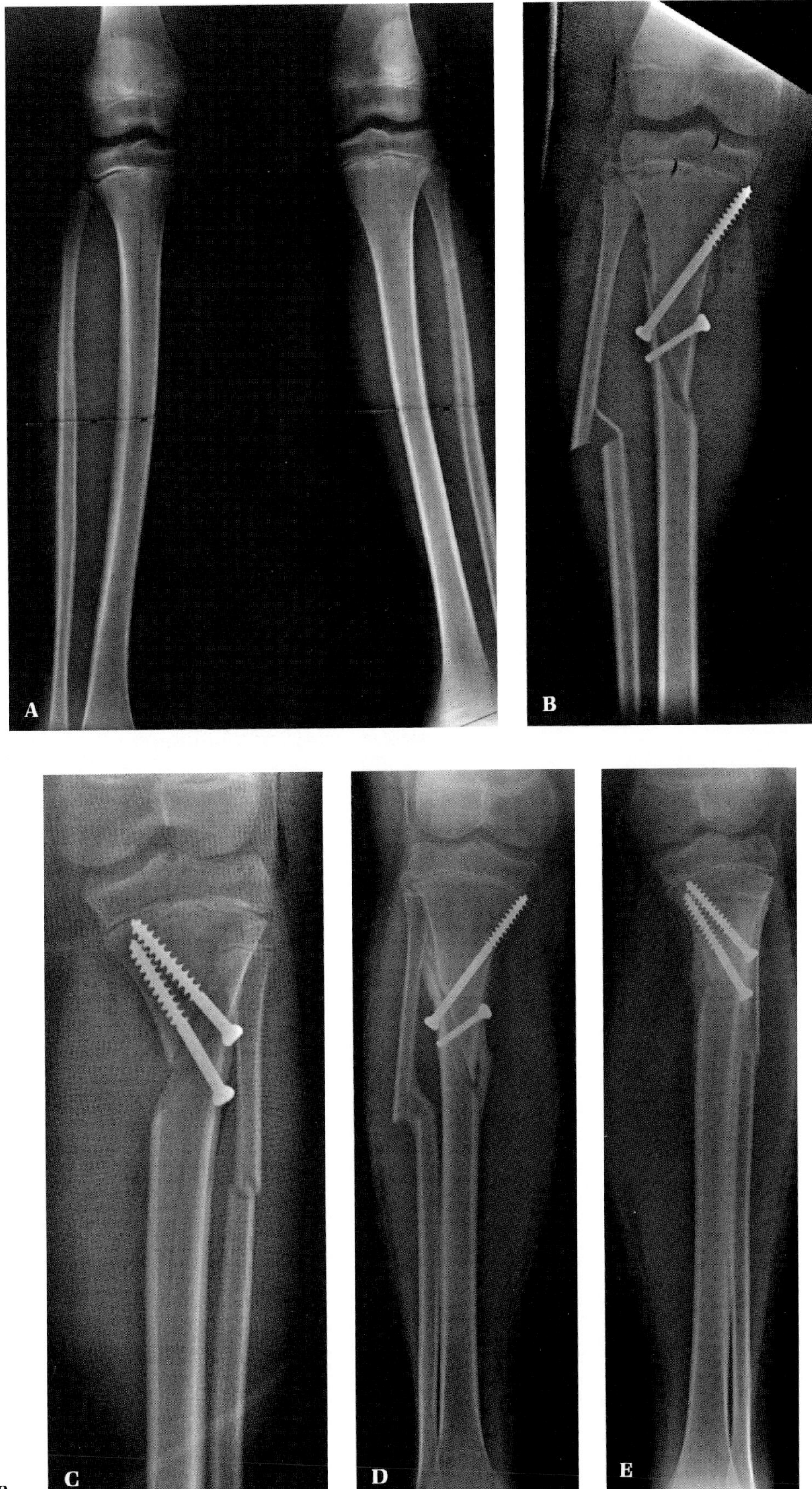

Figure 5–22

5.4 Oblique Coronal Osteotomy of Proximal Tibia

Recently Rab[1] has described an oblique osteotomy of the proximal tibia in the coronal plane to correct the angular and rotational deformities that are seen in Blount's disease. The principle is the same as introduced by MacEwen and Shands[2] for osteotomy of the proximal femur. Correction of varus or valgus requires an osteotomy in the coronal plane. Correction of rotation requires an osteotomy in the transverse plane. Because patients with Blount's disease have both deformities, an osteotomy angled in the frontal plane should correct both components of the deformity. If the cut is made at 45 degrees in the frontal plane, it will correct equal amounts of angulation and rotation. Rab states that this is the usual case in Blount's disease, but has provided a nomogram to help the surgeon determine the angle of the osteotomy when different degrees of varus-valgus and rotation are present. The osteotomy is fixed with a single screw that allows for rotation at the osteotomy site. Thus, the amount of correction can be determined after the drapes are removed and just before cast application. If vascular complications develop in the postoperative period, the cast can be removed and the correction reversed without losing fixation of the osteotomy.

Figure 5–23. The patient is placed on a radiolucent operating table in the supine position. Image-intensifier control is an essential part of this procedure. The surgeon should be certain that he is able to obtain a good lateral view of the tibia. This is essential to confirm the location of the osteotomy and the depth of the saw or osteotomes. The image intensifier can be positioned horizontally over the operating table and moved toward the head or foot of the table when not in use to keep it out of the surgeon's way. Although Rab[1] describes a transverse incision below the tibial tubercle with a separate incision for the fibular osteotomy, the author has continued to use and prefers the oblique incision described for the dome osteotomy of the proximal tibia. The exposure of the tibia is also the same as described for the dome osteotomy. It is important that the exposure be sufficient to allow retractors to be placed behind the tibia. The fibula is divided as described previously.

Figure 5–24. Beginning about 1 cm below the tibial tubercle, a smooth Steinmann pin is drilled into the tibia at the angle chosen for the osteotomy. The angle, depth, and location of this pin should be verified on the lateral image. The point at which the osteotomy cut will reach the posterior cortex should be a safe distance distal to the physeal plate. The saw is now used to create the osteotomy just distal to this pin. The progress of the saw is carefully monitored on the lateral view of the image intensifier. It is not usually possible to complete the osteotomy with the saw because of the saw blade striking the retractors. A narrow saw blade or a small osteotome can be used to complete the osteotomy. The distal fragment should now be manipulated to loosen the periosteum from the posterior surface of the tibia, allowing free motion at the osteotomy site. It is now possible to manipulate the distal fragment and demonstrate the correction of both the varus and the internal rotation.

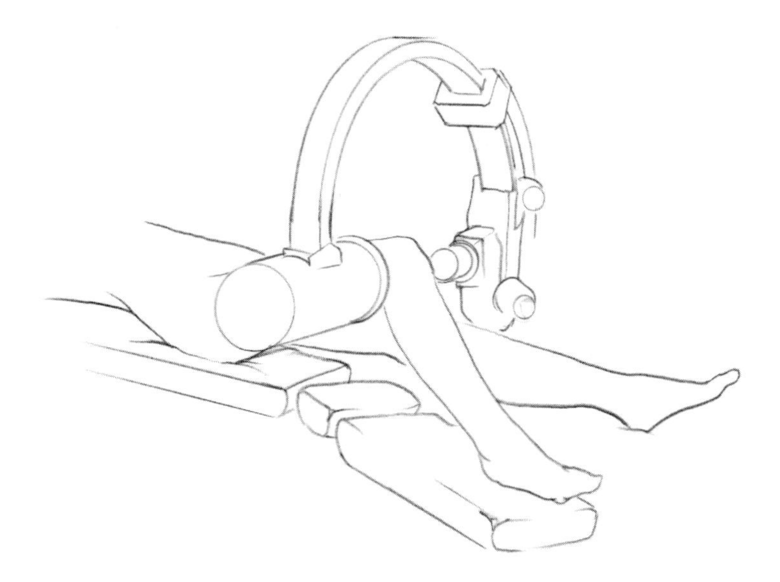

Figure 5–23

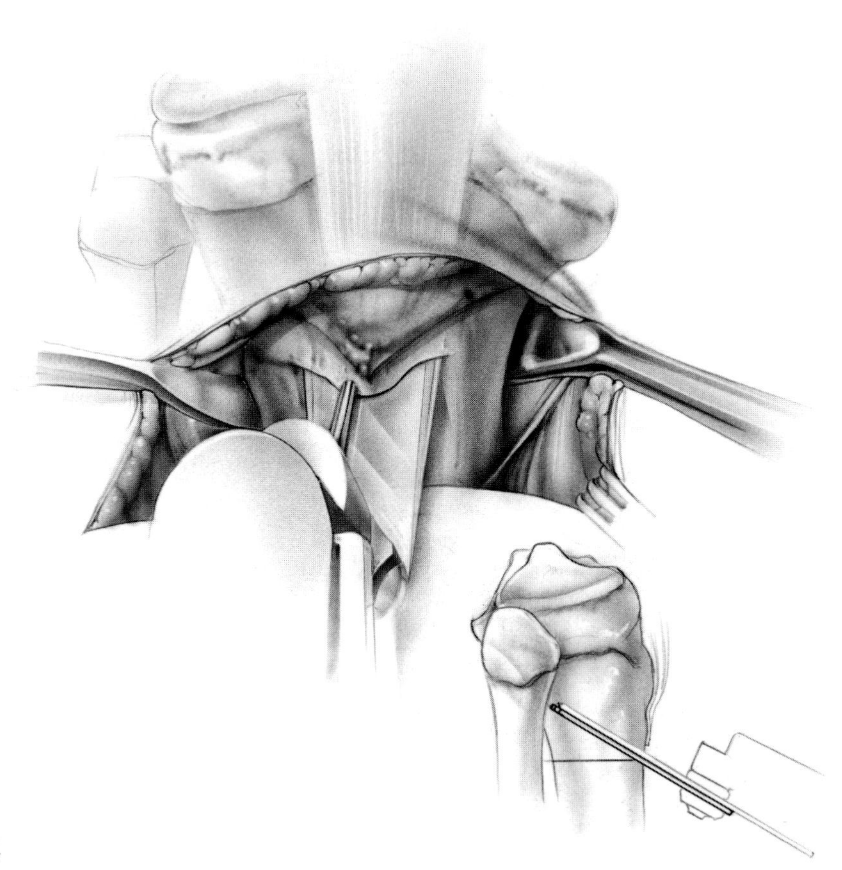

Figure 5–24

Figure 5–25. The osteotomy is now fixed with a single screw that will hold the two fragments together while allowing motion between them in the plane of the osteotomy. This is achieved by first reducing the fragments to their original position, then drilling a screw hole lateral to the tibial tubercle that will penetrate both fragments. The hole in the proximal fragment should be over drilled. It is important for good fixation that the screw penetrate the cortex of the distal fragment. Because this osteotomy will usually be used in smaller children, a 3.5-mm cortical screw is chosen. The screw should not be tightened so as to prevent free motion between the fragments. Before closing the wound, the surgeon should verify that the fragments can move sufficiently to provide the desired correction.

Figure 5–26. After the wound is dressed, the leg is manipulated into correct position for casting. The correct position can be verified by image intensification, or better, a radiograph on a large film that includes the knee joint and the entire tibial shaft.

There is a potential pitfall in determining the final position of the osteotomy that is present in all osteotomies for Blount's disease, but is more difficult to avoid in this technique. Any time the osteotomy is held in the valgus position while the degree of correction is being determined, there are two factors at play that may cause the surgeon to overestimate the amount of correction that has been achieved. First, the knee joint is being opened medially, and in many deformities about the knee lax ligaments are the rule. Second, there may be more correction at the osteotomy site than the fixation will maintain when the force is released. These two factors often lead surgeons to believe that they have achieved more correction at the osteotomy site than they actually have. When the leg is left to lie on the table without being held or after the cast is removed and the patient begins to walk, the problem becomes apparent. The best solution to this problem is to fix the osteotomy rigidly and then force the leg back into varus for visual inspection and while the radiograph is taken. In this osteotomy rigid fixation is avoided; however, if the surgeon is aware of this potential problem it can usually be avoided.

After the position of the osteotomy has been verified and deemed acceptable, a long leg cast is applied. If the knee is kept straight, it is easier both to maintain and verify radiographically the position of the osteotomy. With the knee straight, however, it may not be possible to keep a small child from walking on the leg. After the cast is applied, the position can again be checked with a radiograph. If the correction is not as desired or if a problem with the circulation develops, the cast can be removed, the position of the osteotomy changed, and a new cast applied, all without loosing fixation of the osteotomy site.

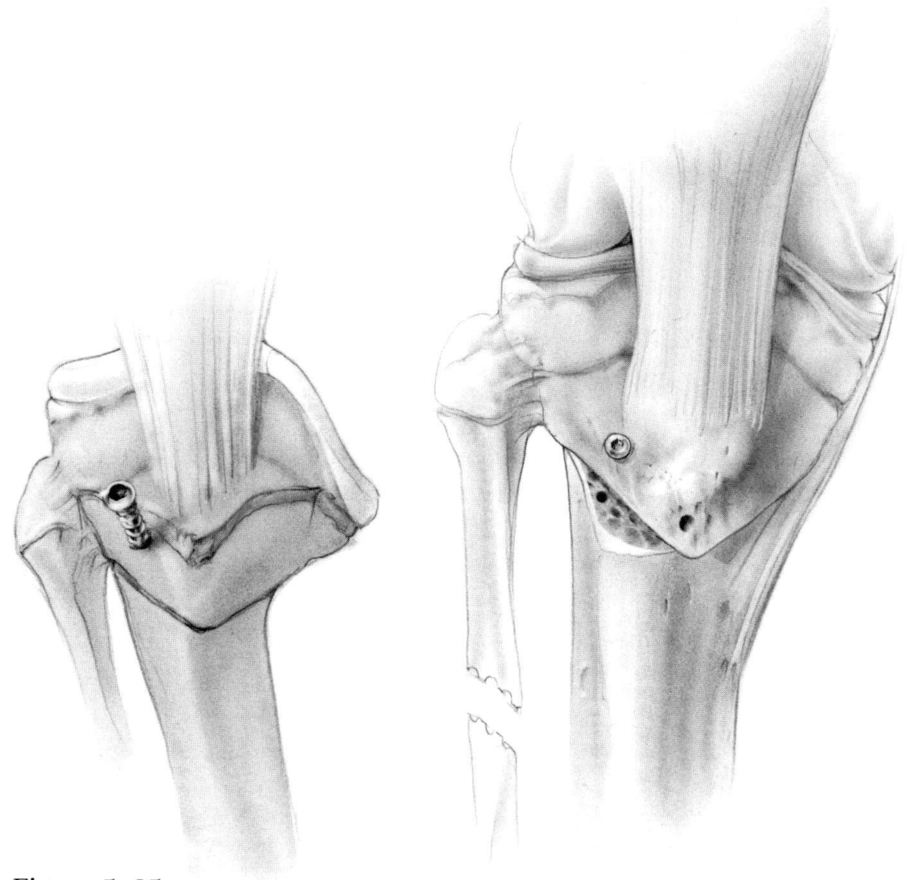

Figure 5–25

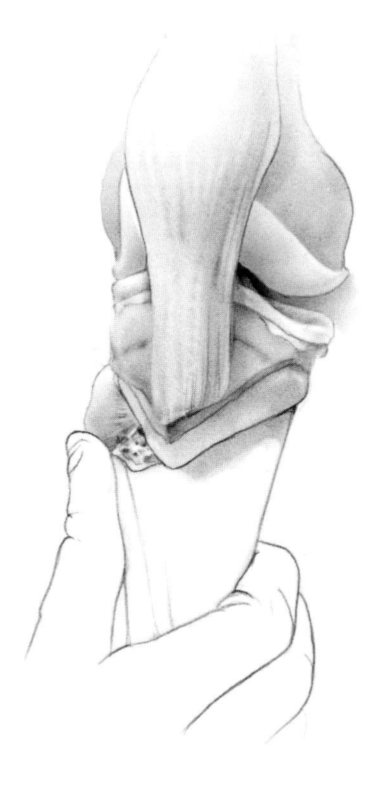

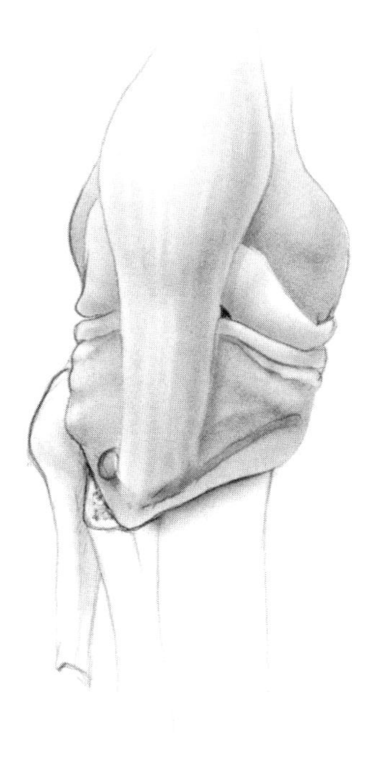

Figure 5–26

Figure 5–27. Anteroposterior radiographs of a 2.5-year-old child with bilateral Blount's disease (***Figure 5–27A***). Image obtained at the time of surgery showing the guide pin in place in the left leg (***Figure 5–27B***). Although this is in the physeal plate, the osteotomy cut was made beneath the pin. Anteroposterior (***Figure 5–27C***) and lateral views of the left leg (***Figure 5–27D***) 3 months following surgery show the correction that was obtained.

POSTOPERATIVE CARE

The drain is removed the day following surgery. The patient is usually ready for discharge within 1 to 2 days following the surgery. Weight-bearing is not permitted. Healing is usually sufficient at 6 weeks to either remove the cast or place the patient in a long-leg walking cast. After cast removal physical therapy is begun to rehabilitate the knee and progression to full weight-bearing is made as rapidly as possible.

REFERENCES

1. Rab GT. Oblique tibial osteotomy for Blount's disease (tibia vara). J Pediatr Orthop 1988;8:715.
2. MacEwen GD, Shands AR Jr. Oblique trochanteric osteotomy. J Bone Joint Surg 1967;49A:345.

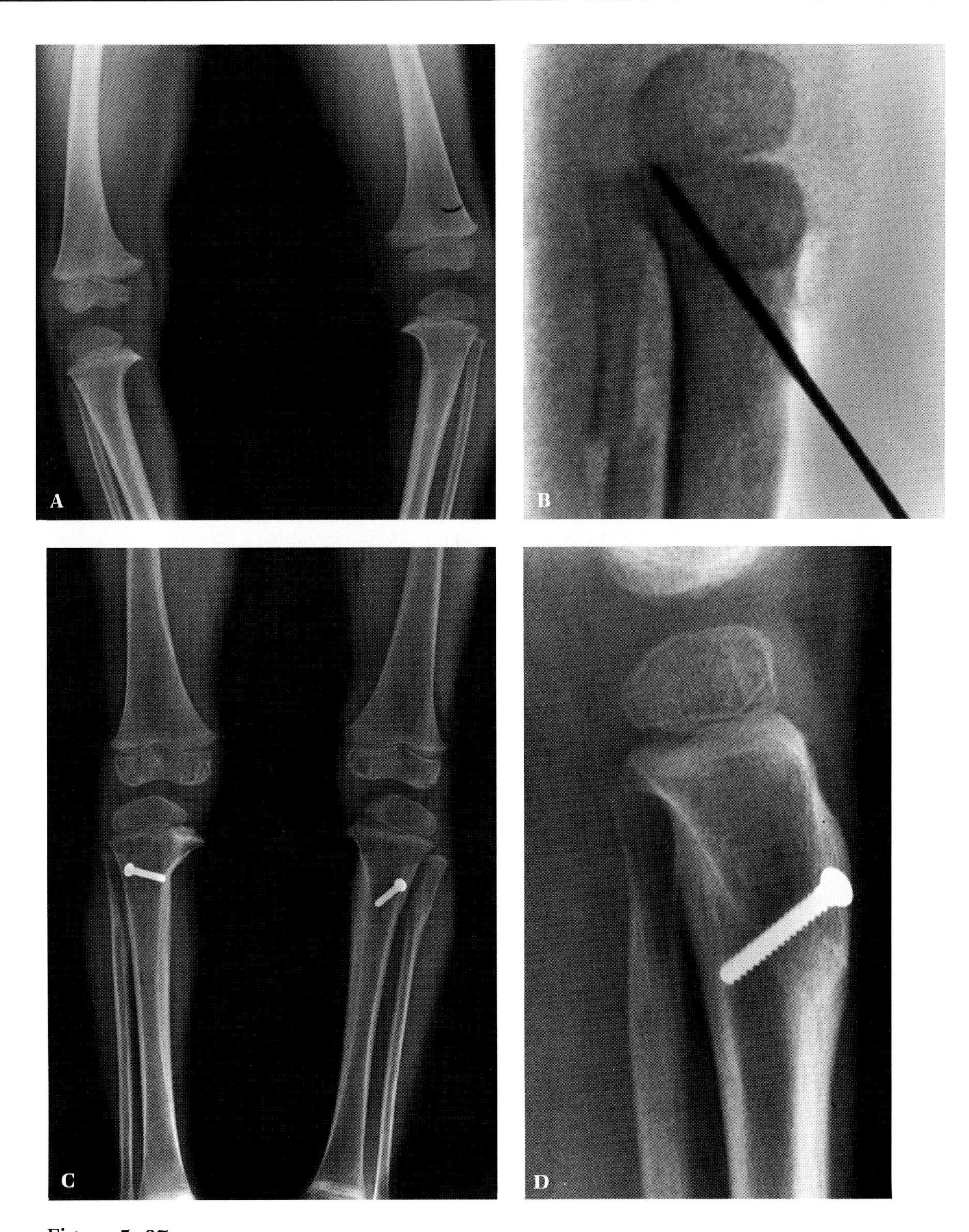

Figure 5–27

5.5
Distal Tibial Osteotomy, Wiltse's Technique

Osteotomy of the distal tibia is an operation that is used more frequently in children than adults. Its need commonly arises from growth disturbances following epiphyseal fracture or from congenital problems of the leg (*eg*, "ball and socket" ankle joint).

Figure 5–28. Wiltse has pointed out that if a simple closing wedge osteotomy is performed for a valgus deformity, malalignment with displacement of the ankle joint and a noticeable prominence of the medial malleolus will result; he has described an osteotomy that avoids this problem.[1] Although this problem can be true of any osteotomy, it is most obvious in the ankle and to a lesser extent in the distal humerus.

Figure 5–29. The calculation of the angles of the osteotomy need not be precise because considerable adjustment is possible in realigning the distal fragment. An approximation of the correct angles of the wedge will create a better fit, improved stability, and more rapid healing, however. The angle of the osteotomy at a^1 should equal the amount of angular deformity of the joint surface, a^2. In addition, the greater the deformity, the further the apex of the osteotomy should be displaced laterally.

Figure 5–30. The approach for this osteotomy is similar to that for an arthrodesis of the ankle but with greater proximal extension. The incision is placed anteriorly between the extensor digitorum longus laterally and the extensor hallucis longus medially where they come together just above the ankle joint. It should extend to the level of the ankle joint and far enough proximally to permit sufficient retraction to expose the entire anterior tibia (***Figure 5–30A***). The superficial peroneal nerve will have emerged from beneath the deep fascia and retinaculum, and care should be taken not to injure it. When the fascia and retinaculum are split, the two tendons are identified and separated (***Figure 5–30B***). The neurovascular bundle will lie lateral to the exposure in the proximal part of the wound. However, it comes to lie anteriorly between the two tendons at the level of the ankle joint. Therefore, care should be taken to retract it medially with the tendon of the extensor hallucis longus. The periosteum is now divided and the entire circumference of the tibia exposed subperiosteally.

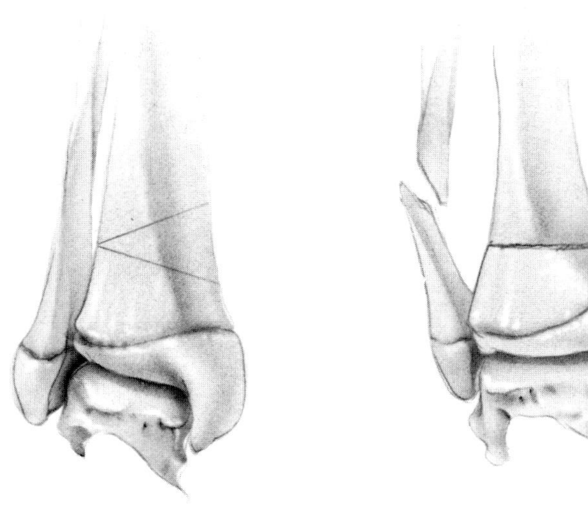

Figure 5–28

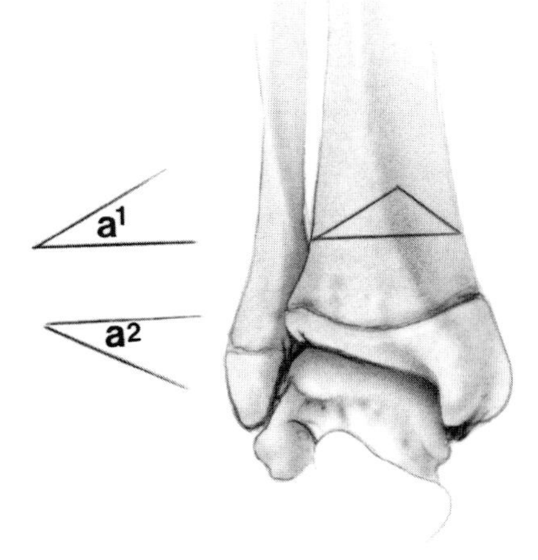

Figure 5–29

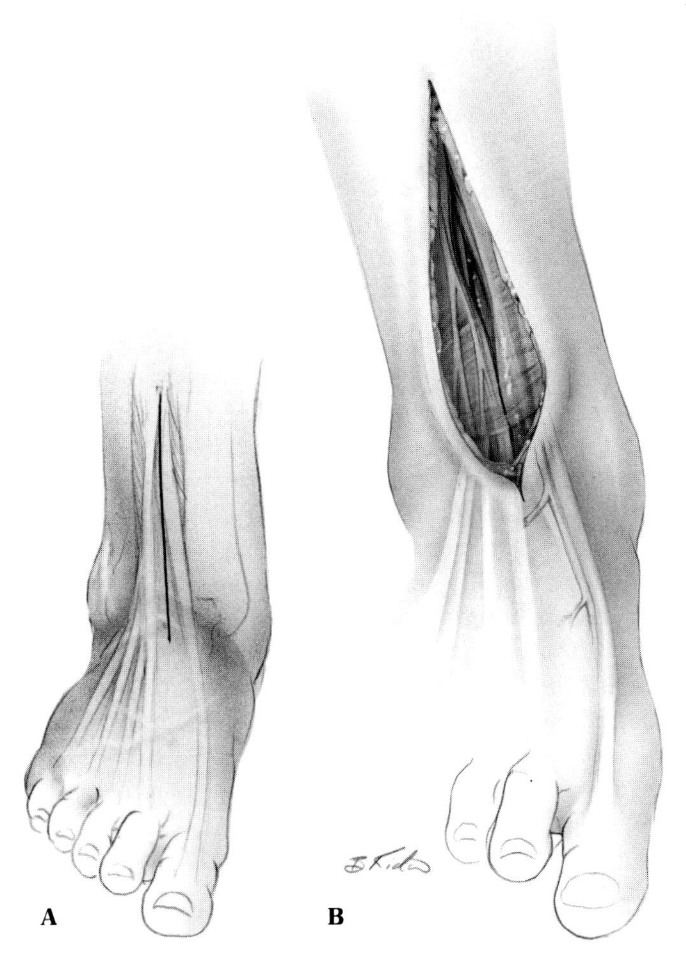

Figure 5–30

Figure 5–31. The fibula is exposed through a small lateral incision and divided obliquely with a power saw.

Figure 5–32. With retractors protecting the tissues, the transverse osteotomy cut is made first with a power saw. The appropriate triangle of bone is then more easily removed, again using a power saw with a smaller blade.

Figure 5–33. The distal fragment is rotated and displaced so that its medial side comes to lie against the medial face of the triangular cut. It is important to verify that the desired correction has been obtained. This can usually be done clinically but is best confirmed with a radiograph that shows the tibial shaft as well as the ankle joint. If further adjustment is necessary either for more correction or better coaption of the fragments, this can be achieved by removing bone with a rongeur. Stabilization of the osteotomy is achieved with a single Steinmann pin drilled from either medial or lateral as seems best. It should engage the opposite cortex.

The wound is closed over a drain, and a short leg cast is applied.

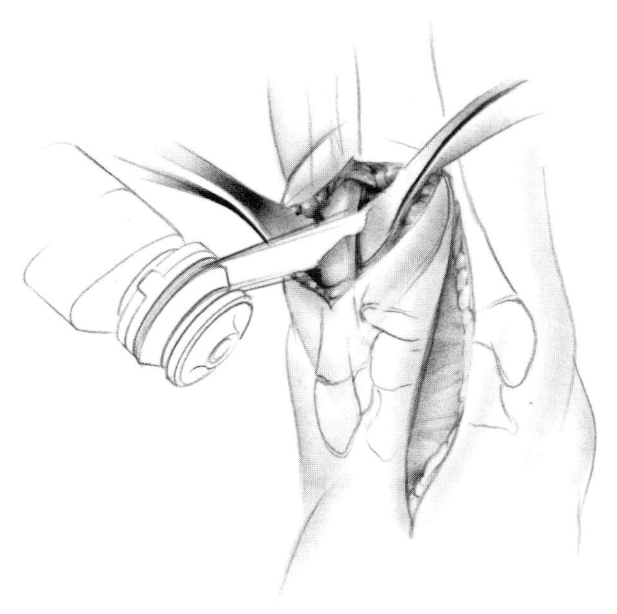

Figure 5–31

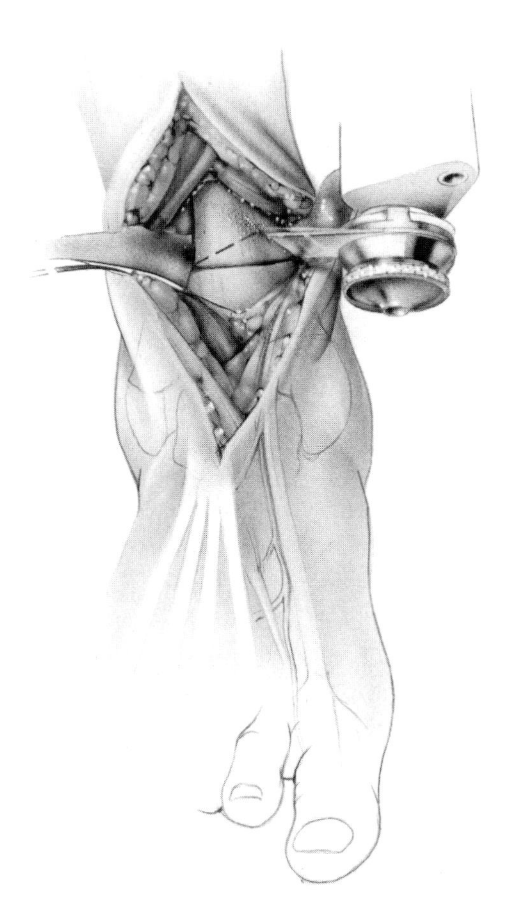

Figure 5–32

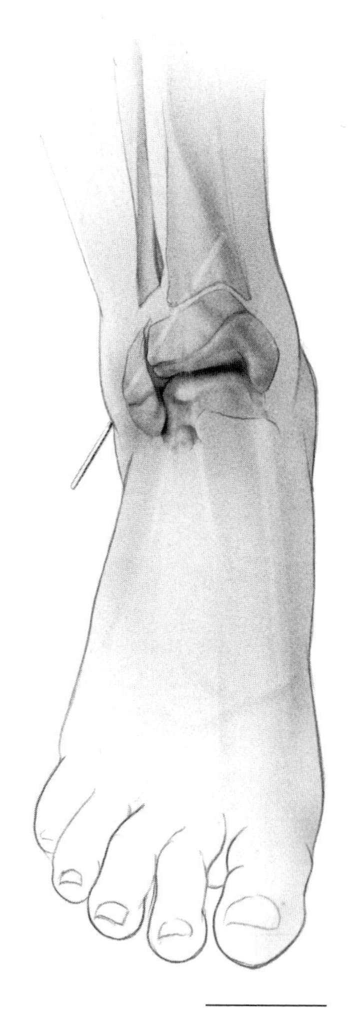

Figure 5–33

Figure 5–34. EW is a 12.5-year-old boy who sustained a severe fracture of the distal tibia and fibula (***Figure 5–34A***). This resulted in a growth arrest of the distal fibula and the lateral side of the distal tibial physis. A bony union also developed between the tibia and fibula (***Figure 5–34B***). The patient underwent a distal tibial and fibular osteotomy as described by Wiltse. In addition, to solve the growth problem, the remainder of the physis of the affected tibia was destroyed, and a distal tibial and fibular arrest was performed on the opposite leg (***Figure 5–34C***).

POSTOPERATIVE CARE

The drain can usually be removed the day following surgery and the patient started on a three-point non–weight-bearing crutch gait. Healing is usually complete in 6 weeks, at which time the cast and pin are removed in the office and the patient is instructed to progress to full weight-bearing.

REFERENCE

1. Wiltse LL. Valgus deformity of the ankle: a sequel to acquired or congenital abnormalities of the fibula. J Bone Joint Surg 1972;54A:595.

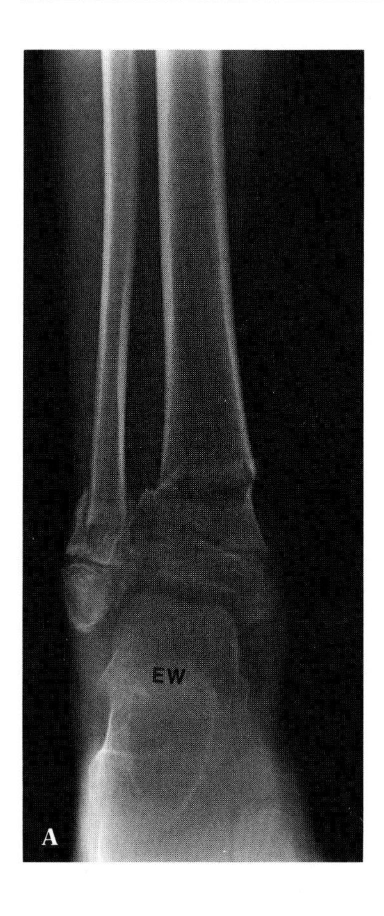

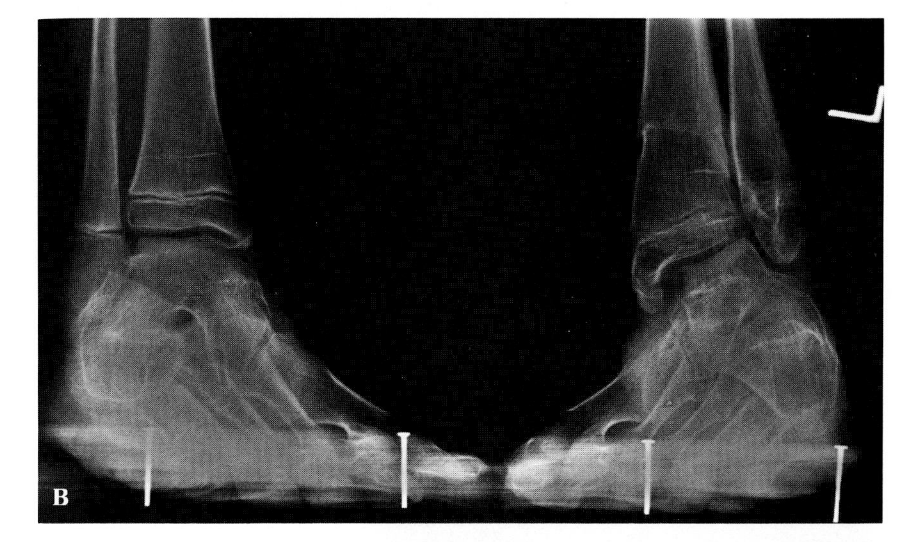

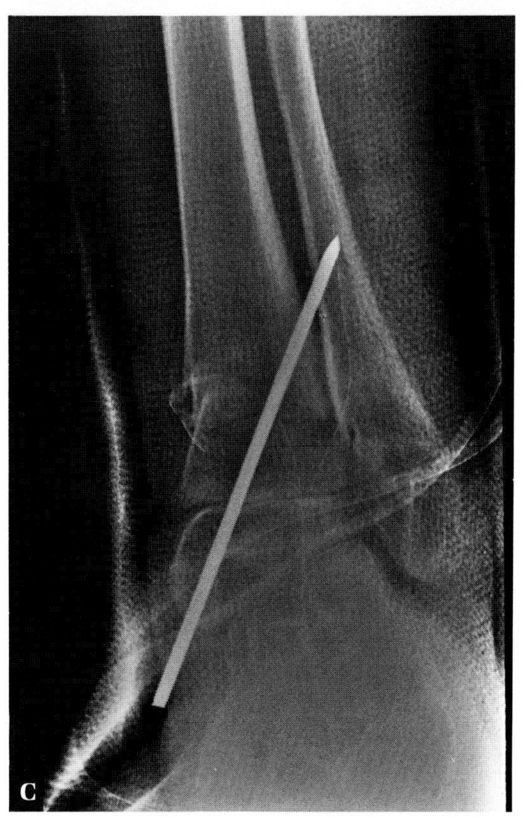

Figure 5–34

5.6
Orthofix Technique of Tibial Lengthening

The advantages and disadvantages of the Orthofix device as compared with other lengthening devices for tibial lengthening are the same as for lengthening of the femur. The basic technique of inserting the screws has been described in the description of femoral lengthening and will not be repeated here. The description of the femoral lengthening showed the use of the dynamic axial fixator, whereas the use of the lengthener will be shown here. The main difference is that the lengthener is more rigid and will not permit correction of rotational or angular deformity.

Figure 5–35. The patient is placed supine on a translucent operating table with a bolster under the hip and a large roll under the knee to aid in positioning the leg. The leg is draped free. The image intensifier is set up on the side of the operated leg. The operation begins by dividing the fibula while seated on the side of the operated leg. The surgeon then moves to the opposite side of the table to insert the screws into the tibia while the image intensifier is positioned on the side of the operated leg. This allows the image intensifier to remain in place to monitor the placement and depth of the screws without disturbing the surgeon. After the pins are inserted and the template is removed, the surgeon may move back to the opposite side of the table to perform the tibial osteotomy because the image intensifier will no longer be required.

Figure 5–36. With the patient positioned as described, the surgeon begins by dividing the fibula. It is necessary to remove a piece of the fibula to delay union. Lengthening will be delayed to allow early callus formation, and if the fibula is merely divided, it is possible that premature union of the fibula will occur before tibial lengthening is completed.

An incision is made over the subcutaneous border of the distal fibula, and a small section of the bone above the syndesmosis is exposed subperiosteally. To stabilize the tibial-fibular syndesmosis, the fibula is fixed to the tibia with a cortical screw. A 3.2-cm drill is used to make a hole that passes through the fibula into the tibia, engaging both the lateral and then the medial fibular and tibial cortex. It must be remembered that the tibia will lie anteriorly to the fibula; therefore, the drill must be aimed in an anterior direction as it is passed from the tibia to the fibula. The holes in the fibula and the tibia are both tapped, and an appropriate-length cortical screw is inserted. This screw should be fully threaded as the object is to hold the fibula in its normal relationship to the tibia. If this screw is lagged or overtightened, it will tilt the distal fibular fragment.

Figure 5–37. The entire circumference of the fibula is exposed subperiosteally 1 cm above the screw. The soft tissues are protected by two small retractors, and a 1-cm section of the fibula is removed with a power saw. The periosteum is approximated to lessen the bleeding, and the wound is closed. A drain can be placed in the subcutaneous space if the surgeon wishes.

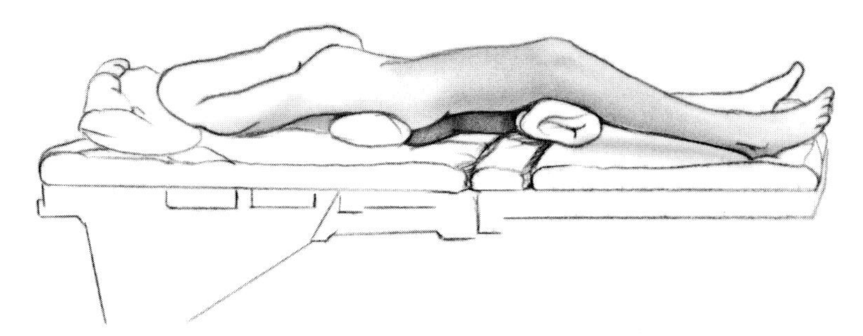

Figure 5–35

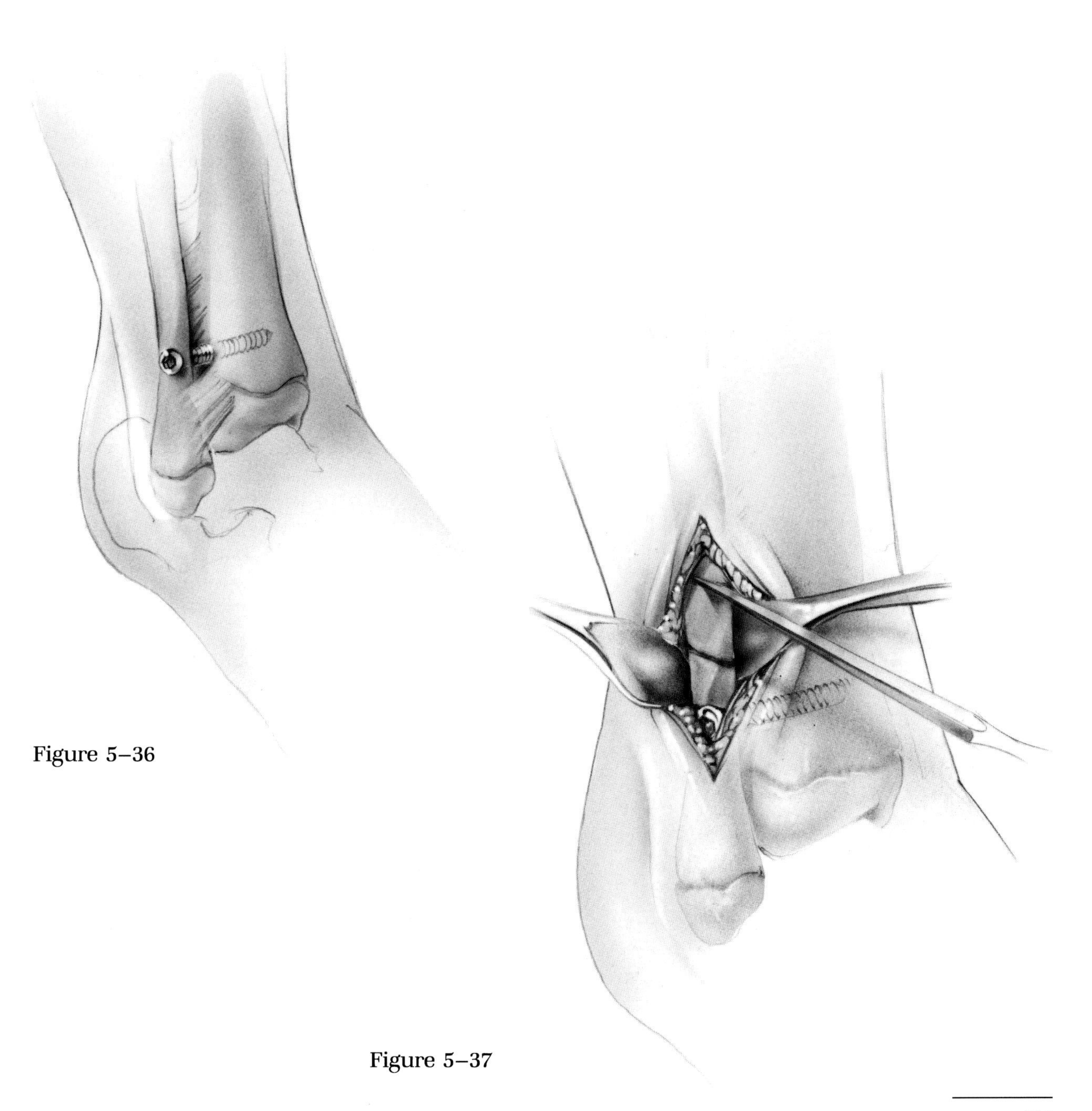

Figure 5–36

Figure 5–37

Figure 5–38. There are two different lengtheners: one that will lengthen 5 cm and one that will lengthen 10 cm. If the 5-cm lengthener is used, the template is fully collapsed; if the 10-cm lengthener is used, the template is fully extended. The case illustrated here is of a smaller child in which the smaller lengthener is used, and thus the template is fully collapsed. Only two screws proximal and two screws distal will be used. In larger children approaching adolescence, it is desirable to use three screws proximal and three screws distal for better fixation and stability.

The template is aligned with the axis of the tibia along its medial face. The proximal screw should be placed about 1 cm distal to the physeal plate of the proximal tibia. The image intensifier is used to identify this location. The most proximal screw is placed first, and the most distal screw is placed second (***Figure 5–38A***). This is different than with fracture fixation because the tibia remains whole, and there is no adjustment for screws placed in different axes with the lengthener. The placement of these two screws is critical because it will determine the position of the lengthener and all of the other screws. No adjustment will be possible.

The remaining screws are now placed as described for the technique of femoral lengthening. The placement of the screws is much easier in the tibia because the bone is subcutaneous. The incision for the screws can be made through the skin and the periosteum with one cut. After all of the screws are placed, the template is removed (***Figure 5–38B***).

Figure 5–39. The osteotomy of the tibia is now performed. A small incision about 2 cm in length is made just lateral to the tibial crest. This incision should start at the level of the most distal of the proximal screws. Through this incision a small area of the tibia 1 cm below the most distal of the proximal screws is exposed circumferentially. This task is aided by using the curved Crego periosteal elevators. Care should be taken not to damage the periosteum.

Multiple drill holes are now made in the tibia. The drill guide can be used to avoid overpenetration of the posterior cortex with damage to the soft tissues posterior to the tibia (***Figure 5–39A***). A small osteotome is used to complete the osteotomy as was described in the technique of Orthofix lengthening of the femur. Completion of the osteotomy can be verified by rotating the distal screws externally (to avoid stretching the peroneal nerve) while holding the proximal screws. The periosteum can be loosely approximated with interrupted absorbable sutures. If desired, a fasciotomy of the proximal part of the anterior compartment can be performed by sliding a scissors distal and proximal to cut the fascia (***Figure 5–39B***). A drain may be used. The wound is closed.

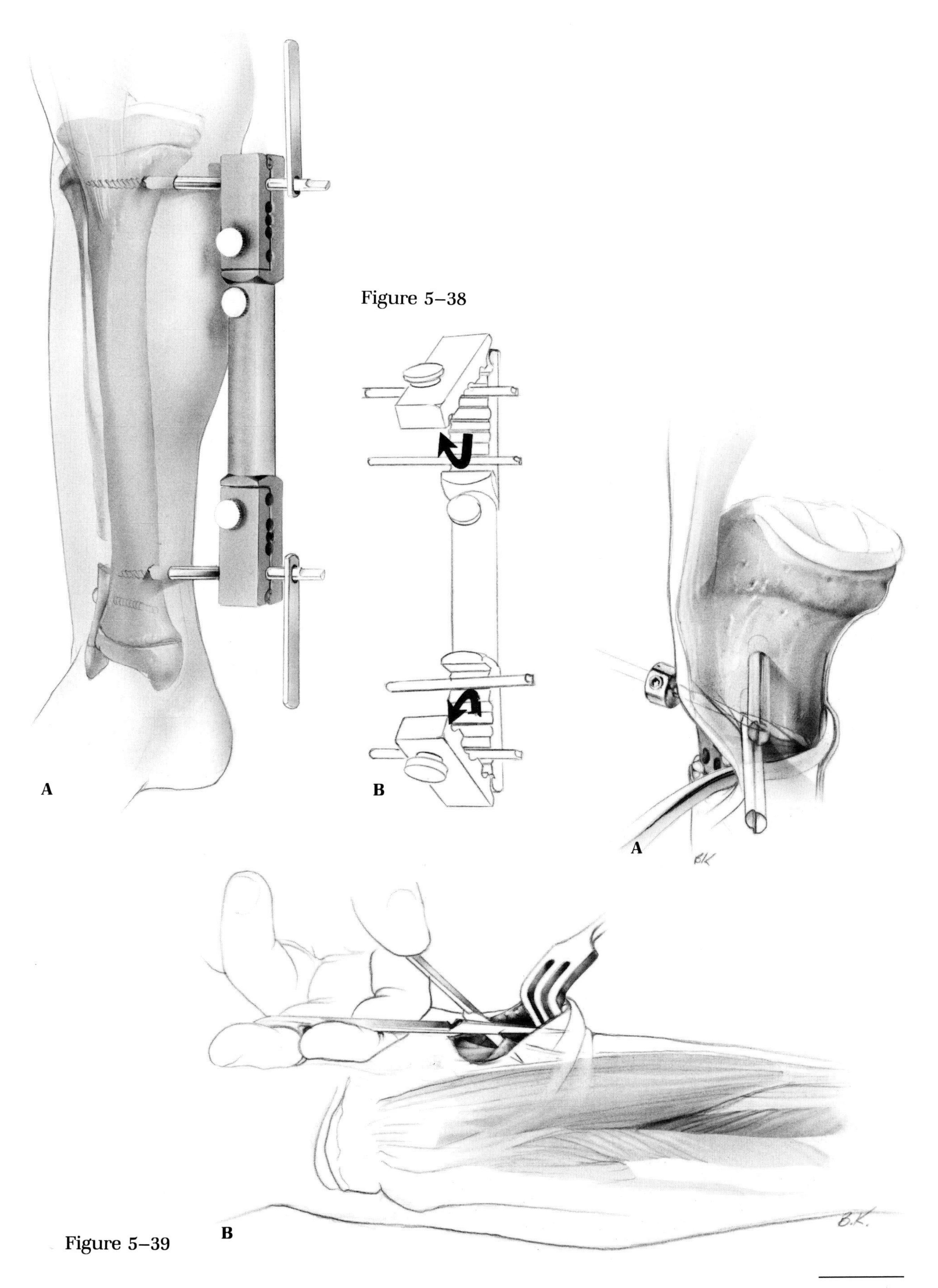

Figure 5–38

Figure 5–39

Figure 5–40. The lengthener is secured to the screws with the holes for the distraction-compression bar facing upward and the body-locking nut facing outward. The distraction-compression bar is attached to the device with the adjusting nut facing toward the patient's head. This is then fully compressed to achieve maximum stability at the osteotomy site. The body-locking nut is tightened. Now the distraction-compression bar is lengthened until it becomes tight. This ensures that when lengthening begins, there will be no slack, and the first turns will distract the bone.

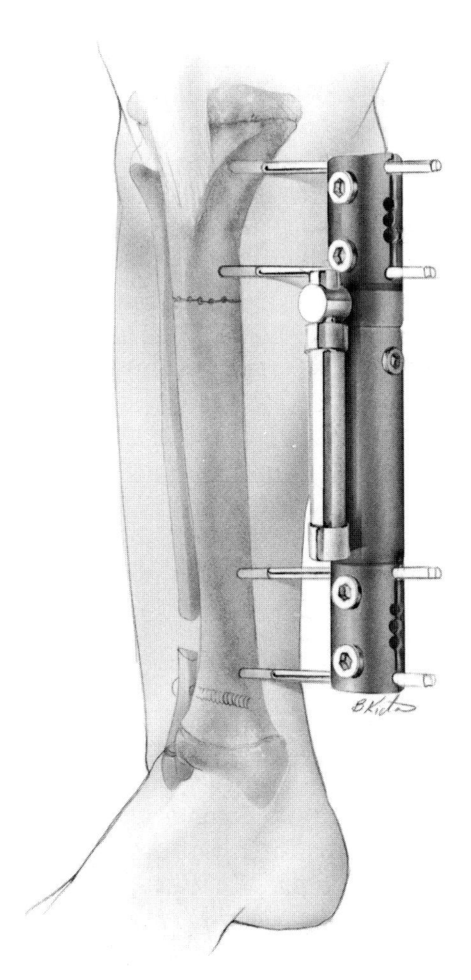

Figure 5–40

Figure 5–41. Lateral radiograph of a 12.5-year-old boy who was born with posterior medial bowing of the tibia (***Figure 5–39A***). He currently has a leg length discrepancy of 4.5 cm projected to be 6 cm at the completion of growth. At 1 week after application of the fixator and osteotomy of the tibia and the fibula, the lengthening was begun (***Figure 5–41B***). Although the osteotomy was done in the diaphyseal region, which is not recommended, the subsequent course demonstrates the remarkable healing of the distracted callus. At 3 weeks (***Figure 5–41C***), the callus formation in the osteotomy gap is not readily apparent on this radiograph. Notice that slight translation of the fragments has occurred. This persisted throughout the lengthening, but it was not considered sufficient to require correction. By 4 months adequate callus fills the gap (***Figure 5–41D***). At 5 months after osteotomy (***Figure 5–41E***), healing is sufficient to remove the fixator. (Courtesy of Charles T. Price, MD.)

POSTOPERATIVE CARE

The day following surgery range of motion exercises for the knee and the ankle are started. The patient can be ambulated as soon as comfortable, usually on the first postoperative day if only the tibia is lengthened. Full weight-bearing can be permitted at this time. Continuous caudal analgesia speeds the postoperative progress and greatly improves the child's attitude toward the operation.

Distraction begins when there is evidence of some callus formation. This will vary between 1 and 2 weeks, depending on the age of the child and the circumstances. Distraction is done by the patient while at home and is monitored as appropriate. At first this may be every week but may be every 3 to 4 weeks later, depending on the family and how well the lengthening is going.

Lengthening is done at a rate of 1 mm per day in four increments. Thus, the patient will turn the distraction bar one quarter turn four times per day. It is important for the surgeon to realize that 1 mm per day is the usual and should serve as a guide. In many children this will be too slow, and premature consolidation may result; in others, a break in the callus may be observed, indicating that the rate of distraction will need to be slowed or even halted for a while.

In tibial lengthening the ankle rather than the knee is the joint that causes the most problems. There are no firm guidelines regarding how much motion must be maintained during lengthening. The author has accepted up to 30 degrees of fixed equinus in adolescents without subsequent problems or the need for corrective surgery. It would seem that if the ankle is anatomically normal it will recover normal function. In those patients with a short fibula, (*ie,* "ball and socket" ankle joint etc), however, the surgeon should probably exercise greater caution.

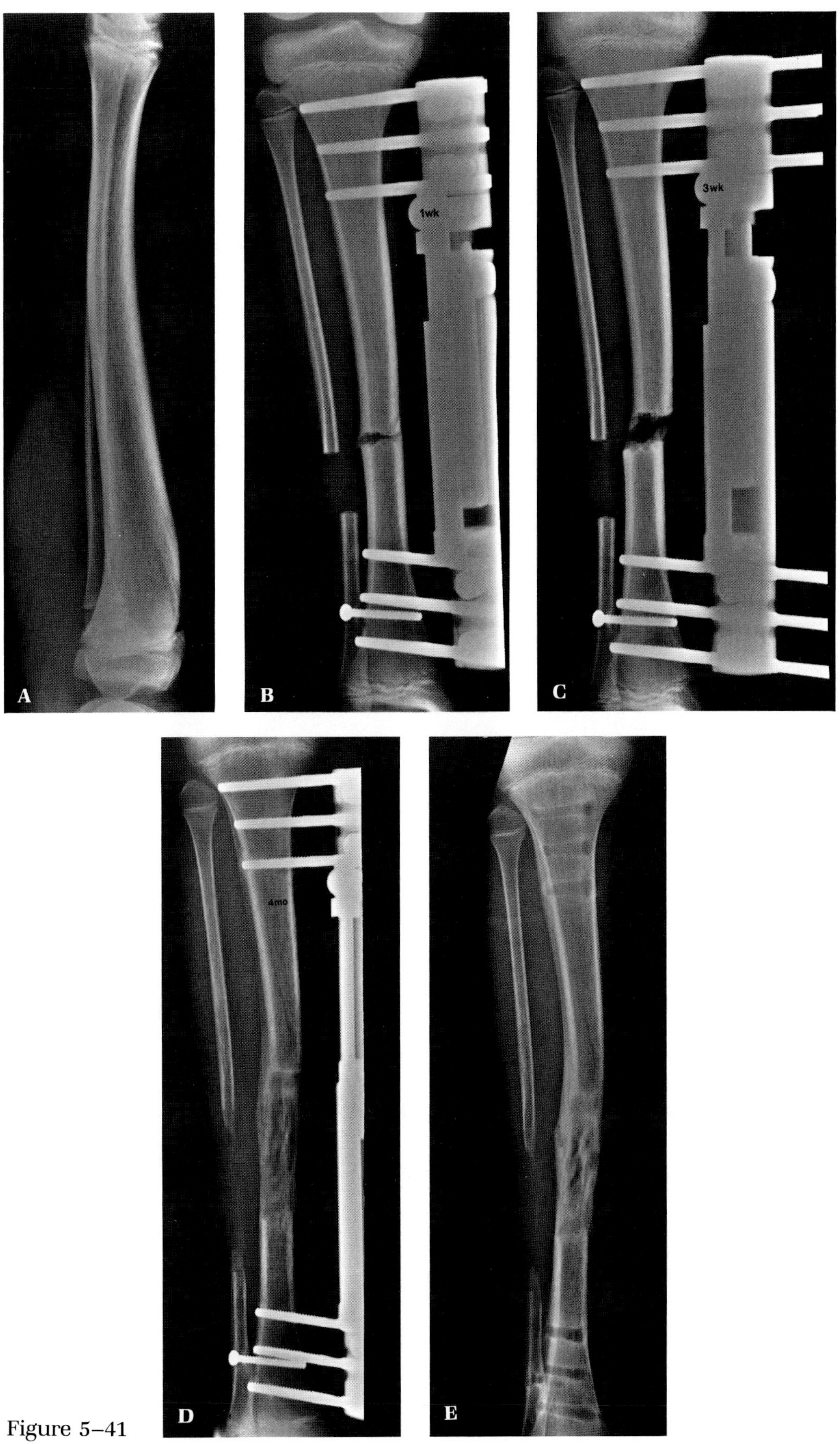

Figure 5–41

Once the desired length has been obtained, the body-locking nut is tightened while awaiting consolidation of the gap. Although in the past it was necessary to await formation of a cortex to loosen the body-locking nut and permit compression of the callus, it is now possible to apply the dynamic-locking collar to prevent shortening while allowing compression of the callus (see discussion on orthofix technique of femoral lengthening).

When there is radiographic evidence suggesting sufficient healing to remove the device, the author prefers to remove the dynamic-locking collar, leave the body-locking nut loose, and permit full unprotected weight-bearing for 2 weeks. If the patient experiences no discomfort and there is no break in the callus on the radiographs, the body of the lengthener is removed while the screws are left in place. The limb is stressed and if there is no discomfort or apprehension, the patient is allowed protected weight-bearing for 24 to 48 hours. If all remains well, the screws are removed, and the patient is progressed to full weight-bearing at the surgeon's discretion.

5.7
Ilizarov Technique of Tibial Lengthening

The Ilizarov method and apparatus for limb lengthening have been widely used by Professor Ilizarov in Russia for 40 years and has been used by some surgeons in Italy for more than 10 years. Experience in the United States, although brief, is more widespread. For this reason, at the time of this writing, there is no large published series of limb lengthening with the Ilizarov technique from a North American center.

The Ilizarov device differs from the Wagner and Orthofix devices in that it consists of rings rather than a unilateral frame, and is connected to the bone by small smooth wires (1.5 and 1.8 mm) that are joined to the rings under tension as opposed to heavier threaded pins that engage both cortices but do not pass through the limb. In mechanical testing the Ilizarov device is the least rigid, allowing more axial motion and shear at the osteotomy gap than the other devices.[1] This is thought by its proponents to promote better bone formation by avoidance of stress shielding.

It is apparent that this lack of rigidity does not sacrifice anything in terms of control of bone fragments. In fact, because of the multiple planes of fixation in both the horizontal and vertical axes, the ability to control the fragments may be better than other fixators. The wide latitude permitted the surgeon in the construction of the frame also allows for correction of angular and rotational deformities to a greater extent than is possible with any other device.

The trade-off for these advantages is a significant learning curve. The insertion of multiple transfixing wires through the limb and the fact that these wires will be pulled through the soft tissues during the lengthening requires a good knowledge of the cross-sectional anatomy. The correction of rotational and angular deformities requires a level of preoperative planning not required by most other surgical procedures. Finally, it is apparent that the apparatus does not eliminate the myriad problems that are encountered in any attempt to lengthen a limb.[2]

The wide and varied application of the Ilizarov device to clinical problems makes it impossible within the scope of this atlas to do more than illustrate a typical case to acquaint the surgeon with its use and general principles.

Figure 5–42. There are two sizes of wire used depending on the size of the patient. In general the 1.8-mm wires will be used in the lower extremity. Wires are also available with an "olive" on the wire. These are used to resist anticipated lateral forces on the bone during the lengthening.

The wires are attached to the rings in a variety of ways. To avoid pressure on the skin and bone, it is important that the wires not be bent to reach the ring but rather adjustments must be made in the way they are attached to the ring so that they are left completely straight. There are different connectors that permit this adjustment in either the horizontal or vertical plane. If the wire passes directly over the hole, a cannulated bolt is used (***Figure 5–42A***). If the wire is passed to the side of the hole, a slotted bolt is used (***Figure 5–42B***). If the wire is above or below the ring, the appropriate bolt is raised above or below the ring with washers (***Figure 5–42C***) or a post can be used (***Figure 5–42D***). This latter technique is most often used to place a single wire through the bone in a plane different from the ring and is called a "dropped wire." It is used in small children in place of a second ring.

Figure 5–43. The wire is first tightened on one side. In doing this the bolt holding the wire should be held with a wrench to prevent it from rotating and bending the wire (***Figure 5–43A***). If this is not done, the bolt will twist the wire and cause it to deviate from its proper position (***Figure 5–43B***).

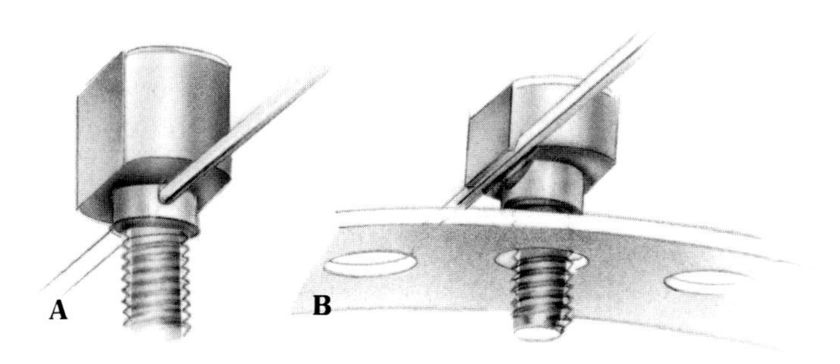

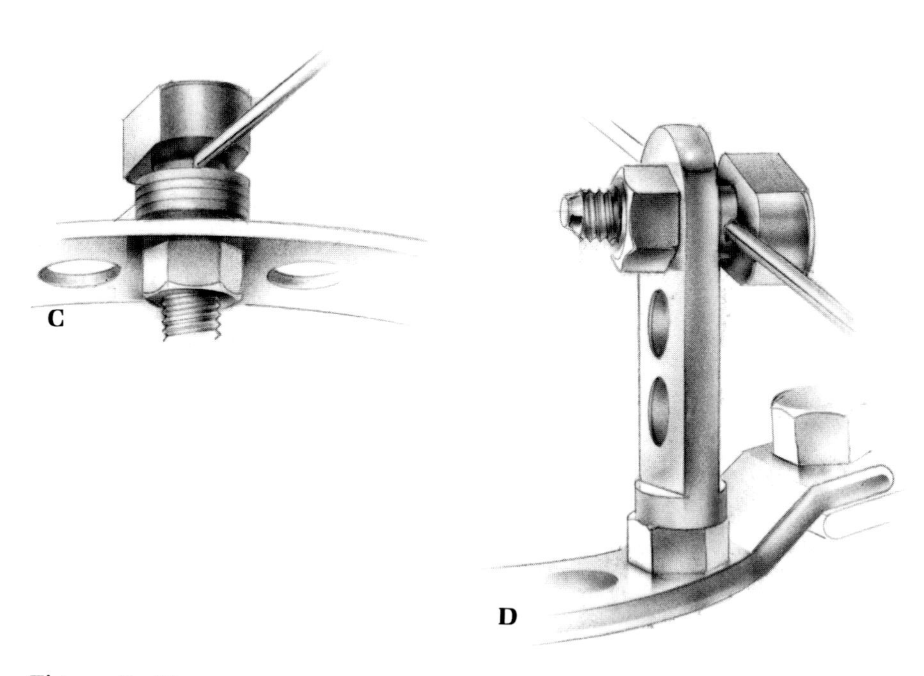

Figure 5–42

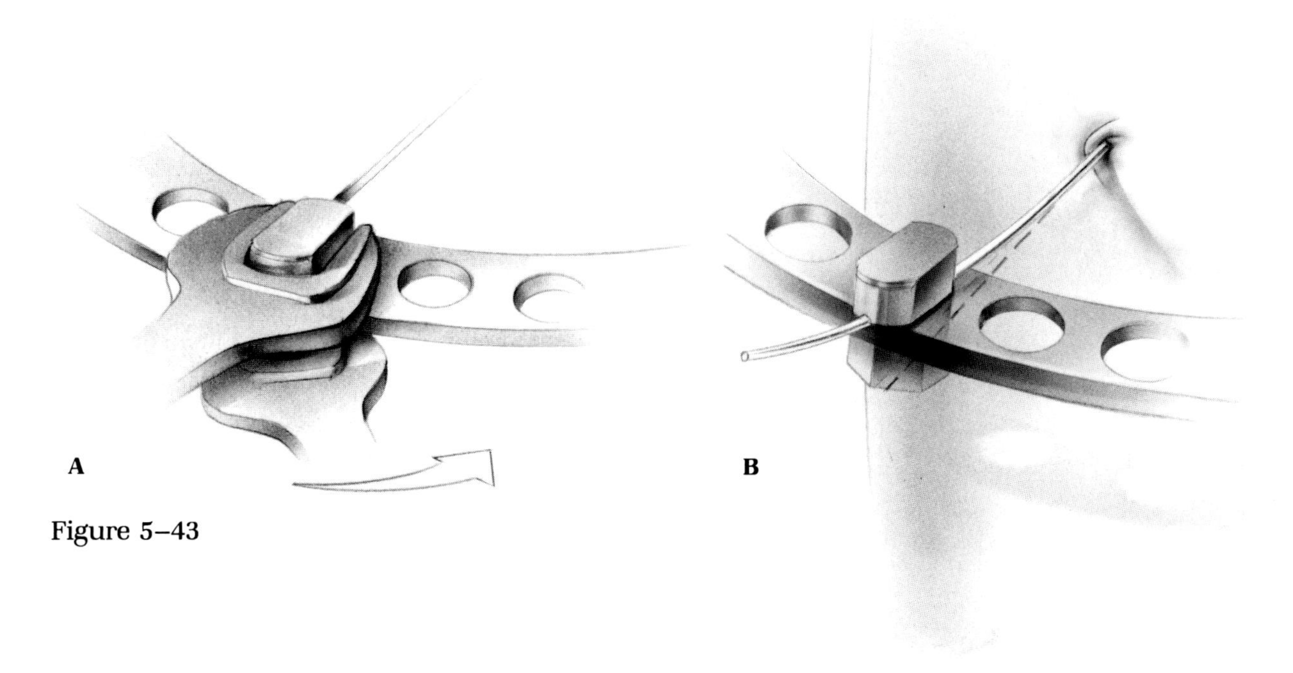

Figure 5–43

Figure 5–44. The wires are tensioned with a tensioning device to approximately 100 to 130 kg of force by observing the markings on the device and are then held by tightening the remaining nut. After each wire is tightened, it should be cut allowing a sufficient length of wire to remain in case there is need to retension the wire. The remaining wire is bent over the ring.

Figure 5–45. As much as possible of the apparatus should be assembled before surgery. In the tibia the entire apparatus can usually be assembled. The most proximal and distal rings should lie just distal and proximal to the physeal plates, respectively.

The rings are connected from half rings that are bolted together. The connections are offset to maintain both halves of the ring in the same plane. The diameter of the completed rings should allow about two finger breadths between the ring and the skin. Five-eighth rings are also available and can be used around the knee to permit more flexion.

Each segment of bone will be fixed to two rings that are rigidly linked by connectors. Initially only two connectors are used to connect these rings to avoid interference with wire placement. After all of the wires are placed, however, additional connectors are added to provide rigidity. The rings that will be closest to the osteotomy should be close together to allow the osteotomy to be done in the metaphysis. In the other segment removed from the osteotomy, the second ring can be further from the first ring for enhanced stability. In joining two rings together it is best to position the rings first with their joints exactly anterior and posterior. The two connectors are then placed on the medial side of these joints, leaving more of the lateral side of the ring free for attachment points for the wires.

These ring assemblies, one proximal and one distal, are now connected with two threaded rods or lengtheners of the correct length. These connectors are placed just lateral to the point where two half rings join to form a complete ring. These connectors will be removed to complete the osteotomy, and the rings will then be joined by four connectors.

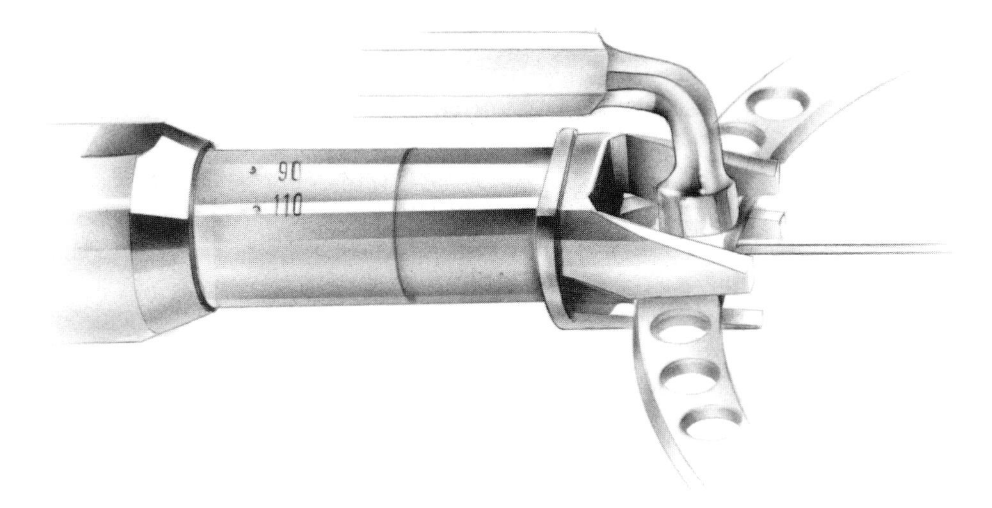

Figure 5–44

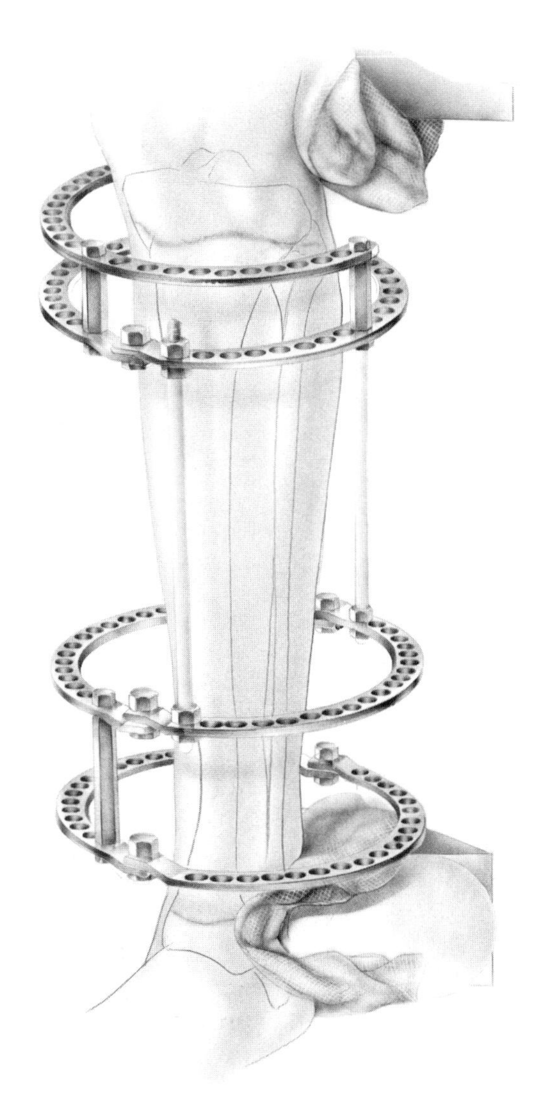

Figure 5–45

Figure 5–46. If it is anticipated that anterior and valgus angulation will occur, the proximal and distal rings will not be assembled parallel to each other. Rather the proximal set of rings will be fixed to the tibia with about 5 degrees of posterior angulation (***Figure 5–46A***). This degree of adjustability in the initial frame is achieved by placing a conical washer on the rods, connecting the two sets of rings with the convex side facing the ring (***Figure 5–46B***). This will allow 7 degrees of motion in either direction. After the osteotomy is completed, the proximal and distal sets of rings will be joined together parallel, thus creating about 5 degrees of recurvatum that will straighten during lengthening. Varus can be built in by directing the fixation wires at a slight angle to the epiphysis (***Figure 5–46C***). Again, when the rings are finally joined parallel to each other, a small amount of varus will be built in that will correct during lengthening. Many surgeons do not think that this step is necessary in most tibial lengthenings, and the subsequent description will not include this feature.

Figure 5–47. The patient is placed supine on the operating table with the limb draped free. A tourniquet is usually not necessary but can be used. The surgery is greatly facilitated by having the limb supported free. The preconstructed frame is placed on the leg.

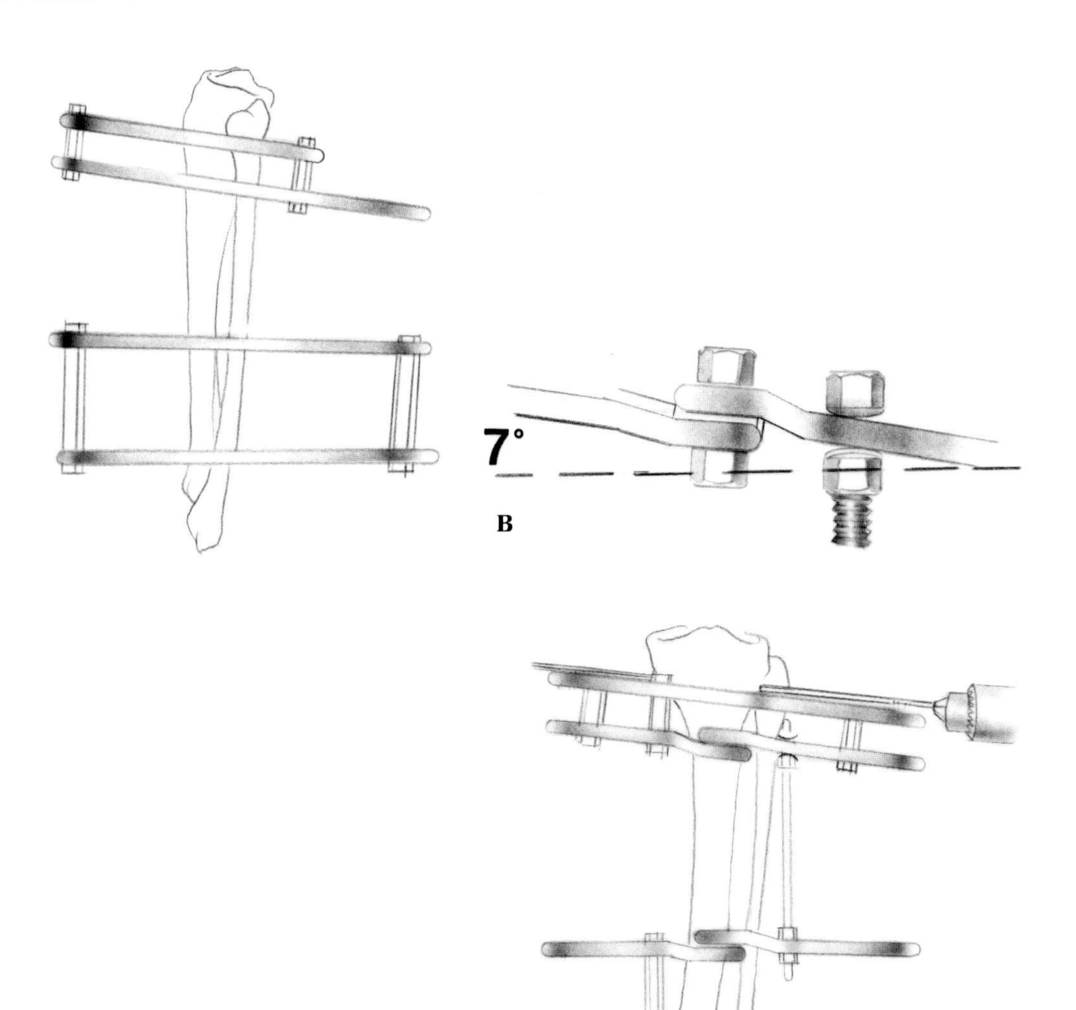

Figure 5–46

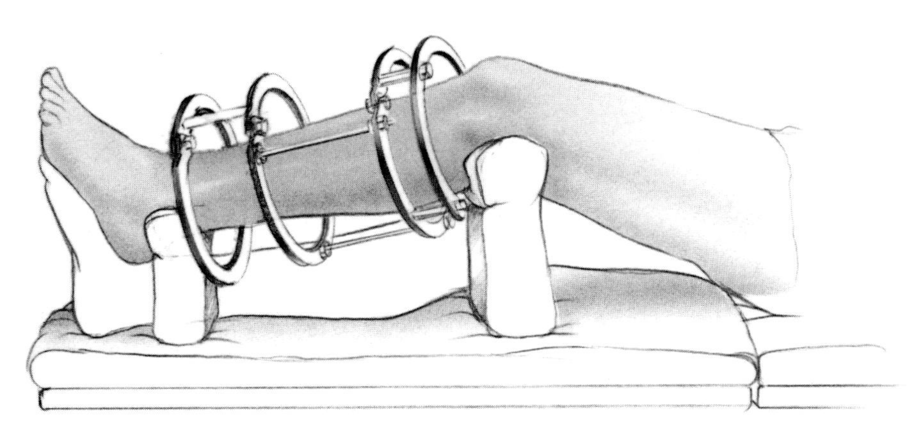

Figure 5–47

Figure 5–48. The first wires placed will both be transverse. They will attach to the most proximal and most distal ring. They should be placed as close to the epiphyseal plate as possible.

First the most proximal transverse wire is placed lateral to medial *(a)*. This wire should be an olive wire. This wire is parallel to the knee joint or proximal physis. Next, the most distal wire is placed just proximal to the distal physis in the same transverse plane *(b)*. This should be an olive wire passing from lateral to medial. It is now possible to secure the frame to the leg by these two wires. Care should be taken to allow sufficient room, about two finger breadths, for the soft tissues. The connecting bar should lie directly over the anterior surface of the tibia, and it should be parallel to the anterior border of the tibia.

The next two wires will be the fibular wires. These will not be olive wires. They will be passed lateral to medial. Proximally, the wire should pass through the fibular head where the peroneal nerve is known to be posterior *(c)*. It should aim anterior and medial almost perpendicular to the medial face of the tibia. Distally, the fibular wire will attach to the more proximal of the two rings so as to avoid pinning the syndesmosis. The direction of this wire will be the same as the proximal fibular wire *(d)*.

The next wires will be parallel to the medial face of the tibia, and will attach to the most proximal and most distal rings. These will be smooth wires passed lateral to medial *(e, f)*.

The final wires will be two transverse olive wires attaching to the more central rings proximal and distal. They will pass medial to lateral *(g, h)*.

After all of the wires, four proximal and four distal, are connected, the two threaded rods or lengtheners that were used to connect the proximal two rings with the distal two rings are removed in preparation for the osteotomy.

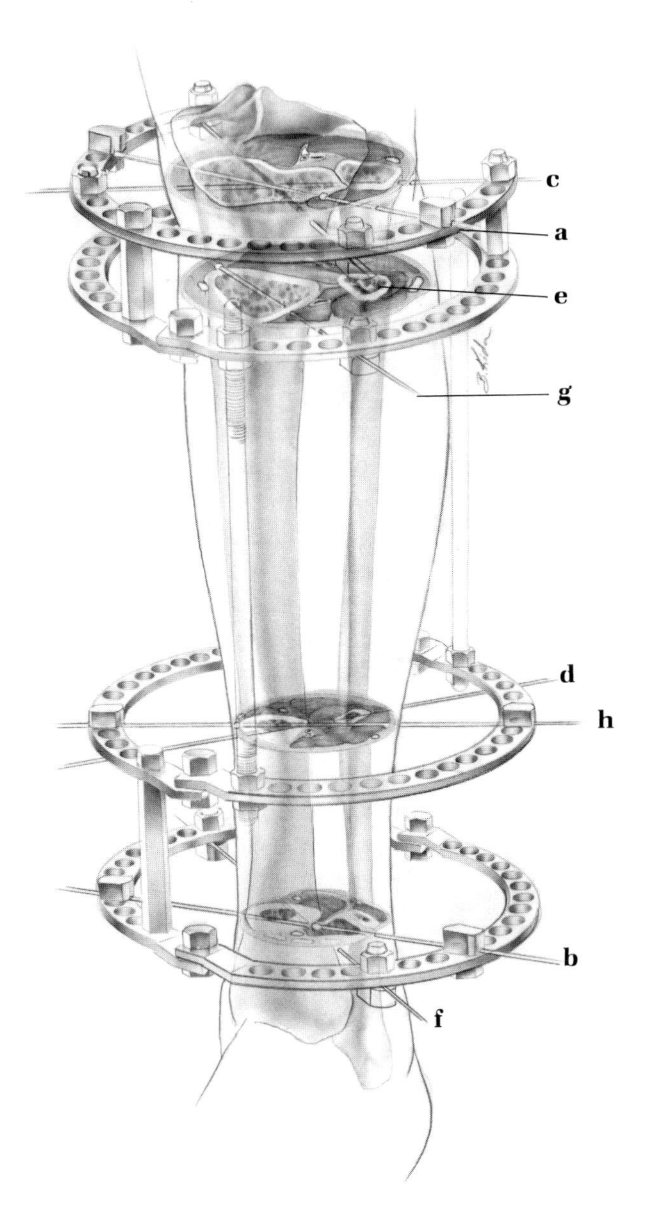

Figure 5–48

Figure 5–49. A principle that is emphasized in the Ilizarov technique is that only the cortical bone is cut, leaving the medullary space with its vessels intact (thus, the terms *compactotomy* or *corticotomy*). This osteotomy should be performed in the metaphysis about 1 cm distal to the wires. Unlike the femoral osteotomy that is performed at the distal end of the bone, the osteotomy of the tibia is done in the proximal tibia.

A small 1- to 2-cm incision is made just lateral to the crest of the tibia. The periosteum is incised vertically, and the medial and lateral surface of the tibia is exposed subperiosteally. Care should be taken to protect the periosteum during the subsequent maneuvers (***Figure 5–49A***).

Using the 1-cm osteotome, a cut is made in the anterior cortex only. The 0.5-cm osteotome is then used to first cut the lateral and then the medial cortex (***Figure 5–49B***). Because it is not possible to cut the posterior cortex without violating the medullary space, it is fractured by placing the osteotome in the posterior medial and posterolateral corners alternately, and twisting it to crack or fracture the posterior cortex (***Figure 5–49C***). To be certain that the osteotomy is complete, the proximal and distal rings are grasped, and the distal rings are rotated externally (relaxing the peroneal nerve). Both the periosteum and the wound are closed.

That this maneuver does not disrupt the medullary blood supply is difficult to believe. In addition, fracturing the posterior cortex in the manner described can lead to propagation of the fracture into one of the pin sites. The technique of the osteotomy described for the Orthofix lengthening would seem preferable because it is not so difficult, avoids this complication of fracture, and does not seem to affect the healing.

The fibula is divided in its midportion, a safe distance from the peroneal nerve. It is advisable to remove a small section of the fibula to avoid premature consolidation.

Figure 5–50. The two sets of rings are now joined by four lengtheners. Additional connectors are added between pairs of rings to increase their rigidity.

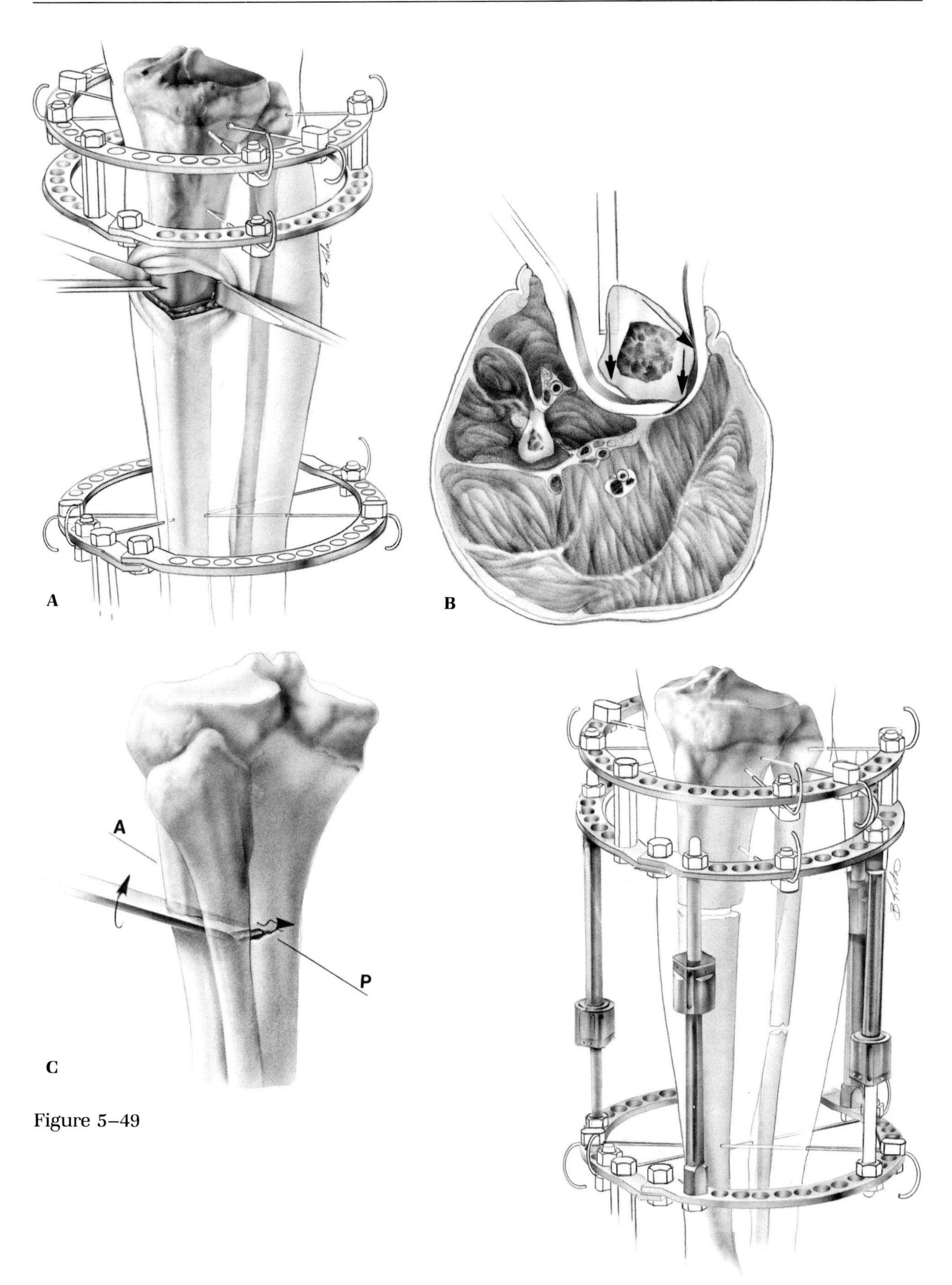

Figure 5–49

Figure 5–50

Figure 5–51. OA is a 10-year-old boy with congenital shortening of the tibia associated with a "ball and socket" ankle joint. Now 3 cm short, his final discrepancy is calculated to be near 6 cm (***Figure 5–51A***). Two months (***Figure 5–51B***) and 4.5 months (***Figure 5–51C***) after lengthening, the amount of correction and the regenerating bone can be seen. Fourteen months after lengthening and 6 months after removal of the apparatus, the maturation of the regenerated bone is apparent (***Figure 5–51D***). (Courtesy Deborah F. Bell, MD, FRCSC.)

POSTOPERATIVE CARE

Physical therapy is started as soon as the patient will tolerate. It is best to start on the first postoperative day with gentle range of motion and progress to weight-bearing on the second or third day. Lengthening of the leg can begin on the third to fifth day for children and later for adolescents and adults. The use of the lengtheners greatly simplifies this because each "click" is equal to a 0.25 turn, or 0.25 mm. Four turns per day produces the recommended amount of lengthening.

It should be noted that 1 mm per day is the usual amount of lengthening. This may have to be increased if premature consolidation is occurring or decreased if there is a break in the callus formation.

When there is radiographic evidence of cortical bone formation in the regenerated bone, consideration is given to removal of the connecting rods and the apparatus. It is best to first remove the lengtheners connecting the two sets of rings. The leg should be stable clinically and free from discomfort with manipulation and weight-bearing. If this is the case, the patient may be allowed to weight-bear with crutches for a few days before removal of the wires. This will allow for reapplication if fracture occurs. Many surgeons prefer to protect the leg in an orthosis for some months after removal of the apparatus.

REFERENCES

1. Paley D et al. Mechanical evaluation of external fixators used in limb lengthening. Clin Orthop 1990;250:50.
2. Paley D. Problems, obstacles, and complications of limb lengthening by the Ilizarov method. Clin Orthop 1990;250:81.

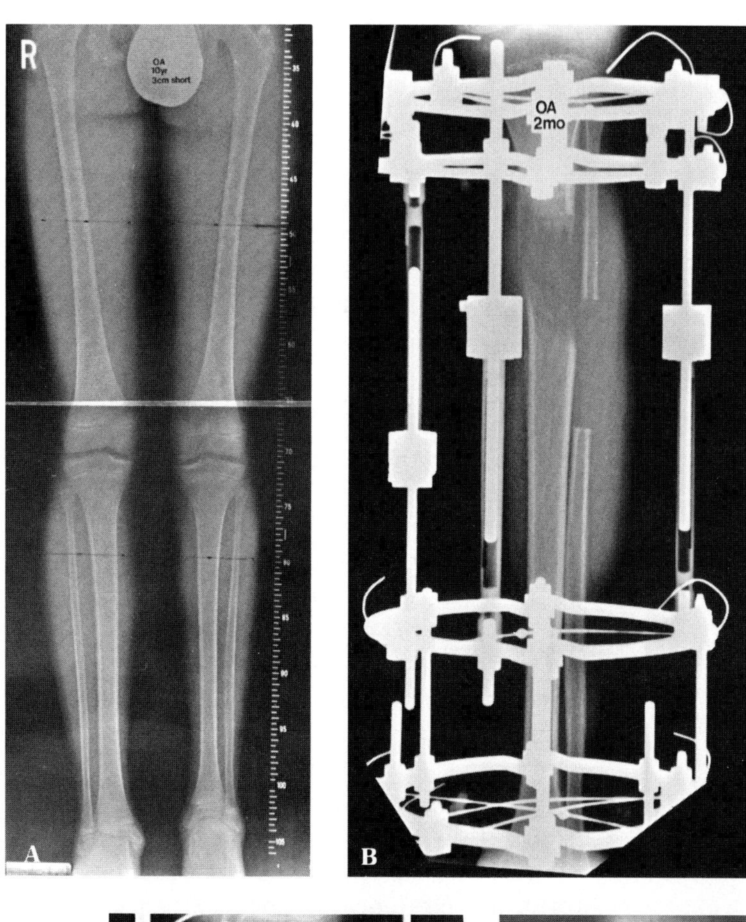

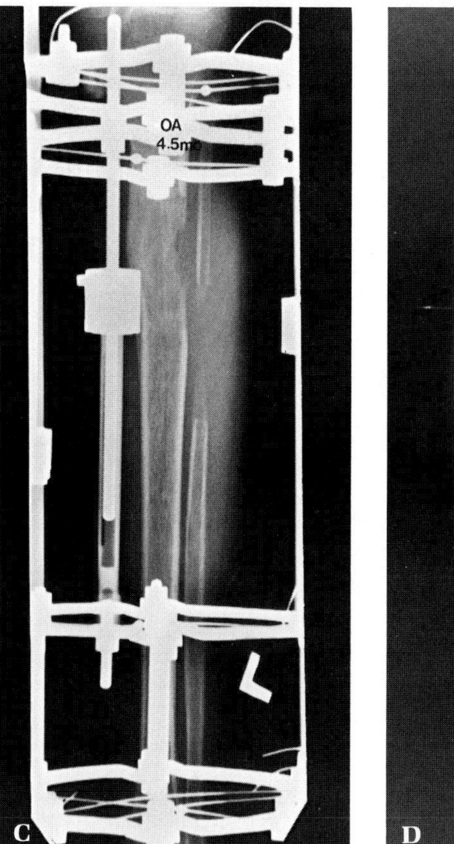

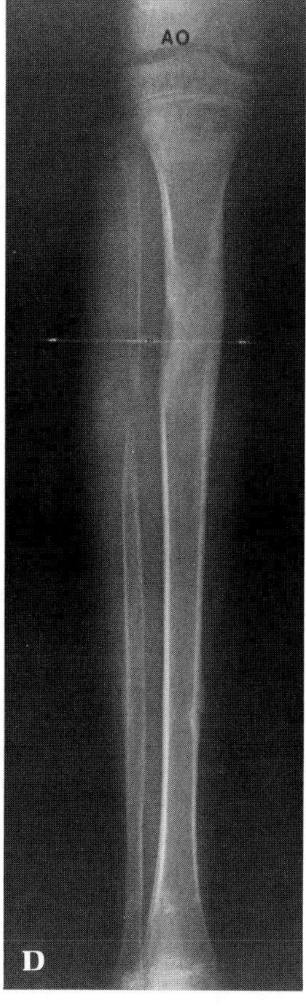

Figure 5–51

5.8 Repair of Congenital Pseudarthrosis of Tibia With Williams's Rod

Congenital pseudarthrosis of the tibia is an uncommon condition characterized by persistent non-union of a pathologic tibial fracture. The unique biologic characteristics of this condition are not well understood. The treatment of this condition entails some form of bone grafting along with fixation of the fragments as the initial treatment.[1]

In addition to the unique biologic characteristics, there are unique mechanical characteristics. Most often the operation is initially performed on small children with open physeal plates. There is an anterior and lateral bowing of the tibia that must be corrected as a part of the treatment. The bone is small and osteopenic. The distal segment is often short, making fixation to the distal segment difficult and insecure. The soft-tissue coverage in the leg of a small child is not great. The fracture may take a long time to heal, necessitating that the fixation serve its purpose for years. Finally, there is a great tendency to refracture, encouraging the surgeon to avoid the stress shielding that occurs under a rigid plate, and the stress riser created by the screw holes that remain when the plate is removed.

All of these factors make intramedullary fixation the ideal choice. The stimulus of weight-bearing is preserved, no stress risers are created in the bone, and the device can cross the ankle into the talus and calcaneus with little morbidity to help secure fixation of a short distal fragment. The problem of rods small enough for the tibia of small children and that can be inserted easily is solved by the Williams's rods, which were originated by Peter Williams of Melbourne, Australia.

The Williams's rods are available by special order from Zimmer (Zimer Co., Warsaw, IN.) and consist of two Steinmann pins threaded on one end. One end is a male thread, and the other is a female thread, allowing the two rods to be joined. The available sizes are $\frac{1}{8}$-, $\frac{3}{16}$-, and $\frac{1}{4}$-inch diameter.

Figure 5–52. The pseudarthrosis is exposed through an anterolateral incision over the midportion of the tibia (***Figure 5–52A***). There is debate among surgeons about what and how much of it is to be excised. Some think that all of the abnormal-appearing tissue and bone should be excised, whereas others would advocate that only sufficient bone be resected to correct the deformity and expose a reasonable medullary canal (***Figure 5–52B***). This author is a convert to the latter camp because some of his worst results have followed radical excision of abnormal soft tissue and bone. There is no evidence that radical excision will enhance the healing, the result perhaps depending more on the natural history of the individual case. If radical excision is performed, however, the surgeon should give some consideration to the blood supply of the distal segment of the tibia.

A pseudoarthrosis of the fibula often coexists. When the fibula is intact, however, it may be necessary to divide it to correct the tibia. If this creates a pseudarthrosis, it does not seem to affect the ultimate outcome. In those cases in which the fibular pseudarthrosis is distal, however, there may be instability of the tibial-fibular syndesmosis and thus the ankle mortice. In such cases, the surgeon should consider stabilization by intramedullary fixation of the fibula with a Kirschner wire or by establishing a bony union between the distal tibia and distal fibula.

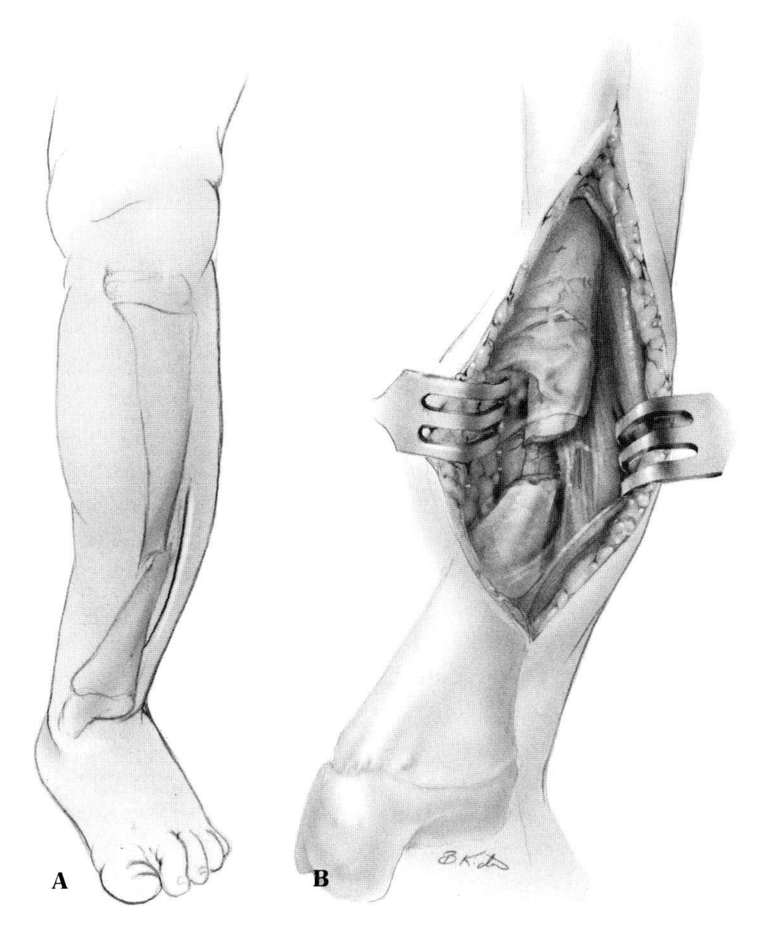

Figure 5–52

Figure 5–53. The Williams's rods of a size that will fit snugly in the medullary canal are joined together forming a very long rod with a point on each end. It may be necessary to drill the medullary canal of the proximal and distal fragment to allow passage of a suitable-sized rod. The rod is first drilled up the proximal fragment through the tight portion of the medullary canal to be certain that the rod will pass and to establish the proper direction for the rod, which in turn will ensure proper alignment of the proximal fragment (***Figure 5–53A***). If any residual bow remains in this fragment, the rod should start anterior and medial. In some cases there will be considerable bow, which will be unacceptable from a mechanical viewpoint as well as making central placement of the rod impossible. In these cases a second osteotomy should be done at the proximal extent of the bow. Minimal periosteal stripping should be done so that this intercalary segment of bone is not completely stripped of periosteum and thus its blood supply.

Next the rod is drilled into the distal fragment, again in such a way as to ensure proper axial alignment of this fragment (***Figure 5–53B***). This can be checked on an image intensifier. This segment of the rod that is drilled into the distal fragment should be the male-threaded portion, which will leave the female end in the tibia. The reasons for this will become obvious in the next steps. When the direction is proved to be satisfactory, the rod is drilled through the physis, the ankle joint, the talus, the calcaneus, and out the bottom of the foot. The drill is now placed on that section of the rod that protrudes from the foot, and the rod is withdrawn until the junction between the two rods is flush with the cut end of the bone.

If it is anticipated that the rod will need to be left in the calcaneus crossing the ankle joint, the foot should be carefully held in the correct anatomic position while the rod is being drilled across it. It is often necessary to leave the rod in the calcaneous in very small children or in cases in which the pseudarthrosis is distal and the fixation in the distal fragment will be insufficient. If the pseudarthrosis is in the midshaft this is not usually necessary. It is desirable, however, to leave the rod across the epiphyseal plate for two reasons: This is the strongest region within the tibia, which aids in fixation, and the extra length of the rod will permit extra growth.

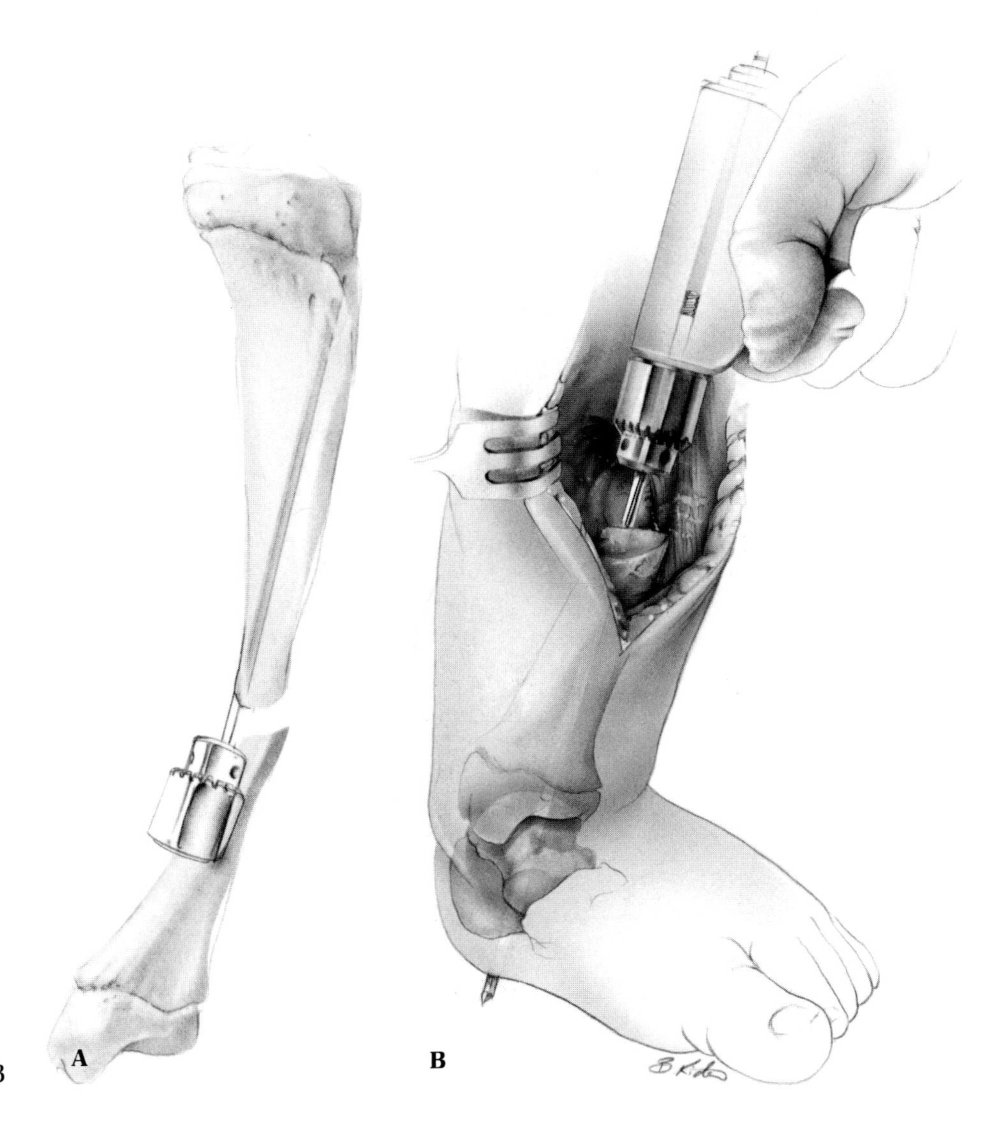

Figure 5–53

Figure 5–54. The rods are now unscrewed, and the proximal portion that is not within the bone is set aside. The tibia is reduced into the correct alignment and held temporarily in position by drilling the rod in the distal segment partway into the proximal segment. Because this is the male end of the rod the threads can be easily cleaned of bone fragments when the rods are joined together again. The female portion of the rod that was removed is placed over the tibia, and the desired length is measured from the threaded end by the aid of an image intensifier. It is usually desirable and not at all harmful to have the rod cross both physeal plates. This extra length will allow for extra growth and provide better fixation as mentioned previously. The extra length of rod that will be discarded is cut from the sharply pointed end in an oblique manner to produce as sharp a point on the remaining rod as is possible.

Figure 5–55. The rod is backed out of the proximal fragment, and the female segment that was just cut to length is reattached. The two joined rods are further withdrawn from the distal fragment until the cut end of the rod is flush with the cut end of the distal fragment. The fragments are reduced with care to hold the correct alignment, and the rod is drilled into the proximal fragment under image-intensifier control until the tip comes to lie within the proximal physis. The leg is again checked for correct alignment, and the image intensifier is used to ascertain that when the rods are unscrewed, the portion remaining will lie at the desired level distally (*ie,* either within the calcaneus or within the distal epiphysis). The distal tibial epiphysis is small in the growing child, and there is not much room for fixation. If the male end with its thin, threaded portion were left in the epiphysis, it would not add much fixation—thus, another reason for leaving the female rod in the tibia. If all is correct, the rod protruding from the foot is unscrewed and removed.

The bone graft is added, and the wound is closed over a suction drain. A cast is applied. It is important that the patient not bear weight for the first several weeks, so if the child is young or the reliability of the parents to enforce bed rest is at all in doubt, a double spica cast can be used to ensure non–weight-bearing. In addition, the chubby legs of small children will require a spica cast for good immobilization.

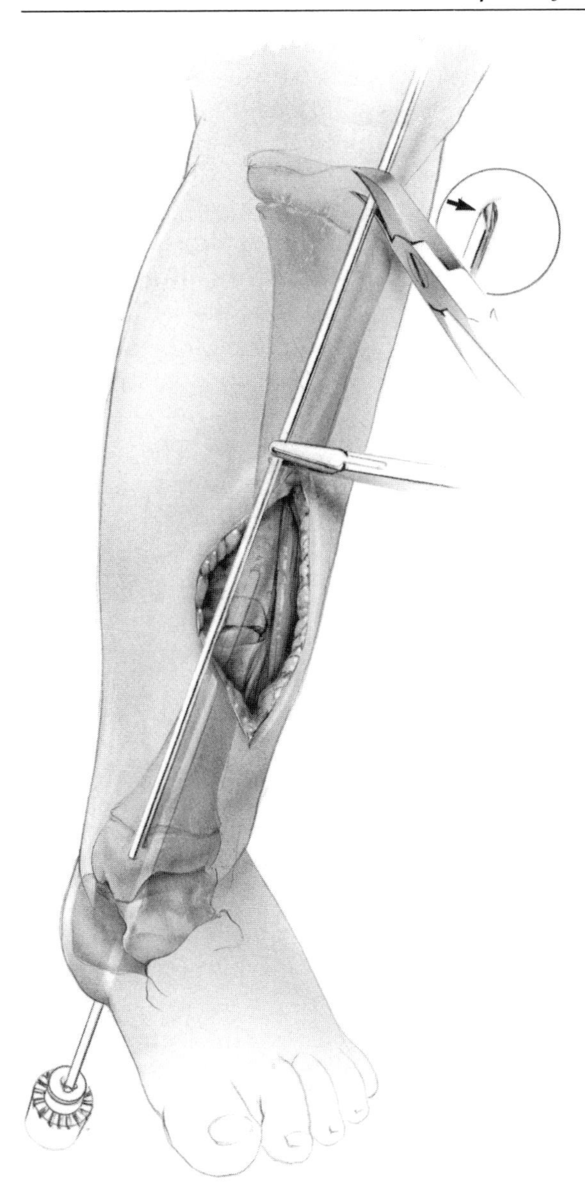

Figure 5–54

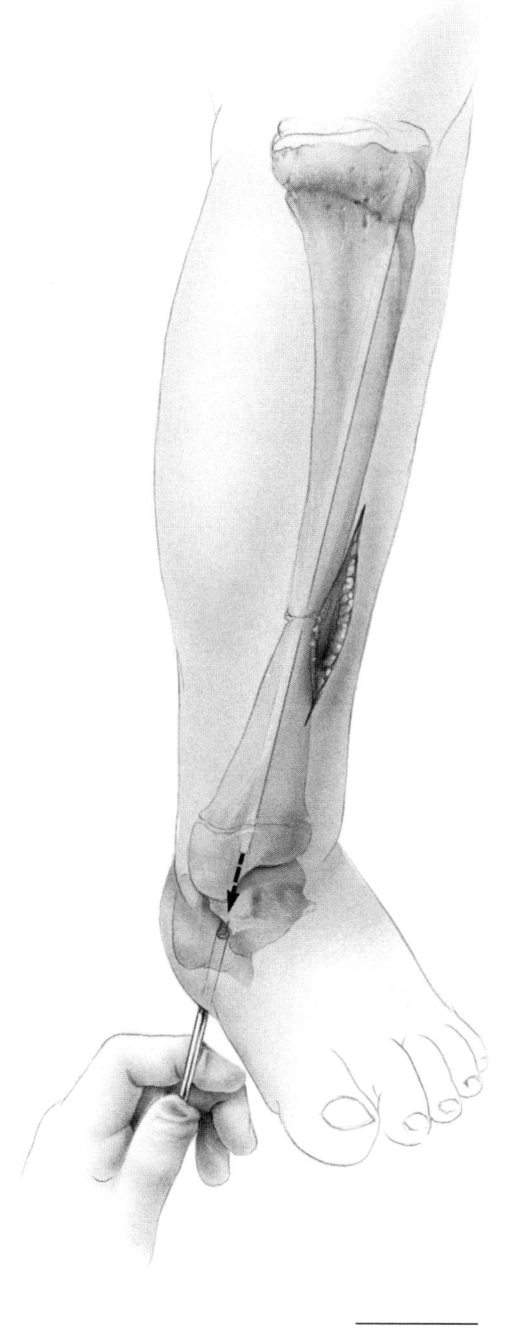

Figure 5–55

Figure 5–56. Pseudarthrosis seen in a 6-year-old girl (***Figure 5–56A, B***). The pseudarthrosis had been present for 2 years, and amputation had been recommended. She was treated with electrical stimulation for 1 year without improvement during this period. Radiographs (***Figure 5–56C, D***) show the result 3 months following surgery. Notice that these rods did not cross the physeal plates and that proximally the rod lies anterior because of residual bow in the proximal fragment. This latter problem could have been improved by an additional osteotomy of the proximal fragment. Four and one-half years later the tibia remains united (***Figure 5–56E, F***). The patient has remained in a solid ankle-foot orthosis during this entire period. The amount of growth at both ends of the bone is illustrated by the distance the physeal plates have moved from the ends of the rod.

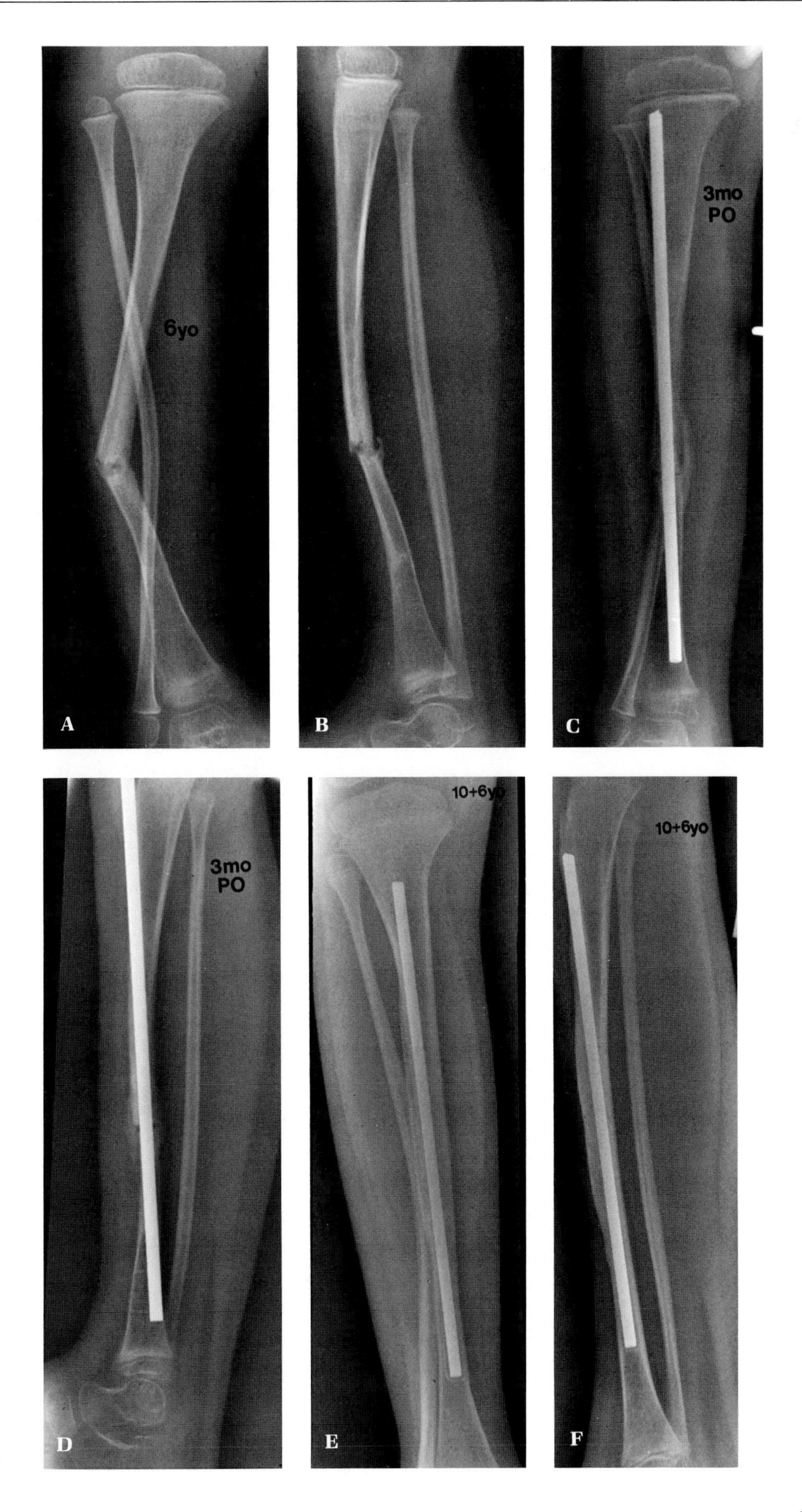

Figure 5–56

POSTOPERATIVE CARE

The drain can usually be removed on the first postoperative day and the patient discharged a day or two thereafter. How long the patient should be kept non–weight-bearing is a more difficult question. In all cases healing will be much slower than an osteotomy through normal bone, and the surgeon is usually forced by reason to permit ambulation before healing is complete. In most cases the author has permitted ambulation by 8 weeks in older children who can be well immobilized in a cast or an orthosis. In small children with their chubby legs, however, 3 months is probably safer. All children regardless of the success of the healing are maintained in an orthosis until skeletal maturity. The orthosis is a solid ankle-foot orthosis that grips the tibial and femoral condyles and has an anterior "clam shell" that maintains a tight fit over the anterior aspect of the tibia.

The patient is periodically monitored radiographically for union as well as the position of the rod. If the distal physis continues to grow (a good prognostic sign), the rod will eventually pull out of the bones of the foot and the ankle joint. This is because of the motion in the foot that loosens the rod distally while it remains fixed proximally. At this point the patient is usually older and an articulated ankle-foot orthosis can be used.

The rod can be left in the tibia indefinitely. If the patient grows to the point that the rod is very short, it need not be replaced as in osteogenesis imperfecta, provided the bone is well healed. If healing is not sufficient, however, the rod should be exchanged for a longer and if possible thicker rod when fixation is jeopardized. The rod is most easily retrieved proximally where it will usually come to lie against the anterior lateral cortex.

REFERENCE

1. Morrissy RT, Riseborough EJ, Hall JE. Congenital pseudarthrosis of the tibia. J Bone Joint Surg 1981;63B:367.

CHAPTER SIX
THE FOOT

6.1 Surgical Correction of Club Foot

Turco[1] popularized the posteromedial release for club foot deformity in the United States in 1971[1] and followed this with a second report in 1979.[2] Since that time there have been numerous articles on the surgical correction of resistant club foot deformity. Unfortunately, a careful reading of all of these articles may not convince the surgeon that one best operative procedure is known. This is due to several factors: Not all club feet are the same and, thus, do not need the same surgery; there is no good classification that would allow a comparison of club feet before or after surgery; there is not always complete agreement between surgeons on what the morbid anatomy of the foot is;[3] and incisions are often confused with what is done beneath the skin. In short, there still remains considerable art to the surgery of resistant club feet.

The surgical release of resistant club foot is discussed as the various components of an operation that the surgeon may choose to use or omit. There is no intention to advocate a particular operation or incision, and the surgeon is left to decide what is needed for each club foot. The techniques that various surgeons bring to the surgical treatment of club foot are so numerous and without published objective evidence of superiority that no one operation can be advocated. The operative steps are described through three separate incisions, although it is recognized that some may prefer one large or two separate incisions.

Figure 6–1. The incisions used vary widely and are more numerous than can be described here. It is important to remember that they have all been used successfully and that what is done beneath the incision is far more important to the result than the incision itself.

Turco[1] described a straight incision that ran from the base of the first metatarsal, under the medial malleolus, until it reached the Achilles tendon (***Figure 6–1A***). He pointed out that a proximal extension of the incision along the Achilles tendon was contraindicated and that no undermining of the wound should be done. Ignoring these two admonitions has led to many wound problems.

Crawford, Marxen, and Osterfeld[4] described an incision used by Giannestras (***Figure 6–1B***). This transverse incision begins on the medial side of the foot over the naviculocuneiform joint. From there the incision passes posteriorly to cross just beneath the tip of the medial malleolus. It continues across the back of the foot over the Achilles tendon at the level of the tibiotalar joint and continues laterally to pass over the lateral malleolus ending at the sinus tarsi. Although many surgeons have abandoned this incision because of wound complications, just as many report using it routinely without problems.

Many surgeons prefer to use two incisions; one posterior and one medial, with a third incision laterally over the calcaneocuboid joint if this is necessary. Carroll has described a medial incision with three limbs (***Figure 6–1C***). The center of the calcaneus, the front of the medial malleolus, and the base of the first metatarsal, marked by the x's, form a triangle. The center part of this incision is parallel with the base of the triangle, whereas the proximal part angles toward the center of the heel, and the distal part crosses over the dorsum of the foot. The posterior incision runs from a point in the midline approximately 4 cm above the tibiotalar joint obliquely to a point midway between the Achilles tendon and the lateral malleolus.

For years the author has used an incision learned from Campos de Pas and his staff in Brazilia, Brazil (***Figures 6–1D, E***). It consists of a separate medial and posterior zigzag incision. The first limb of the medial incision begins above and behind the medial malleolus, and extends forward and downward toward the sole of the foot. The second limb angles distal and dorsal to end over the region of the navicular. The third limb extends distal and plantarward to end at the base of the first metatarsal. The posterior incision is also composed of three limbs. The author has moved this incision to the lateral side of the Achilles tendon rather than placing it on the medial side as originally described. The first limb begins along the posterolateral side of the calcaneus and angles proximal to the lateral border of the Achilles tendon. Two more limbs of equal length extending proximal complete the incision. The advantage of the zigzag incision is that much more side-to-side exposure can be gained with a shorter incision, and as the foot is corrected the tension on the incision is largely eliminated. With this posterior incision it is possible to reach from the posterior tibial tendon medially to well past the peroneal tendons laterally.

If the Cincinnati incision is not used, and it is desired to open the calcaneocuboid joint from the lateral side, there are two choices for the incision. An oblique incision in the skin lines can be made directly over the calcaneocuboid joint (***Figure 6–1F***). If this is used the surgeon must be sure of its placement directly over the joint, or exposure becomes difficult. The second option is a curvilinear incision perpendicular to the calcaneocuboid joint (***Figure 6–1G***). This has the advantage of easier exposure and heals with surprisingly little scarring.

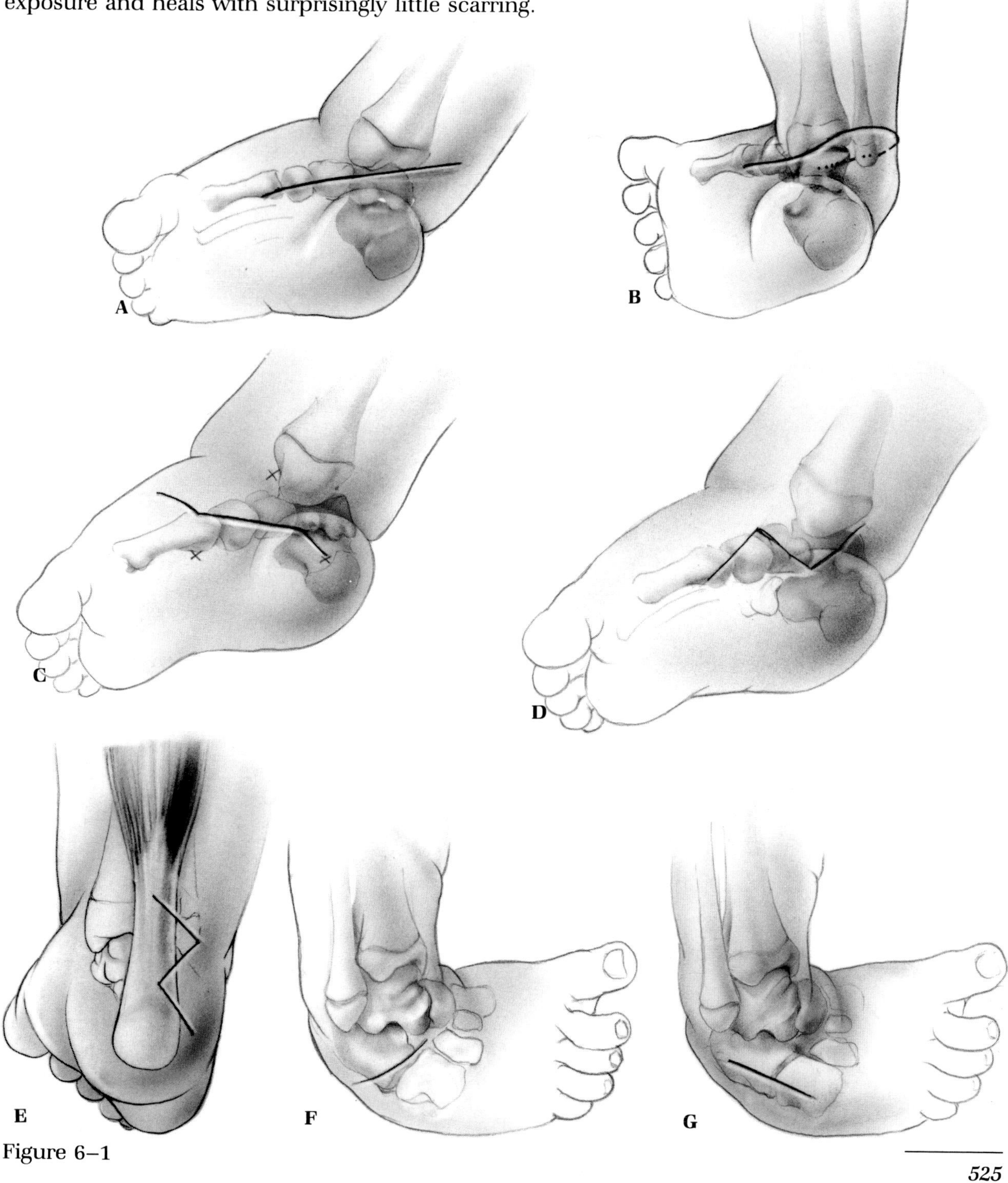

Figure 6–1

POSTERIOR RELEASE

Figure 6–2. The skin is divided sharply down to the Achilles tendon. It is important to preserve the sheath of the tendon. This is best accomplished by leaving the sheath attached to the subcutaneous tissue. Therefore, the incision in the skin and subcutaneous tissue is carried directly down onto the tendon passing through its filmy sheath. The tendon is then exposed circumferentially by gently teasing its sheath away with a small elevator. A large amount of proximal exposure can be achieved by placing the blade of a Senn retractor proximally and pulling upward while "toeing in" on the retractor.

It is now possible to divide the tendon in a *Z* fashion. This starts proximally with a cut in the middle of the tendon. It should be sufficiently long, as it is often surprising how much length is needed in a severe club foot. When the knife reaches the calcaneus, it is turned medially to detach the medial one half of the tendon from the calcaneus. The medial one half is detached to lessen the varus force. With the Senn retractor elevating the skin proximally the lateral one half of the tendon is detached proximally. Both halves are dissected free. The proximal one half can be curled under the skin and subcutaneous tissue proximally where a tunnel was formed. A suture can be passed through the distal one half and attached to a small hemostat to hold it out of the way.

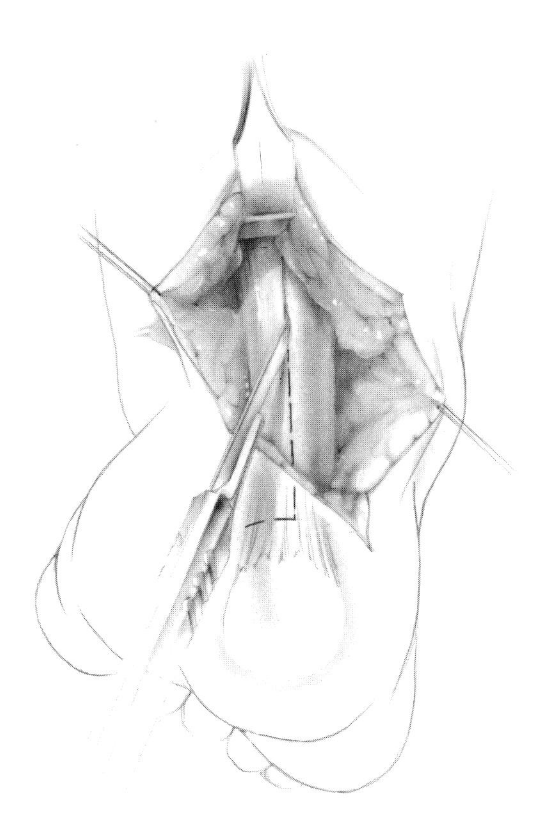

Figure 6–2

Figure 6–3. The next step is to open the posterior compartment. The surgeon may be tempted to do this by spreading with a scissors or hemostat, but this is unnecessarily destructive and can only lead to poor healing and scarring. The posterior compartment is a distinct anatomic compartment and can be opened by incising it with a knife. Starting proximally, the fat under the Achilles tendon is sharply incised in a straight line. As this incision is deepened, the fascial boundary of the compartment is encountered and beneath it more fat in the posterior compartment. Often, after this incision is completed, the anatomic structures in the posterior compartment will come instantly into view. In addition, in the severe club foot, the normal anatomic relationships may not remain. In such cases the incision may come down directly over the posterior tibial nerve as illustrated here. Note the flexor hallucis longus just lateral to the nerve. This structure is the first landmark to identify in the posterior compartment and is easily recognized as the only tendon passing behind the medial malleolus in which the muscle belly extends this low. This is easily remembered as the only muscle with "beef at the heel."

A small periosteal elevator is used to dissect beneath this muscle, staying in close contact with the posterior capsule. This dissection is continued around the medial side of the ankle as far as the posterior aspect of the medial malleolus. The dissection is facilitated by opening the sheath of the flexor hallucis longus distal to the medial malleolus to allow this muscle to be displaced. The neurovascular bundle is elevated with the fatty tissue and need not be disturbed. If a plantar release is to be performed later in the procedure, it is easiest to dissect the neurovascular bundle out at this point to facilitate the plantar release. A Senn or House retractor can be used to retract all of these structures giving a clear view of the posterior capsules from the midline to the medial malleolus (***Figure 6–3B***). Allowing the foot to go into plantar flexion makes this exposure even easier.

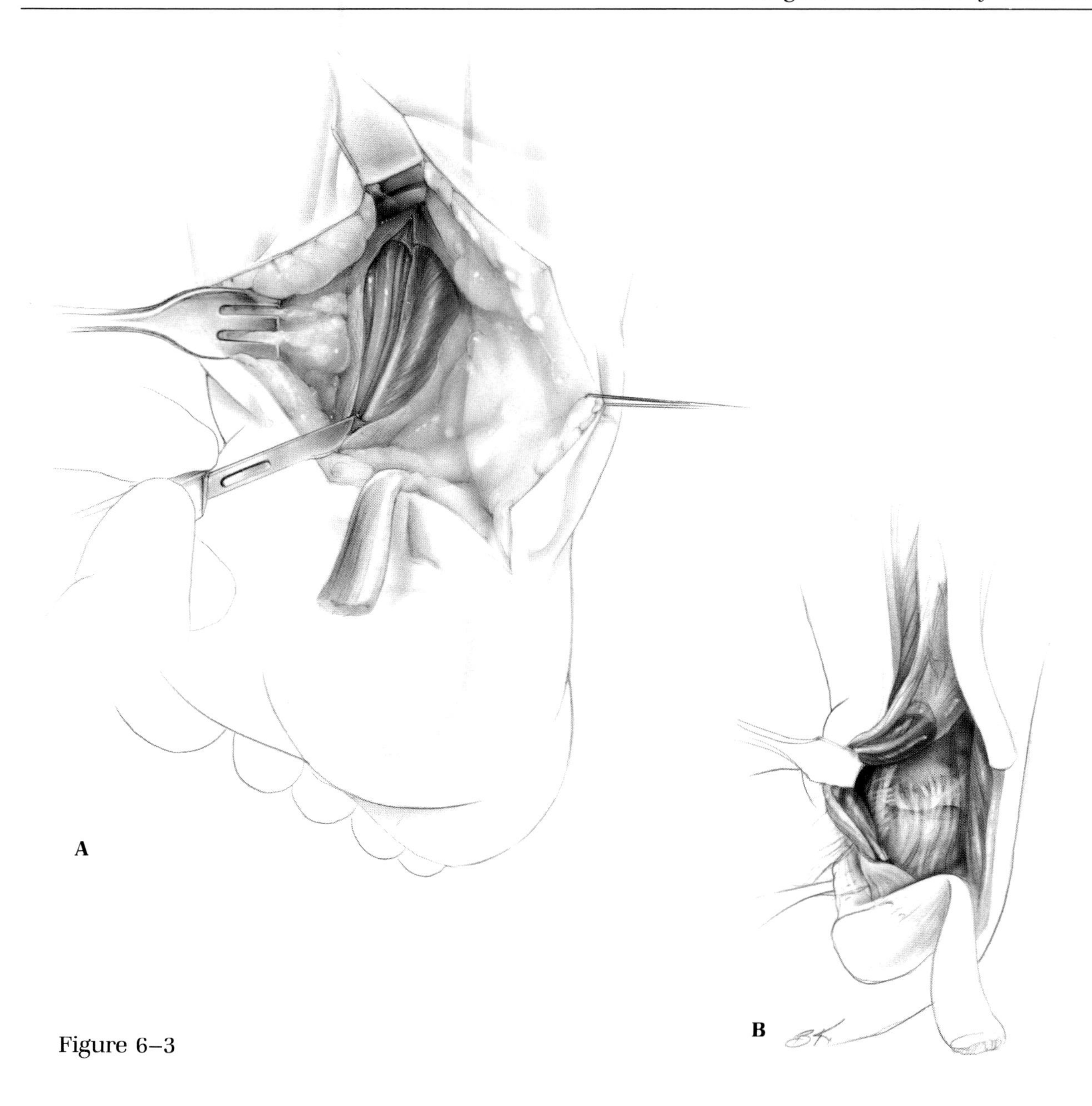

Figure 6–3

Figure 6–4. The lateral side of the capsules must now be exposed in the same manner. This is most easily accomplished by incising the fascia over the peroneal muscle bellies. These muscles are enveloped in fat and fascia lateral to the flexor hallucis longus whose muscle belly is shown exposed along the neurovascular bundle. Once the muscle tissue is identified, a scissors is used to open this fascial envelope around the peroneal muscles and tendons. This incision should be carried to the point where the peroneal tendons curve under the lateral malleolus so that these tendons can be retracted sufficiently to permit a complete division of the calcaneofibular ligament, which lies beneath the peroneal tendon sheath (***Figure 6–4B***). This completes the exposure of the posterior aspect of the tibiotalar and subtalar joint.

Figure 6–5. The capsule is now divided. This is best done with a scissors to avoid cutting the cartilage. The tibiotalar joint can be identified by palpation and inspection while the foot is flexed and extended. The scissors is used to cut into the joint and then with one blade in the joint and the other outside the joint, the capsule is opened around the medial side until the flexor digitorum longus muscle is identified. Two notes of caution: Be sure the neurovascular structures are retracted, and go slowly behind the medial malleolus so as not to divide the flexor digitorum longus and posterior tibial tendons. The peroneal tendons are now retracted, and the incision in the capsule is continued around the lateral side. As the foot is dorsiflexed the dome of the talus will come into view. Cutting the calcaneofibular ligament will usually make the largest difference in the amount of dorsiflexion that is obtained.

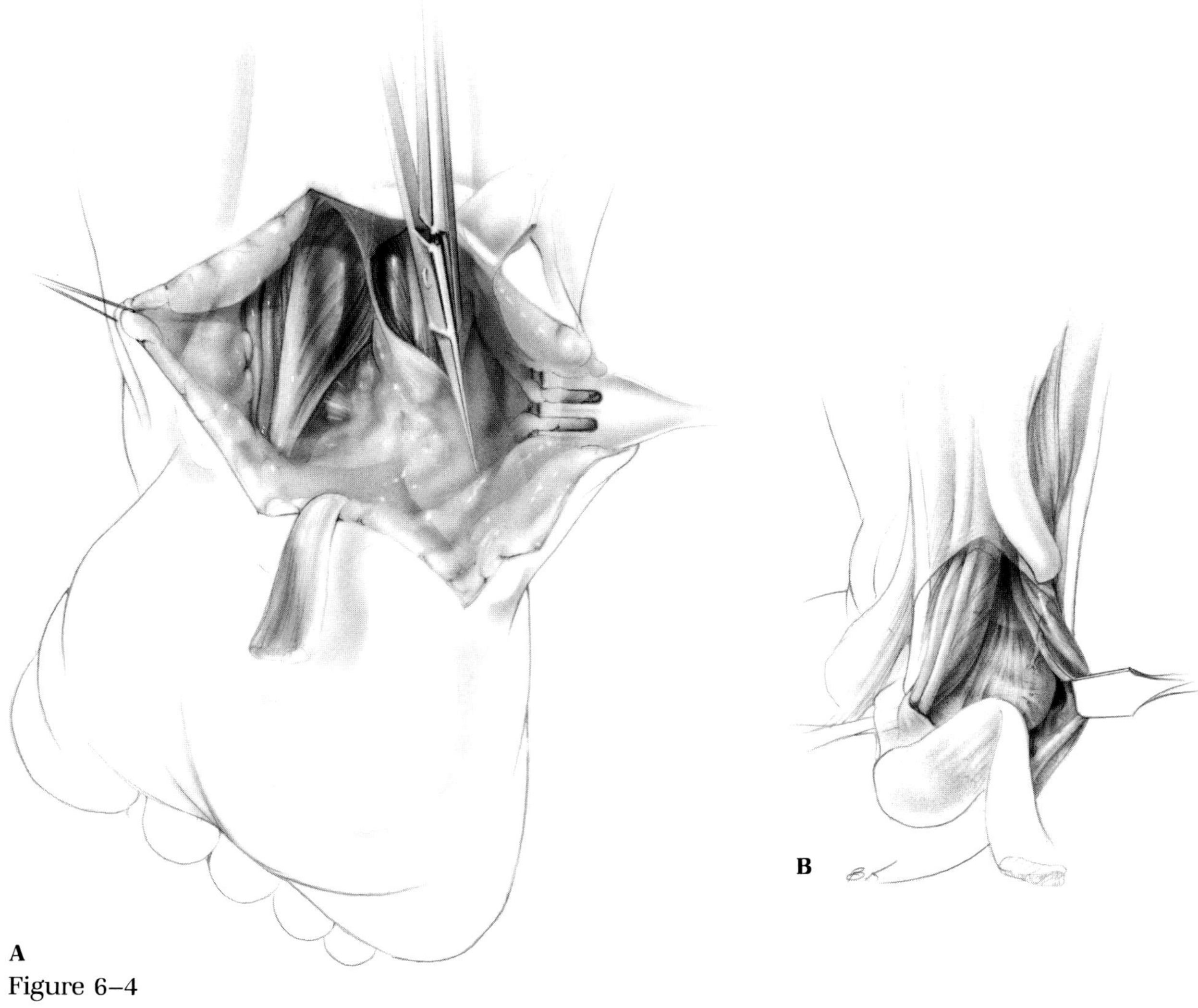

A

Figure 6–4

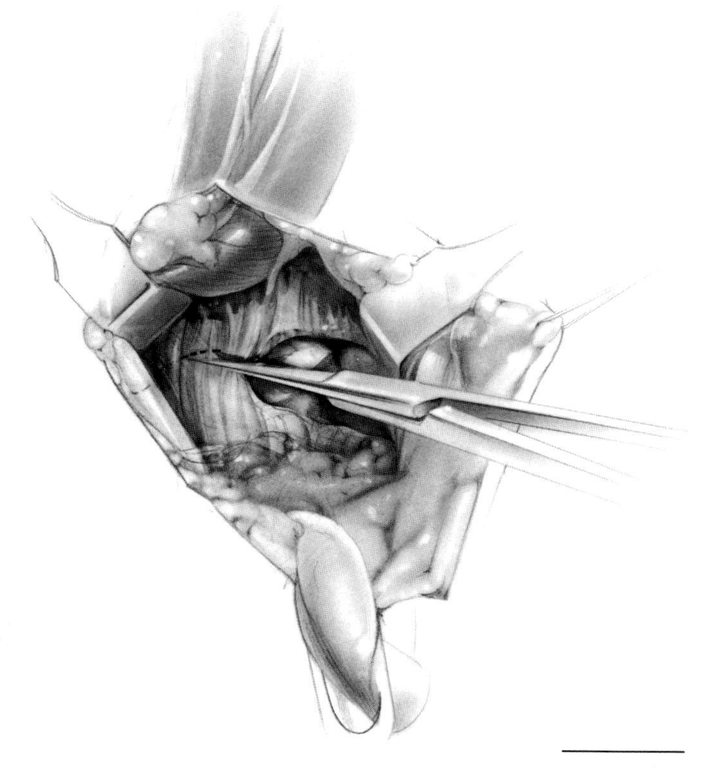

Figure 6–5

Figure 6–6. The subtalar joint is now opened. If it was opened inadvertently first, there is no problem. The subtalar joint will be found very close to the tibiotalar joint posteriorly. Use the scissors to open this capsule and just as before extend the incision in the capsule medially and laterally. On the medial side caution must be used not to cut the flexor hallucis tendon that runs alongside the medial aspect of the subtalar joint. With care this can be retracted out of the way, allowing the subtalar joint to be opened as far medially as was the tibiotalar joint. Extending the capsular incisions this far medially greatly facilitates the medial dissection because the capsulotomies of these joints will make them obvious.

Figure 6–7. Although many illustrations of club foot surgery show the ligaments of the posterior capsule as distinct structures, the surgeon will rarely see them this way as they are merely condensations of the continuous posterior capsule. Occasionally the posterior fibulotalar ligament and the calcaneofibular ligament will stand out, the latter occasionally appearing like a tendon. The geographic cuts in the posterior capsule of the tibiotalar and subtalar joint will divide the ligaments as shown (***Figure 6–7A,*** posterior tibiotalar ligament; ***B,*** posterior talofibular ligament; ***C,*** talofibular ligament; ***D,*** calcaneofibular ligament; ***E,*** deltoid ligament).

It should be noted that the deltoid ligament consists of several parts. One part of the deltoid ligament referred to as the "deep deltoid ligament" (anterior tibiotalar part of the deltoid ligament) is attached to the talus and in the opinion of many should not be divided to avoid the complication of lateral subluxation of the talus. Division of this part of the deltoid ligament is avoided by stopping the capsulotomy of the tibiotalar joint at the posterior aspect of the medial malleolus. If it is desired to divide this portion of the deltoid ligament as a part of the operation, as is done in the procedure described by Goldner,[5] it should be repaired.

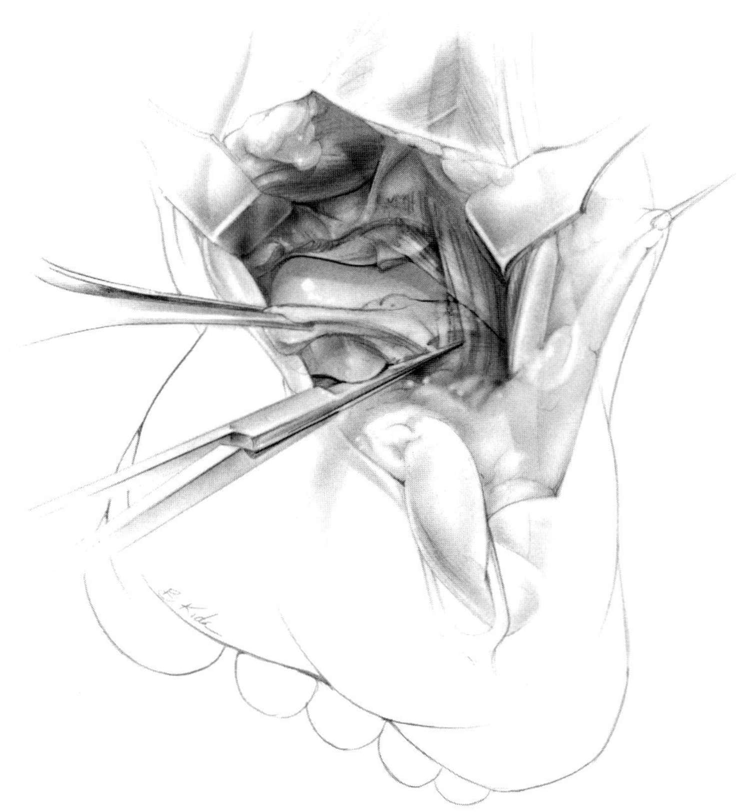

Figure 6–6

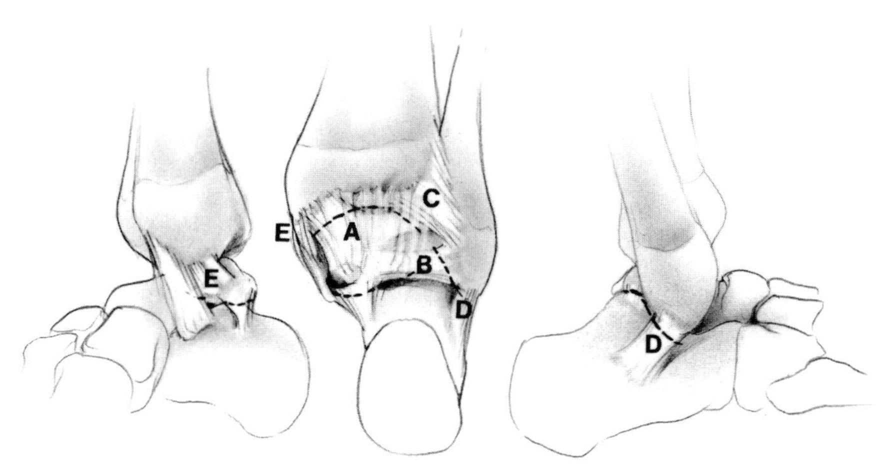

Figure 6–7

Figure 6–8. All that remains posteriorly is to repair the Achilles tendon. This should be done after the completion of the entire release, and after the foot is reduced and fixed with Kirschner wires. To minimize scarring the tendon is repaired end to end with a suture that remains buried in the tendon. Any extra length of tendon is removed to permit an end-to-end repair. The repair should be under modest tension to avoid unnecessary weakening of the gastrocnemius muscle.

MEDIAL RELEASE

Figure 6–9. Despite the fact that this is called a "medial release," much of the operation will occur on the sole of the foot and a lesser part on the dorsum. The key to this part of the operation, like all other surgery, is the exposure. The key to this exposure is the abductor hallucis muscle, which Henry has called the door to the cage; the cage is that space formed by the arch of the skeleton.[6]

After the skin incision is made, it is deepened down to the belly of the abductor hallucis muscle. The dorsal edge of this muscle is then identified and detached all the way back to its insertion on the medial tuberosity of the calcaneus. This muscle is then hinged downward with a small periosteal elevator that dissects it off of the underlying fascia. Be careful in detaching the posterior insertion of the abductor hallucis because the neurovascular bundle will run beneath the muscle in this region. At this point in the dissection very little of the important anatomy is visible because it is all hidden beneath the fascia. The next step will be to expose all of the essential anatomic structures.

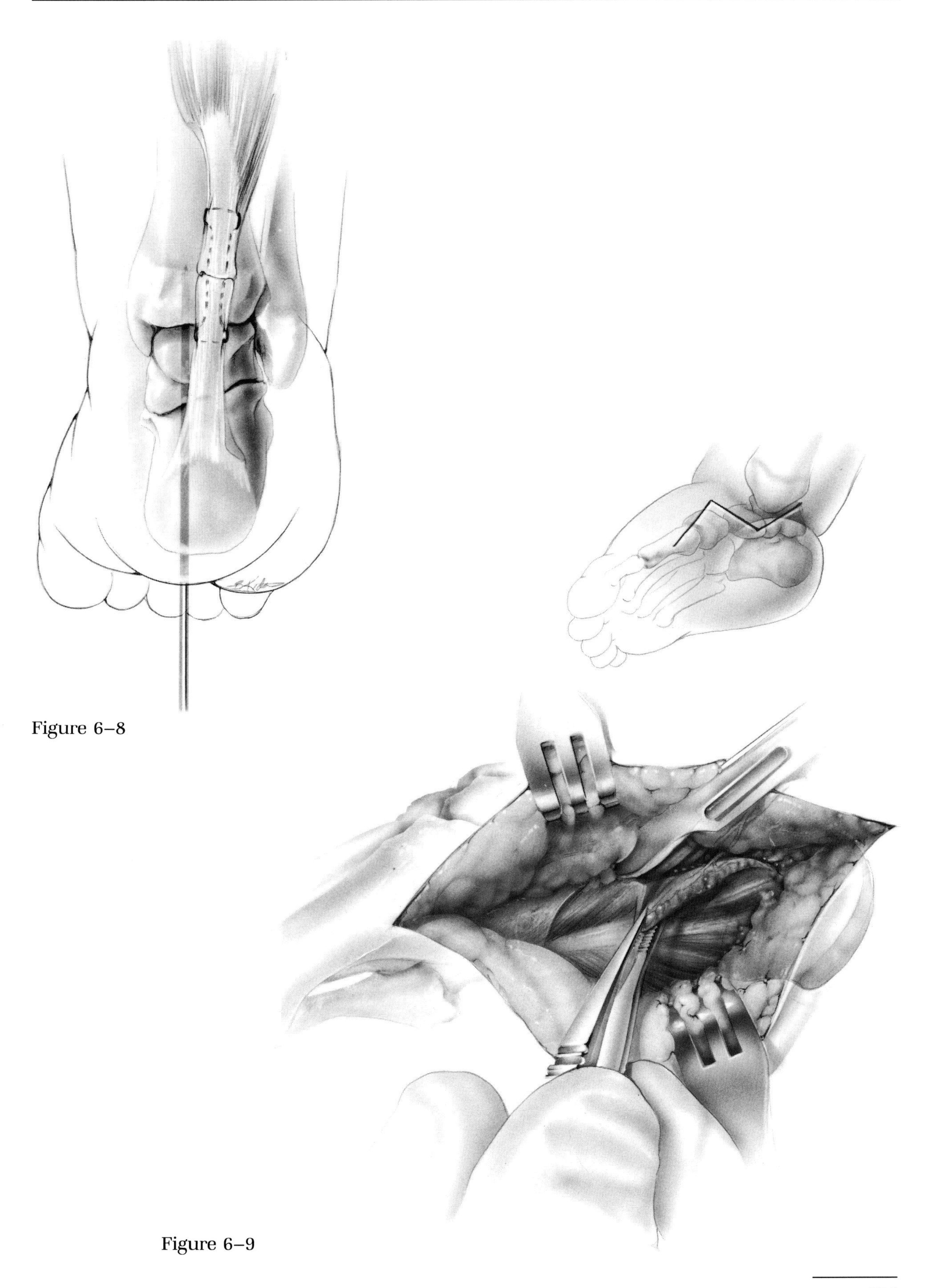

Figure 6–8

Figure 6–9

Figure 6–10. The dissection on the dorsal surface of the foot is the easiest. This part of the dissection is only necessary to open the dorsal capsule of the talonavicular joint and therefore does not have to be extensive. This dissection can be done either with a knife or by spreading with the scissors. The subcutaneous fat is lifted off of the deep fascia covering the bones. The only important structure that needs to be identified is the anterior tibial tendon. This dissection is beneath this tendon staying directly on the bony structure of the dorsum of the foot close to the ankle. Do not unnecessarily divide the small blood vessels that are seen in this area; all that is needed is enough exposure to divide the dorsal capsule of the talonavicular joint (***Figure 6–10B***).

To gain access safely beneath the fascia covering the structures on the sole of the foot, first identify the posterior tibial and the flexor digitorum longus tendons where they run behind the medial malleolus. A small, carefully made, transverse incision extending posterior from the tip of the medial malleolus will cut open their sheaths without cutting the tendons (***Figure 6–10B***). The sheath of the flexor digitorum longus tendon that lies just posterior to the posterior tibial tendon is opened first with a scissors. This sheath will guide the scissors beneath the navicular where the master knot of Henry will be divided. The dissection of the flexor digitorum should be continued distal to the region beneath the metatarsals. The fascia is much thinner after passing the master knot.

The posterior tibial tendon will be dorsal. It is much shorter, seeming to end in the tuberosity of the navicular. Because the navicular is so close to the medial malleolus in an uncorrected club foot, the novice may think that this tendon is missing or may unknowingly transect it at its insertion.

The medial plantar nerve from the posterior tibial nerve will run almost parallel to the flexor digitorum longus tendon in the sole of the foot and will be just volar to it. The medial plantar branch of the posterior tibial nerve can be followed proximally to help identify the neurovascular bundle just posterior to the flexor digitorum longus tendon behind the medial malleolus.

At the completion of this stage of the dissection the following structures are visible: Most volar is the medial plantar branch of the posterior tibial nerve, just dorsal to it and paralleling its course is the flexor digitorum longus, crossing this tendon transversely at the master knot of Henry is the flexor hallucis longus tendon, and splaying out over the tuberosity of the navicular is the insertion of the posterior tibial tendon. If the flexor digitorum longus tendon is retracted, the plantar ligaments, the peroneus longus tendon coming to insert on the base of the first metatarsal, and the medial side of the calcaneocuboid joint can all be exposed, as will be seen later.

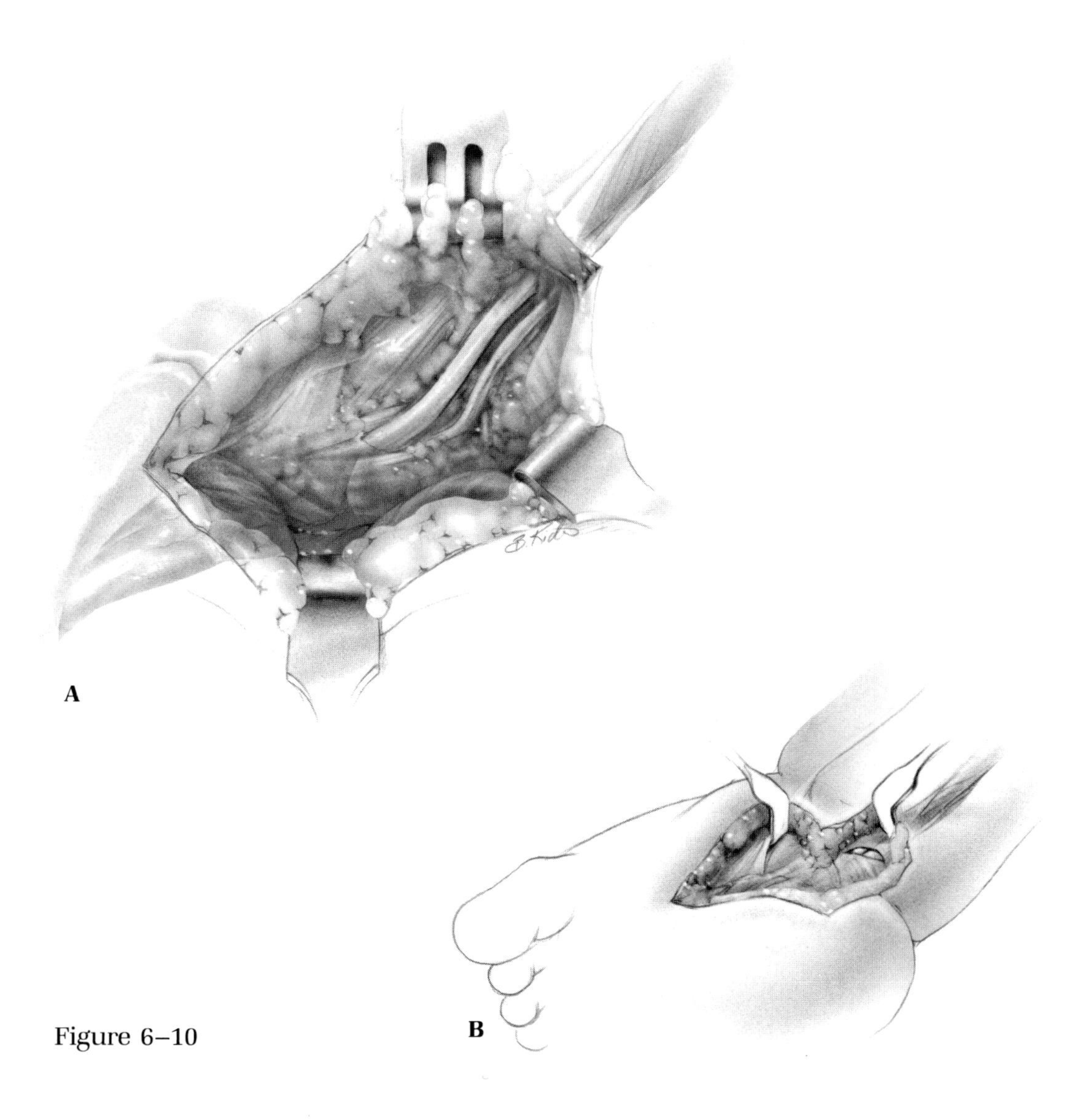

Figure 6–10

Figure 6–11. The posterior tibial tendon is now lengthened. This is actually necessary more to gain release of the talonavicular joint than it is to lengthen the tendon.

The posterior tibial tendon can be lengthened in a Z fashion behind the medial malleolus either through the medial incision or the posterior incision. The author prefers to detach it from its insertion, however. To provide for the extra length of tendon that will be required to lengthen the tendon, one of its insersions distal to the tuberosity of the navicular is identified and detached. These insertions are not easily seen. One major insertion passes down to the sustentaculum tali, whereas another insertion is an almost straight continuation of the posterior tibial tendon that runs beneath the cuneiform bone to the base of the first metatarsal. This one seems preferable.

It is exposed by removing the fascia over it with a small, sharp periosteal elevator. At the same time and by the same method, the peroneus longus tendon, which is coming from the lateral side of the foot to insert into the base of the first metatarsal, should also be identified. (It is shown here as if retracted for clarity but will overlap the extension of the posterior tibial tendon.) This will allow the distal insertion of the posterior tibial tendon to be divided without danger of cutting the peroneus longus tendon. This extension of the posterior tibial insertion is divided as far distal as possible. It is much smaller than the broad insertion of the posterior tibial tendon, which is now detached from the tuberosity of the navicular but is sufficient to reattach the tendon.

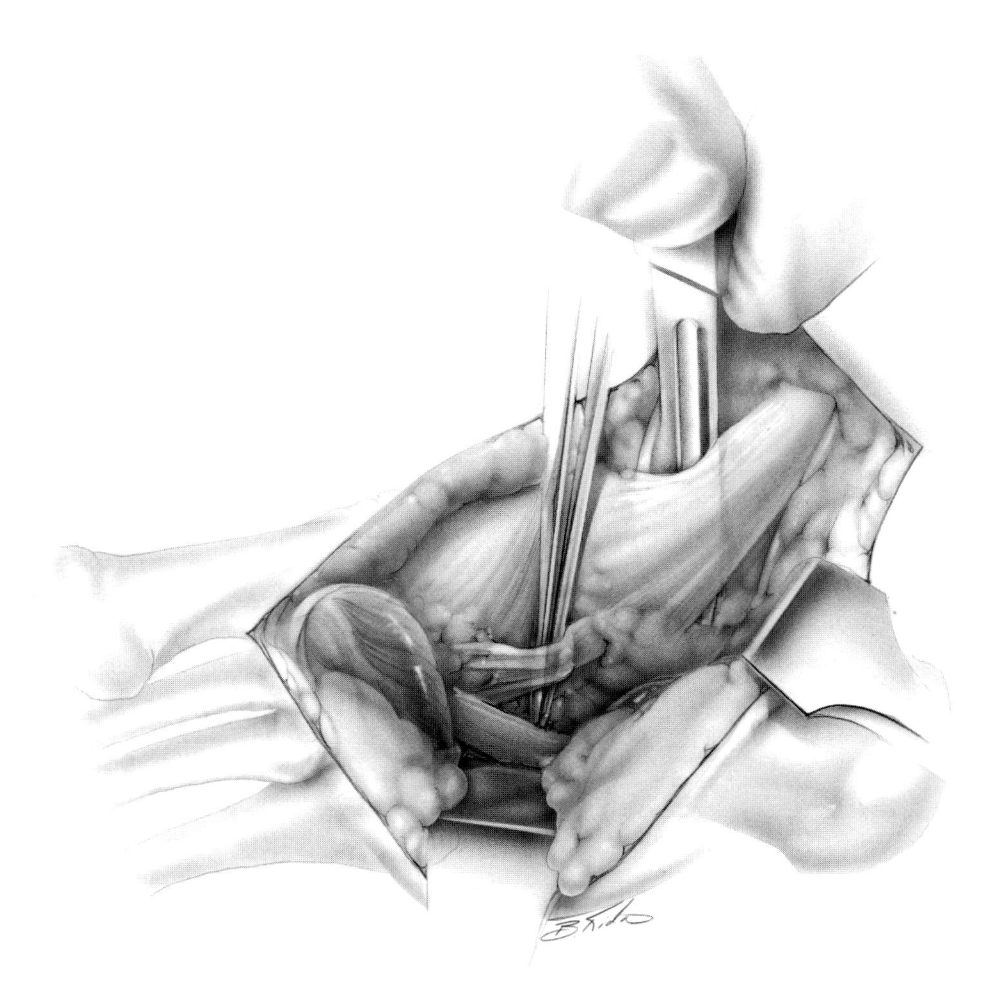

Figure 6–11

Figure 6–12. With the posterior tibial tendon detached it should be easy to identify the talonavicular joint, and it would be in a normal foot. In a club foot it must be remembered that the navicular is displaced medially, however, causing it to lie on the medial side of the neck of the talus and closer than normal to the medial malleolus (***Figure 6–12B***). In addition, the space between the tuberosity of the navicular and the medial malleolus will be filled with dense fibrous tissue. This dense fibrous tissue can be excised with a knife if the surgeon knows the anatomy. Leave a small portion attached to the navicular for reattachment of the posterior tibial tendon.

A scissors is then used to open the talonavicular joint. This joint will be found by directing the scissors distally toward the first metatarsal between the neck of the talus and the navicular (***Figure 6–12B***). The error is to cut transversely across the foot as if the anatomic relationship between the navicular and the talus were normal. This is especially dangerous if done with a knife as it is not difficult to divide the cartilaginous neck of the talus. The navicular is easily retracted by inserting a sharp double-pronged skin hook into it. This exposes the joint and aids in cutting the dorsal and volar capsule. (Much of the capsule has been removed in this drawing for clarity, but this should not be done during the surgery.)

The dorsal aspect of the talonavicular joint is easy to open; however, the volar aspect usually remains tight even after the capsule is cut. To free it, the plantar calcaneonavicular (spring) ligament and the anterior portion of the deltoid ligament inserting into the navicular (tibionavicular ligament) must be divided. Because these ligaments are condensations of the capsules, they will be divided when the capsules between the talus and the navicular dorsally, and the calcaneus and the cuboid volar are opened. This can be done with a scissors or a knife once the surgeon is certain that he or she has identified the joint.

Volar and lateral to the talonavicular joint and almost in line with it is the calcaneocuboid joint (***Figure 6–12C***). It can now be opened.

Because the peroneus longus tendon crosses the most volar and lateral aspect of this joint, it should be retracted. In ***Figure 6–12A*** it is shown as retracted but is seen in its more normal relationship in ***Figure 6–11.*** The medial capsule of the calcaneocuboid joint like all of the others can be opened most safely with a scissors, although some experienced surgeons prefer to use a knife. The lateral aspect of the capsule can be divided by passing a small, sharp, periosteal elevator or similar instrument through the joint and pushing this repeatedly through the lateral capsule while palpating the lateral aspect of the joint through the skin with the opposite hand.

If desired, the remainder of the subtalar joint capsule can now be divided. If the navicular will not slide around the head of the talus but instead opens like a book, it may be necessary to open the lateral side of the calcaneocuboid joint and remove bone from the lateral side. Release of the plantar fascia is another step that aids in the proper reduction of the navicular on the talus.

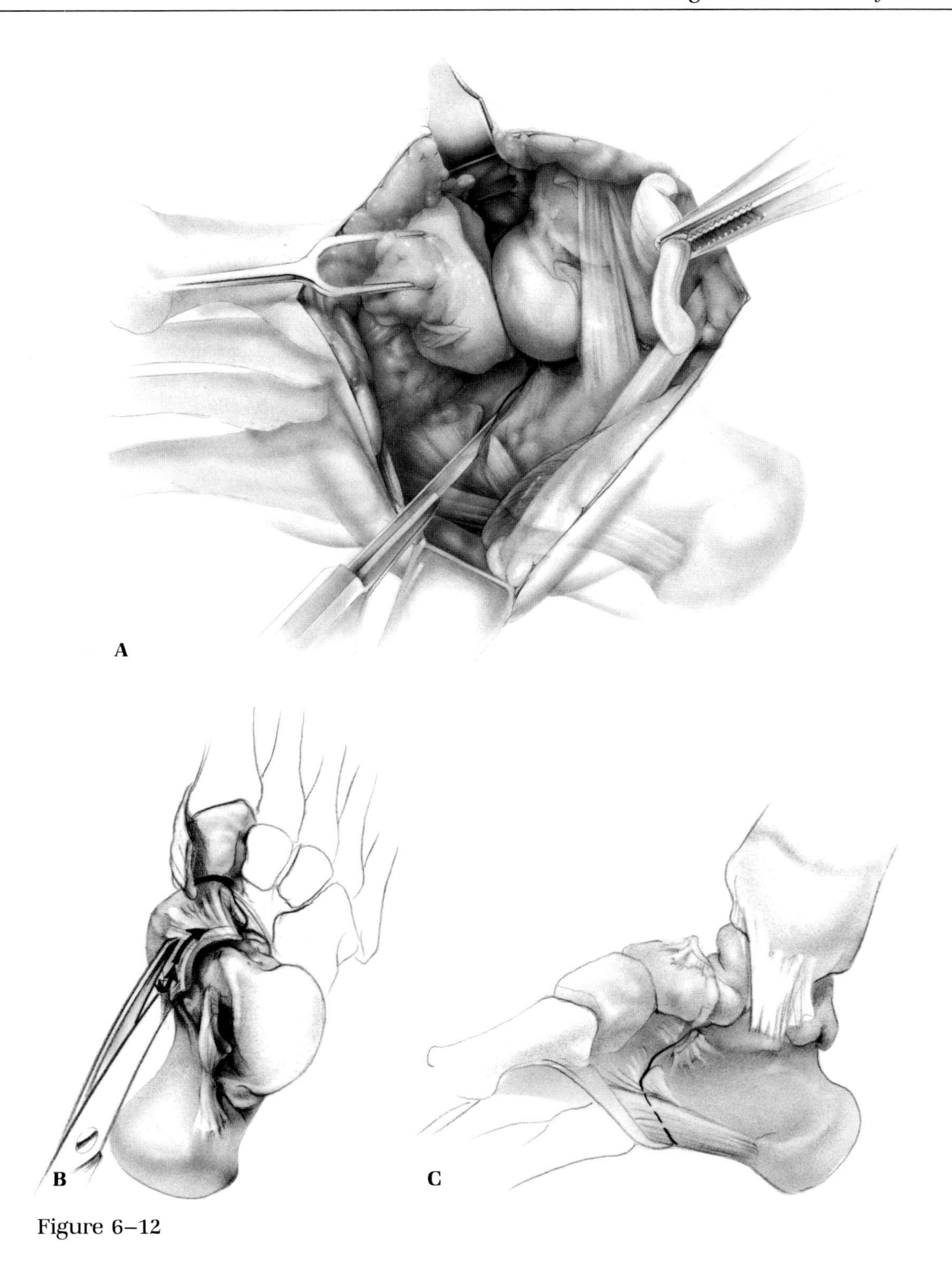

Figure 6–12

Figure 6–13. Another component of the medial release is the division of the plantar fascia and muscles at their insertion into the calcaneus as described by Carroll.[3] The author believes this should be done in most resistant club feet. This part of the operation will be done posterior to the neurovascular structures. The medial plantar nerve is easily identified in the neurovascular bundle. The lateral plantar nerve must also be identified. This can be done by following the medial plantar branch proximally until the lateral plantar branch is found. It will lie posterior to the medial plantar branch and if followed for a short distance will have a course that is more volar and lateral. Both of these branches along with the vascular structures are retracted distally, exposing a fatty space behind them and above the plantar structures that are to be divided.

Figure 6–14. Next, a plane is developed between the volar aspect of the plantar fascia and the subcutaneous tissue extending to the lateral border of the foot. A heavy Mayo scissors is inserted from medial to lateral with one blade in this plane and the other in the fatty space behind the neurovascular structures, and above the plantar fascia and muscles. These structures can now be safely cut off of their insertion into the calcaneus.

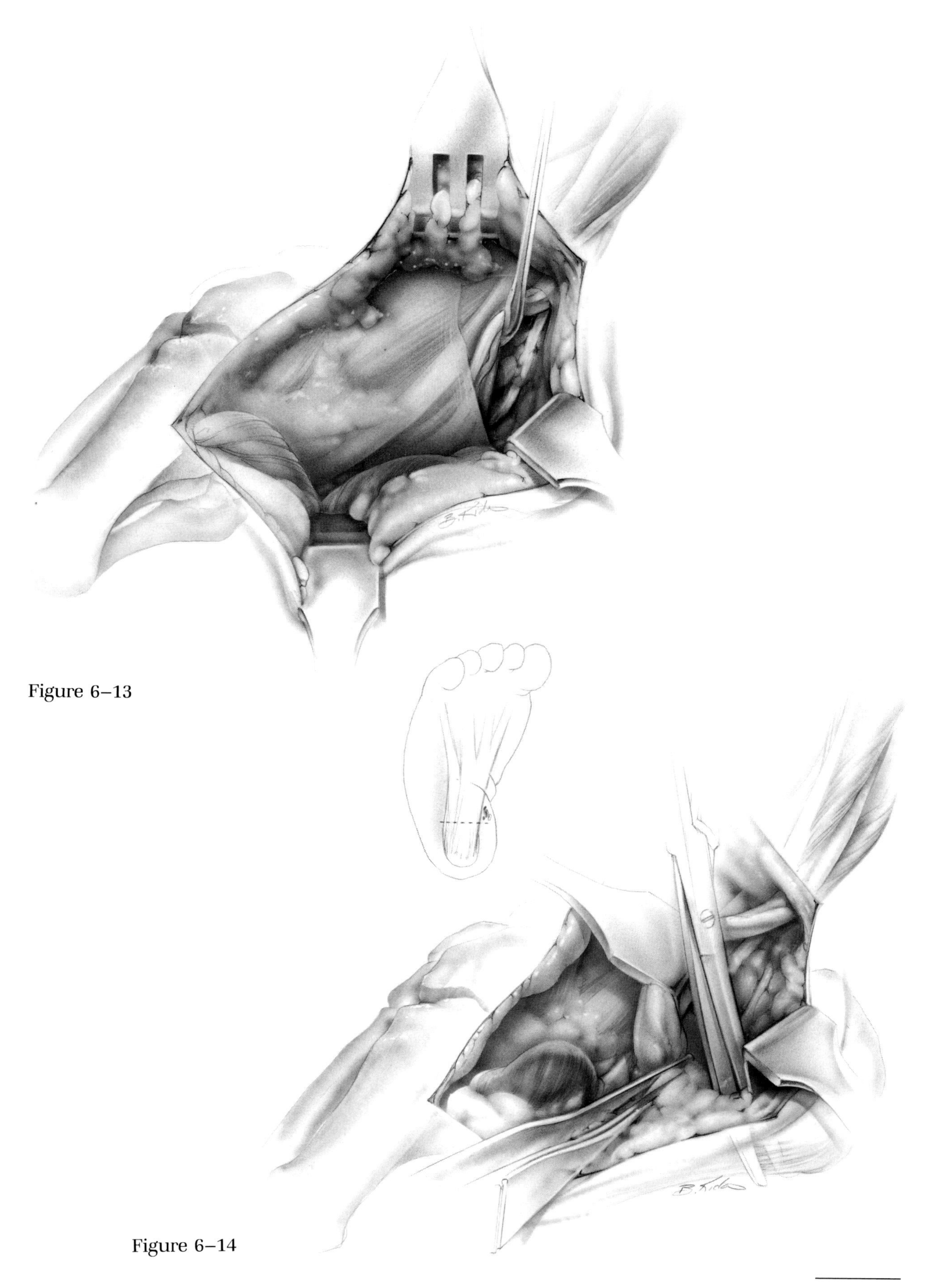

Figure 6–13

Figure 6–14

Figure 6–15. After the release is completed to the surgeon's satisfaction, the correction of the foot should be secured with two small Kirschner wires. The talonavicular joint is reduced first and transfixed with a smooth wire. This may be passed either from distal to proximal, or proximal to distal starting through the posterior exposure. During this step take care to see that the navicular is not displaced dorsally in relation to the head of the talus by keeping the foot dorsiflexed. The wire should not protrude from the talus posteriorly. It should remain protruding through the skin on the dorsum of the foot where a short bend is placed in it.

With the ankle held in neutral, one wire is passed or drilled through the skin of the heel, through the calcaneus and the talus, and into the tibia. The wire is cut off, leaving a short piece to be bent over.

If the surgeon wishes to obtain radiographs of the foot to verify the correction, they are done at this point. The posterior tibial tendon is reattached to the navicular, and the flexor hallucis longus and the flexor digitorum longus are then lengthened and repaired. A technique for this is described next.

Figure 6–16. The flexor hallicus longus and the flexor digitorum longus will need to be lengthened. If they are not, when the ankle is dorsiflexed they will cause severe flexion of the toes. Although these tendons can be lengthened through the posterior incision this may be better accomplished in the sole of the foot where the resulting scar will not restrict the excursion of these tendons. As these two tendons are dissected in the sole of the foot, they will be seen to cross with a variable amount of interconnection. This is why they often move simultaneously.

To achieve this lengthening, the two tendons—flexor digitorum longus and the flexor hallicus longus—are sutured together both proximally and distally. Then both tendons are divided: One just proximal to where they are sutured together distally, and the other just distal to where they are sutured together proximally. These resulting cut ends are then sutured together under the appropriate tension. This is most easily done after the ankle and talonavicular joint are correctly positioned and transfixed with Kirschner wires.

Fine absorbable sutures used to close the skin do not cause undue reaction and obviate the need for removal. A small suction drain can be placed that runs from the posterior operative field, under the medial skin bridge into the medial wound, and out through the skin distal to the medial incision. This will greatly reduce the postoperative swelling.

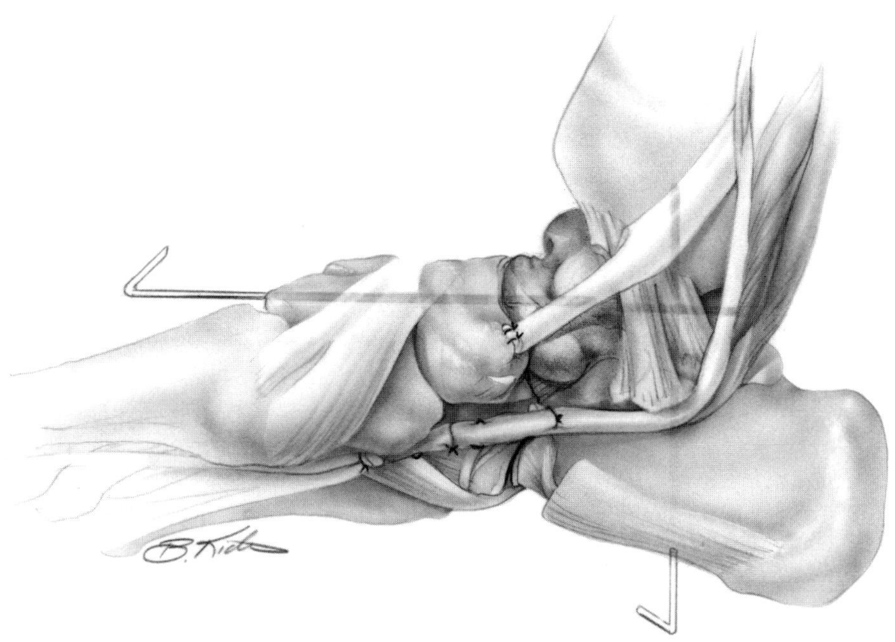

Figure 6–15

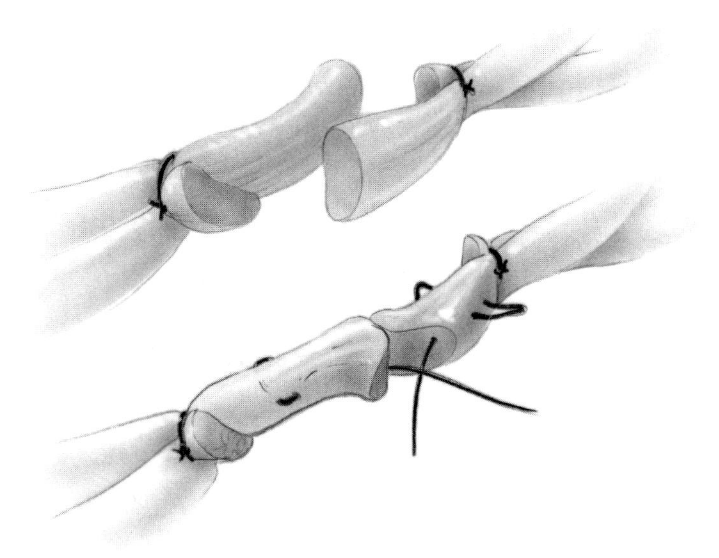

Figure 6–16

LATERAL RELEASE

Figure 6–17. If a lateral release is required, the calcaneocuboid joint can be exposed by use of the Cincinnati incision or either of the other two incisions described.

After dividing the subcutaneous tissue the muscle of the abductor brevis muscle will be seen. This muscle is detached proximally and reflected distally to expose the calcaneocuboid joint. The tendon of the peroneus brevis will run over the volar aspect of the joint and should be freed and retracted volar.

Although numerous methods have been described to shorten the lateral column of the foot, there are three that receive the widest use today. The Lichtblau procedure[7] is based on the assumption that adaptive changes in the calcaneocuboid joint are what prevent adequate reduction. With the medial displacement of the navicular the lateral side of the calcaneus overgrows, and the result is a calcaneocuboid joint that is angled in such a way that the cuboid cannot be laterally displaced on the calcaneus **(*Figure 6–17A*).** The operation, which is recommended for children over the age of 2 years, excises a laterally based wedge from the distal end of the calcaneus. The resulting fibrocartilaginous joint functions well and remains asymptomatic.

Goldner achieves the shortening of the lateral side of the foot by resecting a wedge of bone from the cuboid bone. This preserves the joint surfaces and is more effective than decancelation of the bone **(*Figure 6–17B*).** This operation is used at any age when it is believed necessary by the surgeon.

The final method of achieving lateral column shortening is that described by Evans,[8] who first called attention to the lateral column of the foot. His operation excises a portion from each side of the calcaneocuboid joint. The defect created by the wedge is held closed by staples and is intended to result in fusion **(*Figure 6–17C*).** The operation is not recommended before the age of 4 years; before that age so much of these bones is cartilage, and fusion will not result.

Figure 6–18. Lateral radiograph of a 4-month-old child with uncorrected club foot is shown **(*Figure 6–18A*).** Postoperatively the parallelism between the talus and the calcaneus has been corrected. The pins are shown in place **(*Figure 6–18B*).** The surgeon chose not to transfix the talotibial joint. (Courtesy of Douglas Kehl, MD.)

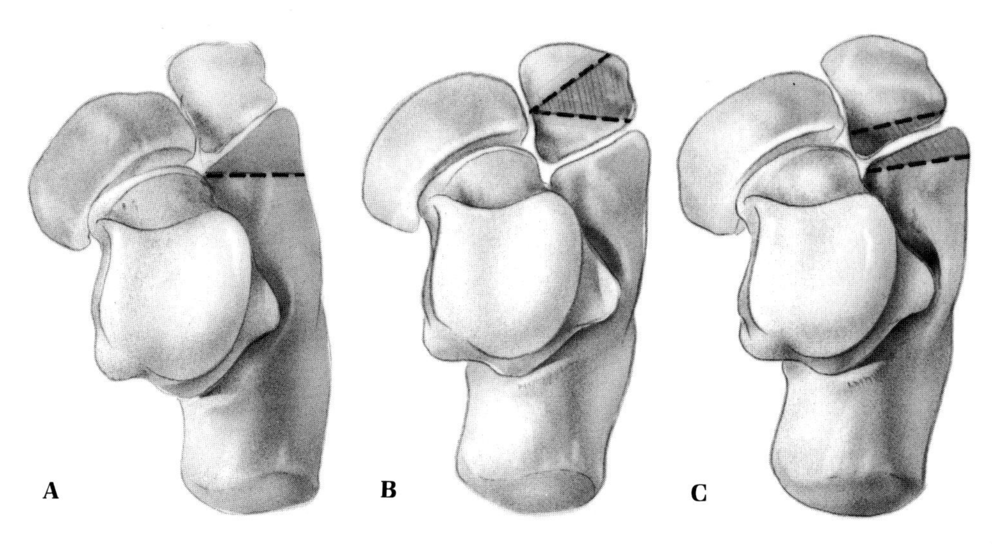

Figure 6–17

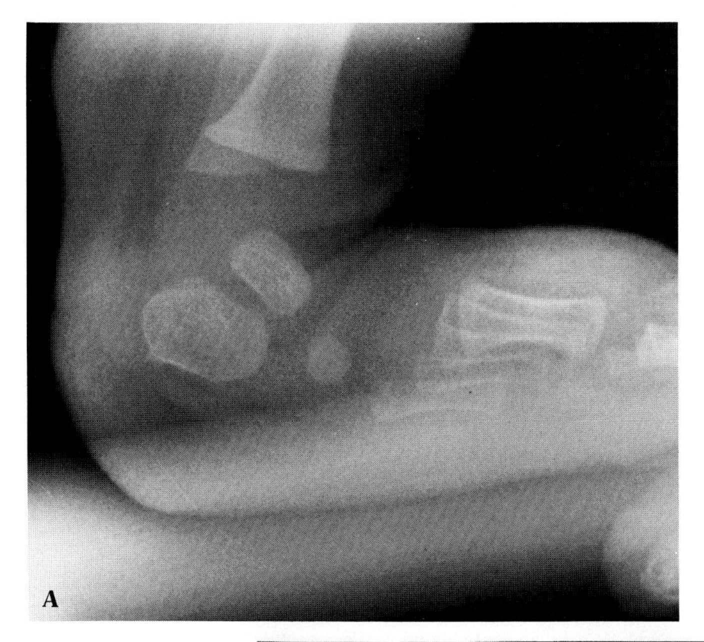

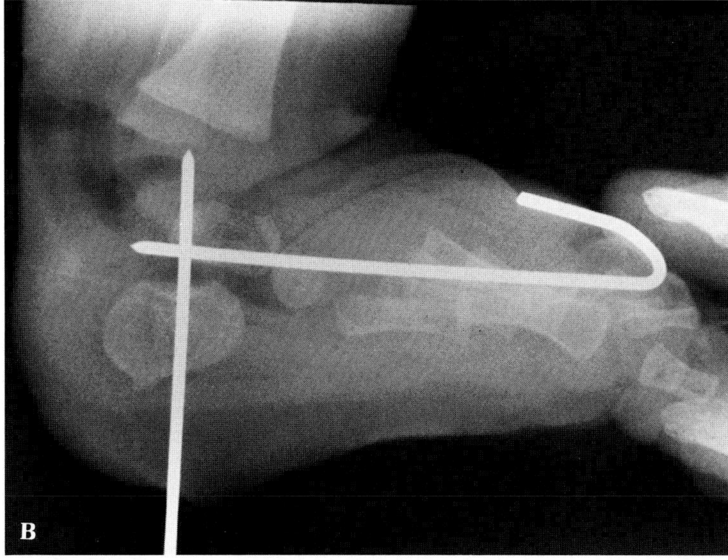

Figure 6–18

POSTOPERATIVE CARE

There are so many dearly held beliefs about what is important in the postoperative management of the club foot that the author can only relate what he does and why (with no more scientific certitude than a surgeon who does something different).

Before closure of the wound a small silastic drain is placed in the wound, running from the posterior wound through the medial wound and out of a small stab wound distal to the medial incision. This drain is removed the day after surgery. At the conclusion of surgery the patient is placed in a long leg cast with the knee bent 90 degrees. This is to allow a loose-fitting cast to be applied without danger of slipping off. At 6 weeks this cast and the pins are removed in the office. There is no manipulation of the foot during this initial 6 weeks as full correction is gained at the operating table and secured with the wires. The use of the two zigzag skin incisions running longitudinal to the direction of tension along with the broad medial area of intact skin prevents any undue tension on the wound.

After removal of the pins, a short leg cast is applied and maintained for an additional 4 weeks. After this is removed the patient is placed in reverse last shoes set at 20 degrees of external rotation on a 6-inch Fillaeur bar. The reverse last shoes are intended to maintain the forefoot correction, whereas the bar promotes inversion and eversion along with some dorsiflexion and plantar flexion as the child flexes and extends the legs. After an additional 3 to 4 months of wear, the shoes and bar are discontinued, and no further specific treatment is given. The patient is seen and evaluated as circumstances dictate. This is usually every 4 months during the first year, and then yearly or biyearly thereafter.

REFERENCES

1. Turco VJ. Surgical correction of the resistant club foot: one stage posteromedial release with internal fixation: a preliminary report. J Bone Joint Surg 1971;53A:447.
2. Turco VJ. Resistant congenital club foot—one-stage posteromedial release with internal fixation: a follow-up report of a fifteen-year experience. J Bone Joint Surg 1979;61A:805.
3. Carroll N. Clubfoot. In: Morrissy RT, ed. Lovell and Winter's Pediatric Orthopaedics, 3rd ed. Philadelphia: JB Lippincott, 1989:931.
4. Crawford AH, Marxen JL, Osterfeld DL. The Cincinnati incision: a comprehensive approach for surgical procedures of the foot and ankle in childhood. J Bone Joint Surg 1982;64A:1355.
5. Goldner JL. Congenital talipes equinovarus—fifteen years of surgical treatment. Curr Pract Orthop Surg 1969;4:61.
6. Henry AK. Extensile exposure. Baltimore: Williams & Wilkins, 1970:303.
7. Lichtblau S. A medial and lateral release operation for clubfoot: a preliminary report. J Bone Joint Surg 1973;55A:1377.
8. Evans D. Relapsed club foot. J Bone Joint Surg 1961;43B:722.

6.2 Excision of Calcaneonavicular Coalition

In 1967 Mitchell and Gibson[1] reported on excision of calcaneonavicular bars that remain symptomatic after conservative treatment as an alternative to the usual treatment of triple arthrodesis. A subsequent report by Cowell[2] in this country in 1970 helped to popularize this approach, and following reports have validated the success of this operation.[3–5] Between 80% to 90% of patients who have excision can expect an acceptable result. Talar beaking has been felt by some to represent arthritis of the talonavicular joint and thus a contraindication to this surgery. It has been pointed out that this change is actually extra-articular, however, and probably due to the excessive motion at this joint, producing traction on the ligaments. It would appear from the reported results that this is not a contraindication to this procedure.

Figure 6–19. The calcaneonavicular bar is approached through the Ollier incision on the lateral side of the foot. The incision should extend from the extensor tendons to the peroneal tendons in a skin crease over the coalition ***(Figure 6–19A)***. It is important that the initial incision be made through the entire layer of skin, subcutaneous tissue, and fascia overlying the extensor brevis muscle without undermining the wound edges. This is very thin skin that must be handled with care.

After the fascia of the extensor brevis muscle is opened, it is elevated proximally off of the muscle itself. This will lead to the fibrofatty tissue in the sinus tarsi. It is not necessary to remove all of this tissue, but only the most distal portion that covers the distal surface of the calcaneus and talus. After exposing the origin of the extensor brevis muscle, an incision is made into this fibrofatty tissue. This incision is made very deep into the depth of the sinus tarsi. This portion of the fibrofatty tissue and the extensor brevis muscle are then dissected distally as a unit exposing the distal talus and calcaneus, the bar connecting the distal end of the calcaneus and the navicular, and the proximal portion of the cuboid ***(Figure 6–19B)***.

Figure 6–20. A hemostat can be put on the fibrofatty tissue to retract it and the extensor brevis muscle out of the way without damaging the muscle that will be used later to fill the area where the bar is excised. At this point the anatomy should be easily visualized, showing the coalition. An understanding of the normal anatomy is important at this point in planning the excision. If too much is excised, the joints will be violated. If too little is excised, motion will not be restored, and the bar may reform. The commonest error is to excise too little bone from the medial side of the bar. It is important that the piece of bone excised be trapezoidal and not triangular. A $\frac{1}{4}$-in straight osteotome is used to excise the bar. Good exposure of the sinus tarsi in its depths where the calcaneus and the talus are in close approximation will aid in directing the osteotome in the correct direction.

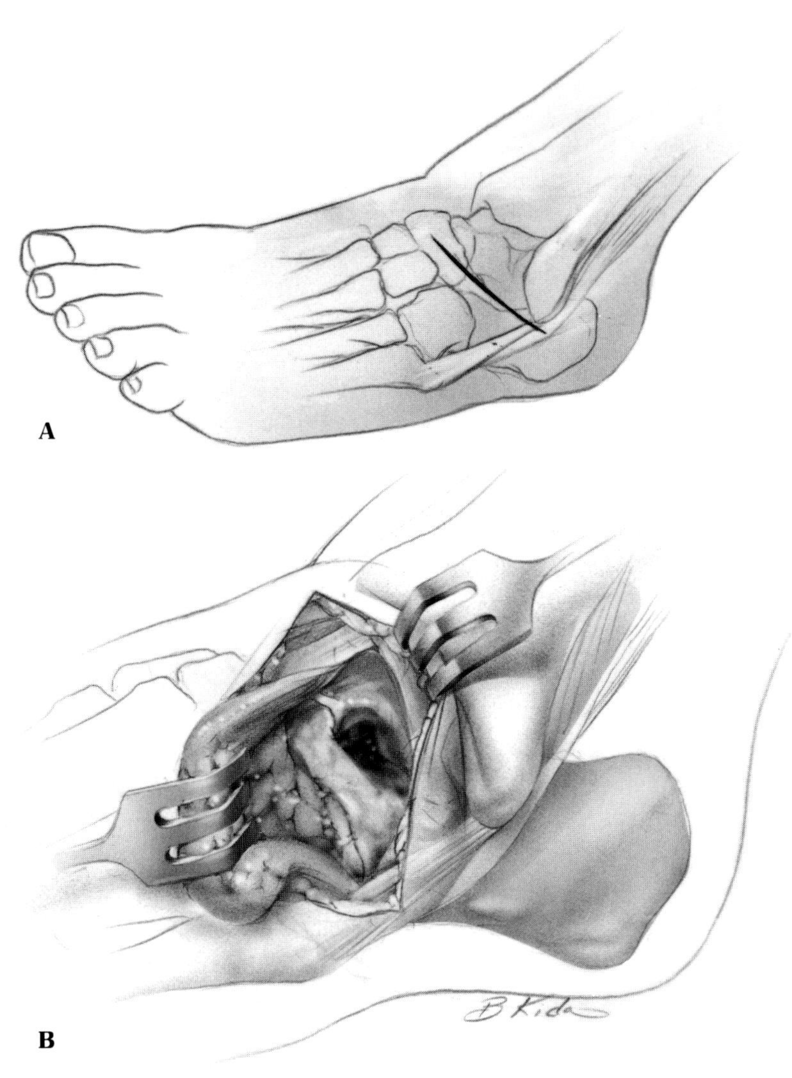

Figure 6–19

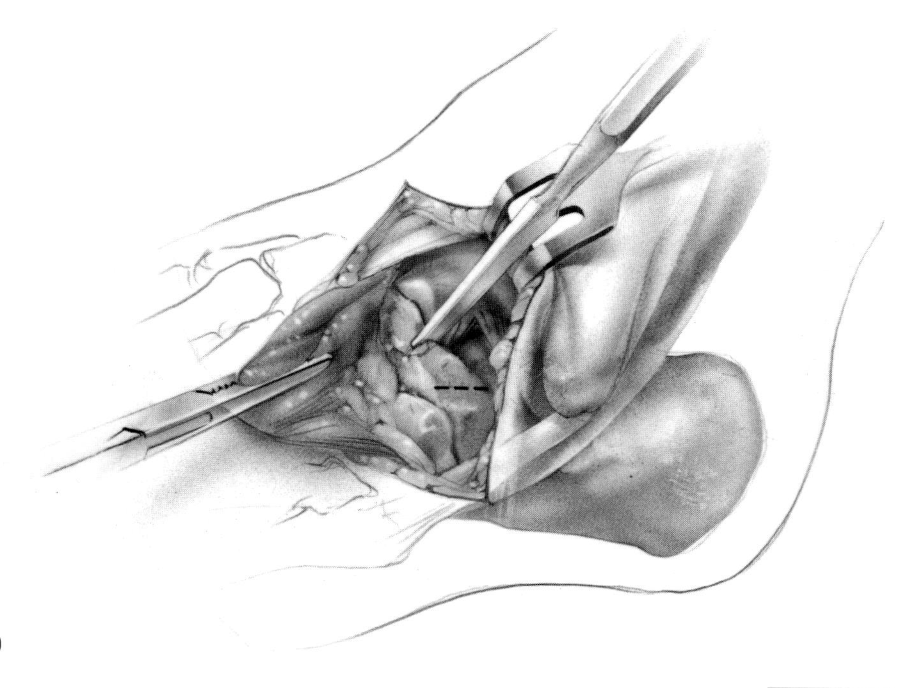

Figure 6–20

Figure 6–21. After the bar is excised, the surgeon should be able to visualize a distinct gap separating the anterior aspect of the calcaneus and the navicular. In addition, examination of the foot should confirm that subtalar motion is restored. It should now be possible to displace the origin of the extensor brevis muscle into this gap between the calcaneus and the navicular that was created by removal of the bar. The excess of fibrofatty tissue that is not needed can be cut off and discarded.

A heavy absorbable suture is threaded through the end of the extensor brevis muscle, and a long, heavy, straight Keith needle is threaded onto each end of the suture.

Figure 6–22. The two straight Keith needles are passed through the gap that was left by the excision of the bar and out through the skin on the medial side of the foot. As the needles emerge, they are passed through a small piece of sterile felt and a sterile button.

A forceps is used to guide the muscle deep into the defect while the suture is pulled through and tied over the button on the medial side of the foot. This should result in the muscle being interposed between the cut ends of the calcaneus and navicular.

The wound is closed with interupted absorbable sutures in the deep layer of muscle fascia and subcutaneous tissue that was carefully preserved at the beginning of the operation. The skin is closed with care to evert the skin edges. A short leg cast is applied.

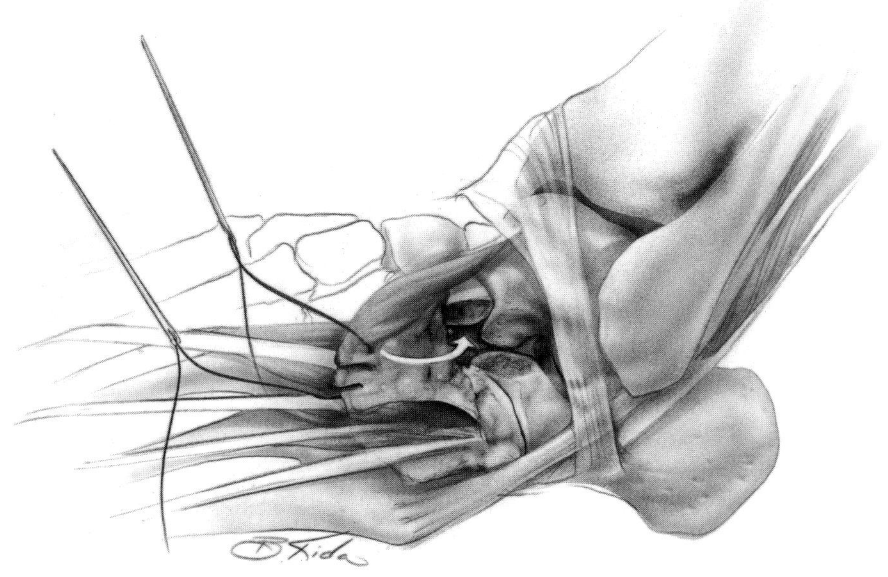

Figure 6–21

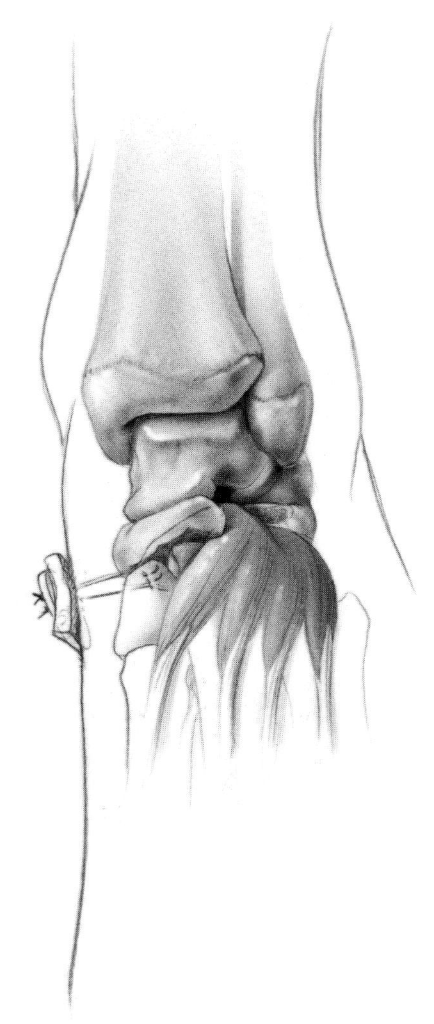

Figure 6–22

Figure 6–23. Oblique radiograph of the foot of a 10-year-old girl with 1 year of foot pain demonstrates an incomplete calcaneonavicular coalition (***Figure 6–23A***). Note the incomplete coalition in the opposite asymptomatic right foot (***Figure 6–23B***). One year after resection of the coalition, no reformation of the bar has occurred (***Figure 6–23C***).

POSTOPERATIVE CARE

Cowell has recommended removal of the cast at 10 days at which time exercises are begun to increase the range of motion in the subtalar joint. Weight-bearing is not permitted until subtalar motion equal to that noted in the operating room is regained. The author has chosen to treat these patients in a short leg walking cast for 3 weeks. When the cast is removed, the patients are shown exercises to increase the subtalar motion and are progressed from a partial weight-bearing crutch gait to full weight-bearing as their symptoms dictate—usually 3 to 4 weeks. If the suture has not broken at the time of cast removal, it is cut flush with the skin, and the felt pad and the button are removed.

REFERENCES

1. Mitchell GP, Gibson JMC. Excision of calcaneo-navicular bar for painful spasmodic flat foot. J Bone Joint Surg 1967;49B:281.
2. Cowell HR. Extensor brevis arthroplasty. J Bone Joint Surg 1970;52A:820.
3. Chambers RB, Cook TM, Cowell HR. Surgical reconstruction for calcaneonavicular coalition: evaluation of function and gait. J Bone Joint Surg 1982;64A:829.
4. Swiontkowski MF, Scranton PE, Hansen S. Tarsal coalitions: long-term results of surgical treatment. J Pediatr Orthop 1983;3:287.
5. Inglis G, Buxton RA, Macniclo MF. Symptomatic calcaneonavicular bars: the results 20 years after surgical excision. J Bone Joint Surg 1986;68B:128.

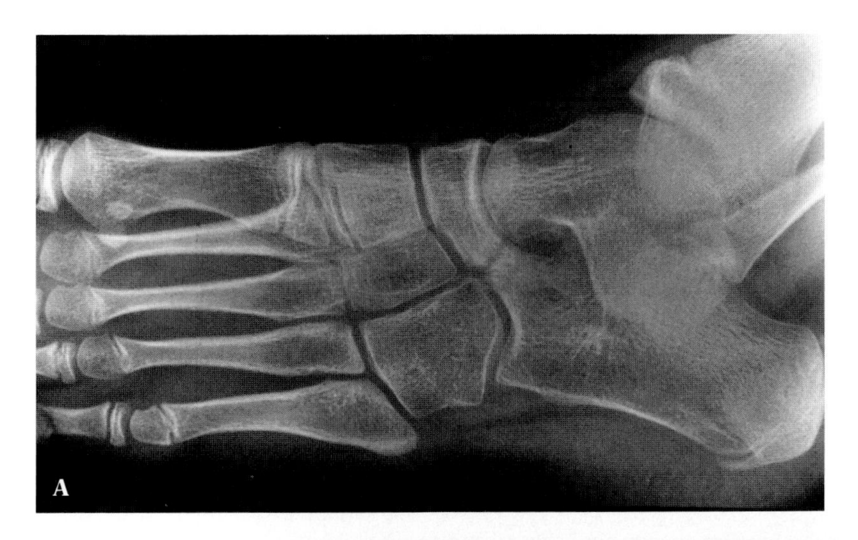

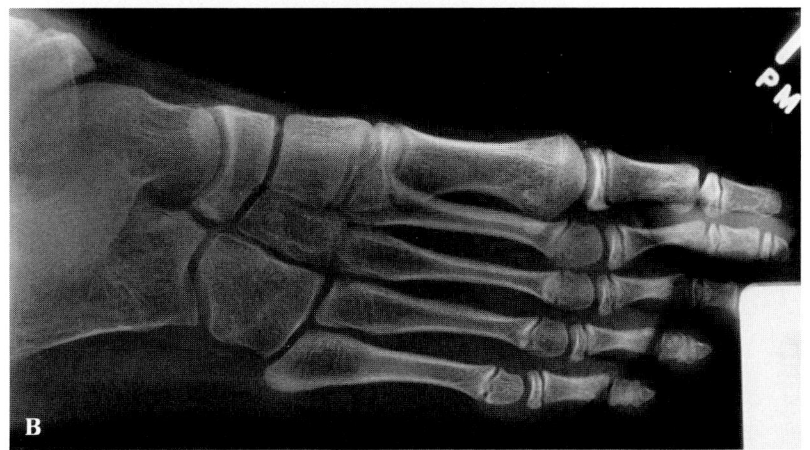

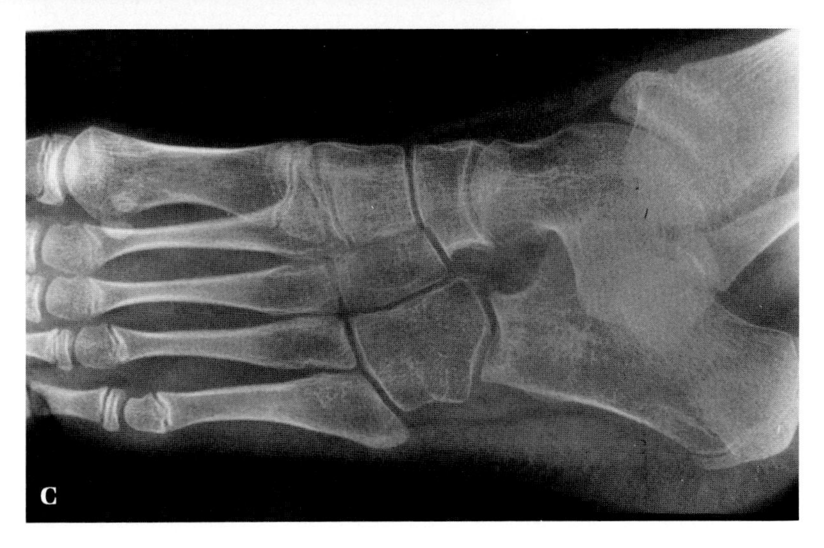

Figure 6–23

6.3
Excision of Talocalcaneal Coalition

Until recently, excision of persistently symptomatic talocalcaneal coalition has not been popular because of the uncertainty of a successful outcome.[1–3] More recently, however, two reports have documented greater success with excision of talocalcaneal coalition.[4,5] This may be due in part to the use of computed tomographic scanning to determine the extent of joint involvement before undertaking surgical excision. Exactly how much of the joint can be involved and a successful result achieved is not known. Scranton[4] recommends that excision not be undertaken if more than 50% of the joint is involved.

Figure 6–24. A slightly curved incision approximately 6 to 7 cm in length is made over the sustenaculum tali following the course of the flexor digitorum longus tendon (***Figure 6–24A***). The incision should extend from the prominence of the navicular to the area posterior to the posterior facet of the subtalar joint. If muscle fibers of the abductor hallucis are encountered, they are reflected plantarward. The flexor retinaculum, which overlies the sustentaculum tali, must be opened to allow the flexor digitorum longus tendon along with the neurovascular bundle to be retracted plantarward. The flexor hallucis longus tendon, which runs just beneath the sustentaculum tali, can also be retracted out of the way. The posterior tibial tendon can be identified running above the sustenaculum tali.

At this point the coalition will still not be apparent as it lies beneath the periosteum and the sheath of the flexor digitorum longus (***Figure 6–24B***).

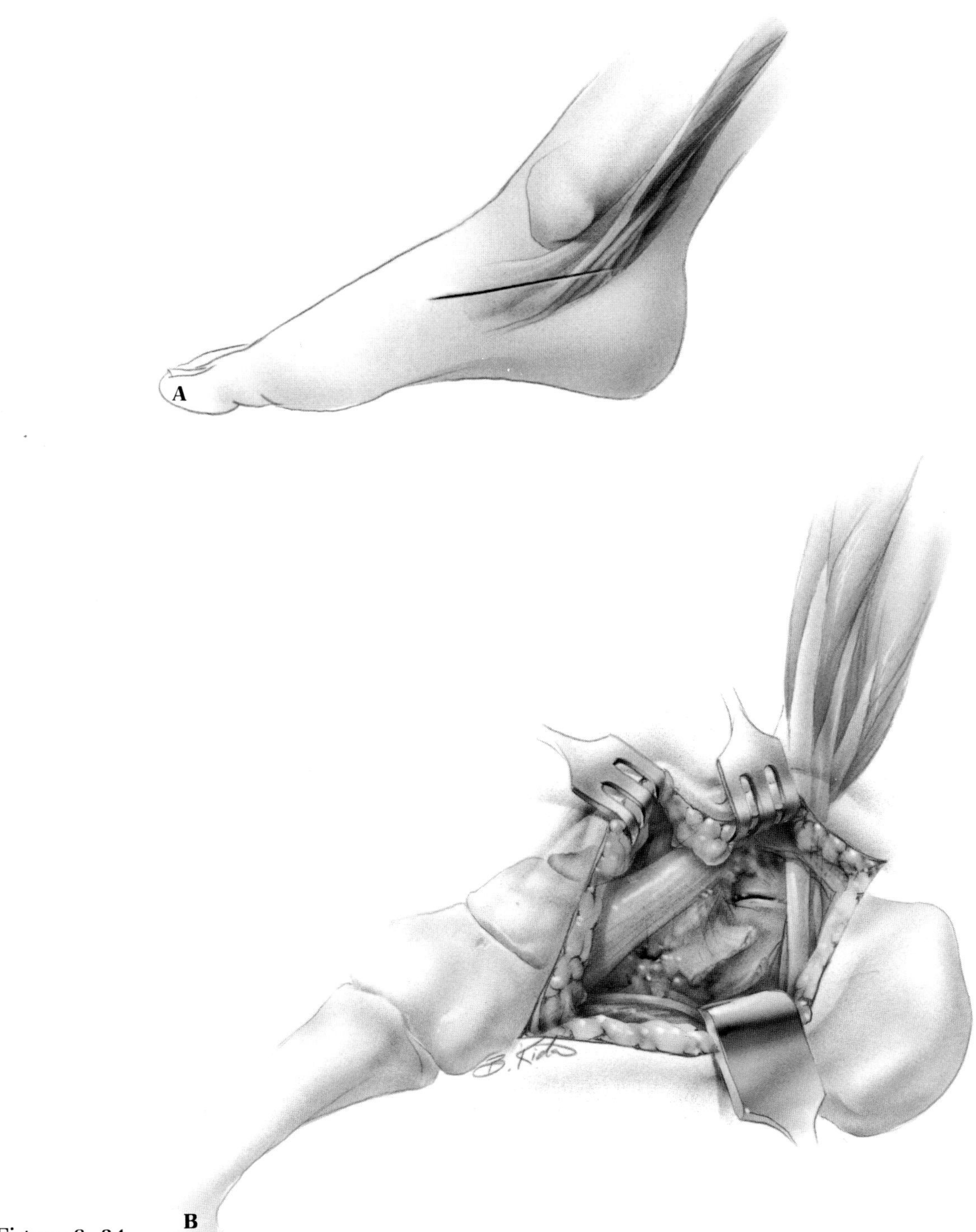

Figure 6–24

Figure 6–25. To expose the coalition and define its anterior and posterior boundaries, an incision is made in the periosteum slightly to the dorsal side of the prominence, which is the sustentaculum tali and the middle facet coalition. The periosteum, including the sheath of the flexor digitorum longus tendon, is elevated off of the bony prominence and reflected volar. This should be done with care for although this periosteum is often very thin, it will be necessary to approximate it later to hold the fat graft in place. This dissection should be carried far enough anteriorly and posteriorly to identify normal joint space. The medial aspect of the coalition and its anterior and posterior boundaries are now identified. The lateral extent of the coalition can be judged from the preoperative CT scans. It is a good idea at this point to test the motion of the subtalar joint. Some slight motion may be observed in the normal parts of the joint that are exposed. This will be useful for comparison after excision of the coalition.

Figure 6–26. To begin the excision of the coalition and preserve as much of the sustentaculum as possible, it is helpful to define the exact location of the coalition within the bony mass. To accomplish this a small osteotome can be used to shave off thin layers of bone until the fibrous or cartilaginous coalition is identified. This is only possible when the coalition is not completely ossified. If it is completely ossified, its removal can be guided by the normal joint surfaces distal and proximal.

Using a small rongeur or a power burr, the coalition is excised. The excision should not be unnecessarily wide and as much of the sustentaculum tali as possible should be preserved. The removal of bone is continued until joint cartilage is visualized anterior, posterior, and in the lateral depths of the excision. At this point subtalar motion should be markedly improved.

Figure 6–27. The final step is to interpose fat between the two bony surfaces. This can most easily be obtained from the area on the dorsal surface of the calcaneus between the posterior facet and the Achilles tendon. This is the reason for the posterior aspect of the incision.

A small amount of fibrofatty tissue is excised from this area. The bony surfaces can be sealed with bone wax to lessen the bleeding that might tend to displace the fat graft. The fat is carefully pushed into the defect created by the excision with care to be sure that it reaches the depth of the excision. It is held in place by approximating the periosteum with small sutures.

The tendons can now be returned to their sheath, which can be approximated with fine absorbable sutures. The subcutaneous tissue and the skin is closed, and a short leg cast is applied.

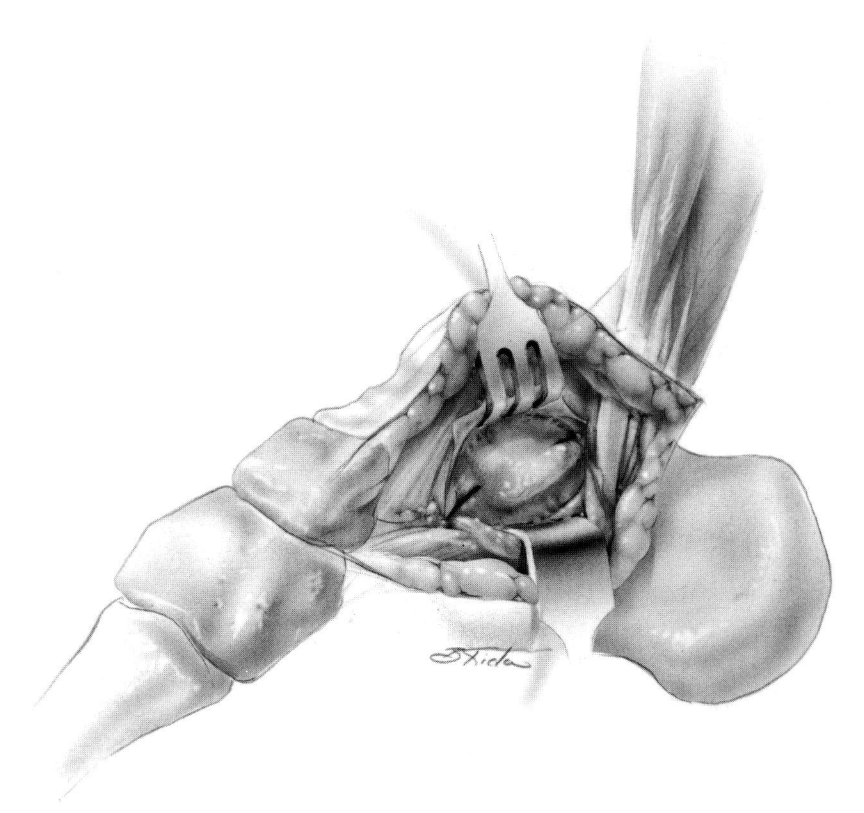

Figure 6–25

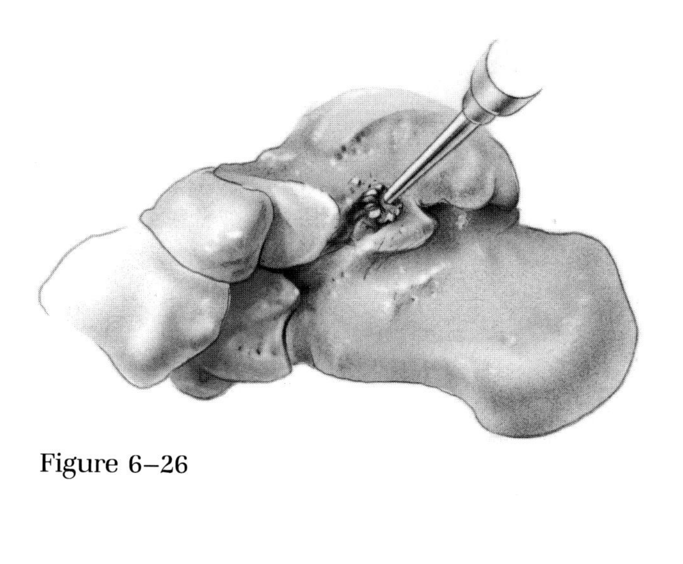

Figure 6–26

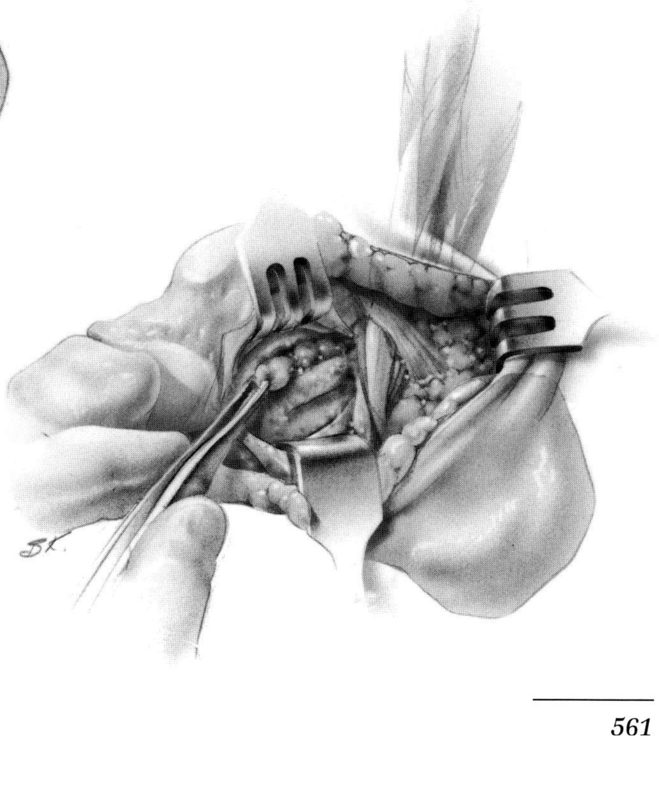

Figure 6–27

POSTOPERATIVE CARE

The patient remains non–weight-bearing for 3 weeks to avoid extrusion of the graft. At that time the cast is removed and the patient is started on a three-point, partial weight-bearing, crutch gait for an additional 3 weeks. Exercises to increase the range of motion of the ankle and subtalar joints can be taught.

REFERENCES

1. Hark FW. Congenital anomalies of the tarsal bones. Clin Orthop 1960;16:21.
2. Jayakumar S, Cowell HR. Rigid flatfoot. Clin Orthop 1977;122:77.
3. Swiontkowski MF, Scranton PE, Hansen S. Tarsal coalitions: long-term results of surgical treatment. J Pediatr Orthop 1983;3:287.
4. Scranton PE Jr. Treatment of symptomatic talocalcaneal coalition. J Bone Joint Surg 1987;69A:533.
5. Olney BW, Asher MA. Excision of symptomatic coalition of the middle facet of the talocalcaneal joint. J Bone Joint Surg 1987;69A:539.

6.4
Osteotomy of Calcaneus for Valgus

Numerous osteotomies of the calcaneus to correct heel valgus have been described. The most popular until recently was the osteotomy described by Dwyer.[1,2] Wound problems resulting from the opening wedge and collapse of the graft have limited the use of this procedure, however. These potential problems are solved, and the same goals achieved by the medial displacement osteotomy of the calcaneus. The operation was first described by Koutsogiannis but attributed to Pridie of Bristol, England.[3]

Figure 6–28. A straight incision is made over the lateral side of the calcaneus. The incision is posteroinferior to the peroneal tendons. It should be long enough to allow exposure of the inferior and dorsal surface of the calcaneus, which actually means that it does not have to be very long. It is important to avoid damage to the sural nerve, which will run slightly inferior to the peroneal tendons.

Figure 6–29. The incision should reach the periosteum of the calcaneus with a minimum of undermining. It should be possible to slide a small retractor (*eg*, a Homann or Chandler retractor) over both the dorsal surface of the calcaneus anterior to the Achilles tendon and under the plantar aspect of the calcaneus. A straight incision is made in the periosteum, and it is elevated for about 5 mm on each side of the incision. The capsule of the posterior facet of the subtalar joint should be visualized but not disturbed. This will ensure that the osteotomy is far enough distal to prevent creation of too small a fragment of the calcaneus.

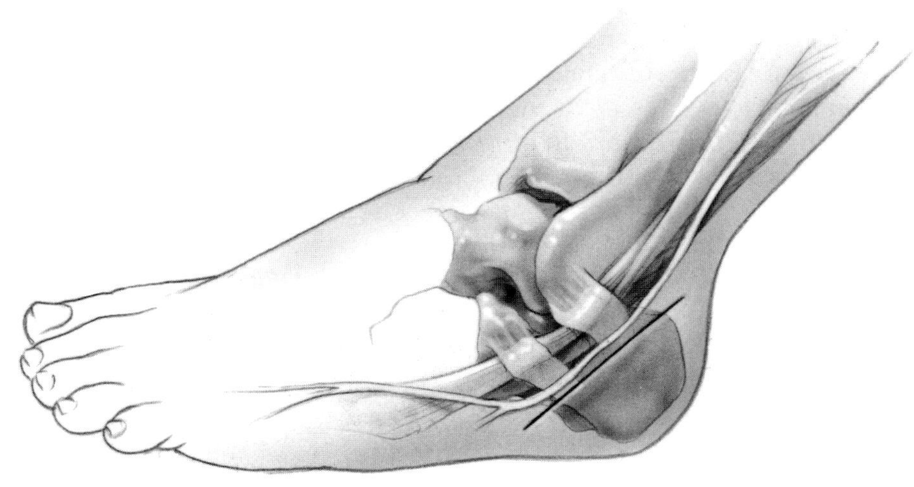

Figure 6–28

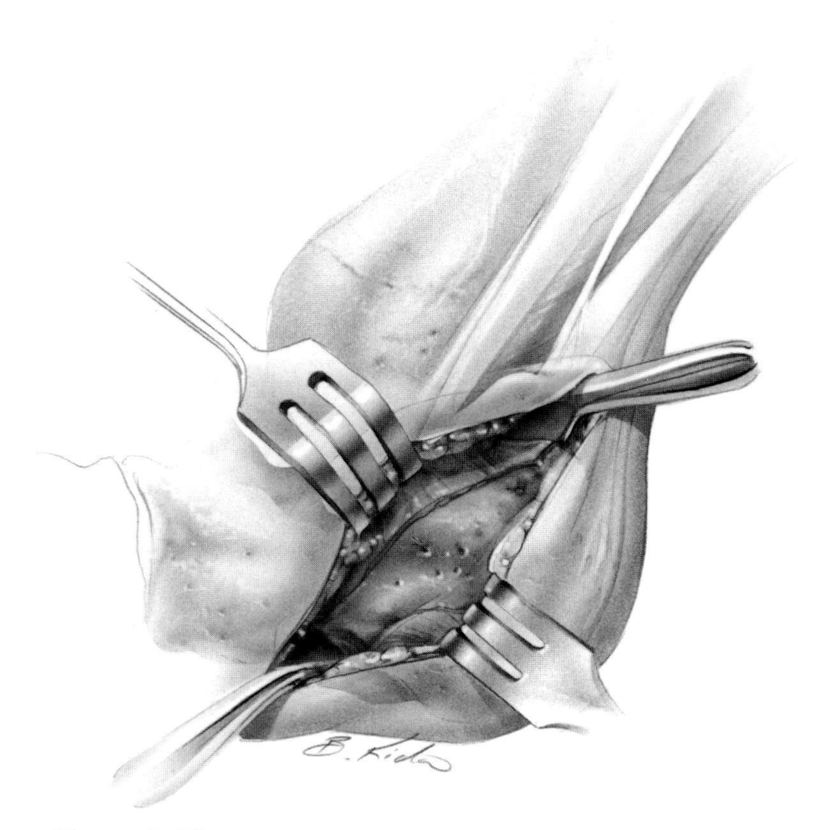

Figure 6–29

Figure 6–30. A broad 1.5-in osteotome or chisel is used to make the osteotomy. The placement and direction of the osteotomy is important. The osteotomy should remain about 1 cm beneath the capsule of the posterior facet of the subtalar joint. The osteotome should be positioned obliquely, parallel with the posterior facet of the subtalar joint (***Figure 6–30A***). As the osteotome is driven across the calcaneus it should remain in the transverse plane or angle slightly toward the subtalar joint (***Figure 6–30B***). If it angles away from the subtalar joint, the fragment will tend to bind as it is displaced, making displacement much more difficult (***Figure 6–30C***). This is analogous to the 10-degree cephalad slope that is used in the Chiari pelvic osteotomy.

Caution must be used in completing the osteotomy through the medial cortex because of the proximity of the posterior tibial vessels and nerve. It is wise to be certain the inferior and superior cortex of the calcaneus are divided first. Then divide the most plantar aspect of the medial cortex and proceed toward the dorsal aspect, which is where the neurovascular bundle is separated from the periosteum only by a thin fascial layer. While dividing the medial cortex, be certain that there is no pressure behind the lateral malleolus that would hold the neurovascular structures against the bone.

Figure 6–31. The large weight-bearing portion of the calcaneus can now be displaced. It is usually necessary to displace it at least one half of the width of the calcaneus. At first this will not seem possible, but with a little perseverance it can be accomplished. A broad stout osteotome or periosteal elevator can be inserted to pry the two fragments apart (***Figure 6–31A***). This will tend to tear the periosteum and separate it from the medial cortex. Strong repeated manipulation of the fragment will also tend to separate the periosteum by stripping it from the bone (***Figure 6–31B***). Since the Achilles tendon and plantar fascia will tend to hold the fragments together when taught, the foot should be held in plantar flexion for all of the manipulations. If a very large amount of displacement is needed, it may be necessary to divide the periosteum. A small lamina retractor can be used to separate the fragments and provide better access while at the same time stretching the medial periosteum taught. Because of the proximity of the neurovascular bundle, the author uses an osteotome for this rather than a sharp knife. Finally, the long plantar ligament can be divided in a similar fashion.

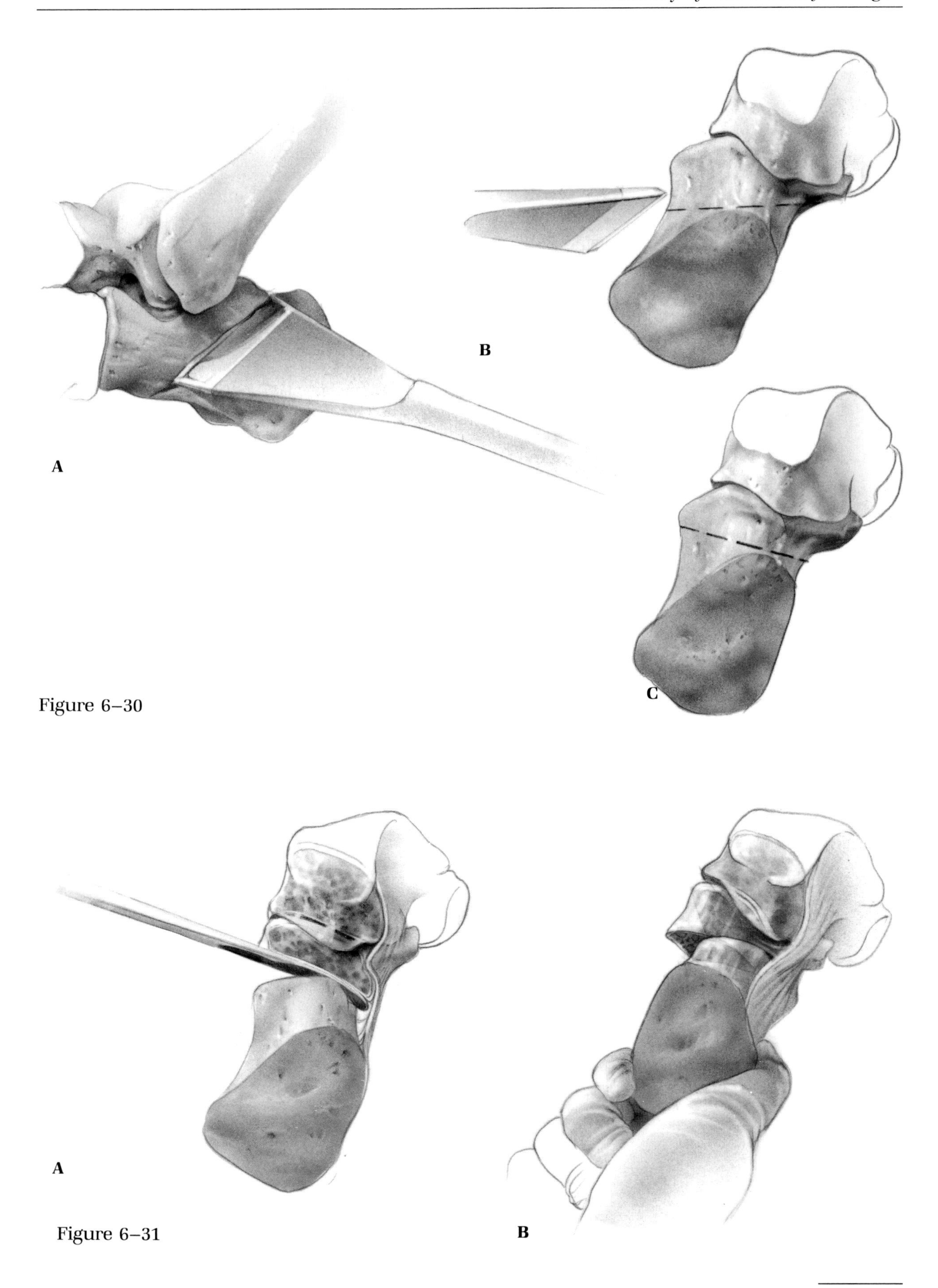

Figure 6–30

Figure 6–31

Figure 6–32. The foot is plantarflexed and the loose fragment of calcaneus is pushed medially. Be certain that it does not displace dorsally. The foot is then dorsiflexed to push the osteotomy surfaces together and maintain the displacement.

To be certain that the displacement is maintained a heavy, smooth, Steinmann pin is drilled from the posterior aspect of the calcaneus distally across the osteotomy site. The pin is cut off, leaving enough protruding through the skin so that it can be easily removed in the office.

It will not be possible to close the periosteum. The deep fascia and the skin are closed with interrupted sutures with care not to damage the sural nerve, and a short leg cast is applied. The portion of the Steinmann pin that protrudes should be well padded in cast padding apart from that used for the foot. This will prevent its being bound to the cast with resulting excessive motion at the pin-skin interface as the foot moves.

Figure 6–33. Preoperative lateral radiograph of the foot of a 13-year-old girl with severe painful flat feet is shown (***Figure 6–33A***). Because of her inability to wear orthotics with her usual shoe wear and only moderate relief with orthotics, she requested surgical correction. The immediate postoperative radiograph demonstrates the pin holding the displacement (***Figure 6–33B***). A larger pin could have been used, and it could have been inserted further. The pin was withdrawn at 2 weeks and the cast changed. The healing is complete at 6 weeks (***Figure 6–33C***).

POSTOPERATIVE CARE

The patient is non–weight-bearing on the operated foot for 2 weeks. Then the cast is removed in the office, and the pin is removed from the bone. A short leg walking cast is applied for 4 weeks while the patient gradually resumes full weight-bearing as tolerated. Six weeks after surgery there should be radiographic evidence of complete healing, and immobilization is discontinued.

REFERENCES

1. Dwyer FC. Osteotomy of the calcaneum in the treatment of grossly everted feet with special reference to cerebral palsy. In: Huitieme congres internationale de chirugie orthopedique. New York, September 4–9, 1960. Societe Internationale de Chirugie Orthopedique et de Traumatologie. Brussels: Imprimerie des Sciences, 1960:892.
2. Dwyer FC. Treatment of relapsed club foot by insertion of a wedge into the calcaneum. J Bone Joint Surg 1963;45B:67.
3. Koutsogiannis E. Treatment of mobile flat foot by displacement osteotomy of the calcaneus. J Bone Joint Surg 1971;53B:96.

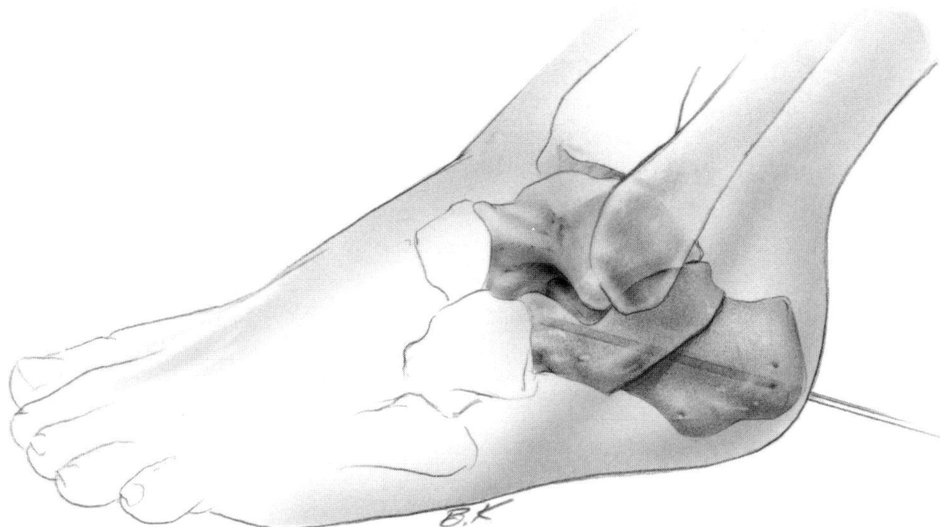

Figure 6–32

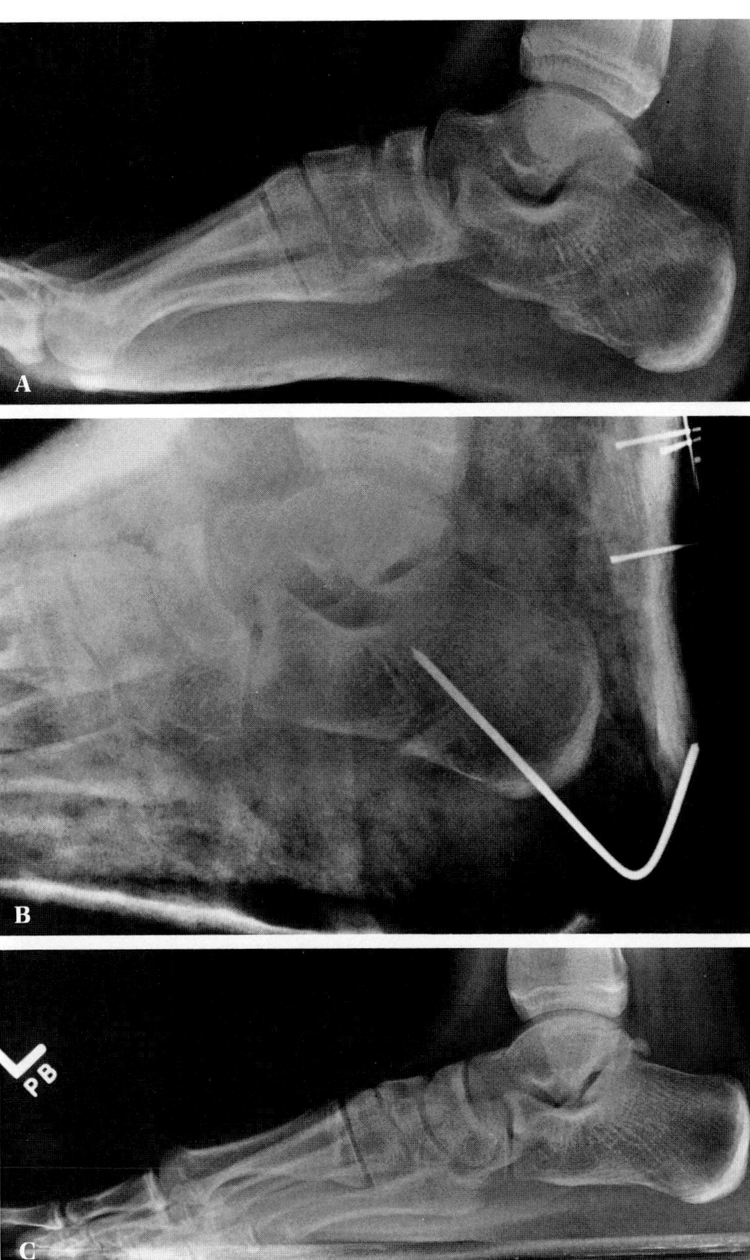

Figure 6–33

6.5 Plantar Release and Metatarsal Osteotomy for Cavus Foot

Although correction of cavus deformity of the foot was common in the treatment of patients with the residuals of poliomyelitis, it is now a much less common procedure. Today cavus deformity of the foot is usually seen as the result of a variety of conditions: degenerative neurologic diseases with Charcot-Marie-Tooth disease being the most common, relapsed club foot, traumatic neurologic injury, or idiopathic cavus foot. In addition to consideration of muscle imbalance, possible progression, and other factors related to the etiology, the most important factor in deciding the treatment is the components of the deformity and their rigidity.

The operation described here is the procedure that the author finds indicated most often in the treatment of cavus deformity. Its successful application assumes one very important factor. The hindfoot must be flexible. It must not have a fixed varus deformity. The calcaneus must be able to move to neutral or preferably beyond into valgus. Most cavus feet will appear to have a varus deformity in stance. This may be due to a depressed first metatarsal that creates what might best be described as a fixed pronation of the forefoot. In stance the first and fifth metatarsal heads can contact the floor only if the heel is in varus. The flexibility of the heel (*ie,* its ability to move into valgus) can be demonstrated by what has come to be called the Coleman block test.[1,2]

Although percutaneous division of the plantar fascia has often been recommended, this will not be sufficient for most feet with significant cavus deformity. In most feet it will be necessary to release not only the plantar fascia but also the origin of the intrinsic muscles of the foot from the calcaneus and the plantar ligaments. Although many different approaches have been recommended, the most versatile is the plantar dissection described by Bost, Schottstaedt, and Larsen.[3] An osteotomy of the first metatarsal can be accomplished through a distal extension of the incision.

Figure 6–34. A curvilinear incision is made along the medial side of the foot from the midportion of the first metatarsal to the posterior tuberosity of the calcaneus (***Figure 6–34A***). This incision should be placed just dorsal to the plantar skin, which is usually distinguishable from the thinner skin that covers the dorsum of the foot. The incision is carried directly through the skin and subcutaneous tissue without undermining until the belly of the abductor hallucis muscle is encountered. The dorsal flap of skin and subcutaneous tissue is then elevated to expose the dorsal edge of the abductor hallucis muscle.

The dorsal edge of this muscle is then detached by sharp dissection and reflected plantarward (***Figure 6–34A***). It is important to carry the detachment far enough posterior so that the origin of the abductor hallucis muscle is detached from the medial tuberosity of the calcaneus. Care should be taken here not to cut carelessly too deeply to avoid damage to the neurovascular bundle. After this muscle is completely reflected, all of the structures of the foot that are to be divided lie shrouded beneath the deep fascia.

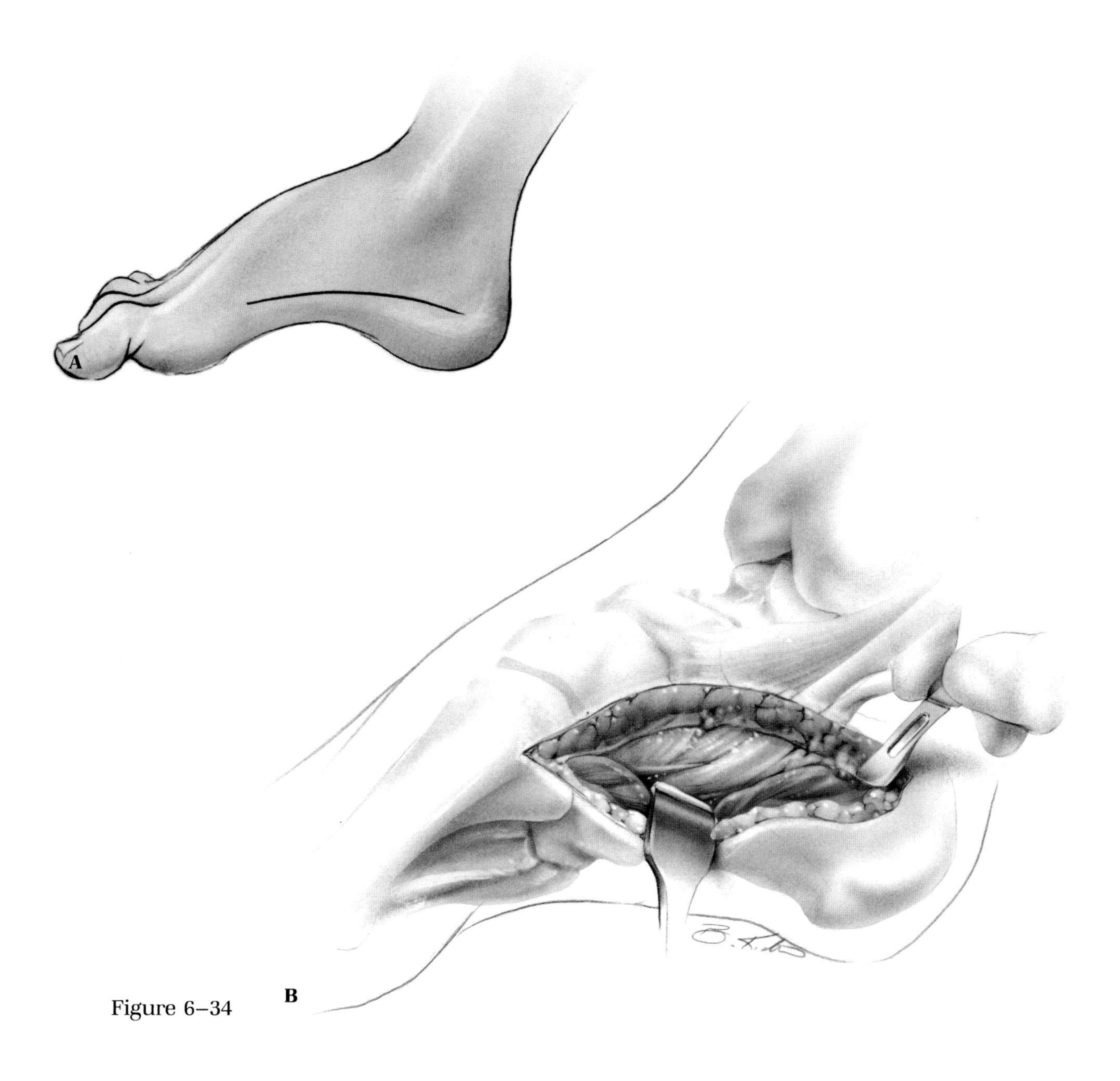

Figure 6–34

Figure 6–35. The structures that are to be protected are dissected free in the following order. First the flexor digitorum longus is identified just posterior to the tip of the medial malleolus. A small transverse incision in this region will enter the sheath of both the flexor digitorum longus and the posterior tibial tendon, which lies just anterior to it. The sheath of the flexor digitorum longus is opened distally, cutting the master knot of Henry and allowing this tendon to be retracted out of the way.

Next the neurovascular bundle is located posterior to the flexor digitorum longus. The posterior tibial nerve is dissected until its bifurcation into the medial and lateral plantar branch is identified. The lateral plantar branch will come off of the posterior tibial nerve and run laterally toward the plantar aspect of the foot. If this lateral plantar branch is not identified, it may inadvertently be cut. The medial plantar branch (on the forceps), and the posterior tibial artery and its accompanying veins are dissected distally so that they too may be retracted along with the flexor digitorum longus. At this point additional muscle attachments to the medial tuberosity of the calcaneus may be divided under direct vision. Also note the tendon of the flexor hallucis longus running under the tendon of the flexor digitorum longus. This tendon will also be released when the master knot of Henry is divided. With all of these structures identified and retracted out of the way, a plane on the dorsal surface of all of the muscles inserting into the calcaneus can be developed by blunt dissection.

Figure 6–36. A plane is now developed between the plantar fascia and the subcutaneous skin of the heel pad. This must extend from the medial to the lateral side of the foot.

Figure 6–37. With the medial and lateral plantar nerves retracted distally and dorsally, a heavy scissors can now be used to divide all of the large muscle originating from the medial and plantar surface of the calcaneus. This will include the abductor hallucis, the flexor digitorum brevis, the abductor digiti minimi, and the quadratus plantae (flexor accessorius). One blade of the scissors is passed in the plane that was developed between the plantar fascia and skin, and the other blade is passed over the dorsal surface of the muscles in the interval posterior to the retracted artery, nerves, and tendons. The surgeon should feel the blades of the scissors near the lateral skin. After these structures are divided a finger can be passed into the gap to be sure that no tight attachments are left.

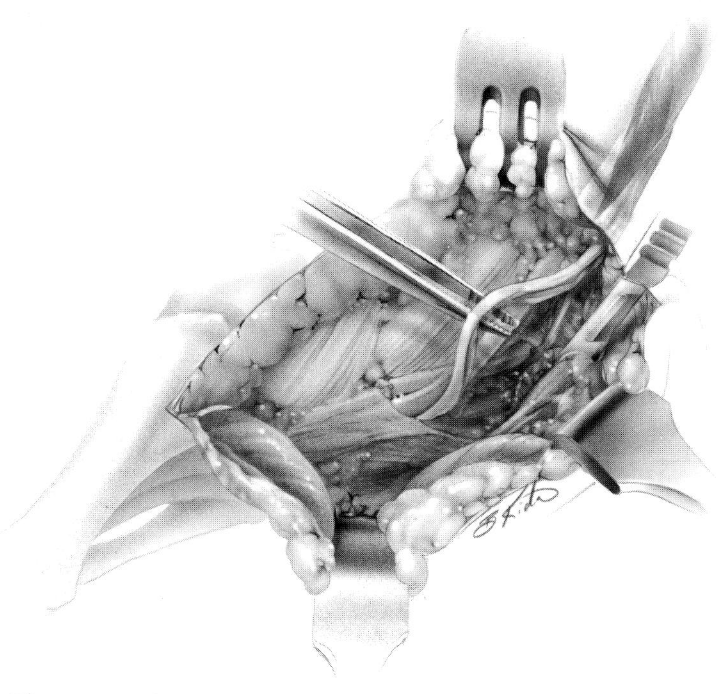

Figure 6–35

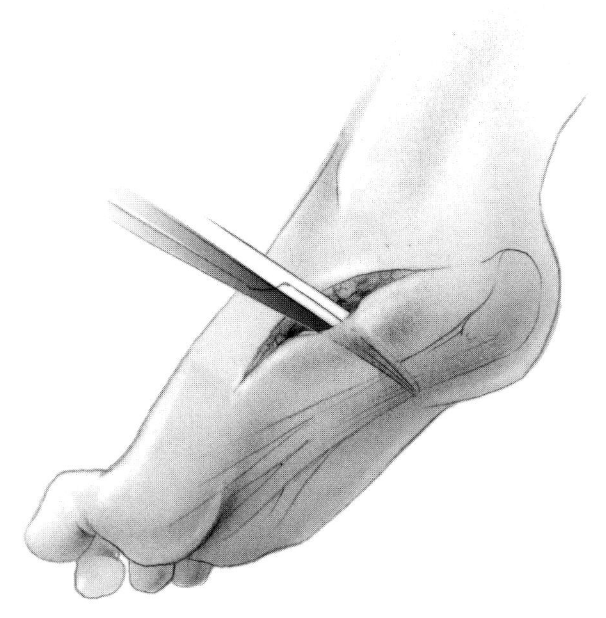

Figure 6–36

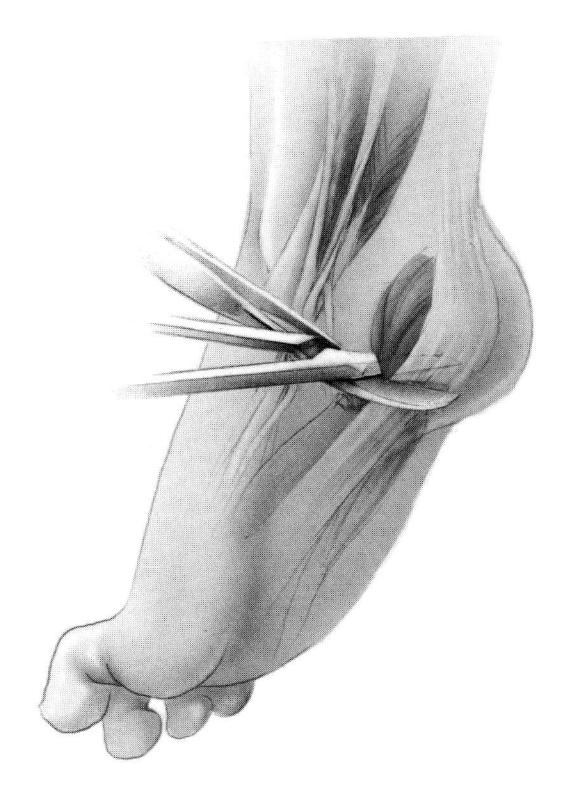

Figure 6–37

Figure 6–38. A broad periosteal elevator is used to dissect this mass off of the bone. This should be done extraperiosteally. Care should be taken to be sure that the long plantar ligament is not missed. It may be necessary to divide this with a knife. Through this extensive exposure the calcaneocuboid ligament and the calcaneonavicular ligament may also be divided. This is most easily achieved by opening the volar capsules of these joints.

Figure 6–39. The proximal portion of the first metatarsal is exposed in the distal aspect of the incision. The periosteum is incised on the dorsomedial aspect of the bone, and the proximal portion is exposed subperiosteally. Two small Homann retractors are placed to protect the soft tissues.

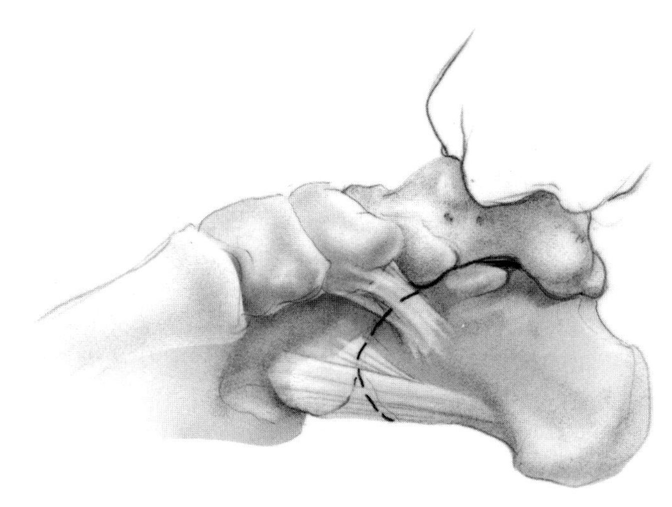

Figure 6–38

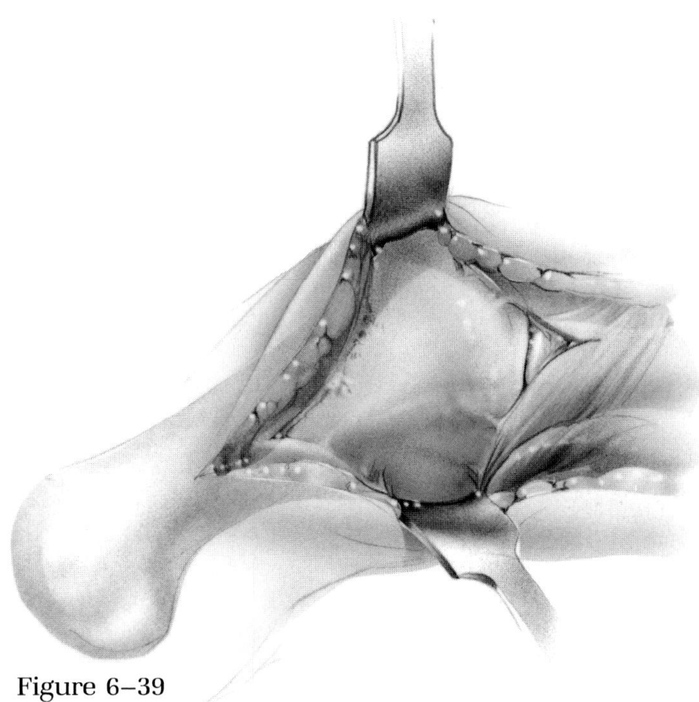

Figure 6–39

Figure 6–40. A dome-shaped osteotomy is then made so that the distal fragment can be rotated dorsally. This may be done with a special saw that is designed to make crescentic cuts or by connecting properly placed drill holes with an osteotome. The dorsal corner of the distal fragment is removed so that rotation of the distal fragment is not obstructed (***Figure 6–40B***). When the desired position is achieved, it can be fixed with a smooth Kirschner wire that is left protruding through the skin for easy removal when healing is complete. Before closure a small suction drain is placed throughout the length of the wound. A short leg cast is applied with the foot in the position of correction that can be obtained without great force.

Figure 6–41. Preoperative standing lateral radiograph of a 15-year-old boy with bilateral cavus feet resulting from Charcot-Marie-Tooth disease is shown (***Figure 6–41A***). His heel would correct into valgus. Six weeks after plantar release and first metatarsal osteotomy, there is sufficient healing of the osteotomy to allow weight-bearing (***Figure 6–41B***).

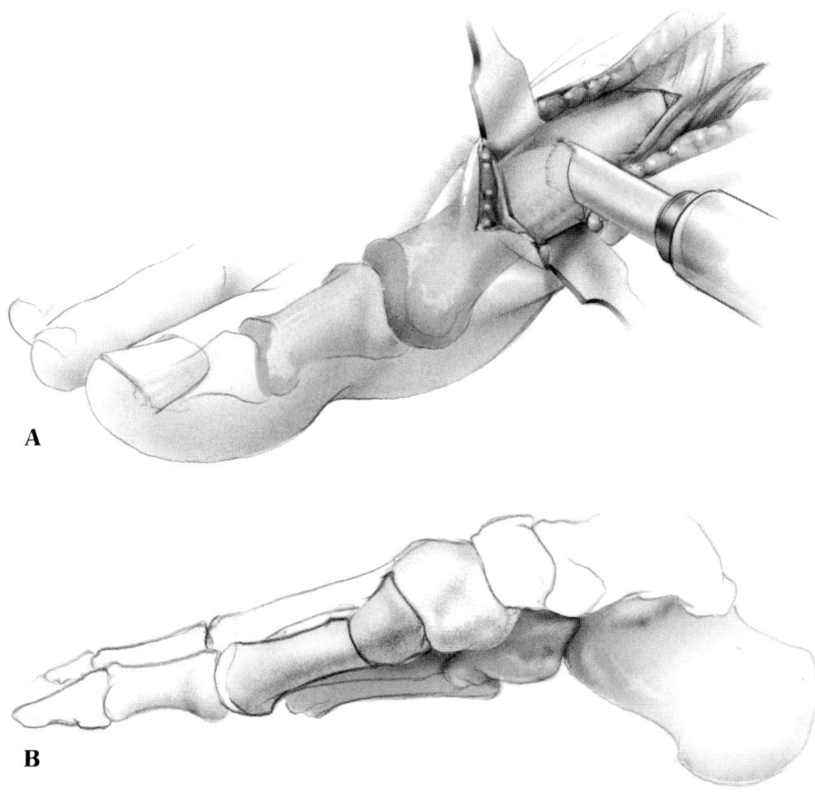

Figure 6–40

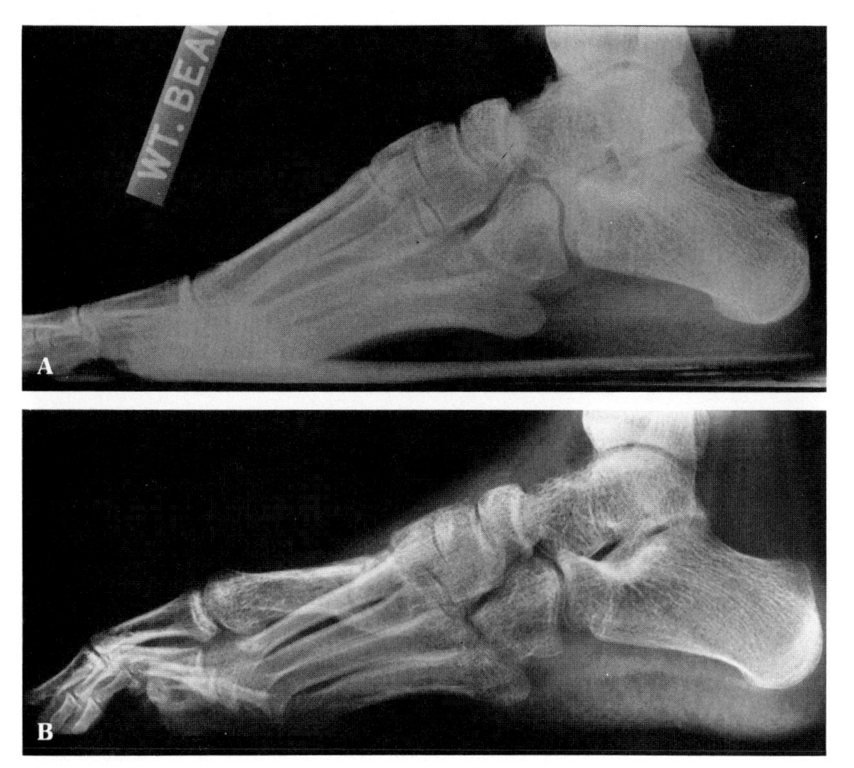

Figure 6–41

POSTOPERATIVE CARE

If full correction is not obtained at the time of surgery (which is usual) plans should be made to change the cast periodically during the first 6 weeks to obtain further correction. Correction of the cavus should not put any stress on a properly placed incision. Care should be taken not to push up on the first metatarsal if an osteotomy has been performed. Weight-bearing can begin as soon as tolerated if no osteotomy has been performed or at 6 weeks if it has. The wire fixing the osteotomy should be removed before weight-bearing. If required, tendon transfers may be done at the same time as the plantar release. If lengthening of the Achilles tendon is required, however, this should wait 6 weeks or until the cavus is maximally corrected. If the Achilles tendon is lengthened at the same time, it will not be possible to apply a corrective force to the plantar structures.

REFERENCES

1. Coleman SS, Chestnut WJ. A simple test for hindfoot flexibility in the cavovarus foot. Clin Orthop 1977;123:60.
2. Meehan PL. The cavus foot. In: Morrissy RT, ed. Lovell and Winter's Pediatric Orthopaedics, 3rd ed. Philadelphia: JB Lippincott, 1989:973.
3. Bost FC, Schottstaedt ER, Larsen LJ. Plantar dissection: an operation to release the soft tissues in recurrent or recalcitrant talipes equinovarus. J Bone Joint Surg 1960;42A:151.

6.6
Midfoot Osteotomy for Cavus Deformity

Removal of a dorsally based wedge from the tarsal bones to correct a fixed cavus deformity with its apex in the midfoot was described by Cole.[1] It is best used only when the problem is bilateral because it shortens the foot. This disadvantage is offset by preservation of the metatarsal-tarsal joints distally, and the talonavicular and calcaneocuboid joints proximally. As this operation only corrects the cavus deformity, the absence of fixed heel varus is necessary prerequisite. The operation should be preceded by a plantar release.

Figure 6–42. The operation may be done either through one long midline incision or two separate incisions, one over the dorsomedial aspect of the navicular and first cuneiform bone, and the second over the cuboid bone in line with the fourth metatarsal. The author prefers the single midline incision in line with the interval between the second and third metatarsal. The incision must extend from the dorsal aspect of the talar neck distally as far as the middle of the metatarsals. Through this incision the entire area of the osteotomy can be exposed subperiosteally without interference from the anterior or posterior tibial tendons. It is also easier to visualize the osteotomy when seen through this single incision.

Figure 6–43. After the skin and subcutaneous tissue are divided the interval between the extensor tendons to the second and third toes is developed. The neurovascular bundle will lie between the extensor tendons to the second and great toe. In developing this interval care should be taken to interrupt as few vessels as possible. The arcuate artery coming off of the dorsalis pedis artery will run laterally at the level of the tarsal-metatarsal joints. If this is identified an effort to preserve it should be made.

Figure 6–44. After this interval is developed, the periosteum is incised from the talonavicular joint to the tarsal-metatarsal joint in line with the incision. Sharp dissection is used to detach the periosteum from the region of the joining capsules and a periosteal elevator used to separate the periosteum from the bones. Persistence is needed to develop the medial and lateral extent of the exposure. Medially the dissection should go completely around the joint of the navicular and first cuneiform bone, and laterally it should go completely around the cuboid bone. This dissection will expose the joints between the navicular proximally and the cuneiform bones distally. Most of the cuboid bones should be exposed, but the joints proximal and distal do not need to be entered. Sufficient bone on each side of these joints should be exposed to permit the correct-size wedge to be removed.

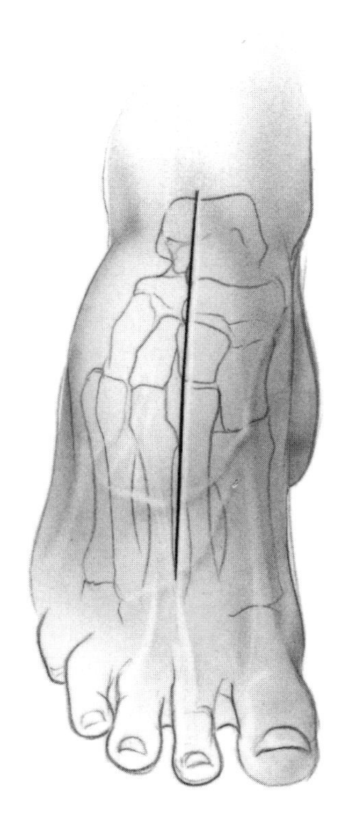

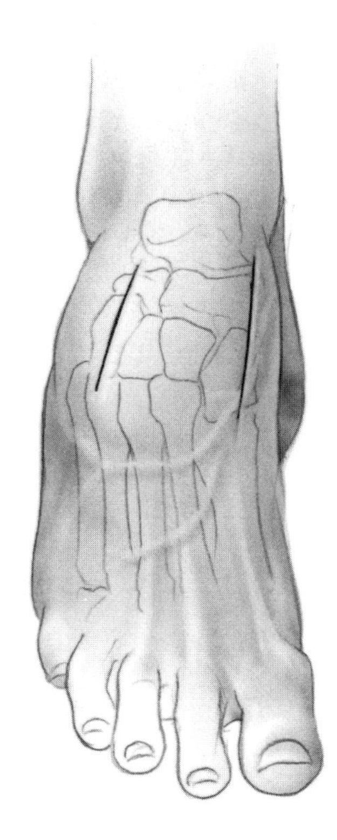

Figure 6–42

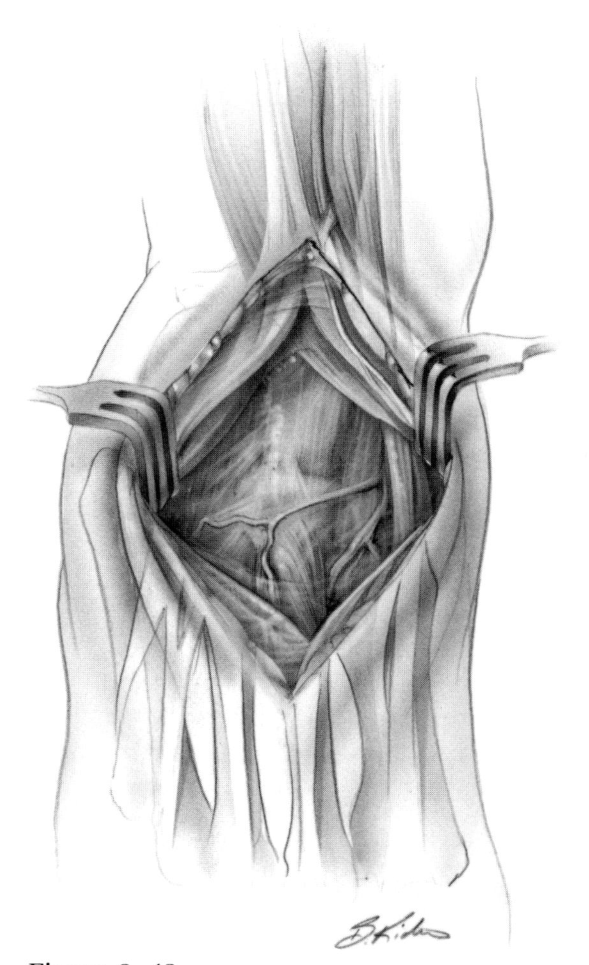

Figure 6–43

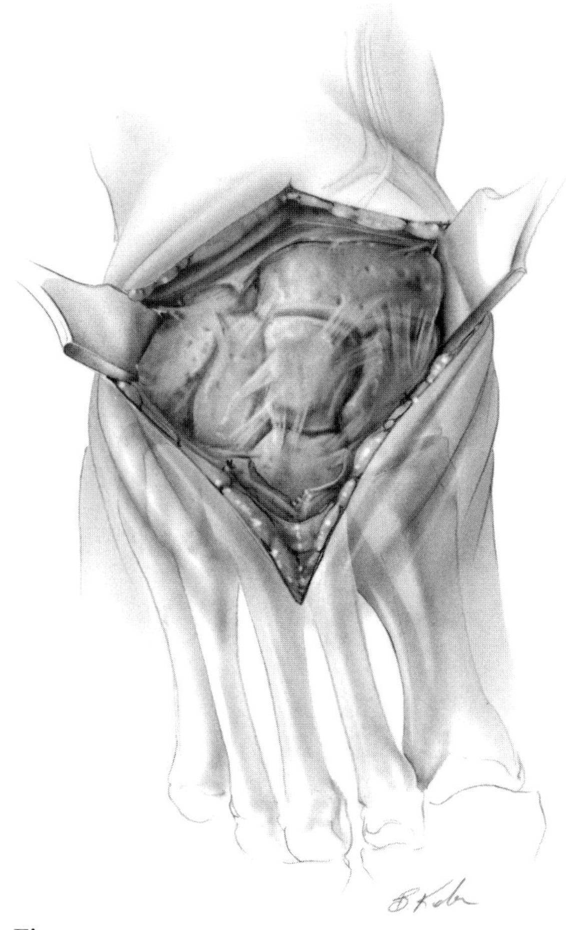

Figure 6–44

Figure 6–45. The osteotomy is now performed using a large 1.5-in osteotome or chisel. The proximal cut is made first, encompassing the distal portion of the navicular and a portion of the cuboid bone. This cut is estimated to be perpendicular to the hindfoot axis. The distal osteotomy is made in the proximal portion of all three cuneiform bones and the distal portion of the cuboid bone. It is made perpendicular to the axis of the forefoot. Note that unlike the remainder of the osteotomy, the joints on either side of the cuboid bone are not entered. Rather, the wedge is removed entirely from the cuboid bone. To avoid excessive shortening of the foot, the osteotomies should be fashioned so that no gap of bone is present at the apex of the wedge.

Figure 6–46. The osteotomy is closed by elevating the forefoot. It is possible to rotate the distal segment if desired. Often the first metatarsal will be more depressed than the others. This can be corrected by externally rotating the forefoot. By the same token, care should be taken not to produce an unintended malrotation.

The osteotomy may be fixed with either two Steinmann pins or staples. The dorsal surface of the cuneiform bones will usually be higher than the navicular, and this may make staple fixation more difficult. Secure fixation with Steinmann pins is not so easy as it may first appear. It is easy for the medial pin to pass too far plantarward. The medial pin is inserted first. It must start in the first metatarsal at an oblique angle directed dorsally and laterally.

The pin can be started at this oblique angle more easily if a small stab wound is made over the starting point, and a small hole is made in the metatarsal with a drill. This will prevent the Steinmann pin from slipping. This pin should engage the first metatarsal, the first cuneiform bone, the navicular, and the talus. The lateral pin is started distal to the flare at the base of the fifth metatarsal and is aimed medial and slightly dorsal, crossing the cuboid bone and entering the calcaneus. The ends of the pins are left protruding outside of the skin.

The periosteum is usually quite tattered at this point but should be approximated as best it can. A small flat silicone drain can be placed in the wound, although the author has not found this very effective. A well-padded nonwalking short leg cast is applied.

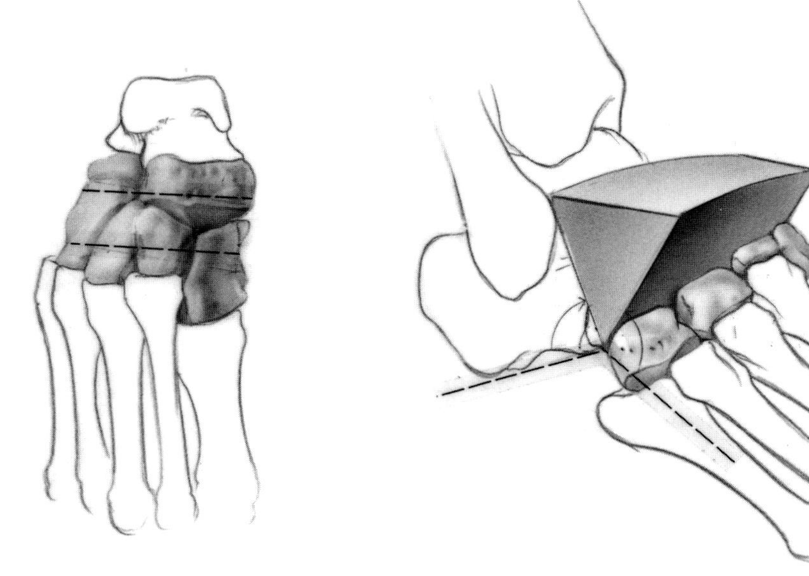

Figure 6–45

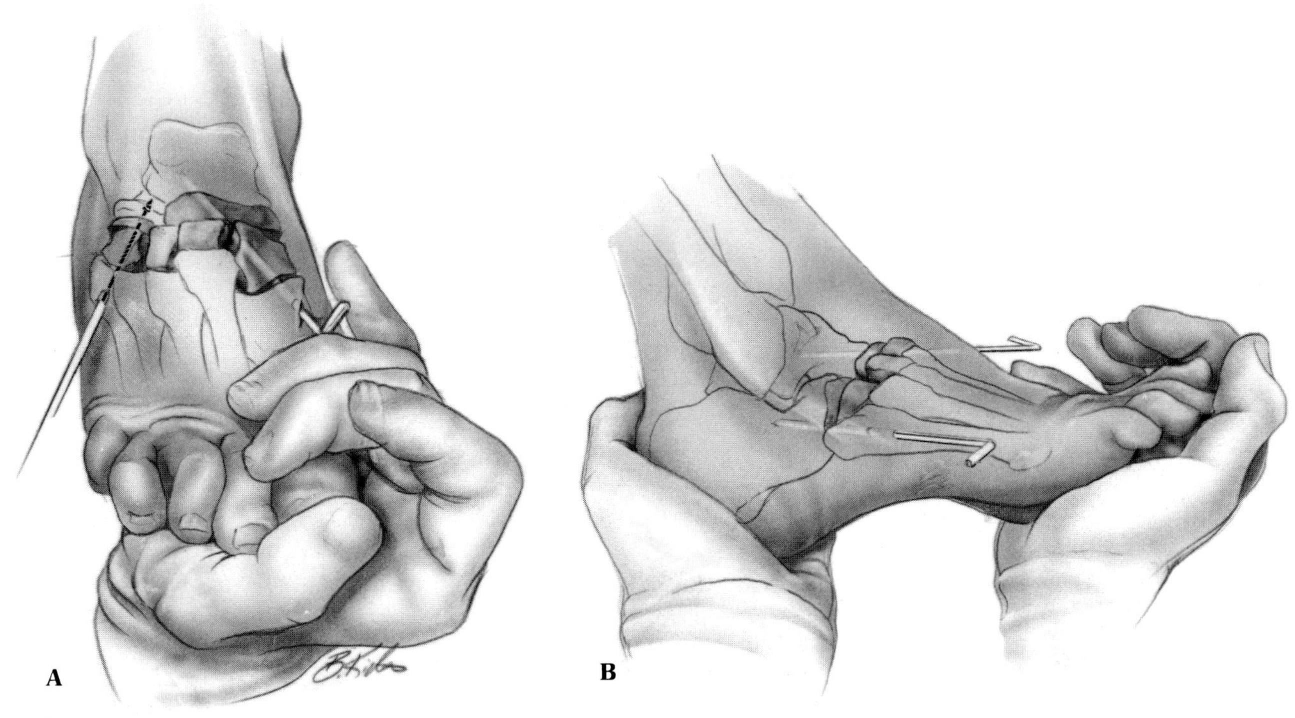

Figure 6–46

Figure 6–47. Anteroposterior (***Figure 6–47A***) and standing lateral (***Figure 6–47B***) radiographs of a 15-year-old boy with rigid symptomatic idiopathic cavus feet. The heel is in neutral in stance. The anteroposterior view 6 weeks after midfoot osteotomy shows the pins before removal (***Figure 6–47C***). The bone that was resected can be seen by comparing this radiograph to ***Figure 6–47A.*** The pins were removed, a short leg cast applied, and weight-bearing begun. Healing was complete at 12 weeks postoperatively.

POSTOPERATIVE CARE

The foot is kept elevated for the first few days. The patient is then ambulated with a three-point non–weight-bearing crutch gait for 6 weeks. At 6 weeks the cast and the pins are removed in the office. A short leg walking cast is applied, and the patient is permitted full weight-bearing for an additional 4 to 6 weeks, at which time healing should be complete.

REFERENCE

1. Cole WH. The treatment of claw-foot. J Bone Joint Surg 1940;22:895.

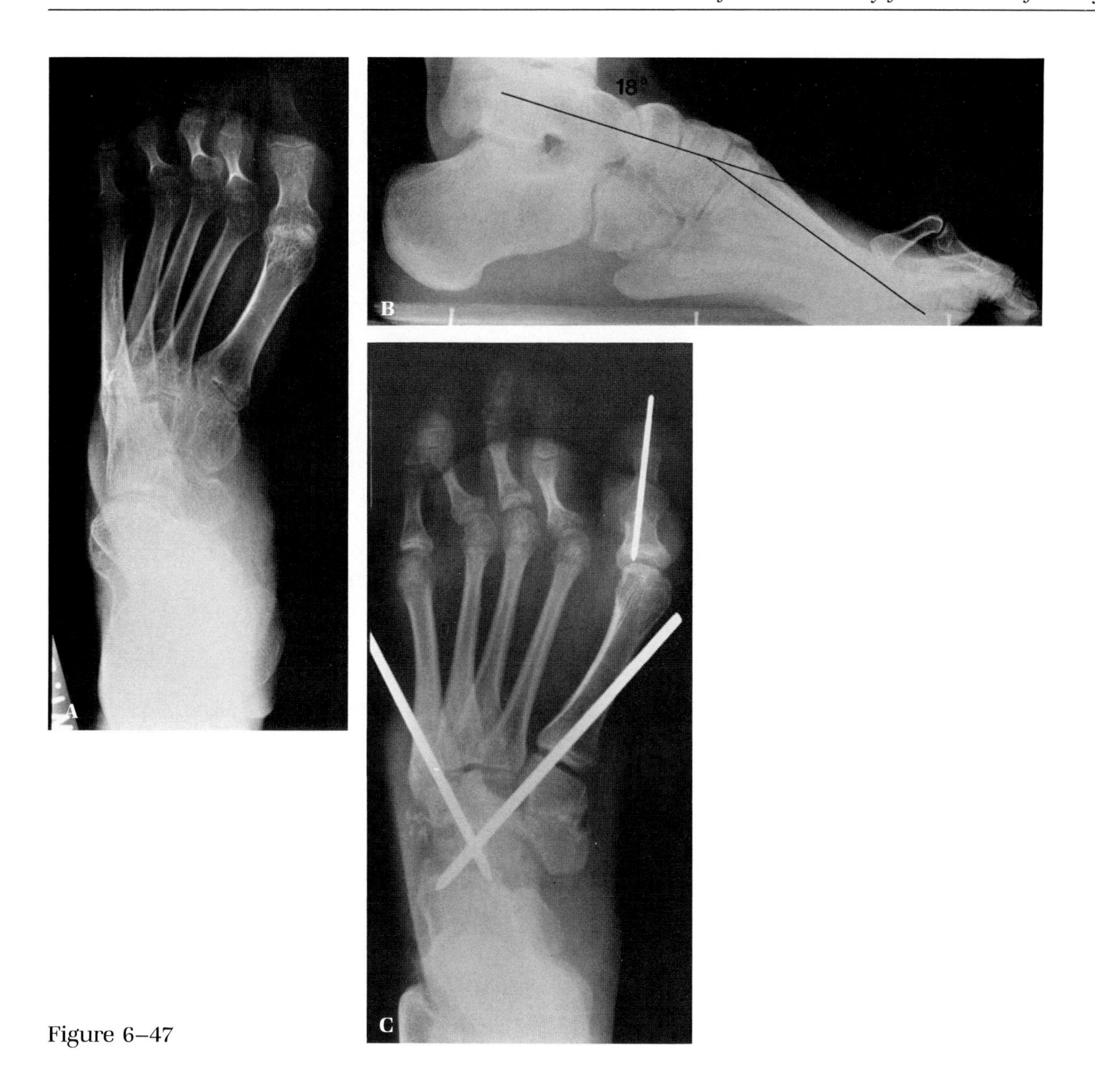

Figure 6–47

6.7 Triple Arthrodesis

The origin of the operation commonly known as triple arthrodesis is attributed to Hoke.[1] As originally described, he resected the head and neck of the talus after resecting the talocalcaneal joint. The foot was displaced posteriorly, and the resected bone was reshaped and reinserted. In 1978 Duncan and Lovell[2] reported on 109 cases of the Hoke triple arthrodesis in which the head and neck of the talus were removed and replaced as originally described with the addition of calcaneocuboid joint resection. The original description of the triple arthrodesis as we know it today was described by Ryerson.[3] In this classic operation he added resection of the calcaneocuboid joint to resection of the talonavicular and talocalcaneal joints. He did not remove the head and neck of talus. Lambrinudi[4,5] described a resection of bone that is designed to correct a dropped-foot deformity. Several reports evaluate these procedures on patients with poliomyelitis,[6] residual of club foot,[7] progressive neuromuscular disease,[8] and arthrogryposis.[9]

In concept the operation is deceptively simple. The three aforementioned joints are resected separating the foot into three movable segments: the forefoot, the calcaneus, and the talus and ankle mortice. If the correct wedges of bone are resected, the position of the foot will be correct when the bony surfaces are apposed. In practice this can be a difficult task.

The operation should be performed within 1 year or at most 2 years of skeletal maturity. In the young child much of the bone is composed of cartilage. Resection of enough cartilage to obtain good bony apposition is difficult in the young child. In addition, this resection will slow the growth of the resected bones. This growth arrest combined with an operation that in itself shortens the foot may result in unacceptable shortening of what may already be a short foot.

Figure 6–48. The surgeon should give some thought to the wedges of bone to be removed and in particular the amount of bone to be removed before beginning the operation. The author has never found it very helpful to plan precise wedges with cutouts once the operation has begun, however. Visualizing the actual foot at surgery and making the osteotomy cuts to create the wedges as described below seems much more practical and accurate.

The commonest deformity for which triple arthrodesis is performed today is fixed varus deformity. To correct this deformity, a laterally based wedge of bone is removed from each of the joints to be resected. Conceptually two wedges of bone at right angles to each other will be removed. The wedge that will allow correction of the forefoot will excise the talonavicular and calcaneocuboid joints. To achieve correction to a neutral position the distal cut will be perpendicular to the long axis of the forefoot, and the proximal cut will be perpendicular to the longitudinal axis of the calcaneus (***Figure 6–48A***). When these two surfaces are opposed, the forefoot should be straight.

To correct the varus of the hindfoot a laterally based wedge must be removed from the subtalar joint. To correct the heel to a neutral position the proximal cut from the undersurface of the talus should be perpendicular to the long axis of the tibia (or parallel with the ankle mortice), whereas the distal cut from the superior surface of the calcaneus should be parallel with the bottom of the heel (***Figure 6–48B***). When these two surfaces are opposed the heel should be in neutral.

A triple arthrodesis for fixed valgus deformity is among the most difficult. This is because medially based wedges created using the same principles described earlier must be removed from the lateral side (***Figure 6–48C***). This task is made easier if all of the joints are widely opened by extensive capsulotomies and cutting the interosseous ligament of the subtalar joint. A small laminectomy retractor can be used to hold the joints open.

Calcaneocavus deformity is the most uncommon indication for triple arthrodesis. In this circumstance a posteriorly based wedge is removed from the subtalar joint, which allows correction of the calcaneus. A dorsal wedge is removed from the talonavicular and calcaneocuboid joints to allow the forefoot to be dorsiflexed (***Figure 6–48D***).

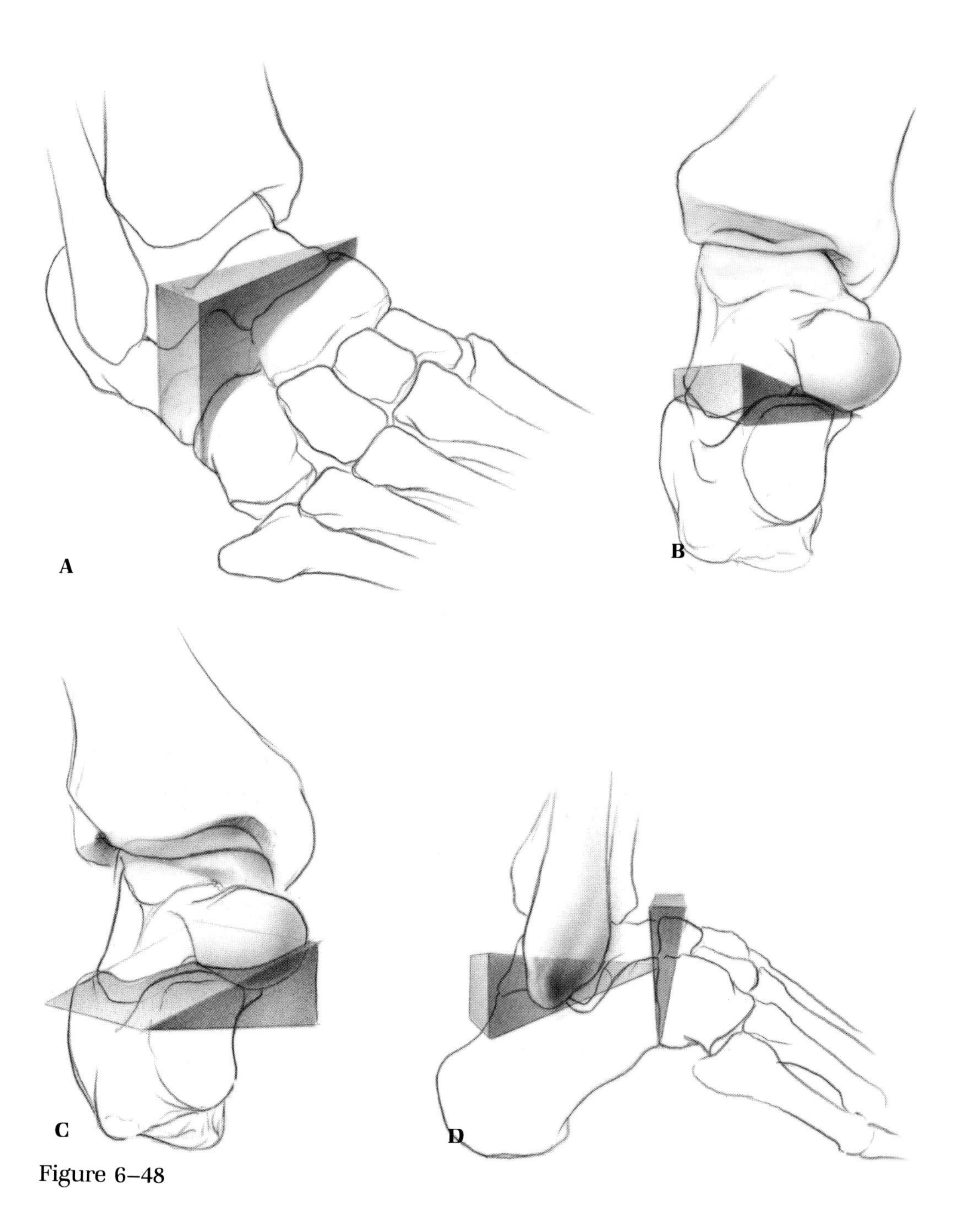

Figure 6–48

Figure 6–49. The operation will be illustrated for the commonest deformity: Varus. The patient is placed on the operating table with a sand bag under the hip on the side to be operated, thus bringing the lateral side of the foot into better position. A small sterile sand bag or other support is placed under the medial side of the foot. This will support the foot while the joint surfaces are cut. The incision is a straight lateral incision that crosses the lateral side of the talonavicular joint and the distal end of the calcaneus. It should extend from just medial to the most lateral extensor tendons dorsally to just past the peroneal tendons volarly. There should be no undermining of the skin edges. Once the fascia over the extensor brevis muscle is incised, the proximal insertion of this muscle is found and the muscle elevated to expose the lateral capsules of the calcaneocuboid and talonavicular joints. The fibrofatty tissue is removed from the sinus tarsi, exposing the lateral aspect of the subtalar joint. (This exposure is described in more detail in the Grice extra-articular subtalar arthrodesis.)

Figure 6–50. The talonavicular and calcaneocuboid capsules are widely incised exposing the joint surfaces. It will be helpful to removal of the bone wedges of the subtalar joint if as much stripping as possible of the capsule of the subtalar joint is accomplished. This can be done by sliding a curved periosteal elevator (*eg,* a Crego) around the lateral and then posterior aspect of the subtalar joint. After this, as much of the capsule of the subtalar joint as can be visualized is incised, the interosseous ligament is divided, and a large bone skid is used to pry the joint open. This will give the surgeon an excellent view of the two bony surfaces of the subtalar joint that are to be excised.

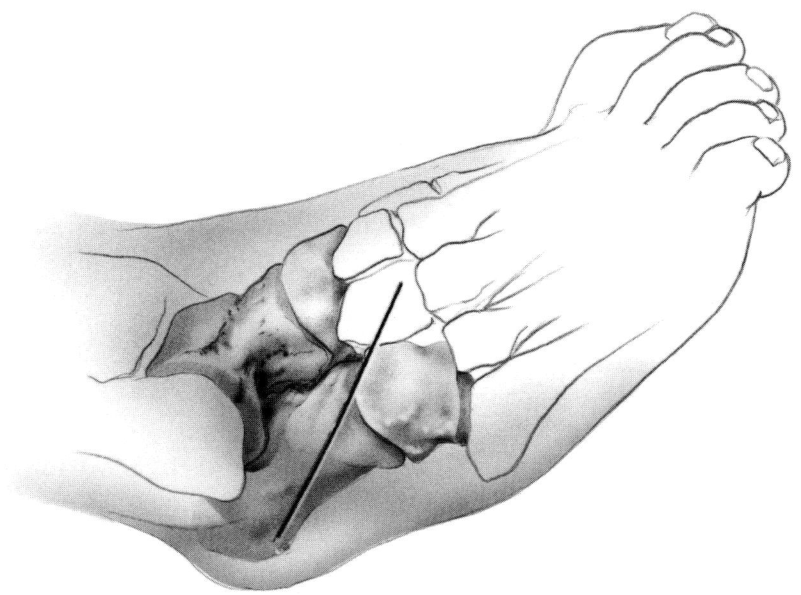

Figure 6–49

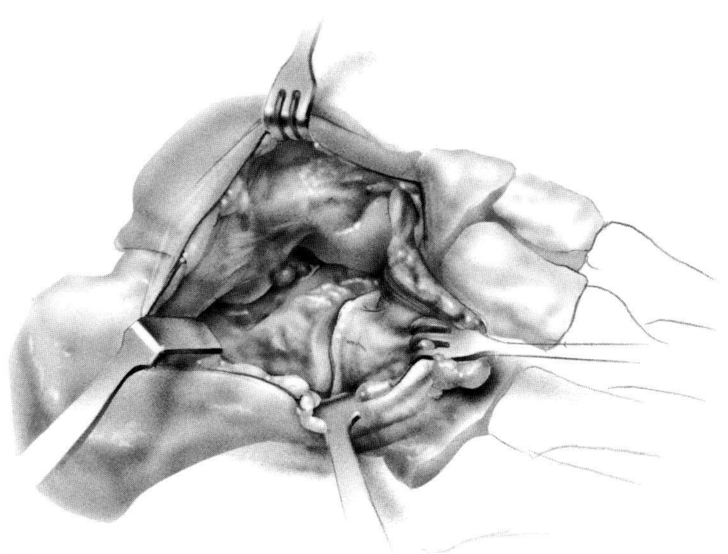

Figure 6–50

Figure 6–51. The wedges of bone are now excised. The subtalar joint is done first. Most of the bone for the correction should be removed from the calcaneus. It is better to use a chisel than an osteotome for these cuts. The chisel with its flat surface as opposed to the double-beveled surface of an osteotome is easier to keep on a straight course (***Figure 6–51A***).

The cut into the dorsal surface of the calcaneus should be parallel to the bottom of the heel (***Figure 6–51B***) while the cut in the bottom of the talus should be parallel with the ankle mortice from medial to lateral (***Figure 6–51C***). It is best to make the most proximal and distal aspects of these cuts first and the middle portion in between last. This is because the middle part will be the most difficult to remove with remaining capsule attached to the prominent sustenaculum tali and the most worrisome to cut through with the neurovascular bundle in close proximity.

If these cuts are made correctly, when the two cut surfaces are opposed, the heel will be in neutral regarding varus and valgus.

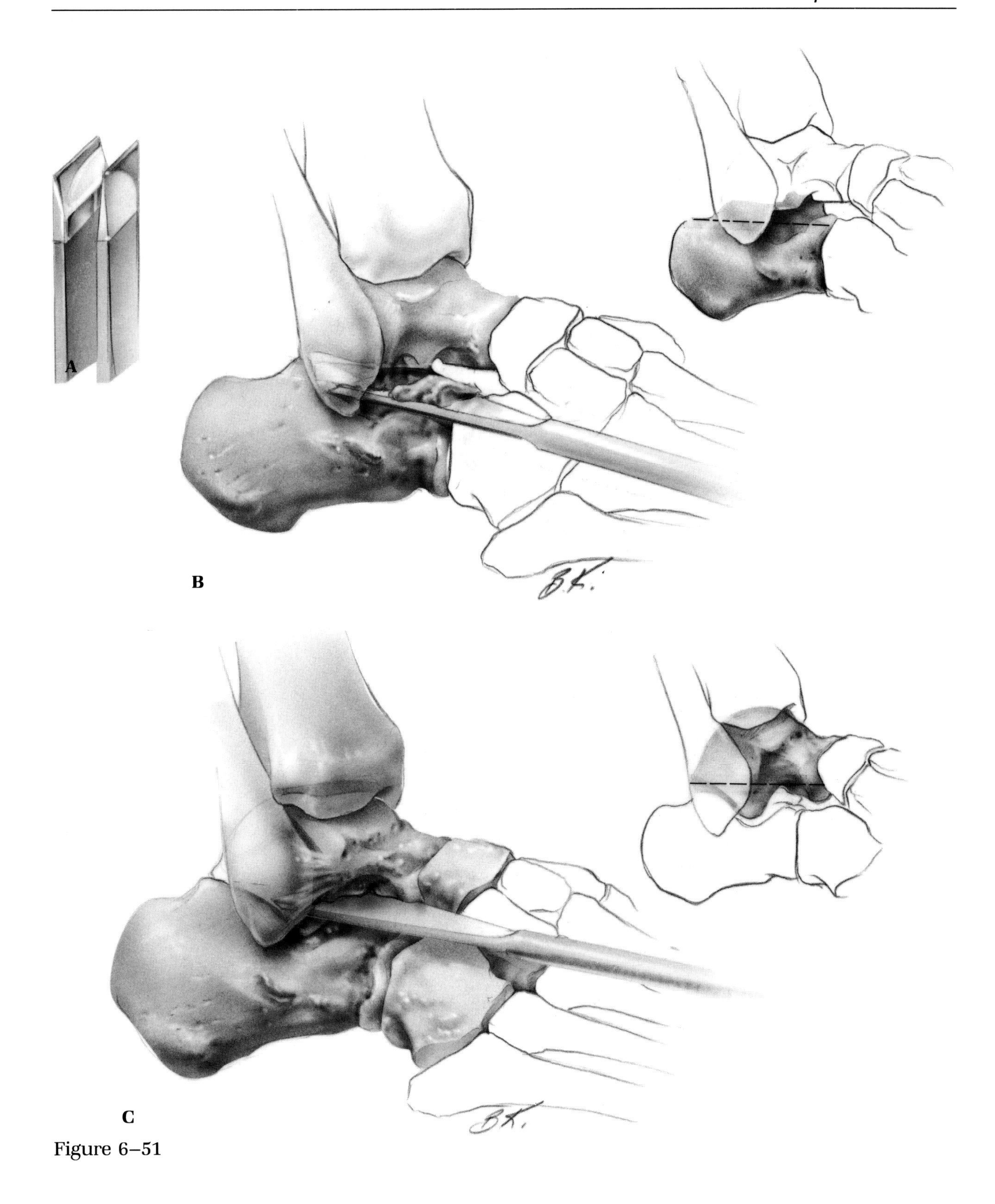

Figure 6–51

Figure 6–52. The same principle is used in aligning the forefoot. The cuts in the navicular and the cuboid should be perpendicular to the longitudinal axis of the forefoot (***Figure 6–52B***), whereas the cuts in the distal talus and calcaneus should be perpendicular to the longitudinal axis of the hindfoot or calcaneus (***Figure 6–52C***).

Figure 6–53. When the wedges are removed the foot is placed in the corrected position, and the surfaces are inspected. Good coaption should be present to ensure prompt healing. The external contour of the foot should be inspected to be certain that the desired alignment has been achieved. If all is as desired, each of the joints is held together with a staple. The author has found the power staple driver to be an ideal tool for this. A drain is placed in the wound and brought out distally where it can easily be removed. A well-padded short leg cast is applied.

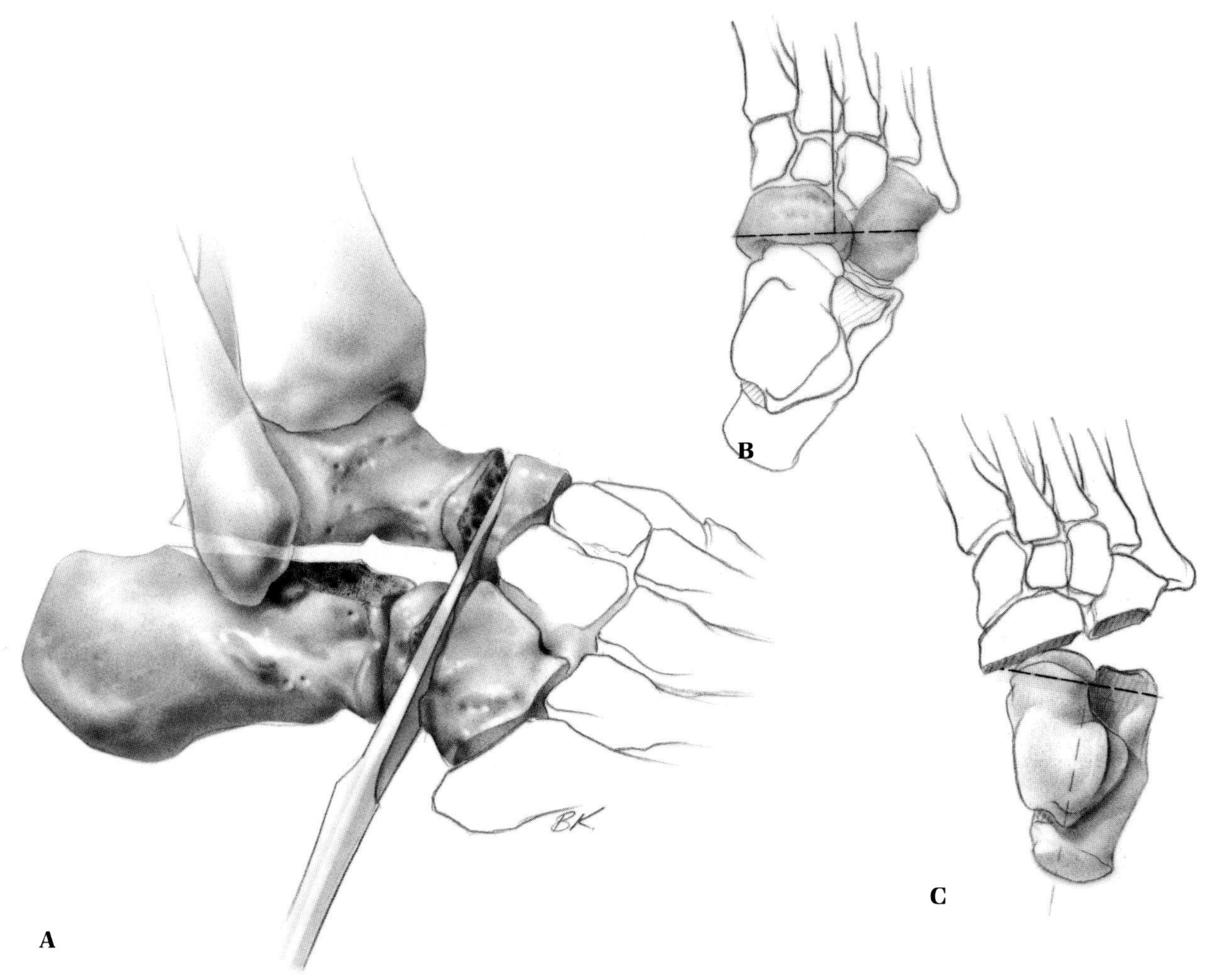

Figure 6–52

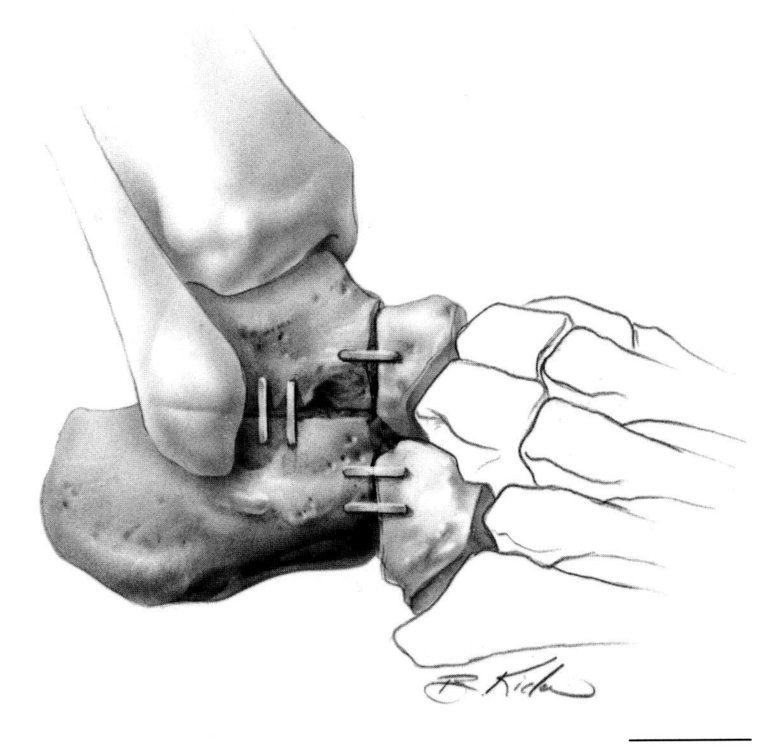

Figure 6–53

Figure 6–54. Anteroposterior (***Figure 6–54A***) and lateral (***Figure 6–54B***) radiographs of a 16-year-old boy with a rigid cavus foot with the heel fixed in varus secondary to Charcot-Marie-Tooth disease. At 6 weeks there is still not trabeculation across the lines of joint resection; however, healing is sufficient to permit weight-bearing in a short leg cast (***Figure 6–54C***). At 12 weeks healing is complete, and no further cast protection is needed (***Figure 6–54D***).

POSTOPERATIVE CARE

The immediate postoperative period is usually characterized by significant discomfort. For this reason continuous epidural analgesia is a nice adjunct to the postoperative management. It can be continued for the first 2 to 3 days while the patient is maintained at bed rest with the foot elevated. The patient is then discharged on a three-point non–weight-bearing crutch gait. At 6 weeks the cast is removed, and radiographs are obtained to monitor the progress of the healing. At this time healing is usually sufficient to permit application of a short leg walking cast for an additional 4 to 6 weeks, after which healing should be complete as evidenced by obliteration of the osteotomy cuts, and cast immobilization can be discontinued.

REFERENCES

1. Hoke M. An operation for stabilizing paralytic feet. Am J Orthop Surg 1921;3:494.
2. Duncan JW, Lovell WW. Hoke triple arthrodesis. J Bone Joint Surg 1978;60A:795.
3. Ryerson EW. Arthrodesing operations on the feet. J Bone Joint Surg 1923;5:453.
4. Lambrinudi C. New operation on drop-foot. Br J Surg 1927;15:193.
5. Hart VL. Lambrinudi operation for drop-foot. J Bone Joint Surg 1940;22:937.
6. Patterson RL, Parrish FF, Hathaway EN. Stabilizing operations on the foot: a study of the indications, techniques used and end results. J Bone Joint Surg 1950;32A:1.
7. Herold HZ, Torok G. Surgical correction of neglected club foot in the older child and adult. J Bone Joint Surg 1973;55A:1385.
8. Levitt RL, Canale ST, Cooke AJ Jr., Gartland JJ. The role of foot surgery in progressive neuromuscular disorders in children. J Bone Joint Surg 1973;55A:1396.
9. Drummond DS, Cruess RL. The management of the foot and ankle in arthrogryposis multiplex congenita. J Bone Joint Surg 1978;60B:96.

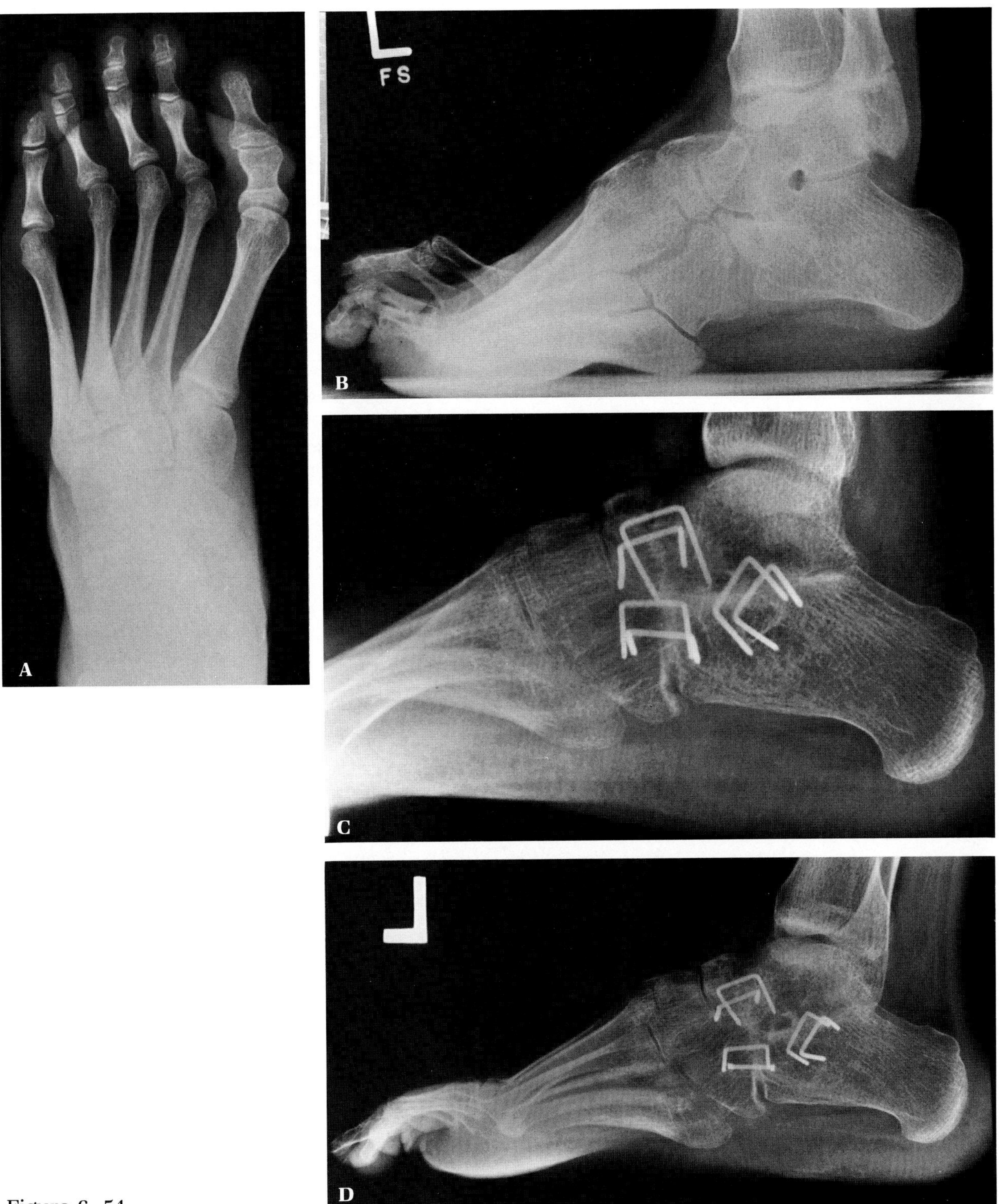

Figure 6–54

6.8 Grice Extra-articular Subtalar Arthrodesis

The extra-articular arthrodesis of the subtalar joint that was devised by Grice[1] was initially used in the treatment of children with polio.[1] Today, however, it finds its commonest application in the treatment of valgus deformity in other paralytic conditions affecting the foot, most notably cerebral palsy. Because the arthrodesis is extra-articular it does not disturb the growth of the bone and does not necessitate the removal of large amounts of articular cartilage that would be required to expose the cancellous bone in an immature child. The Grice procedure is commonly recognized among experienced orthopaedic surgeons as an operation that is difficult to perform correctly and that has a significant failure rate.[2–4] Non-union, overcorrection and undercorrection, and displacement of the graft are among the commonest problems.

The procedure is designed as a bone block to prevent eversion of the calcaneus with consequent valgus deformity. The foot must be correctable to a neutral position before the operation can be considered. In addition, any equinus deformity must be corrected before the Grice procedure. A common error is to perform a subtalar stabilization when there is instability in the ankle joint. This problem is most often encountered in children with spina bifida and can be avoided by assessing the ankle joint with a standing radiograph before surgery. The bone graft is best taken from the iliac crest. If taken from the tibia as originally described, it can result in fracture, and if taken from the fibula, it can result in fibular shortening and a subsequent valgus deformity at the ankle.

Figure 6–55. The incision is a straight obliquely placed incision over the sinus tarsi, which follows the normal skin lines as described in the excision of the calcaneonavicular coalition (***Figure 6–55A***). The incision is carried directly down to and through the deep fascia layer, which overlies the origin of the extensor brevis muscle. This fascia is then divided and undermined proximally to expose the origin of the muscle and the fibrofatty tissue filling the sinus tarsi as well as the peroneal tendons that are freed and retracted plantarward. When the wound is closed, approximation of this deep fascia will also approximate the thin skin lessening the tension on it and minimizing wound problems.

At this point the inexperienced surgeon may be somewhat disoriented regarding where the bony landmarks lie and begin by removing the fibrofatty tissue from the sinus tarsi with a knife and rongeur. If the surgeon knows where the bone lies under the soft tissues, however, it is easier to excise the fibrofatty tissue that fills the sinus tarsi and elevate the muscle as a single distally based flap as illustrated by the solid line (***Figure 6–55B***). With a knife an incision is made down to the bone, first starting on the dorsal surface of the calcaneus just proximal to the calcaneocuboid joint. This incision is carried proximal and then dorsal along the medial side of the body of the talus onto the inferolateral side of the talar neck, where the incision now turns distal until it reaches the talonavicular joint.

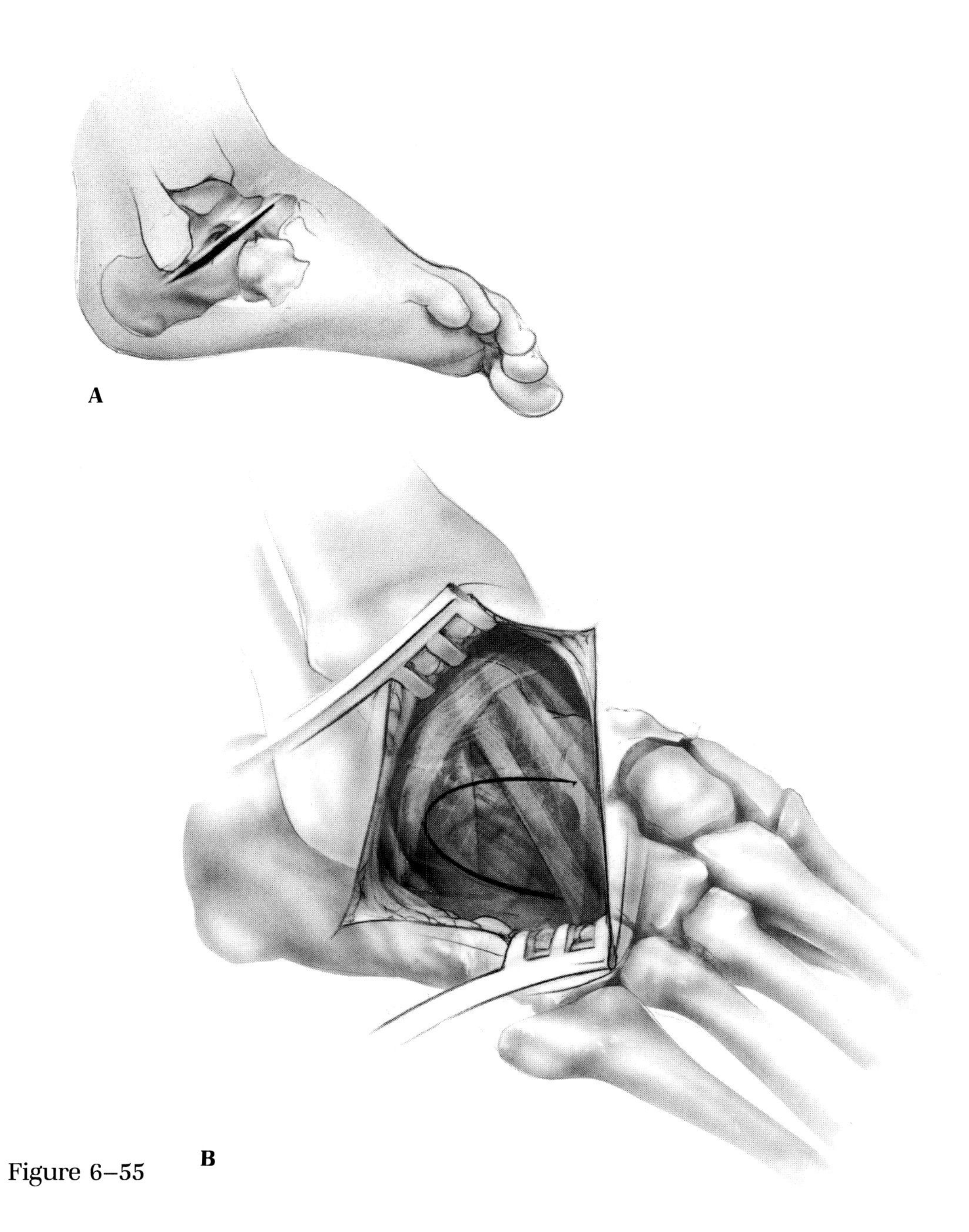

Figure 6–55

Figure 6–56. This U-shaped incision is deepened to excise all of the material from the sinus tarsi. If this is done as described, the fibrofatty tissue will remain attached to the muscle and can be retracted by a hemostat. Any remaining soft tissue that obscures the bony anatomy can be excised with a rongeur or curette (***Figure 6–56A***). During this exposure the subtalar joint may be opened, but this is of no consequence. The surgeon should now be able to clearly visualize the neck of the talus, which forms the roof of the sinus tarsi, and the dorsal surface of the calcaneus, which forms the floor of the sinus tarsi (***Figure 6–56B***). The exposure as illustrated shows the calcaneocuboid joint and the talonavicular joint capsules exposed. This is shown for better orientation of the anatomy but should be avoided if possible because it is not a necessary part of the exposure.

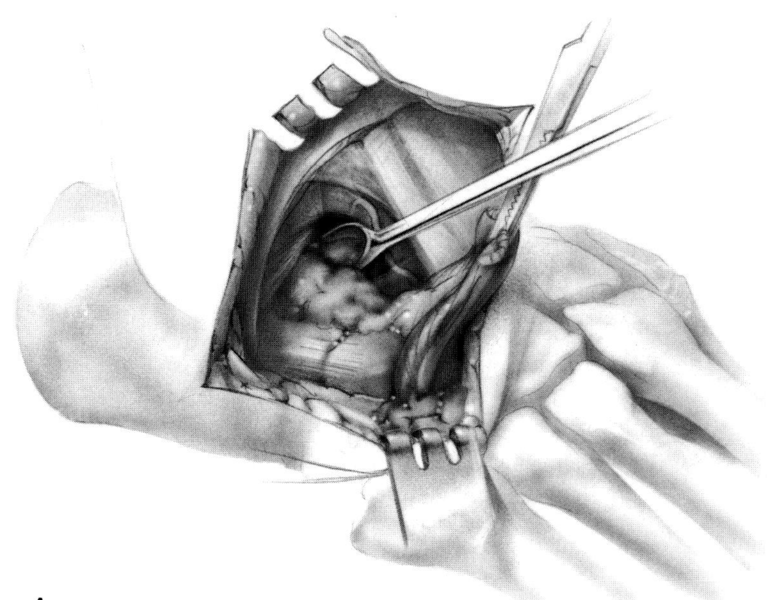

A

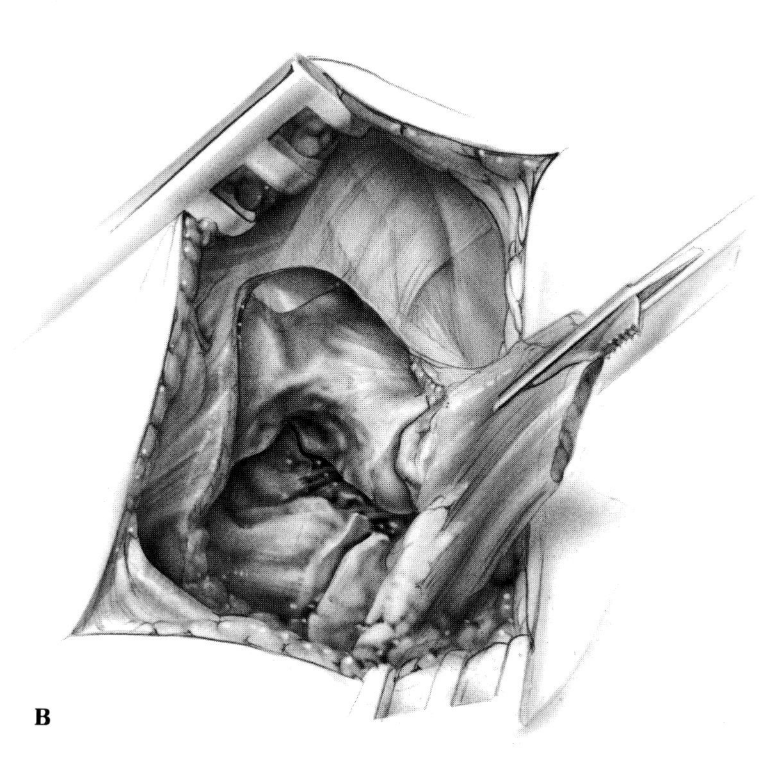

B

Figure 6–56

Figure 6–57. An osteotome can be used to determine both the correct size of the graft and its location. With the foot in equinus, the calcaneus is inverted, opening the sinus tarsi. Osteotomes of various sizes can be placed in the sinus tarsi while the foot is dorsiflexed and everted. Inspection of the foot at this point will give the surgeon an idea of what the position of the foot will be with various-sized grafts. When the foot is dorsiflexed, the osteotome (and subsequently the graft) should lie in a direct line with the tibia.

Figure 6–58. When the correct location for the graft is determined, a small channel is cut into the neck of the talus and the dorsal surface of the calcaneus with a narrow osteotome. As originally described, this cut should not go completely through the cortex into the cancellous bone as it would collapse into the cancellous bone with resulting loss of correction. This in part may account for the problem of non-union. When he was still using this procedure, the author cut these channels completely through the cortical bone in all but the most lateral area where the graft would fit. The graft is then shaped in such a fashion that its lateral portion will fit over this cortical rim while the remainder of the graft can sink into the cancellous bone.

Figure 6–59. The bone graft is taken from the anterior iliac crest just behind the anterosuperior iliac spine. The graft is now shaped to fit into the channels. The approximate height of the graft can be judged by the size of the osteotome that produced the desired correction (***Figure 6–59B***). It should be left slightly longer than measured because it can always be trimmed but not added to.

The graft is put into place by plantar flexing and inverting the foot, placing the graft, and then dorsiflexing and everting the foot. With the graft firmly held in place, the foot is carefully inspected to be certain that the correction is as desired. It is best to leave slight valgus to ensure against the worse complication of producing varus.

The wound is closed by trimming the excess fibrofatty tissue from the sinus tarsi away and bringing the extensor brevis muscle back over the sinus tarsi. The deep fascia layer is closed followed by skin closure. All the time an assistant must hold the foot dorsiflexed and everted to prevent displacement of the graft. It is possible to fix the subtalar joint with a Steinmann pin if desired. A short leg cast is applied with the foot still held in the corrected position.

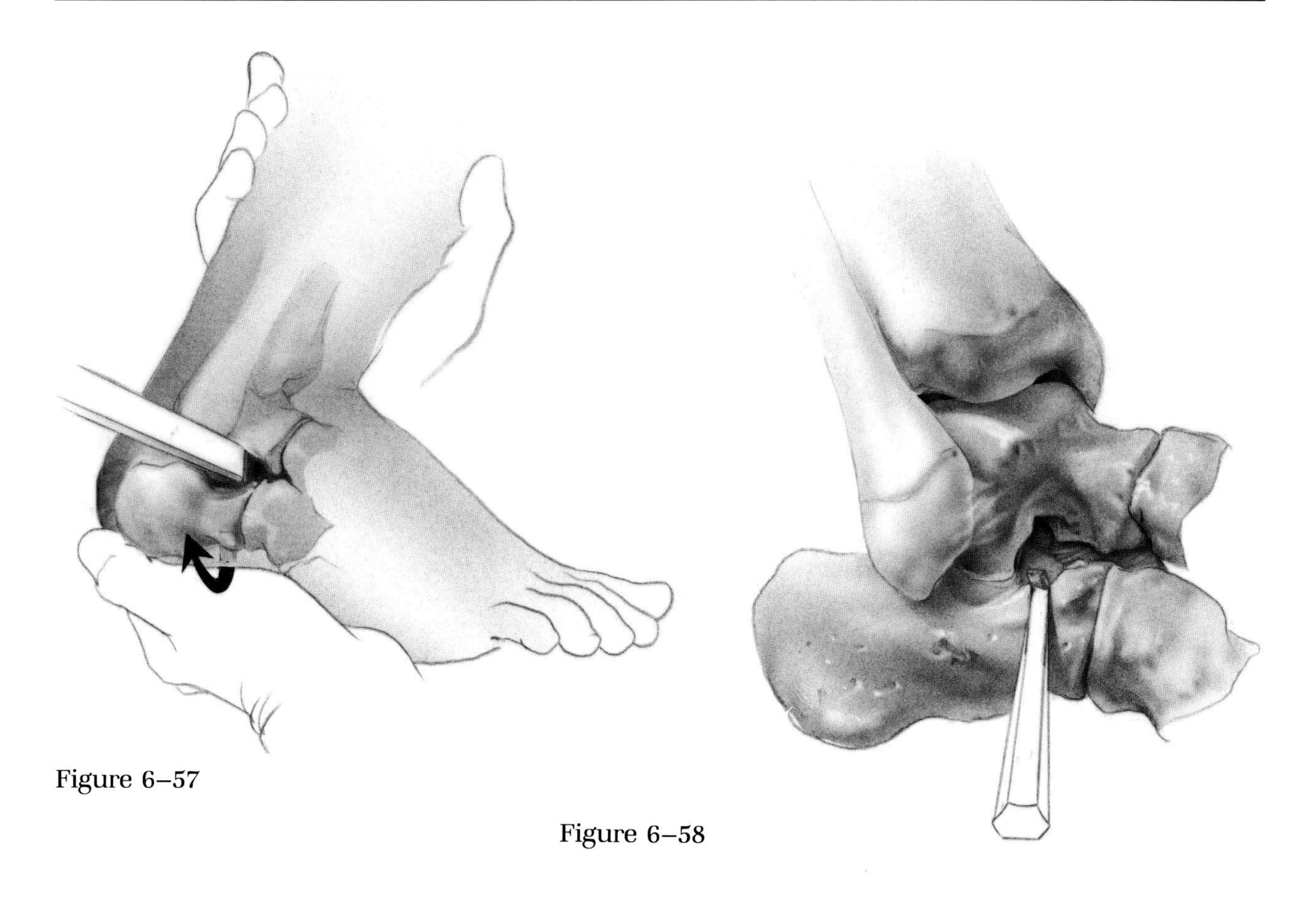

Figure 6–57

Figure 6–58

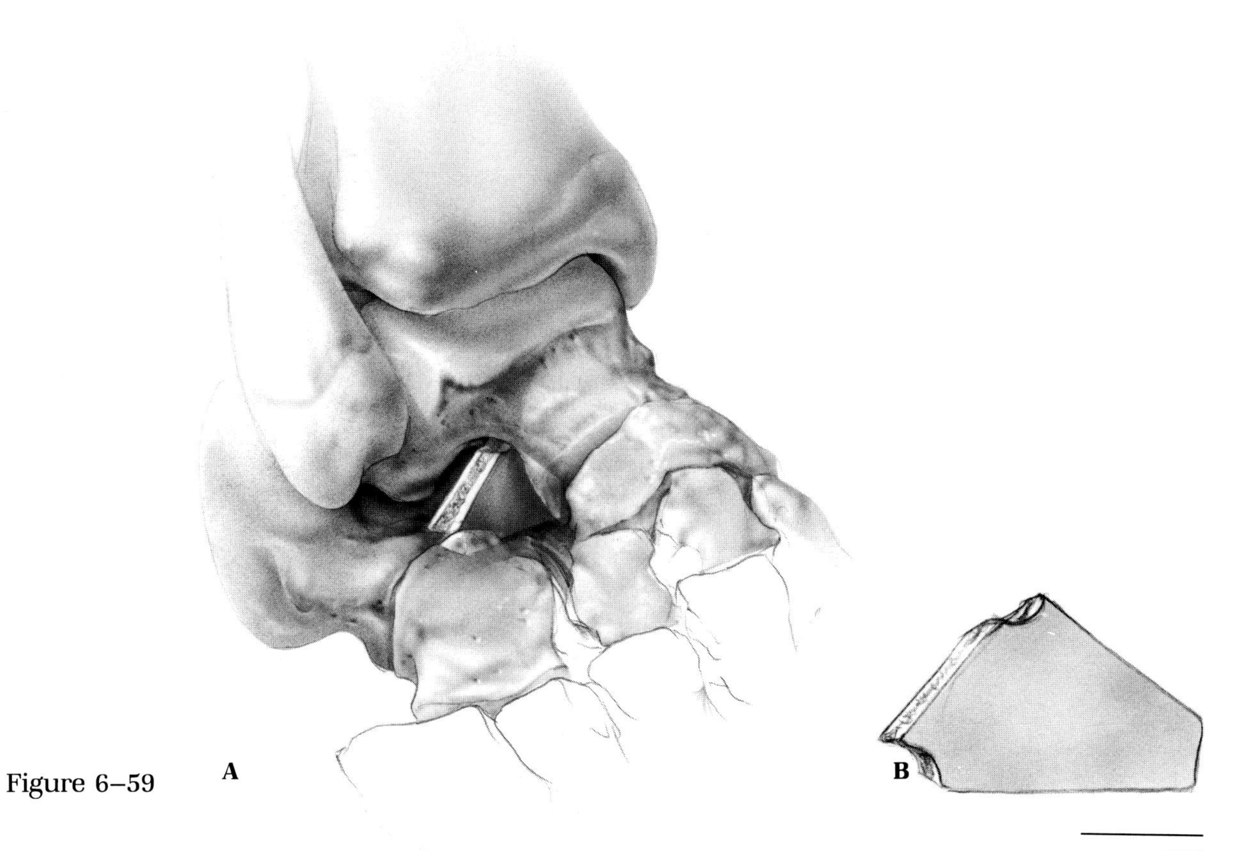

Figure 6–59 A B

POSTOPERATIVE CARE

The cast should be left in place until the graft has solidly united. This may take 10 to 12 weeks. During this time the patient should not bear weight. After roentgenographic confirmation of healing of the graft, the patient is started on range-of-motion exercises for the ankle and progressed from a partial weight-bearing crutch gait to full weight-bearing as tolerated.

REFERENCES

1. Grice DS. An extra-articular arthrodesis of the subastragalar joint for the correction of paralytic flat feet in children. J Bone Joint Surg 1952;34A:927.
2. Pojllock JH, Carrell B. Subtalar extra-articular arthrodesis in the treatment of paralytic valgus deformities: a review of 112 procedures in 100 patients. J Bone Joint Surg 1964;44A:533.
3. Ross PM, Lyne DE. The Grice procedure: indications and evaluation of long-term results. Clin Orthop 1980;153:194.
4. Moreland JR, Westin WG. Further experience with Grice subtalar arthrodesis. Clin Orthop 1986;207:113.

6.9 Subtalar Arthrodesis: Dennyson and Fulford Technique

Numerous variations of the Grice technique of extra-articular subtalar arthrodesis have been tried to circumvent the problems inherent in the technique. The most popular of these is the technique of Dennyson and Fulford, also called the Princess Margaret Rose technique, using cancellous bone for more certain and rapid healing, and a screw for internal fixation of the subtalar joint.[1]

Figure 6–60. The surgical approach and exposure are the same as for the Grice procedure. After this is completed a small osteotome or curette is used to remove cortical bone from the undersurface of the talar neck and the dorsal surface of the calcaneus. This decortication should be confined to the medial aspect of the sinus tarsi because it is important to preserve the cortical bone laterally where the screw will pass.

Figure 6–61. Next it is necessary to expose a small area on the dorsal surface of the neck of the talus as this is where the screw must start. The interval between the extensor digitorum longus and the neurovascular bundle is the correct interval through which to approach the talus. This can be done by extending the lateral incision further medial and further retracting the skin as illustrated here, or by making a second small longitudinal incision directly over the area.

The foot is held in the desired position relative to dorsiflexion and inversion. The appropriate-sized drill for the screw to be used is drilled through the neck of the talus in a posterolateral direction. It is important that the screw not pass directly through the center of the talus and calcaneus as this will be too close to the axis of rotation of the subtalar joint resulting in poor fixation. This is one of the problems of the Batchelor technique of subtalar arthrodesis.

Most often the best screw is a 4.5-mm cortical screw. It should pass through the calcaneus to emerge through the lateral cortex near the plantar surface. The drill can be seen passing through the sinus tarsi and should enter the calcaneus posterolateral to the area of decortication. The length of the screw can be measured from the length of the drill bit that is in the bone. The drill is removed and the appropriate-size screw is inserted and tightened (***Figure 6–61B***). The subtalar joint should now be secured in the correct position.

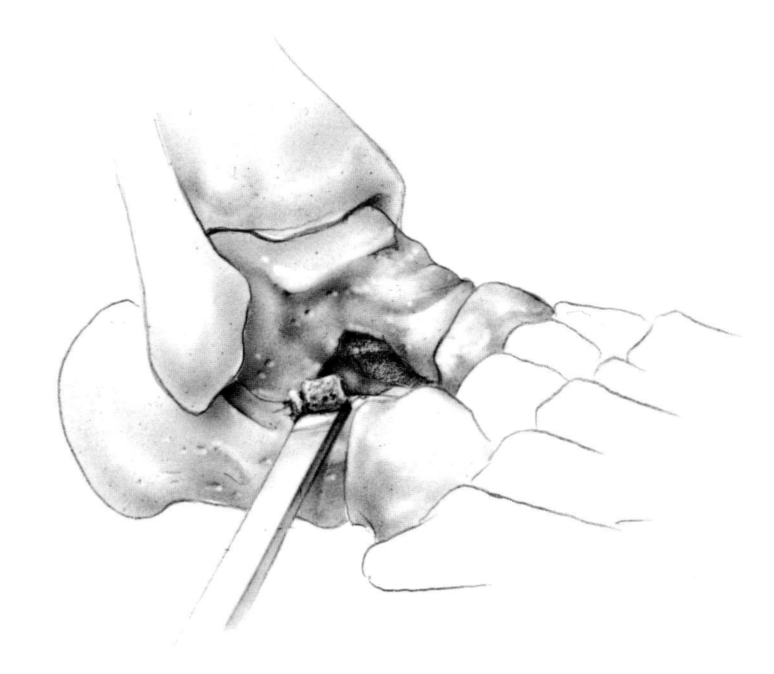

Figure 6–60

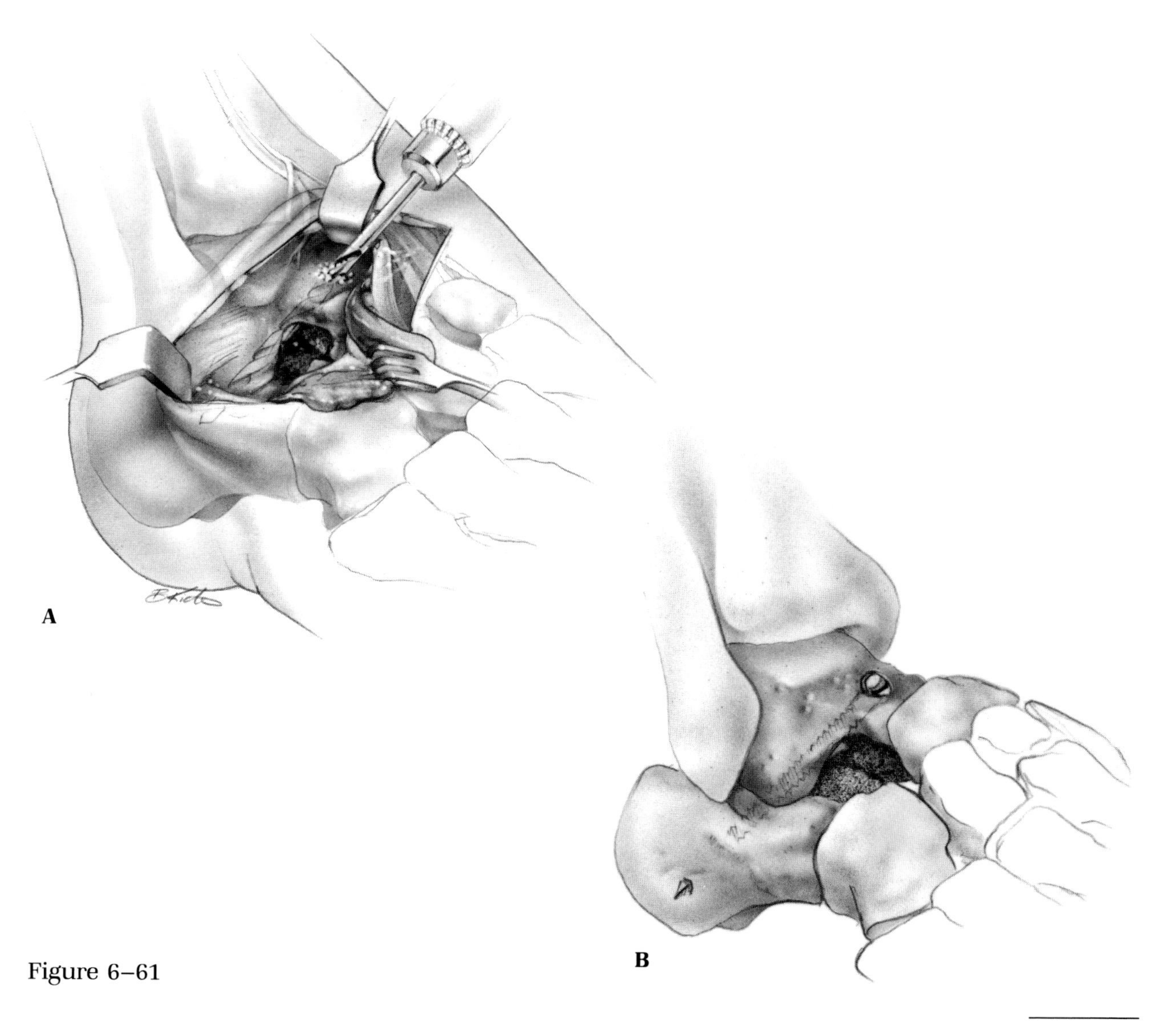

Figure 6–61

Figure 6–62. Following completion of fixation cancellous bone graft is obtained from the iliac crest in the region of the antero-superior iliac spine and is packed into the sinus tarsi.

The wound is closed as described in the Grice procedure by first closing the fascia layer to aid in holding the bone graft in place.

Figure 6–63. Standing lateral radiograph of the foot of a 8+5-year-old girl with juvinile rheumatoid arthritis is shown (***Figure 6–63A***). The foot has been developing an increasing valgus deformity with pain for the past 2 years. The foot can be corrected to neutral. Intraoperative radiographs demonstrate the proper placement of the screw (***Figures 6–63B, C***) before the bone graft being placed. Six months later when the patient is admitted for screw removal, the consolidation of the bone graft producing an extra-articular bone block can be seen (***Figure 6–63D***). Note the subsequent narrowing of the posterior facet of the subtalar joint.

POSTOPERATIVE CARE

Healing is usually complete in 6 to 8 weeks. Although Dennyson and Fulford did not specify when weight-bearing was permitted, the author has usually chosen to keep the patient non–weight-bearing for the first 3 weeks. At that time the cast is changed, and walking is permitted.

REFERENCE

1. Dennyson WG, Fulford GE. Subtalar arthrodesis by cancellous grafts and metalic internal fixation. J Bone Joint Surg 1976;58B:507.

Figure 6–62

Figure 6–63

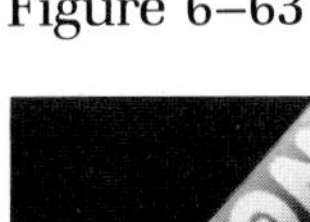

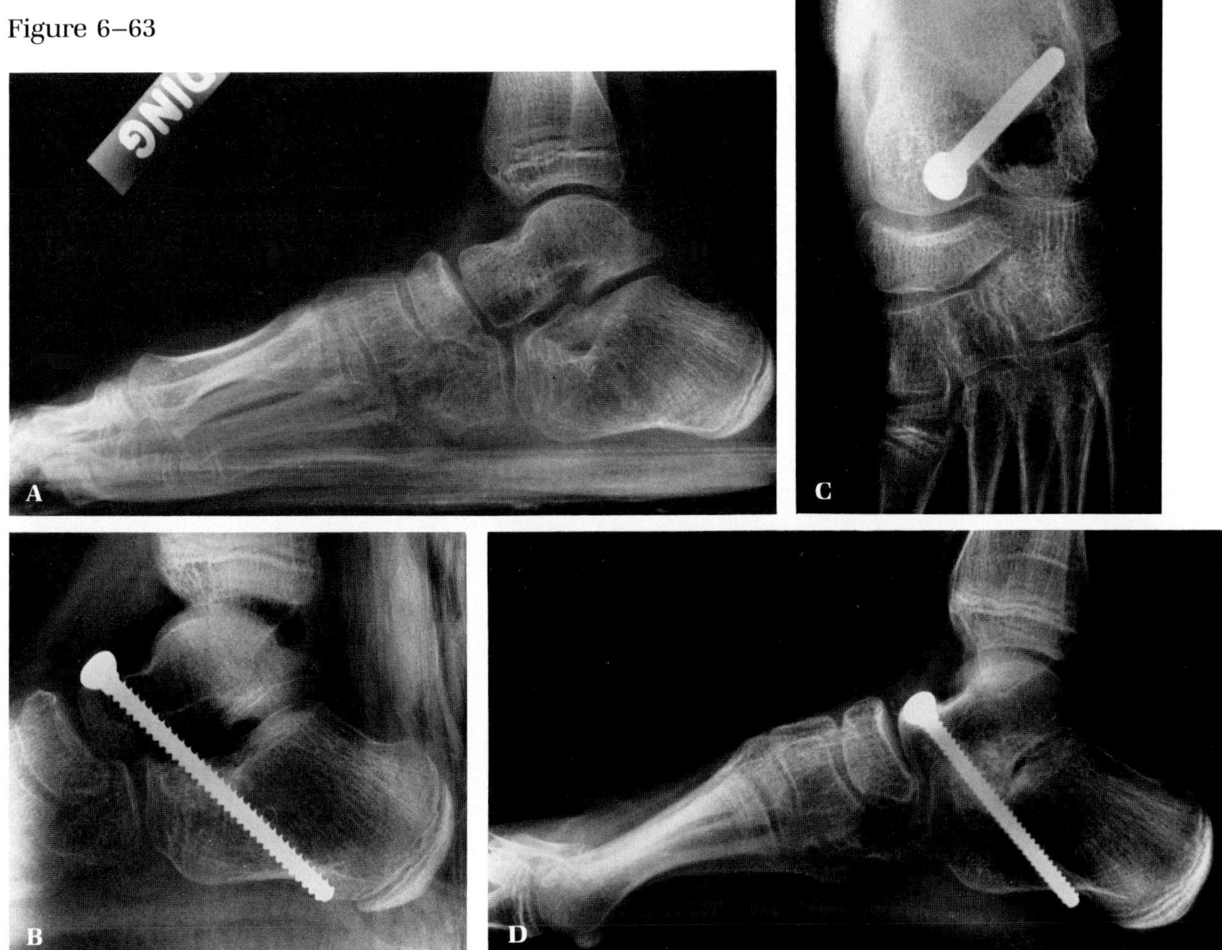

6.10
Mitchell Bunionectomy

In the adolescent, hallux valgus is more often accompanied by metatarsus primus varus than in the adult.[1] In this author's experience, metatarsus primus varus is almost always present in the adolescent with hallux valgus, and his major surgical disappointments have been where a metatarsal osteotomy was not performed. Therefore, correction will usually entail the removal of the exostosis, correction of the hallux valgus, and realignment of the first metatarsal.

Although the removal of the exostosis and the soft-tissue repair to correct the valgus of the great toe are standard, there are many methods described for correction of the metatarsus primus varus. Most surgeons seem to have their favorite method, but other considerations such as whether the metatarsal is short or long should also play a role in the choice of the procedure.

The Mitchell procedure, first described by Hawkins, Mitchell, and Hedrick in 1945,[2] displaces the metatarsal head laterally by means of a step cut just behind the metatarsal head. Although this procedure has a good record, it is technically demanding if the reported complications of avascular necrosis of the metatarsal head, non-union, malunion, and excessive shortening are to be avoided. Because some shortening of the first metatarsal is inevitable with this procedure, it is best used on those patients with a first metatarsal that is longer than the second metatarsal.

Figure 6–64. The incision is placed on the dorsal-medial side of the first metatarsal. It should extend from the flare of the proximal phalanx proximally three quarters of the way up the metatarsal. The incision is then deepened directly down to the periosteum and capsule, with care not to harm the dorsal or plantar branch of the nerve.

Figure 6–65. A V incision with the base on the proximal phalanx is now made in the capsule of the metatarsophalangeal joint. The two limbs of the V should be far enough apart and positioned such that when the capsule is repaired it will not tend to pull the toe into dorsiflexion or plantarflexion. This can occur if the base of the V on the phalanx is too far dorsal or plantar. This flap is elevated from proximal to distal by blunt and sharp dissection. In addition, the periosteum is elevated from the distal one half of the metatarsal. Care should be taken to leave the lateral attachments of capsule and periosteum because this is the sole remaining blood supply of what will become the distal fragment.

Figure 6–66. At the completion of the elevation of the capsular flap the joint will be open and the exostosis will be exposed. There is usually a clear demarcation between the exostosis and the actual metatarsal joint surface. This demarcation is a groove often referred to as Clark's groove. It is important to resist the temptation to remove too much bone with the exostosis as this may leave the medial side of the metatarsal head deficient.

A $\frac{1}{2}$-in osteotome is placed in Clark's groove and directed proximally in line with the metatarsal shaft. In the adolescent this exostosis is not usually large, and a large portion of it will consist of cartilage and fibrous tissue. This is a potential problem if a proximal opening-wedge osteotomy using the exostosis as graft is planned.

Figure 6–67. After the exostosis is removed the holes are drilled through which the suture will be passed to secure the osteotomy. The positioning of these holes will determine the location of the osteotomy, and therefore should be placed with care. The first hole is placed 1 cm behind the joint surface and toward the medial cortex, whereas the second hole is placed 1 cm proximal to the first hole and toward the lateral cortex. The holes are drilled from the dorsal aspect of the metatarsal and should be kept perpendicular to the axis of the shaft.

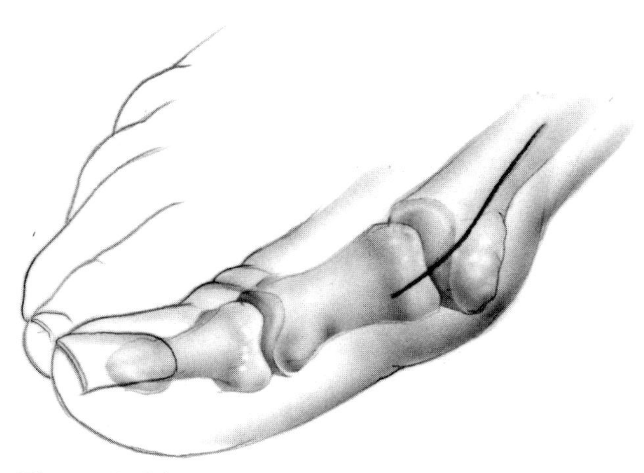

Figure 6–64

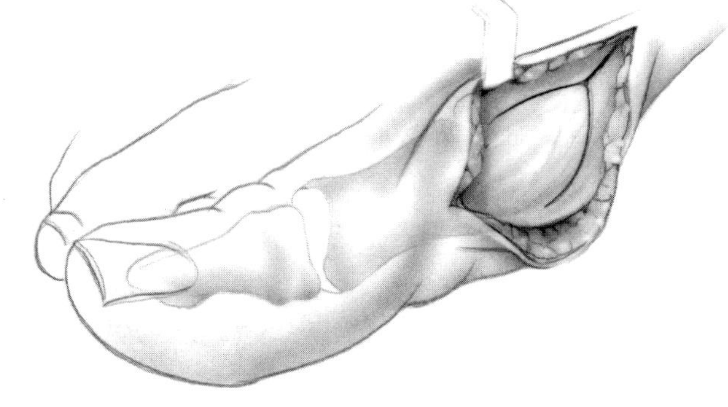

Figure 6–65

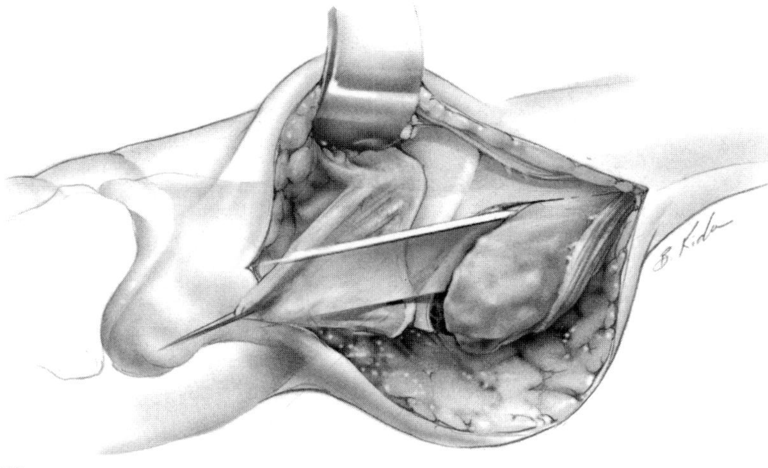

Figure 6–66

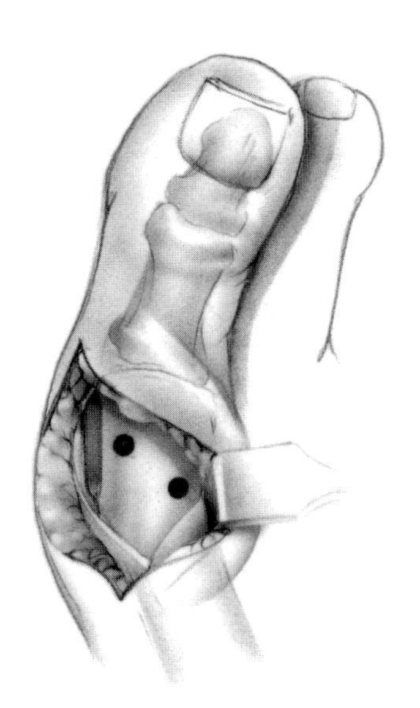

Figure 6–67

Figure 6–68. The suture that will hold the osteotomy can be passed at this point. A large, strong absorbable suture on a large needle is used. The needle is straightened some and is passed through the holes by the end that the suture attaches to rather than the sharp end. This way it will have less tendency to catch in the cancellous bone in the hole. Because it will be easier to tie the suture on the dorsal aspect of the metatarsal, the suture is passed through the first hole dorsal to plantar and through the second hold plantar to dorsal. The suture is left loose so that it will not be cut while performing the osteotomy. If the surgeon wishes the suture can be passed after the osteotomy is performed.

Figure 6–69. The osteotomy is created by first removing a small wedge of bone from the medial two thirds of the metatarsal midway between the two holes. If the distal cut is angled distally to produce a trapezoid, more tilt of the metatarsal head will be gained with less shortening.[3] It is important to keep this wedge small enough to avoid excessive shortening but with enough step-off to produce stability when the metatarsal head is displaced.

In addition, it is critical that the cuts be perpendicular to the longitudinal axis of the metatarsal. If this is not accomplished correctly, the metatarsal head may be plantarflexed or dorsiflexed, resulting in metatarsalgia of the first or second metatarsal heads, respectively.

After the wedge is created, the more proximal cut is completed through the metatarsal shaft, completing the osteotomy.

Figure 6–70. The distal fragment is displaced laterally, locking the step of bone on the proximal fragment over the lateral side of the proximal fragment. When judged to be satisfactory, the suture is tied, securing the osteotomy.

Figure 6–71. The capsular flap is now pulled proximally and the correction of the hallux valgus observed. It should not require excessive tension on this flap to correct the hallux valgus. This flap is in essence a Y to V advancement. It is sutured to the capsule and periosteum. The wound is closed without a drain.

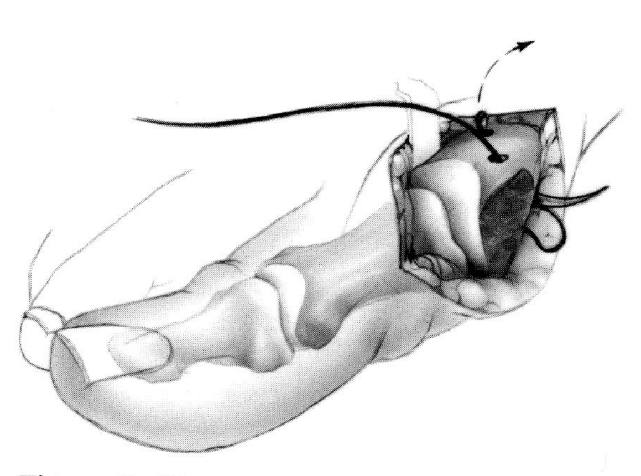

Figure 6–68

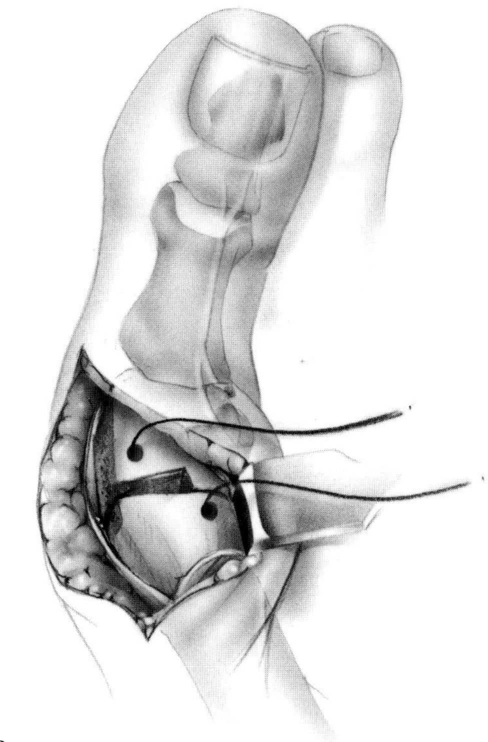

Figure 6–69

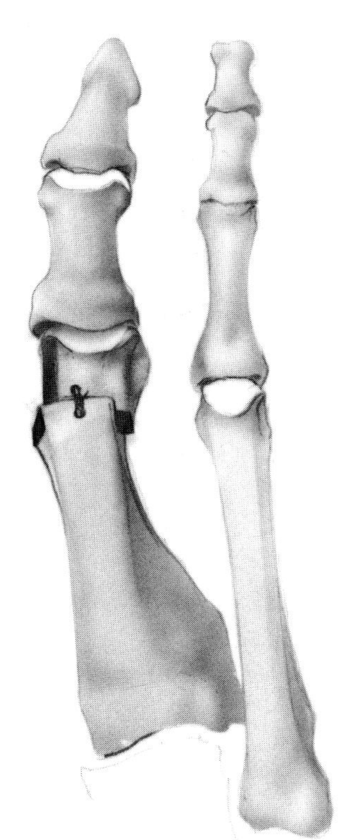

Figure 6–70

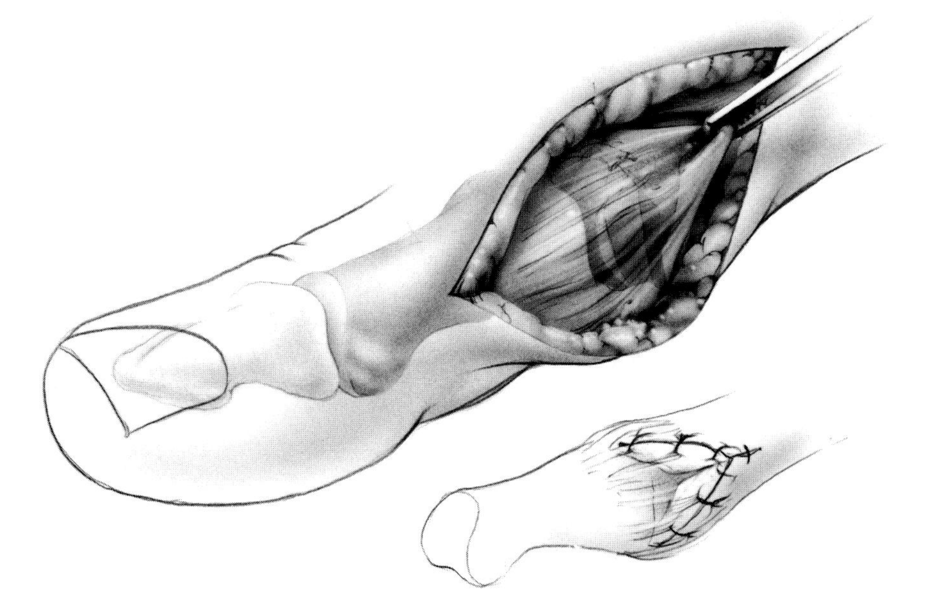

Figure 6–71

Figure 6–72. Preoperative radiograph of the right foot of a 10-year-old child with bilateral symptomatic bunions (***Figure 6–72A***). Note the metatarsus primus varus in addition to the hallux valgus. It is very unusual for a child of this age to be symptomatic. Correction at 6 weeks is demonstrated (***Figures 6–72B, C***).

POSTOPERATIVE CARE

Most surgeons have their favorite postoperative bunion dressing. It is important to note, however, that the average adolescent does not behave like the average adult during the postoperative period. Therefore, the usual type of semirigid bunion dressing is used only for the first week until the swelling and soreness are gone. Then a short leg cast is applied. It should be well-molded around the forefoot, and hold a soft bolster between the first and second toe to take any tension off of the capsular repair. This cast is worn for 6 weeks, at which time the osteotomy is usually healed sufficiently to permit full, unprotected weight-bearing. While in the cast, the patient may be permitted crutch-protected weight-bearing.

REFERENCES

1. Mann RA. Surgery of the foot, 5th ed. St. Louis: CV Mosby, 1986:69.
2. Hawkins FB, Mitchell CL, Hedrick DW. Correction of hallux valgus by metatarsal osteotomy. J Bone Joint Surg 1945;27:387.
3. Hammond G. Mitchell osteotomy-bunionectomy for hallux valgus and metatarsus primus varus. In: Instructional Course Lectures, vol 21. The American Academy of Orthopaedic Surgeons. St. Louis: CV Mosby, 1972:246.

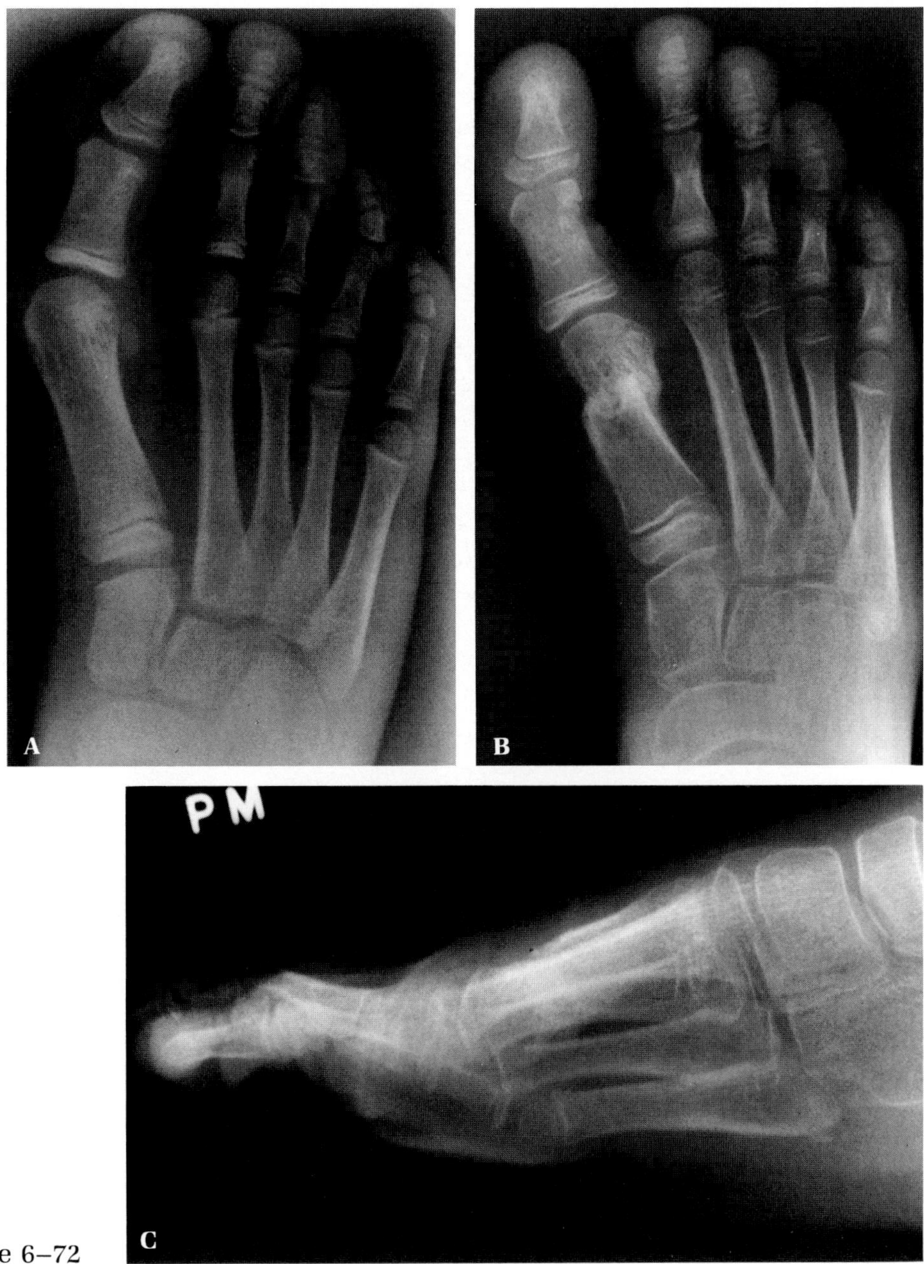

Figure 6–72

6.11 Proximal Metatarsal Osteotomy and Bunionectomy

The proximal osteotomy aims to achieve the same goals as the distal osteotomies (*eg*, the Mitchell osteotomy). The advantages of the proximal osteotomy is that shortening is little to none, the possibility of avascular necrosis of the metatarsal head is avoided, and the fixation is arguably securer. Excision of the exostosis and correction of the hallux valgus are performed in the same manner as described in the Mitchell osteotomy.

Figure 6–73. The operation can be performed through one long incision that is simply a proximal extension to the incision used for the Mitchell procedure (***Figure 6–73B***)**;** the removal of the exostosis and repair of the hallux valgus can also be done through a distal incision, whereas the osteotomy is done through a separate more dorsally placed proximal incision (***Figure 6–73C***)**.** The former will be illustrated for clarity.

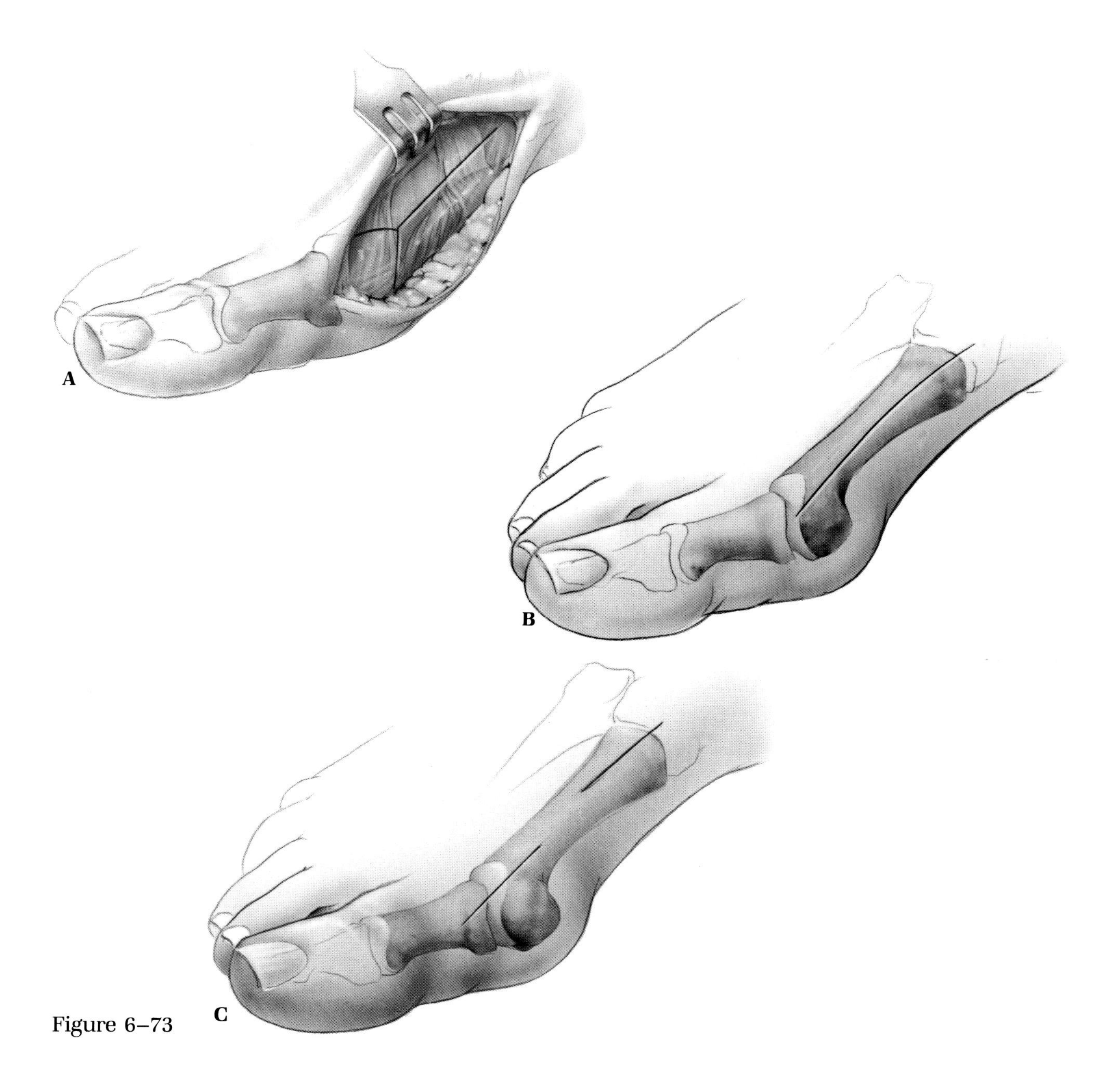

Figure 6–73

Figure 6–74. The periosteum is stripped from the proximal metatarsal to expose the bone 1 cm distal to the metatarsocuneiform joint. Periosteal stripping can be minimized by using two small, sharp, pointed, Homann retractors under the periosteum at the osteotomy site.

Although the osteotomy can be performed by connecting multiple drill holes with a small osteotomy, a powered crescentic osteotomy saw can accomplish this much easier and with less loss of bone. When using this saw it needs to be emphasized that the blade has a very small excursion. If the saw is held still, and worse if it is pressed too hard into the bone, the blade will not move, but rather the saw will vibrate undetectably in the surgeon's hand. Therefore, when the cut is being made the saw should be kept moving in an arch, which describes the desired osteotomy, and it should not be pushed too hard into the bone. Copious irrigation should also be used to avoid excessive heating of the bone.

Figure 6–75. Whether the osteotomy should be concave on the proximal or distal fragment is a matter of debate. Mann believes that the proximal surface should be concave.[1] This will tend to displace the proximal part of the distal fragment medially while the metatarsal head is displaced laterally (***Figure 6–75B***). The author prefers to place the concave surface on the proximal fragment. This will tend to displace the entire shaft laterally as well as tilt the metatarsal head laterally (***Figure 6–75C***). To allow the rotation to occur, the lateral corner of the concave surface should be removed. This is easily accomplished with a small rongeur.

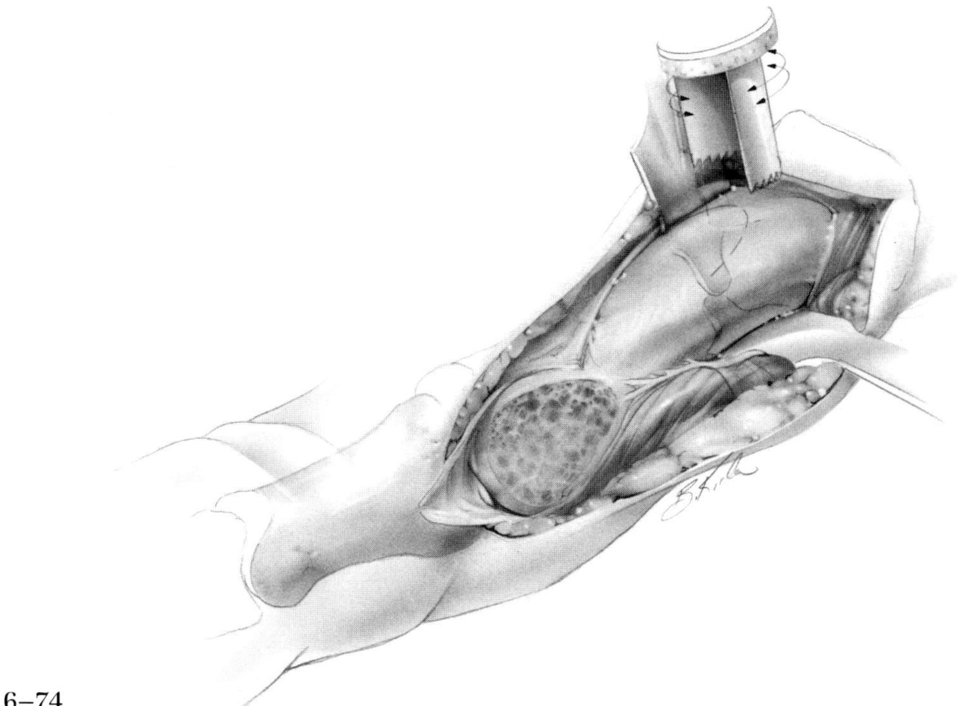

Figure 6–74

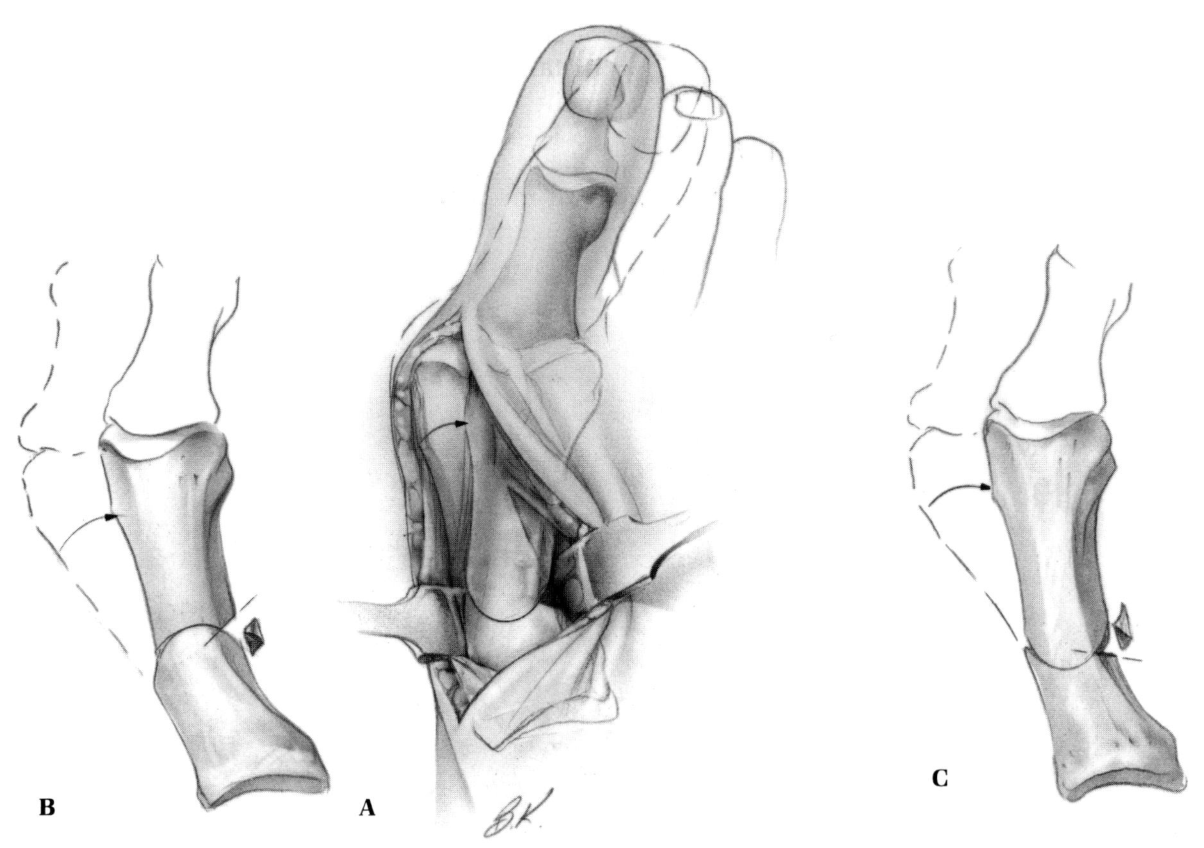

Figure 6–75

Figure 6–76. The osteotomy can be held by several methods of fixation, but none is so simple as a suitably strong Kirschner wire or Steinmann pin. The difficulty of starting this pin at the desired angle through thick cortical bone is avoided by drilling a hole in the lateral aspect of the metatarsal shaft 1 cm distal to the osteotomy. If two incisions are used this can be done through a small stab wound. This pin will usually pass into the base of the more proximally situated second metatarsal. It can be continued into the cuneiform bone. A small length of the pin is left out of the skin so that the pin can be easily removed.

The repair of the capsule to correct the hallux valgus is completed, and the wounds are closed.

Figure 6–77. Anteroposterior view of the right foot of a 13+2-year-old girl who had painful bunions secondary to metatarsus primus varus is shown (***Figure 6–77A***). Twenty months later proximal metatarsal osteotomy and bunionectomy were performed because of the inability to provide relief by modification of the shoe wear that was acceptable to the patient. Six weeks after the surgery (***Figure 6–77B***), the correction of the metatarsus primus varus and removal of the bunion are seen.

POSTOPERATIVE CARE

The postoperative care is the same as for the Mitchell procedure. (See section 6.10.)

REFERENCE

1. Mann RA. Surgery of the foot, 5th ed. St. Louis: CV Mosby, 1986:95.

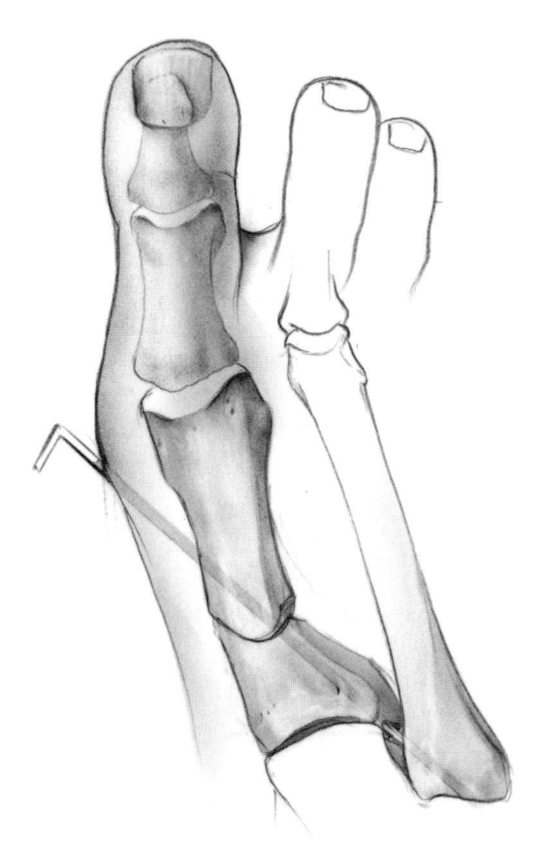

Figure 6–76

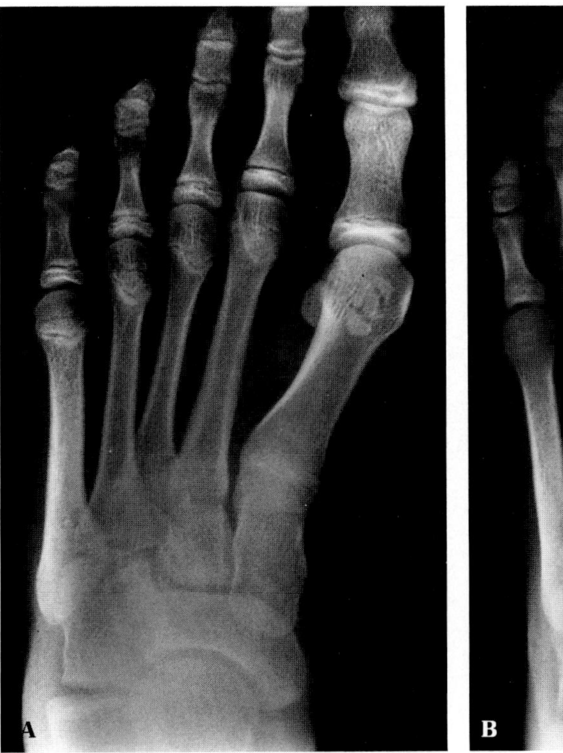

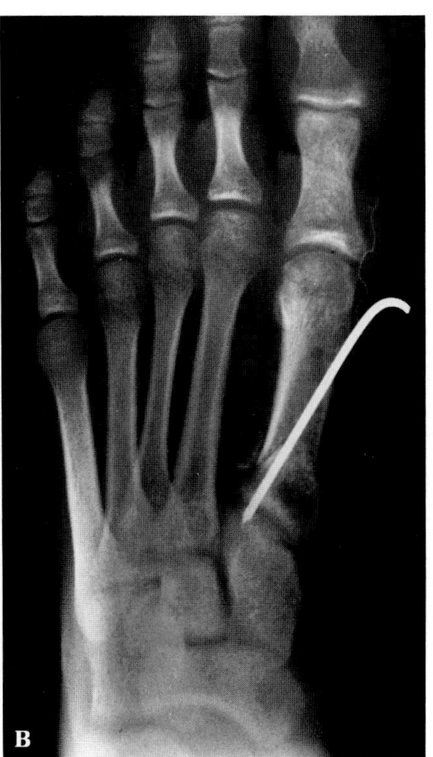

Figure 6–77

6.12 Open Lengthening of Achilles Tendon

Lengthening of the Achilles tendon is one of the commonest operations in pediatric orthopaedics. Traditionally, the operation is performed by completely exposing the tendon. Once exposed the tendon can be completely divided in a Z manner and then sutured together at a longer length. This is indicated when it is also necessary to open the posterior aspect of the subtalar or tibiotalar joint.

Because of the unique anatomic arrangement of the fibers in the tendon, it is also possible to perform a lengthening while leaving the fibers in continuity.[1] Within the portion of the tendon that is exposed for lengthening, the fibers rotate 90 degrees. Thus, as described by White, if the anterior two thirds of the tendon are divided just above its insertion into the calcaneus, and its medial two thirds are divided at the proximal extent of the tendon, the two bundles of fibers will slide past one another as the foot is dorsiflexed. Although initially described as percutaneous technique, this is most often done open.

Figure 6–78. An open lengthening of the Achilles tendon is most easily performed with the patient prone. With an assistant to hold the leg, however, it is possible to perform the operation with the patient supine if this position is dictated by other procedures that are performed at the same time.

The skin over the Achilles tendon is thin, and this in turn can lead to problems in the healing of the wound. The incision should not be placed over the thin skin directly posterior to the Achilles tendon. Incisions with curves are not necessary and can only lead to further problems. The incision should be placed on the medial side on the ankle just anterior to the Achilles tendon. This skin has a good layer of subcutaneous tissue and will pose no problems for wound closure or healing.

Figure 6–79. The incision is carried through the dermis and into the subcutaneous fat. The knife then angles slightly posterior, cutting directly into the sheath of the Achilles tendon. The sheath around the tendon is composed of multiple layers of thin, filmy tissue. In one small area of the incision, before all of the subcutaneous fat is divided, care is taken to deepen the cut to penetrate every layer of this filmy tissue.

At this point a small forceps is used to lift this filmy sheath from the tendon, and one blade of a scissors is passed between it and the tendon. The remainder of the incision is now opened with this scissors cutting through the subcutaneous fat and tendon sheath together. In so doing, the tendon sheath is left attached to the subcutaneous fat. This will preserve the sheath, and as the subcutaneous tissue is closed the sheath will also close without the need for sutures in it.

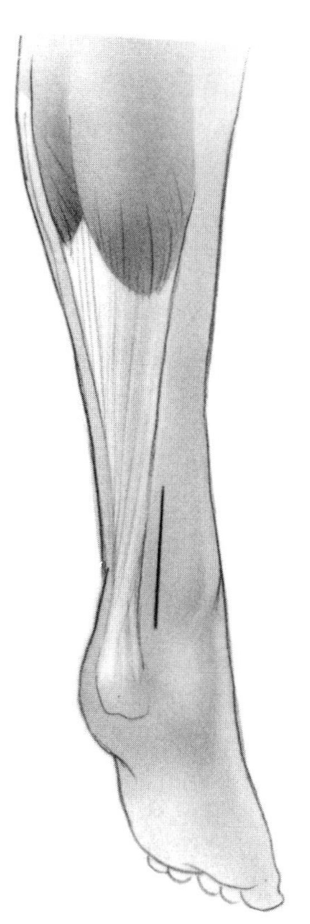

Figure 6–78

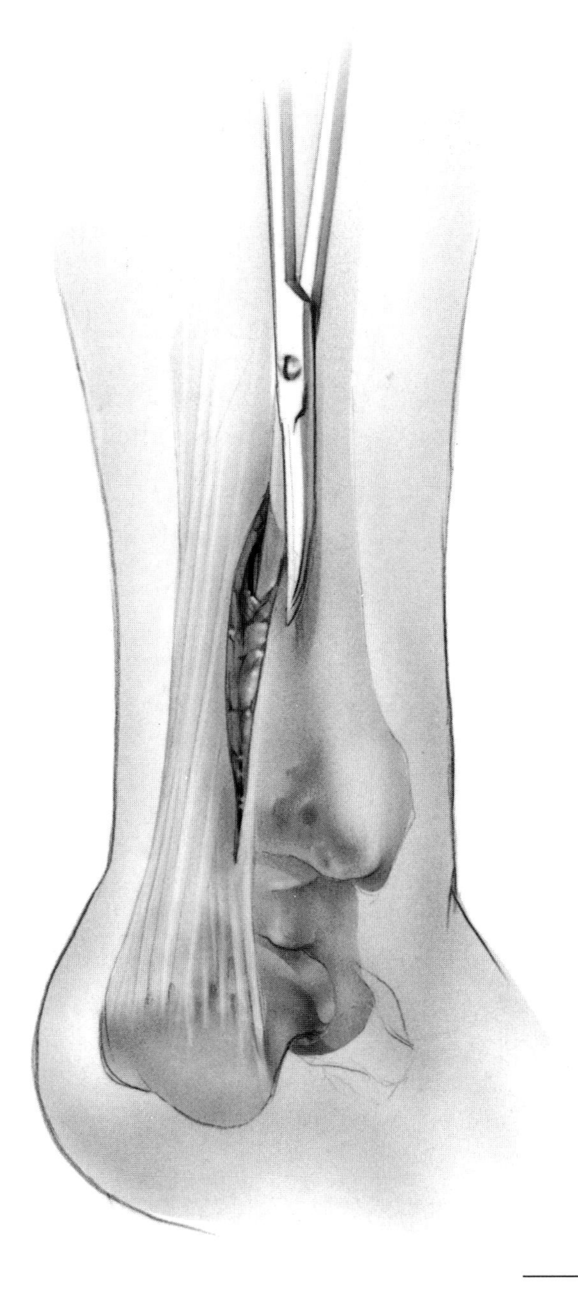

Figure 6–79

Figure 6–80. If a sliding lengthening is to be performed the first incision will be placed just above the attachment of the tendon into the calcaneus. Starting on the anterior surface or undersurface of the tendon, the anterior two thirds of the fibers are divided almost completely across to the lateral side.

Figure 6–81. Next, the medial two thirds of the tendon are divided proximally. This cut should be done as far proximal to the distal cut as is possible while remaining in the purely tendinous portion of the tendon. As this cut is made, the foot is held in dorsiflexion to produce tension on the tendon. Shortly after one half of the tendon is divided, the foot should start to go into dorsiflexion as the two halves of the tendon start to slide past one another. It is not usually necessary to suture the tendon as it should remain in continuity and further undesired lengthening is prevented by the cast.

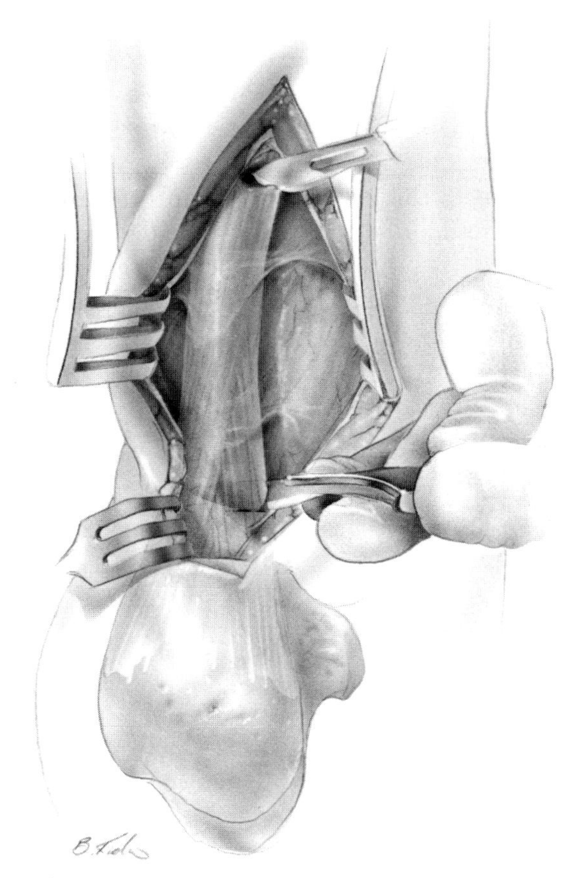

Figure 6–80

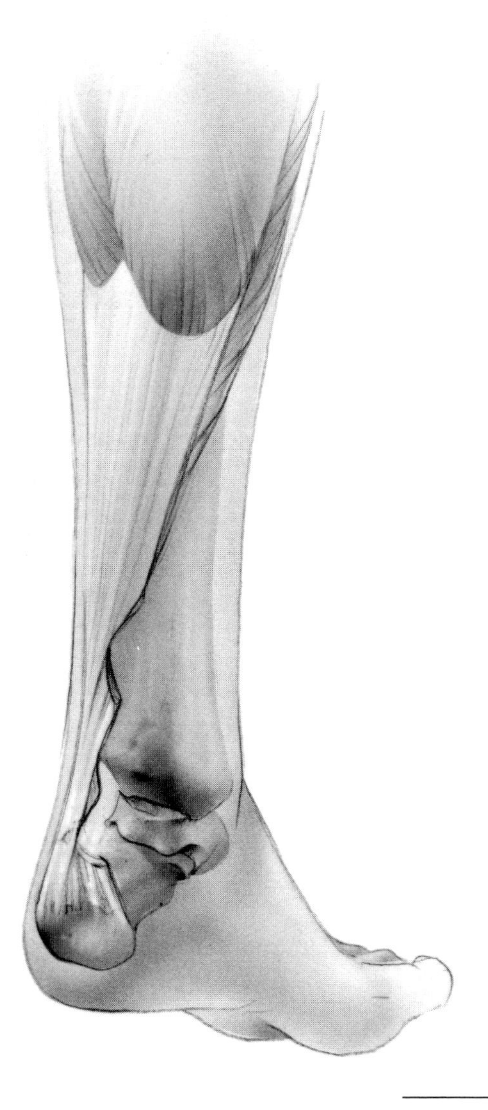

Figure 6–81

Figure 6–82. If it is desired to perform a Z lengthening, it is easiest to start the incision at the proximal extent of the tendon. The blade of a number 15 knife blade is inserted completely through the tendon, and with a sawing motion is drawn distally, producing a division down the middle of the tendon. As the knife reaches the insertion to the calcaneus, it is turned 90 degrees, and the distal and medial one half of the tendon is detached from the calcaneus. The knife is then reinserted into the proximal extent of the longitudinal cut that was made previously and turned laterally, dividing the proximal lateral one half of the tendon.

Figure 6–83. The foot can now be dorsiflexed to the desired position. With an assistant holding the foot in the correct position, the surgeon determines where the tendon should be sutured. This may be done by overlapping the two ends of the tendon and suturing them side to side. (***Figure 6–83A***). It is also possible, especially in the smaller child, to cut off the excess length from one or both sides and perform an end-to-end repair with a buried suture (***Figure 6–83B***). This technique minimizes the amount of foreign body (suture) and thus should minimize inflammation in the tendon sheath. Care should be taken that the tendon is sutured under moderate tension to avoid significant weakening of plantar flexion and a consequent calcaneus gait.

The wound is now closed with a fine, interrupted, absorbable suture in the subcutaneous tissue and subcuticular suture in the skin. Although the fact that the gastrocnemius muscle crosses the knee joint would call for a long leg cast, this is rarely necessary. A short leg cast is applied with the foot in the desired position.

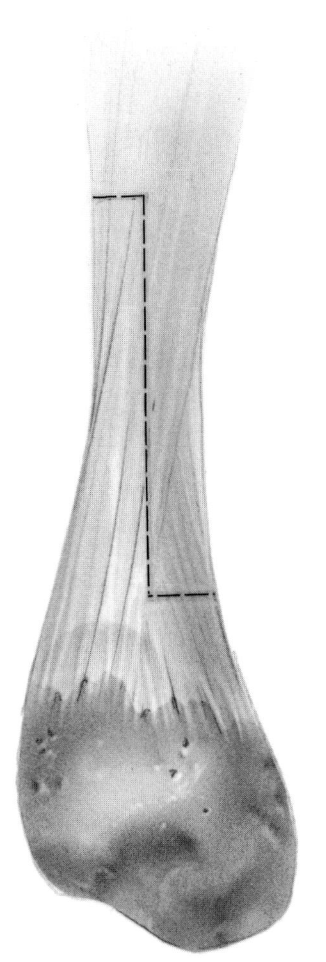

Figure 6–82

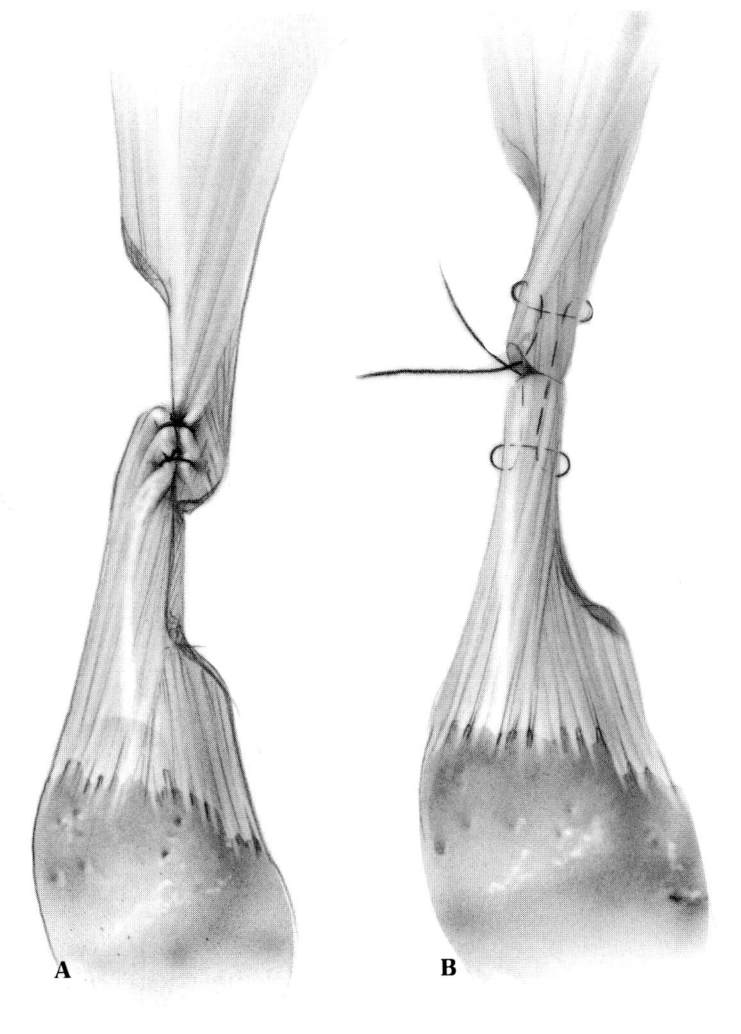

Figure 6–83

POSTOPERATIVE CARE

The procedure is usually performed as an outpatient procedure. The parents are requested to keep the foot elevated for 2 to 3 days, after which the patient may begin ambulation in the cast. The cast can safely be removed at 6 weeks, at which time the tendon should be completely healed.

REFERENCE

1. White WJ. Torsion of the Achilles tendon: its surgical significance. Arch Surg 1943;46:784.

6.13 Percutaneous Lengthening of Achilles Tendon

Percutaneous lengthening of the Achilles tendon has several advantages over open lengthening and, in the opinion of the author, almost no disadvantages. It can be performed at any age and can be done for a repeat lengthening of the tendon. There is no incision, and the postoperative pain is considerably less.

Percutaneous Achilles lengthening is best done with a tenotomy knife. This is a small, specially shaped knife that is designed for percutaneous tenotomy. It is shaped so that it can be stabbed through the skin. It is not so sharp as the disposable surgical knife blades and is thus far less likely to cut the skin.

Although the tenotomy can be done with two cuts in the tendon as described by White,[1] it is most easily done by placing three cuts in the tendon.

Figure 6–84. The tendon will be divided in three places. The medial one half of the tendon will be divided at both the proximal and the distal extent of the tendon, and the lateral one half will be divided midway between the two medial cuts. The location of the entry portals is just above the insertion into the calcaneus, at the most proximal portion of the tendon before it becomes muscular, and midway between these two.

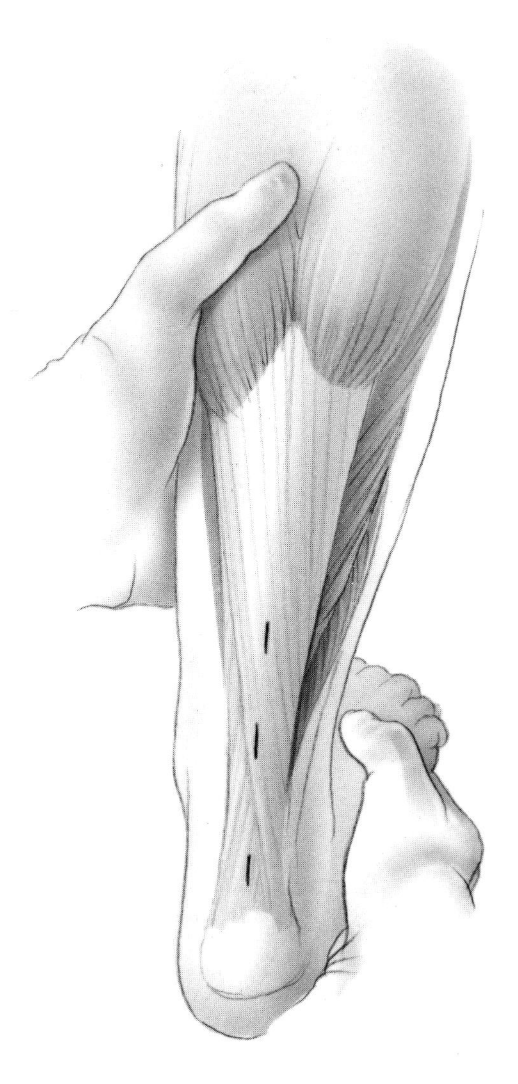

Figure 6–84

Figure 6–85. The three sequential steps in cutting the tendon are illustrated (***Figures 6–85A, B***). *Step 1:* The tenotomy knife is pushed directly through the skin and the tendon, keeping the blade oriented longitudinally with the tendon. (It is easier to make the initial stab wound in the skin with a number 15 disposable surgical blade.) *Step 2:* The blade of the knife is rotated 90 degrees toward the part of the tendon that is to be divided. *Step 3:* The surgeon drops his or her hand to bring the blade of the knife under the portion of the tendon that is to be cut. Using a sawing motion, a portion of the tendon is cut. The knife will be cutting toward the skin. If the surgeon keeps his or her finger directly over the portion of the tendon being cut, he or she will feel the blade of the knife when the cut is completed. The knife will not be so sharp that it cuts through the skin as a disposable knife blade would.

Figure 6–86. The most proximal and distal cuts should be made first and the middle cut last. If the middle cut is made before the proximal and distal cuts, either the proximal or distal segment may lengthen as tension is kept on the tendon. When the middle cut is made, the foot should go into dorsiflexion and the tendon fibers start to slide. A small dressing is placed over the stab wounds, and a short leg walking cast applied.

POSTOPERATIVE CARE

The surgery is performed as an outpatient surgery. The parents are requested to keep the foot elevated for 24 to 48 hours, after which the patient may resume ambulation. Mild narcotic analgesic may be needed for the first night. The cast can be removed in 6 weeks.

REFERENCE

1. White WJ. Torsion of the Achilles tendon: its surgical significance. Arch Surg 1943;46:784.

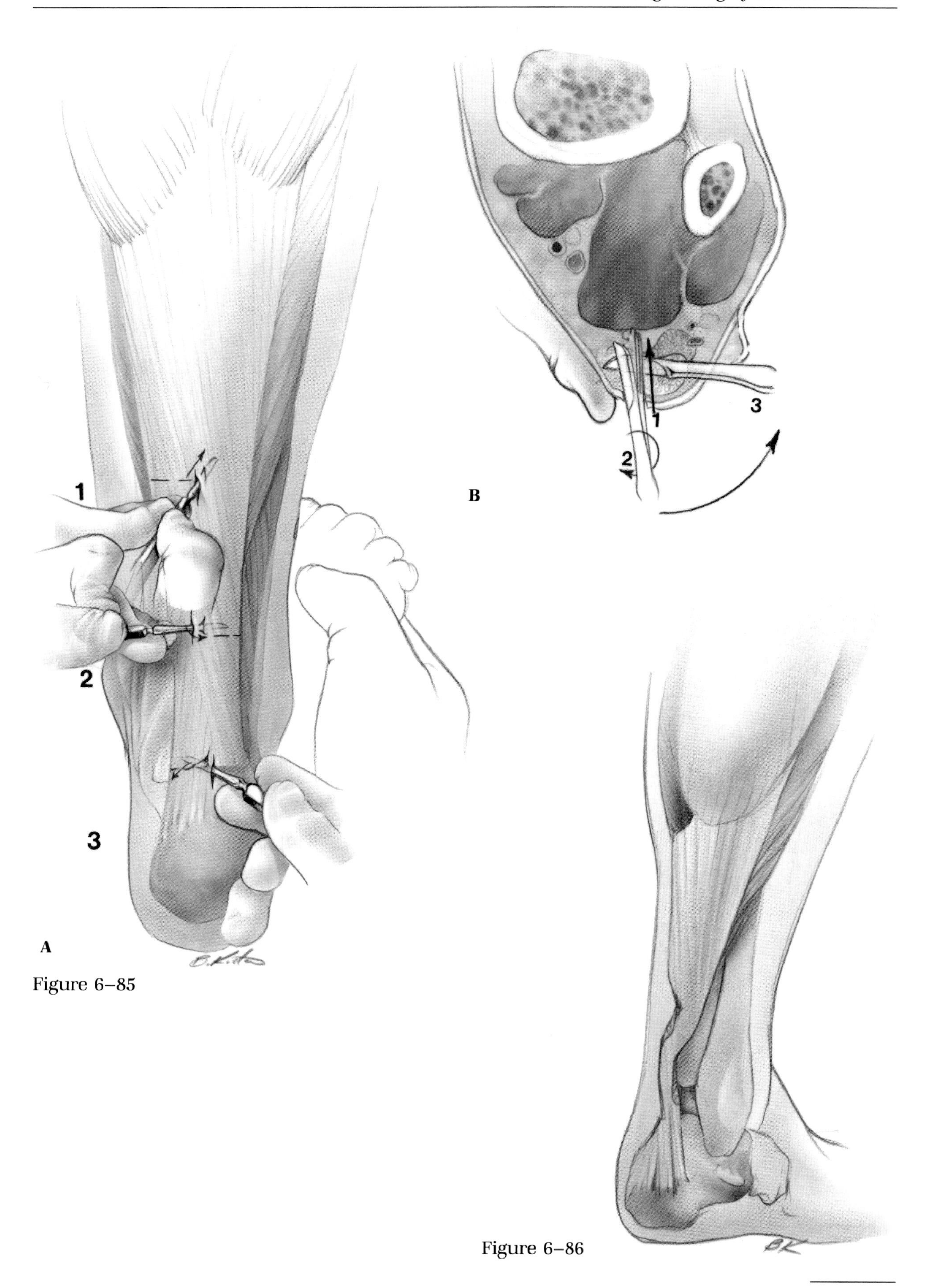

Figure 6–85

Figure 6–86

6.14 Split Posterior Tibial Tendon Transfer

Spasticity of the posterior tibial tendon is recognized as a frequent cause of hindfoot varus in cerebral palsy. This is usually associated with equinus deformity, producing the typical equinovarus foot. Many operations have been described for the treatment of varus from this cause including lengthening, rerouting of the tendon anterior to the medial malleolus, anterior transfer of the tendon through the interosseous membrane, tenotomy, and lengthening. All have been associated, however, with a significant incidence of complications ranging from recurrence to collapse of the foot.

In 1977 Kaufer[1] described splitting the posterior tibial tendon and transferring one half of it to the lateral side of the foot. His goal was to use part of the spastic muscle to balance the foot rather than to transfer the entire spastic muscle or eliminate its function entirely. Green, Griffin, and Shiavi in 1983,[2] and Kling, Kaufer, and Hensinger in 1985[3] further described the technique and their results.

It is important to be certain that it is the posterior tibial tendon and not the anterior tibial tendon that is the deforming force. This can usually be determined by observation of the child in gait. The foot will usually be in equinus as well as varus. The foot remains in varus during the entire swing cycle, and the lateral side of the foot strikes the floor first. The posterior tibial tendon rather than the anterior tibial tendon will be seen to be taught. There should be no fixed deformity. A percutaneous lengthening of the Achilles tendon can be done at the beginning of the procedure to correct the equinus component if it exists.

Figure 6–87. The patient is placed supine on the operating table. Placing a large sand bag under the hip on the side to be operated will make operating on the lateral side of the foot easier and will not interfere with the medial part of the procedure. Kling et al[3] describe using two large incisions; however, the author prefers the four smaller incisions as described by Green et al[2] (***Figure 6–87A***). The first incision is directly over the insertion of the posterior tibial tendon extending from just distal to the tip of the medial malleolus to the insertion of the tendon on the navicular.

Through this incision the inferior one half of the posterior tibial tendon is split and detached (***Figure 6–87B***). It is advisable to detach one of the plantar extensions of the tendon as described in the medial release of club foot. This will be useful in securing the tendon at the conclusion of the operation. The foot is everted to pull as much of the tendon into the wound as possible, and the tendon is split as far proximal as possible. A portion of the tendon sheath should be left intact to hold the remaining tendon in place behind the medial malleolus.

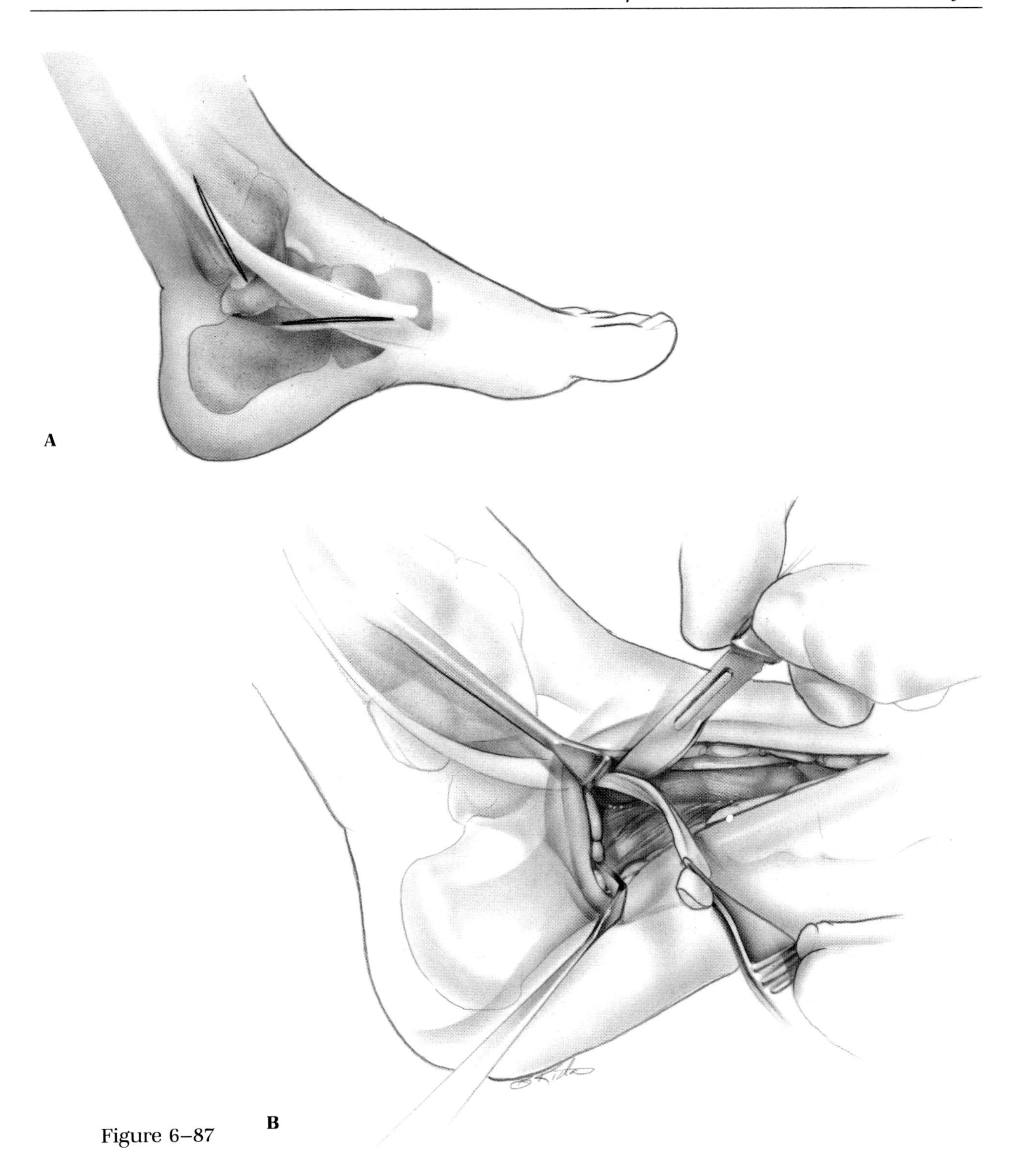

Figure 6–87

Figure 6–88. The second incision is made over the course of the posterior tibial tendon along the posterior border of the tibia beginning 1 cm above the medial malleolus and extending for approximately 4 cm. The foot is now inverted to permit the distal part of the tendon to be drawn into this wound. It is usually possible to identify the most proximal division of the tendon that was accomplished through the first wound. When the split in the tendon is identified, the incision into the tendon is continued to divide it as far proximal as possible. Caution must be used because in many children this is not a large tendon, and it can be difficult to divide it into two equal halves. When the division is complete the split portion of the tendon is drawn into this wound.

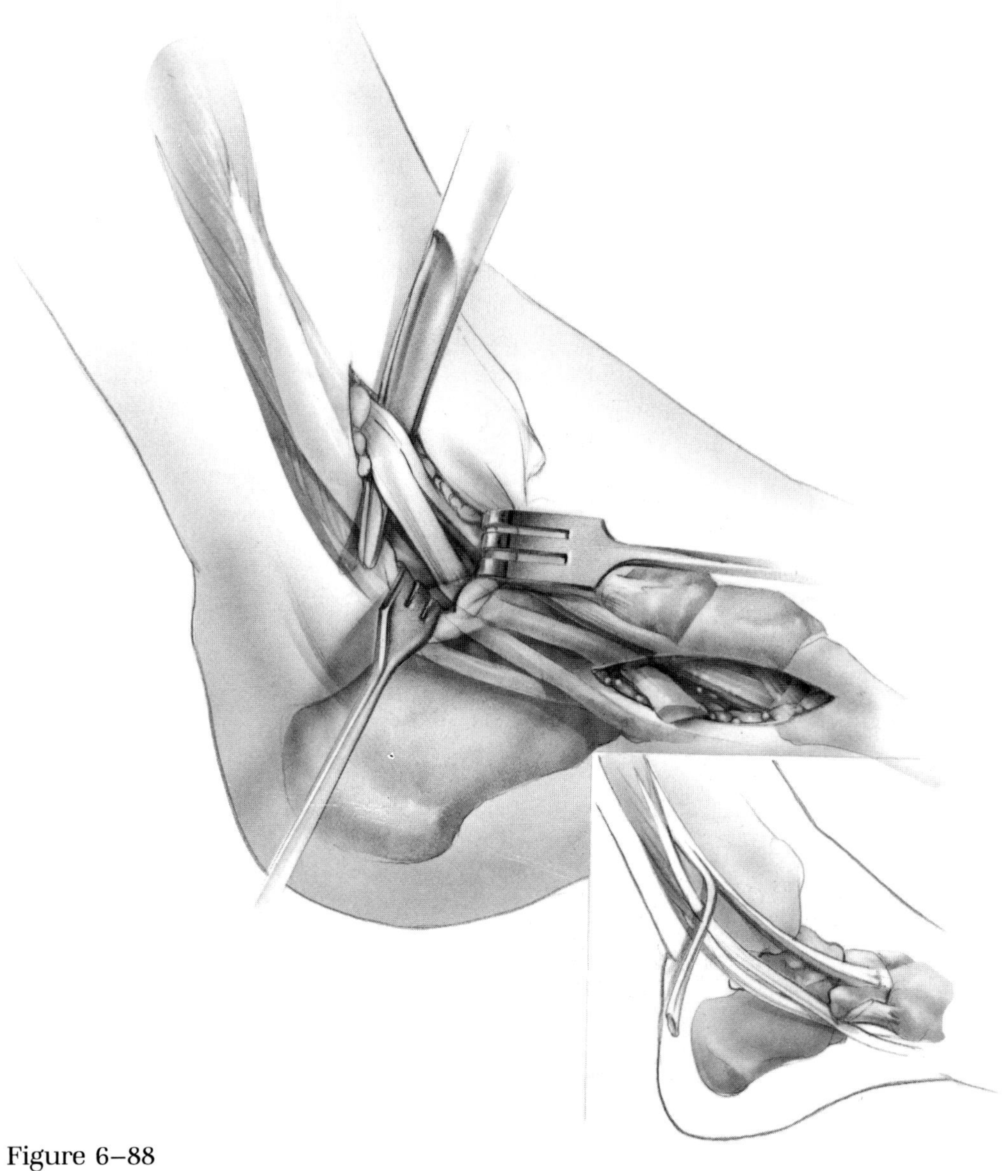

Figure 6–88

Figure 6–89. The third incision is made behind the lateral malleolus. It should extend from near the distal portion of the malleolus proximally for about 4 cm. The peroneal tendons are exposed and the peroneus brevis tendon identified. The peroneus brevis muscle is the smaller, and most superficial and movable of the two peroneal tendons. Confirmation can be made after the next incision is made.

The next task is to pass the split portion of the posterior tibial tendon from the medial side of the leg to the lateral side. In doing so it is important that the tendon remain in contact with the posterior surface of the tibia and anterior to the neurovascular structures (***Figure 6–89B***). The author finds it easier to start the tendon passer on the medial side, where it is certain that it is in contact with the posterior surface of the tibia. After pulling the tendon through, its direction should be checked to be certain that it takes a relatively straight course. An error is to not split the tendon far enough proximally so that it takes off from the muscle belly at an acute angle.

At this point the two medial wounds should be closed.

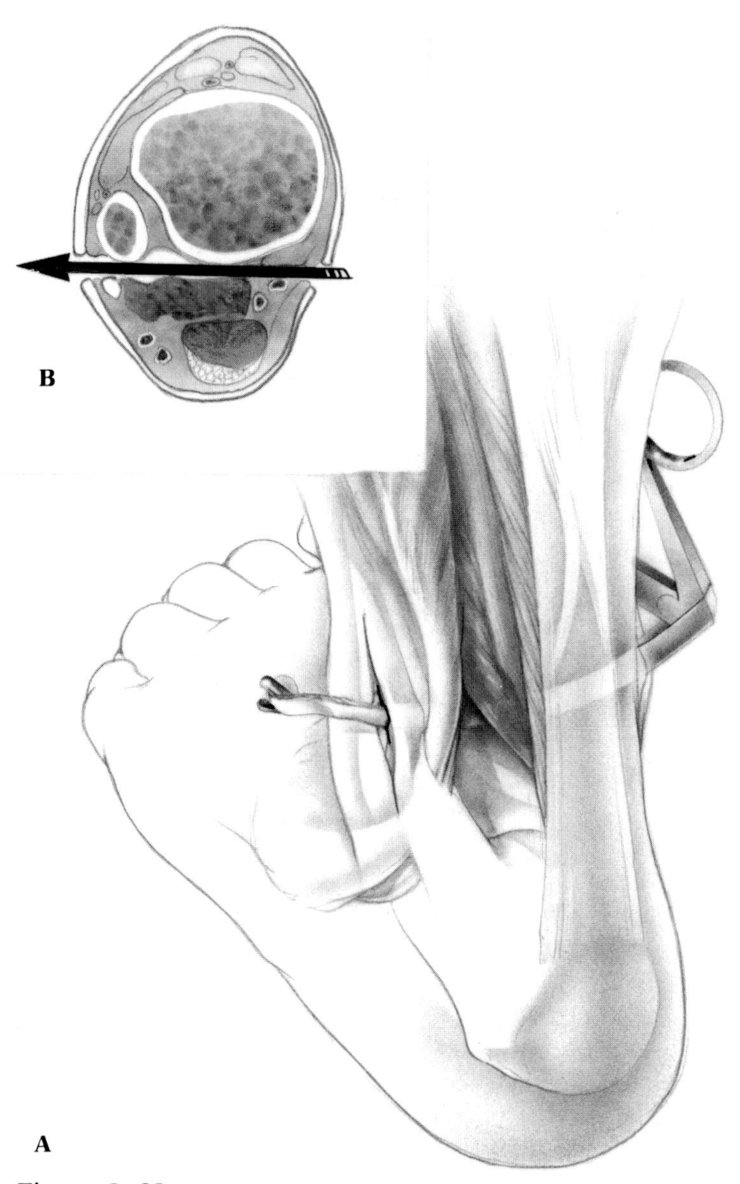

Figure 6–89

Figure 6–90. The final incision is made along the course of the peroneus brevis tendon from just distal to the tip of the lateral malleolus to a point just proximal to the base of the fifth metatarsal. The peroneus brevis muscle is exposed.

The split portion of the posterior tibial tendon is now passed behind the lateral malleolus, under the retinaculum holding the peroneal tendons in place, and into the sheath of the peroneus brevis tendon.

At this point the proximal wound is closed, leaving only the distal wound to close after the tendon is secured.

The split portion of the posterior tibial tendon is now woven through two or three small splits in the peroneus brevis tendon. Care should be taken to adjust the tension in the transfer. With the foot held in a neutral position of varus-valgus, the portion of the posterior tibial tendon is pulled firmly and sutured to the peroneus brevis tendon, where it passes through it. The final suture should secure the end of the posterior tibial tendon to the strong tissue of the insertion of the peroneus brevis tendon. It is here that the surgeon will appreciate the few extra minutes to get all of the possible length on the posterior tibial tendon. This wound is now closed.

POSTOPERATIVE CARE

The author does not use a long leg cast for this procedure or for an Achilles tendon lengthening in an ambulatory child. This does not affect the result, does not result in greater discomfort, and allows the child to ambulate sooner and easier. The cast is maintained for 6 weeks. After the cast is removed, the child is placed in a brace if indicated or allowed unrestricted ambulation if it is not. The author's requirement for no brace is that the child can actively dorsiflex the foot to neutral. It is very unusual for a child with equinovarus deformity owing to cerebral palsy to be able to do this, and bracing is usually required for at least 1 year.

REFERENCES

1. Kaufer H. Split tendon transfers. Orthop Trans 1977;1:191.
2. Green NE, Griffin PP, Shiavi R. Split posterior tibial-tendon transfer in spastic cerebral palsy. J Bone Joint Surg 1983;65A:748.
3. Kling TF, Kaufer H, Hensinger RN. Split posterior tibial-tendon transfers in children with cerebral spastic paralysis and equinovarus deformity. J Bone Joint Surg 1985;67A:186.

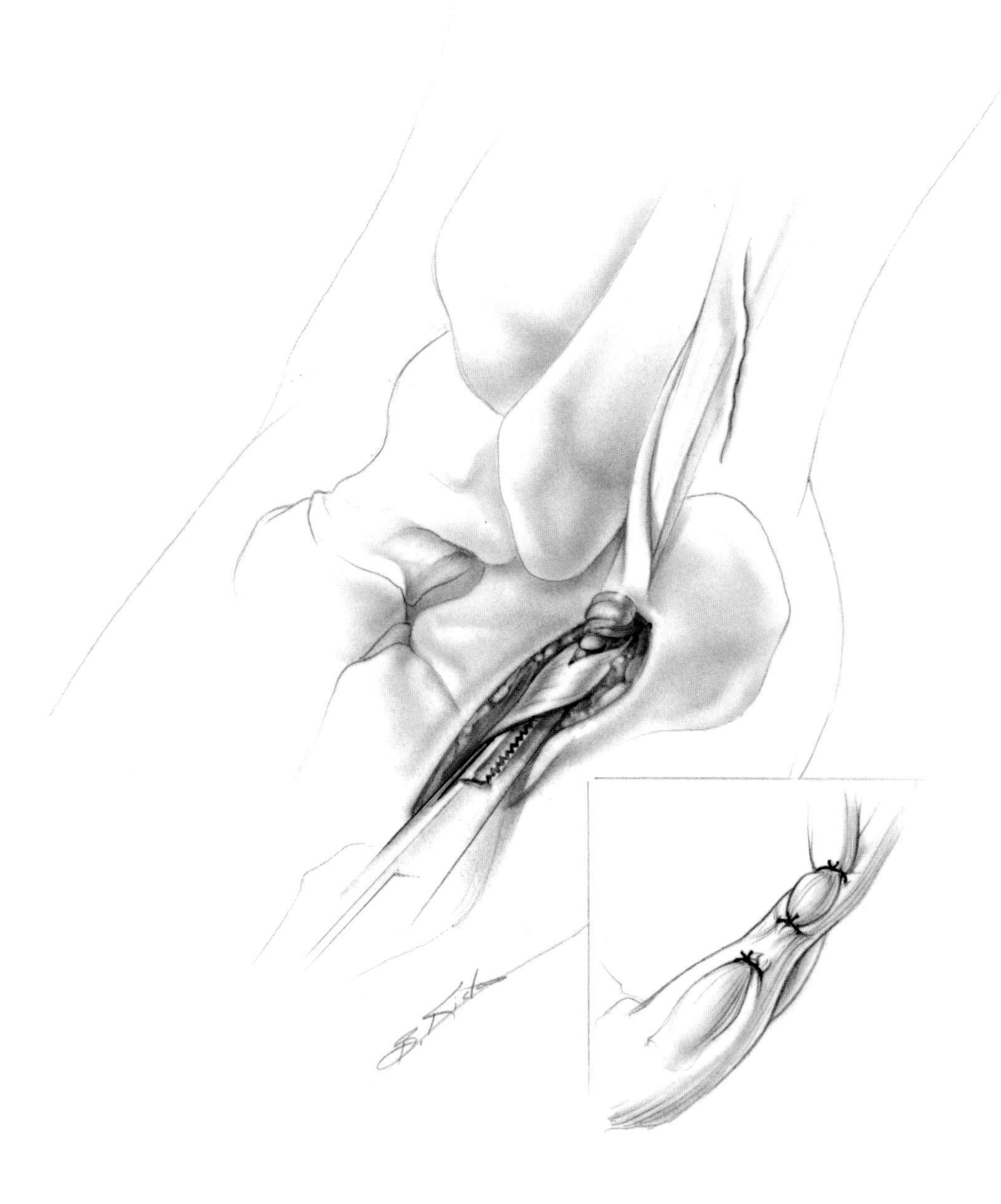

Figure 6–90

6.15
Anterior Transfer of Posterior Tibial Tendon

Transfer of the posterior tibial tendon to the dorsum of the foot has been recommended in the treatment of many conditions: cavovarus deformity as seen in Charcot-Marie-Tooth disease or Duchenne muscular dystrophy, recurrence of forefoot deformity in club foot, and conditions that weaken dorsiflexion of the foot (*eg*, polio and traumatic injuries). This transfer accomplishes two goals. First, it will remove the posterior tibial tendon as a deforming force. Second, it will augment dorsiflexion of the foot. It is important to realize that the posterior tibial muscle cannot substitute for the anterior tibial muscle. The reasons for this are numerous: The muscle is required to act out of phase after the transfer, it will be difficult to establish proper tension in the transferred muscle, and although the posterior tibial muscle is stronger than the anterior tibial muscle, its excursion is less.[1] With these facts in mind the decision is often between transfer and tenotomy of the posterior tibial tendon. In Charcot-Marie-Tooth disease in which the posterior tibial tendon often remains strong for a considerable period, transfer to augment dorsiflexion makes sense, whereas in Duchenne muscular dystrophy in which progression of muscle weakness in all muscles is much more rapid and bracing will be required regardless of the surgery, tenotomy makes more sense.

Two techniques have been described for transfer of the posterior tibial tendon to the dorsum of the foot. One technique routes the tendon around the medial side of the tibia and through the anterior compartment of the leg to the dorsum of the foot. This technique does not appear to be in wide use at the present time. The second technique is to transfer the tendon through the interosseous membrane into the anterior compartment and then onto the dorsum of the foot. This is the technique that will be described here.

Figure 6–91. The first incision extends along the course of the posterior tibial tendon distal to the tip of the medial malleolus **(*Figure 6–91A*).** The tendon can be identified as a distinct structure in its sheath in the proximal part of the wound at the tip of the medial malleolus. From there it will fan out into its broad insertion. It is important to recognize that deep to and blending with the insertion of the posterior tibial tendon is the anterior tibiotalar and tibionavicular ligaments, which are portions of the deltoid ligament. In detaching the posterior tibial tendon, these ligaments should be left undisturbed by avoiding the tendency to take as much of the tendon as can be dissected off of the bone **(*Figure 6–91B*).** Extra length, not thickness, is what is needed. This can be obtained by dissecting and detaching the plantar insertion of the tendon, which inserts on the plantar surface of the first and second metatarsal. This continuation of the posterior tibial tendon is not at first apparent and must be exposed by removing the fascial tissue that covers it. This extension of the tendon, one of its many insertions, will be considerably smaller than the proximal portion of the tendon.

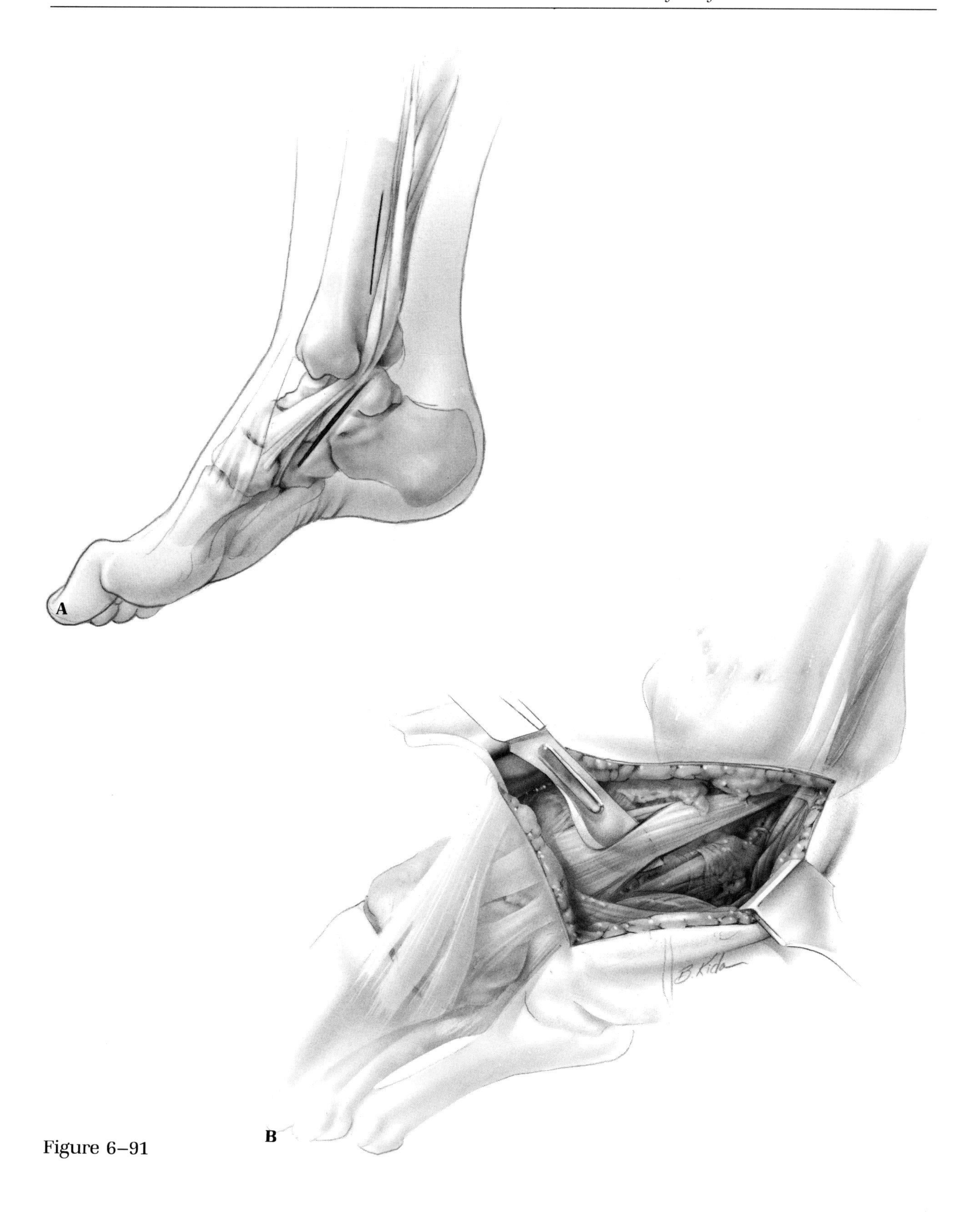

Figure 6–91

Figure 6–92. The next incision is made behind the posterior border of the tibia (***Figure 6–91A***). This incision should begin at approximately the midportion of the leg and extend as far distal as is necessary to free the tendon. The posterior tibial muscle and tendon should lie just beneath the deep fascia just behind the posterior border of the tibia. They can be identified by pulling on the distal end of the tendon, where it has been freed at the ankle. Once exposed, a moist sponge is used to grasp the muscle and pull it into the proximal wound. (Placing a hemostat under the tendon and pulling upward can stretch and damage the muscle tissue if there is much resistance to pulling the tendon into the wound.) Pulling the tendon into the more proximal wound will be resisted by the attachments of the paratenon, which can be divided blindly. Blunt dissection can be used to free the muscle belly for a distance proximally, but not so far as to disrupt the blood and nerve supply.

Coleman[2] eliminates this incision. He removes a large window from the interosseous membrane anteriorly (to be described next), and pulls the muscle belly and tendon through this window from the posterior compartment.

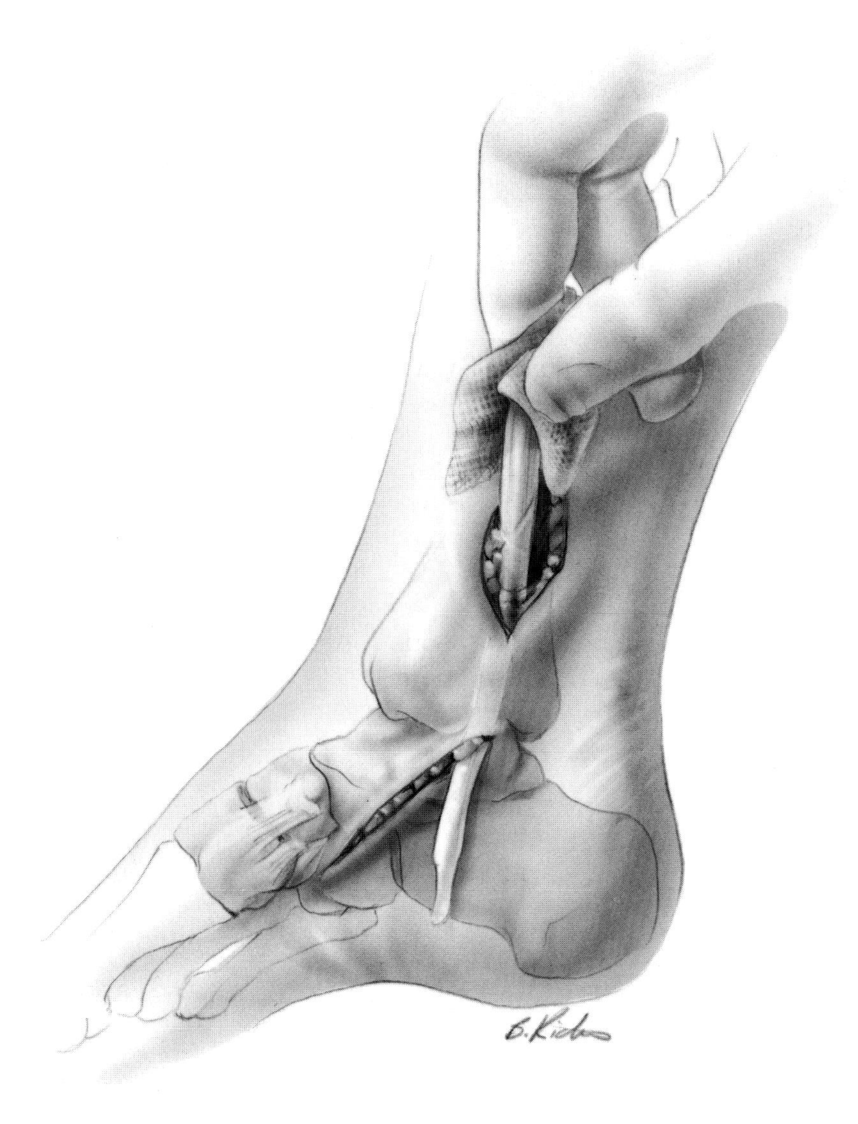

Figure 6-92

Figure 6–93. A proximal incision is made over the anterior muscle compartment of the leg, lateral to the tibial crest, and extends from the midportion of the leg distally (***Figure 6–93A***). To permit adequate exposure, it will need to be approximately 6 to 7 cm in length. The deep fascia over the anterior tibial muscle is opened. A periosteal elevator is used to elevate the anterior tibial and extensor hallucis muscle as well as the neurovascular bundle off of the lateral surface of the tibia and the interosseous membrane. This is done extraperiosteally. With these structures safely retracted out of the way, as large a segment as possible of the interosseous membrane is removed (***Figure 6–93B***). The posterior tibial muscle will lie on the opposite side of this membrane.

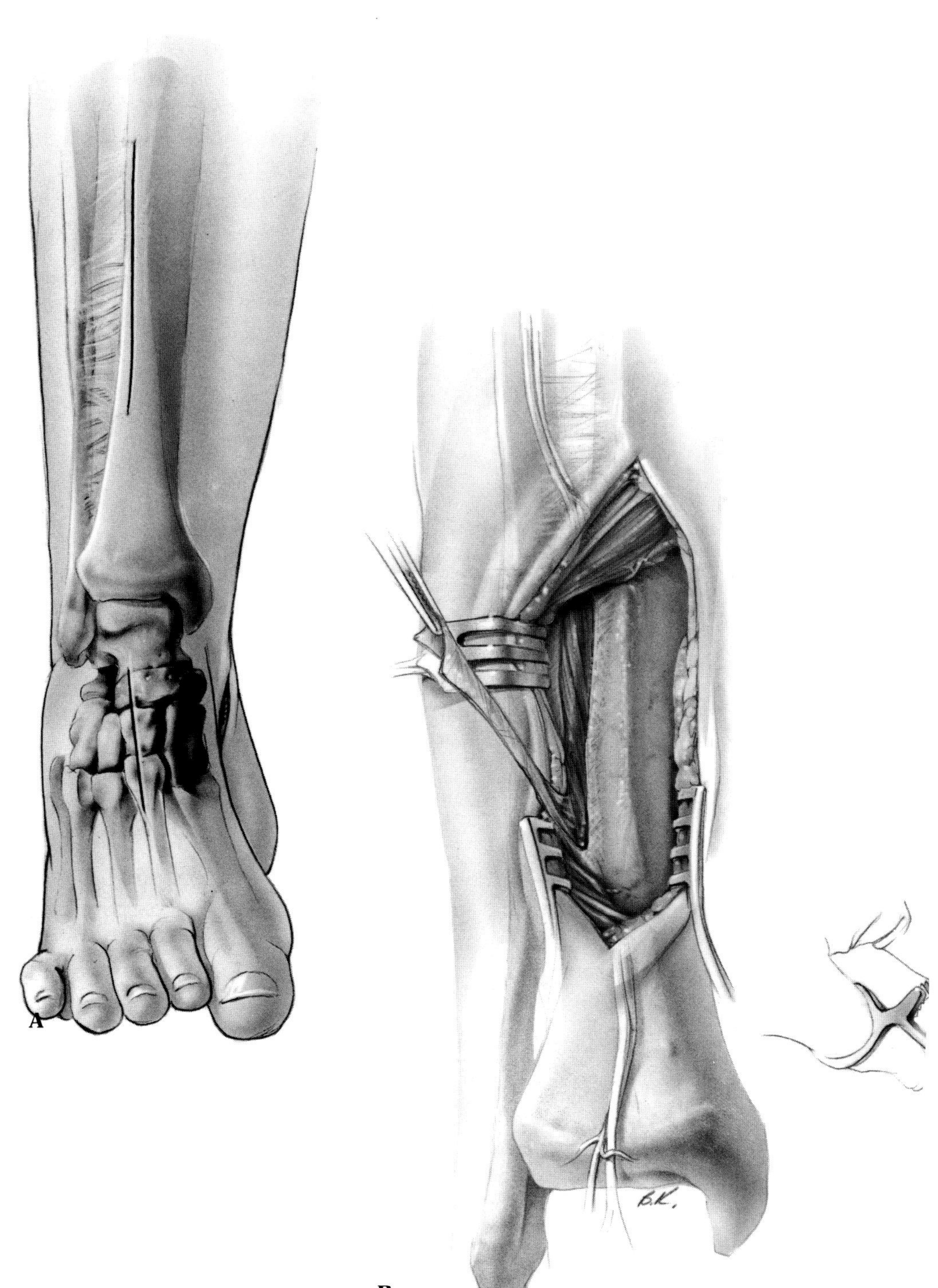

Figure 6–93

Figure 6–94. The final incision is placed over the second or third cuneiform bone and the proximal portion of the corresponding metatarsal, depending on where the surgeon wishes to place the tendon. After the bone is exposed and identified, the periosteum is elevated, and a drill is used to make a hole completely through the bone. It should be large enough for the tendon to pass through. It is for this reason the author prefers to use a cuneiform bone rather than a metatarsal bone.

Figure 6–95. The tendon can now be passed from the posterior compartment to the anterior compartment. To accomplish this a tendon forceps is passed from the anterior compartment into the posterior compartment and out of the proximal wound along the medial border of the tibia. The forceps should be kept close to the posterior surface of the tibia. The distal end of the tendon is grasped and pulled into the anterior compartment. At this point care should be taken to be sure that the window in the interosseous membrane is large enough, and is placed such that the posterior tibial muscle and tendon have a straight line of pull.

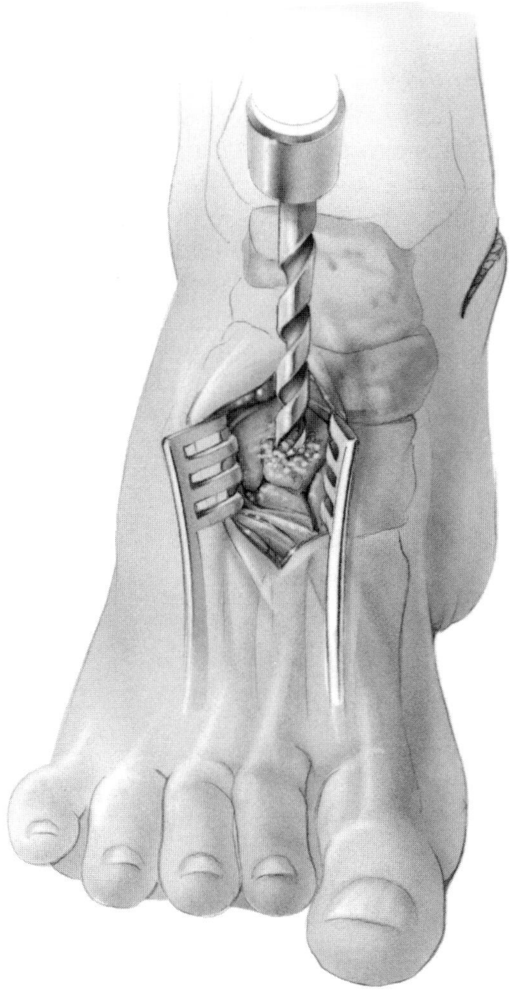

Figure 6–94

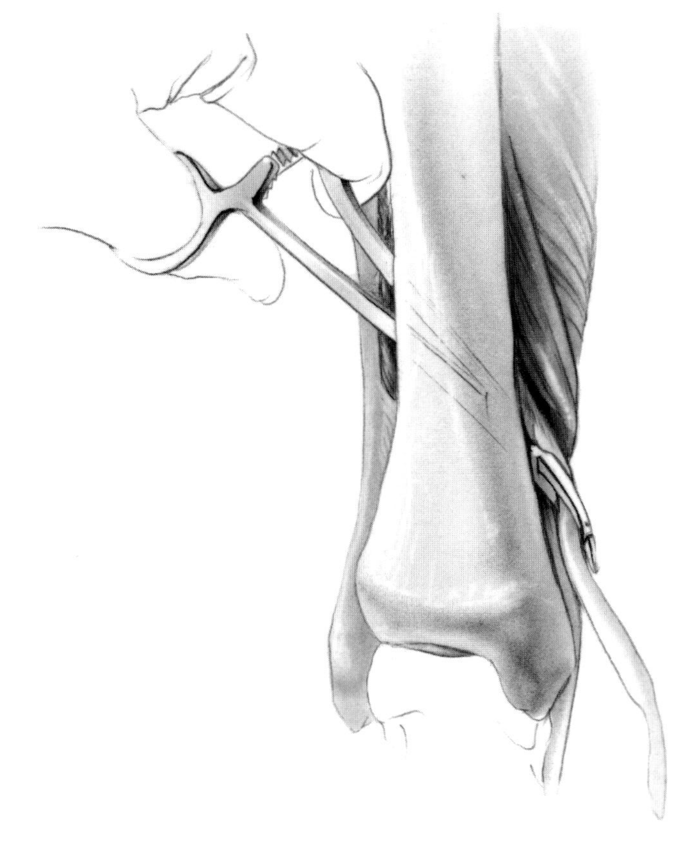

Figure 6–95

Figure 6–96. A heavy absorbable suture is now woven through the end of the tendon. This can be done in such a way as to narrow the end of the tendon to make its passage through the hole in the bone easier (***Figure 6–96A***). A flat malleable tendon passer is then passed beneath the extensor retinaculum of the ankle (***Figure 6–96B***). Both ends of the suture, which is attached to the tendon, are passed through the hole in the tendon passer, and the tendon is then drawn into the distal wound. Pulling on the distal end of the tendon should demonstrate an absence of bow stringing of the tendon at the ankle and indicate that it has been passed beneath the retinaculum.

The first three incisions are now closed.

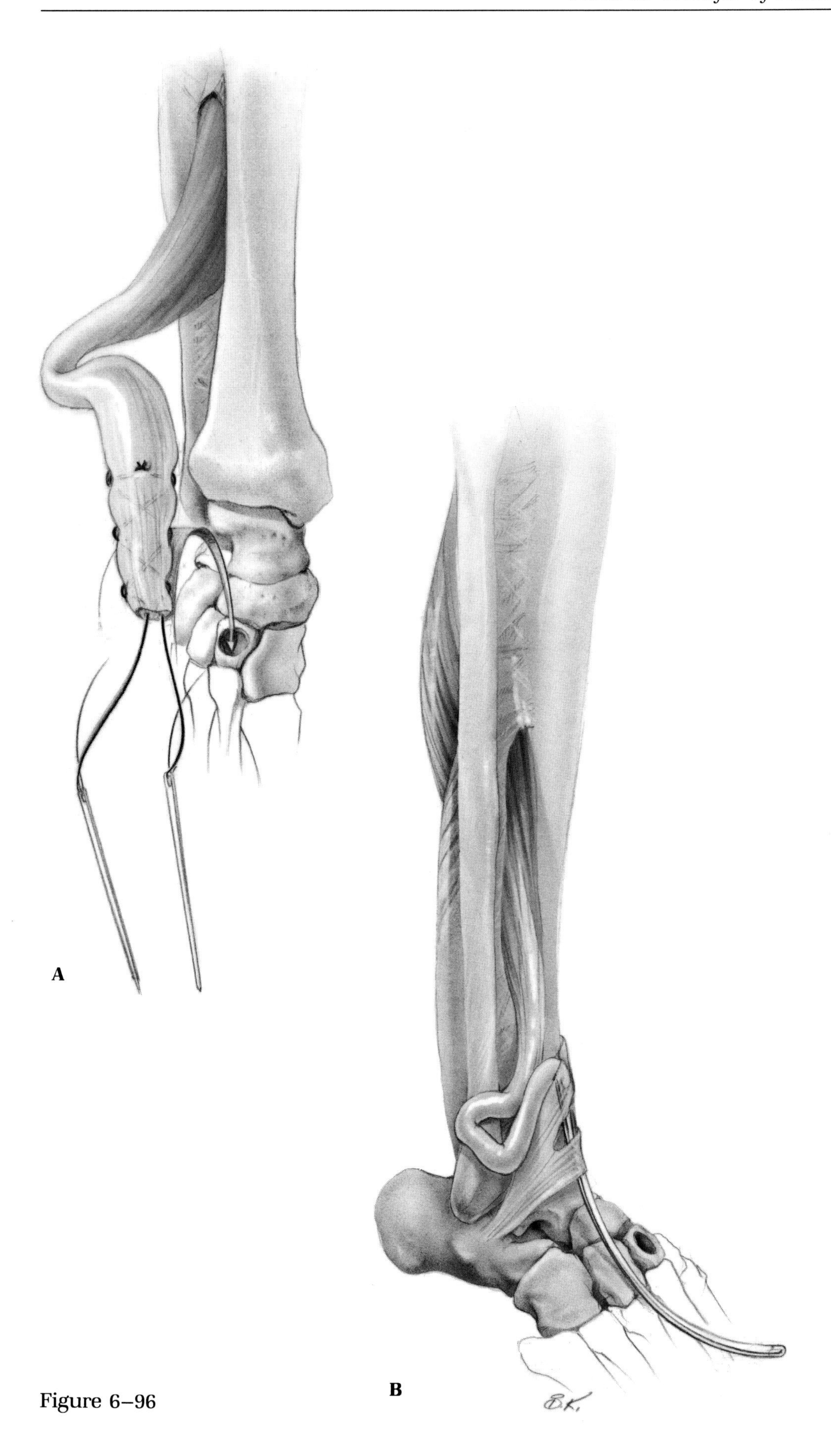

Figure 6–96

Figure 6–97. Each end of the suture in the tendon is threaded on a large, straight, Keith needle. Both of these needles, held together, are passed through the hole in the bone and out through the sole of the foot (***Figure 6–97A***). As the needles emerge from the sole of the foot, they are passed through a piece of sterile felt or sponge rubber, and then through the holes of a button (***Figure 6–97B***).

With the foot held in the corrected position, the sutures are pulled while the tendon is guided into the hole. A common and significant problem at this point is that the tendon will not pass smoothly through the hole in the bone. If this occurs the surgeon may think that he or she has pulled the tendon tight, when in reality, it remains too loose to provide any effective force. To correct the problem, be sure the hole is large enough and that no extraneous portions of the tendon have not been trimmed off. When satisfied that the tension is correct, tie the sutures over the button. This should not be done with excessive force, or pressure necrosis of the underlying skin may result. The periosteum on the dorsum of the cuneiform bone is sutured over the tendon.

While an assistant holds the foot in the corrected position, the wound is closed. A short leg cast is applied. No drains are necessary.

POSTOPERATIVE CARE

The patient remains in a short leg cast for 6 weeks. A long leg cast is not necessary because the muscle does not cross the knee joint. The patient may be ambulatory in the cast.

The care after the cast is removed will depend on factors relating to the disease itself (is bracing necessary?) and the beliefs of the surgeon (does intensive therapy to retrain the muscle improve the result?).

REFERENCES

1. Silver RL, Garza J de la, Rang M. The myth of muscle balance: a study of relative strengths and excursions of normal muscles about the foot and ankle. J Bone Joint Surg 1985;67B:432.
2. Coleman SS. Complex foot deformities in children. Philadelphia: Lea & Febiger, 1983:237.

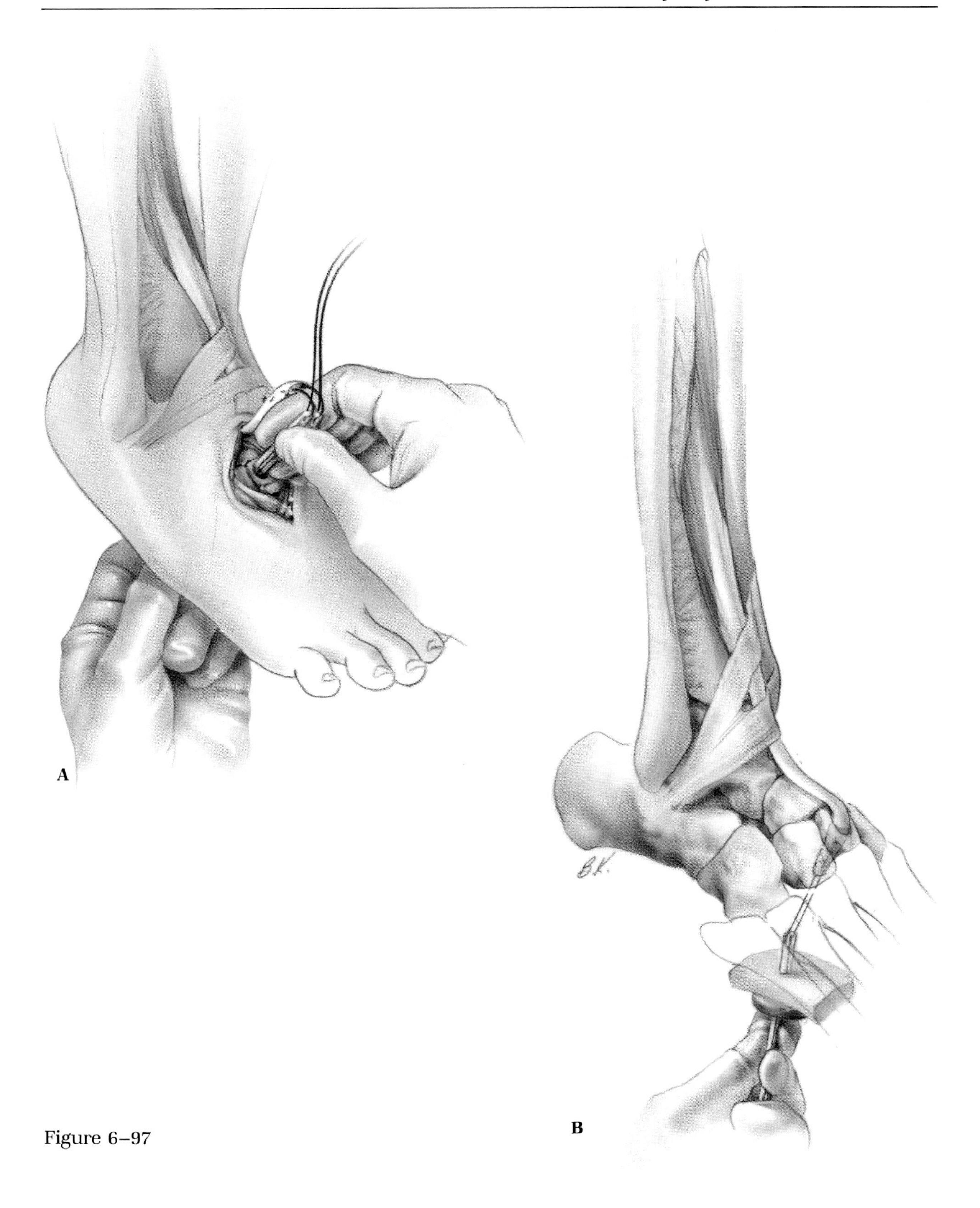

Figure 6–97

CHAPTER SEVEN UPPER EXTREMITY

7.1 Woodward Repair of Sprengel's Deformity

Congenital high scapula, commonly known as Sprengel's deformity, is not a common condition. It can be seen in all degrees of severity. The author has seen numerous children as a result of the school screening programs with minor degrees of scapular elevation and smaller scapulae on one side. Such minor degrees of high-riding scapulae need no treatment and are not usually associated with other developmental abnormalities about the shoulder. At the other end of the spectrum is the child diagnosed at birth or shortly after. The physician recommending surgical correction and the parent making the decision should realize that the deformity will usually become worse with growth. This can be difficult when the child is between 4 and 8 years of age, the ideal time for optimum correction.

It is important to recognize that the condition is the result of a problem during the 9th to 12th week of gestation; therefore, other organs may be affected as well as those structures about the shoulder girdle.

An understanding of the pathologic anatomy is important to the correction of the deformity and the avoidance of complications. The scapula is shorter in its vertical height than the opposite normal scapula and is more concave anteriorly to fit the convex shape of the superior aspect of the thoracic cage. In addition, the supraspinous portion of the scapula is usually tilted forward, and its superior medial portion may be larger. It has been pointed out that the clavicle may also be higher and shorter, lacking its usual anterior convexity.[1] In approximately one third of the cases there will be an omovertebral bone connecting the superior medial angle of the scapula to the posterior elements of the fourth and fifth cervical vertebra. This may be bone, cartilage, or fibrous tissue. Finally, the muscles of the shoulder girdle are usually affected, with hypoplasia of the trapezius and rhomboids being the commonest problem.

Two operations for the correction of Sprengel's deformity have stood the test of time and today are the most commonly used. The Green procedure[2–4] detaches the muscles from the scapula, whereas the Woodward procedure[5] detaches the origins of the trapezius and rhomboids from the spinous processes. The author has had experience with both procedures and finds the Woodward procedure to be easier (but not easy), and to produce the same results with less hospitalization and morbidity.

One of the most important complications is a radial nerve palsy owing to compression of the brachial plexus between the clavicle and the first rib when the scapula is pulled down. Some authors have advocated division or morcelation of the clavicle to prevent this complication.[1,6] This is an effective measure, but the more important question is which patients need it? Because the incidence of this complication is low,[2,5,7,8] especially in young children, the author has used this only in children older than 8 years of age or in those younger children with an unusually severe deformity. If a nerve palsy is noted following the Woodward procedure, division of the clavicle can still be done.

Figure 7–1. The patient is positioned prone. The arm and the shoulder on the affected side should be draped free. It may also be helpful if the entire posterior thorax is in the sterile field so that the level of the opposite scapula can be observed. Is also helpful if the head is positioned as if looking straight ahead. The incision should be in the midline and extend from the level of the upper cervical spine (C1–2) and extend to the lower thoracic spine (T9–10).

The incision is deepened through the subcutaneous tissue and is undermined on the affected side. This dissection should be carried far enough laterally to identify the lateral border of the trapezius muscle in the inferior aspect of the wound, the lateral border of the scapula in the midportion, and far enough to allow exposure of the medial one half of the supraspinous portion of the spine of the scapula in the superior portion.

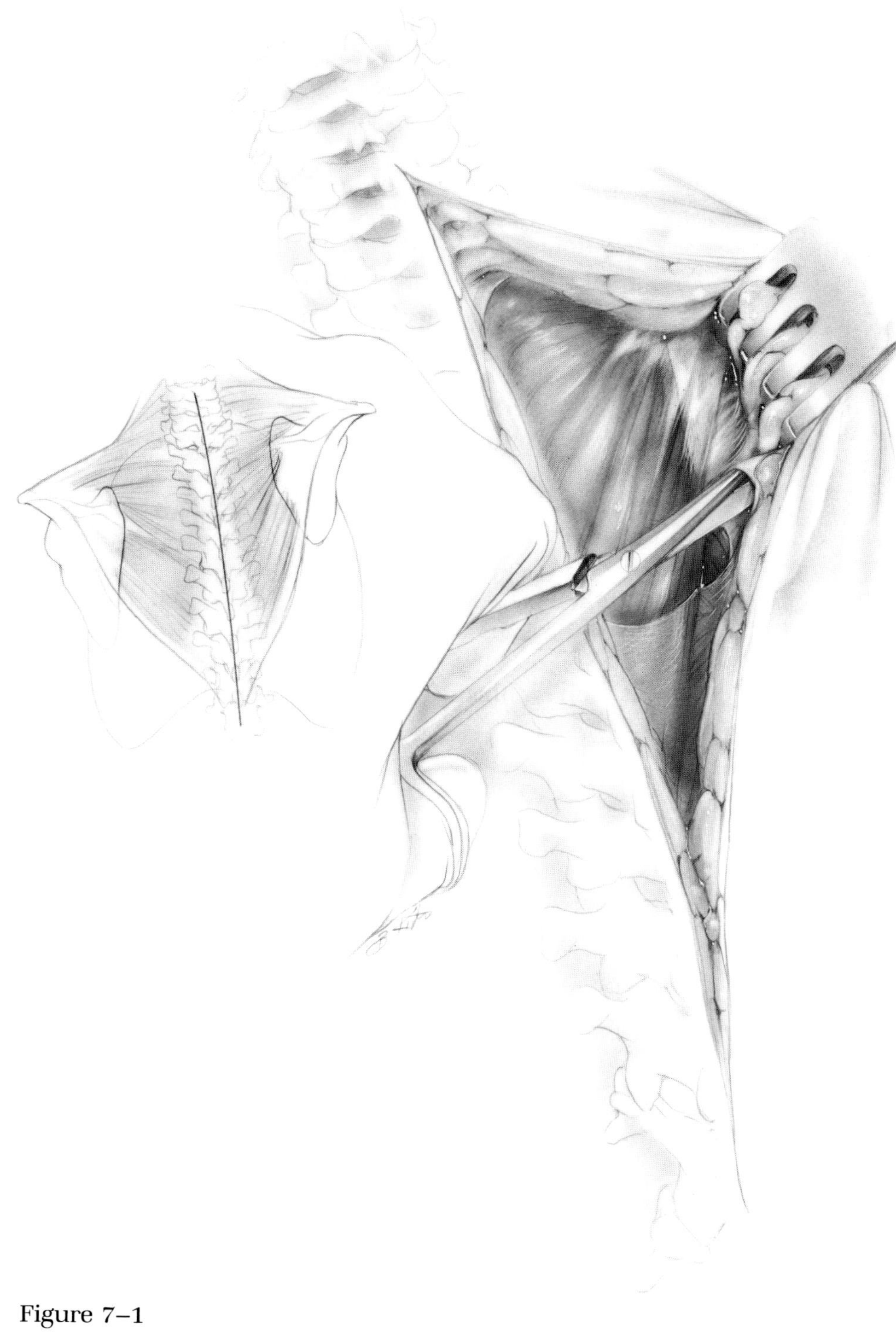

Figure 7–1

Figure 7–2. Although Woodward described detaching the trapezius and rhomboid muscles by directly detaching their origins from the midline, this is virtually impossible because they blend inseparably with all of the other muscle origins at the midline. First identify the lateral border of the trapezius muscle in the inferior aspect of the wound, and by blunt finger dissection separate it from the well-defined thoracolumbar fascia and the latissimus dorsi muscle, which covers the serratus and erector spinae muscles. Now its origin is more easily identified and can be detached without cutting into the deeper muscle layers. This detachment of the trapezius is begun distally and extends to the level of the fourth cervical vertebra, where it can be cut transversely to complete its release. After the trapezius muscle is detached and reflected laterally, the rhomboid muscles attaching to the scapula are identified. Blunt finger dissection can be used to separate them from the underlying deep fascia, aiding in detaching them from their origins like the trapezius muscle.

Although this dissection is rather straightforward in an adult cadaver, it is much more difficult in a 4-year-old child with hypoplastic muscles and abnormal fibrous bands. Nevertheless, this step is the key to the exposure and thus the procedure.

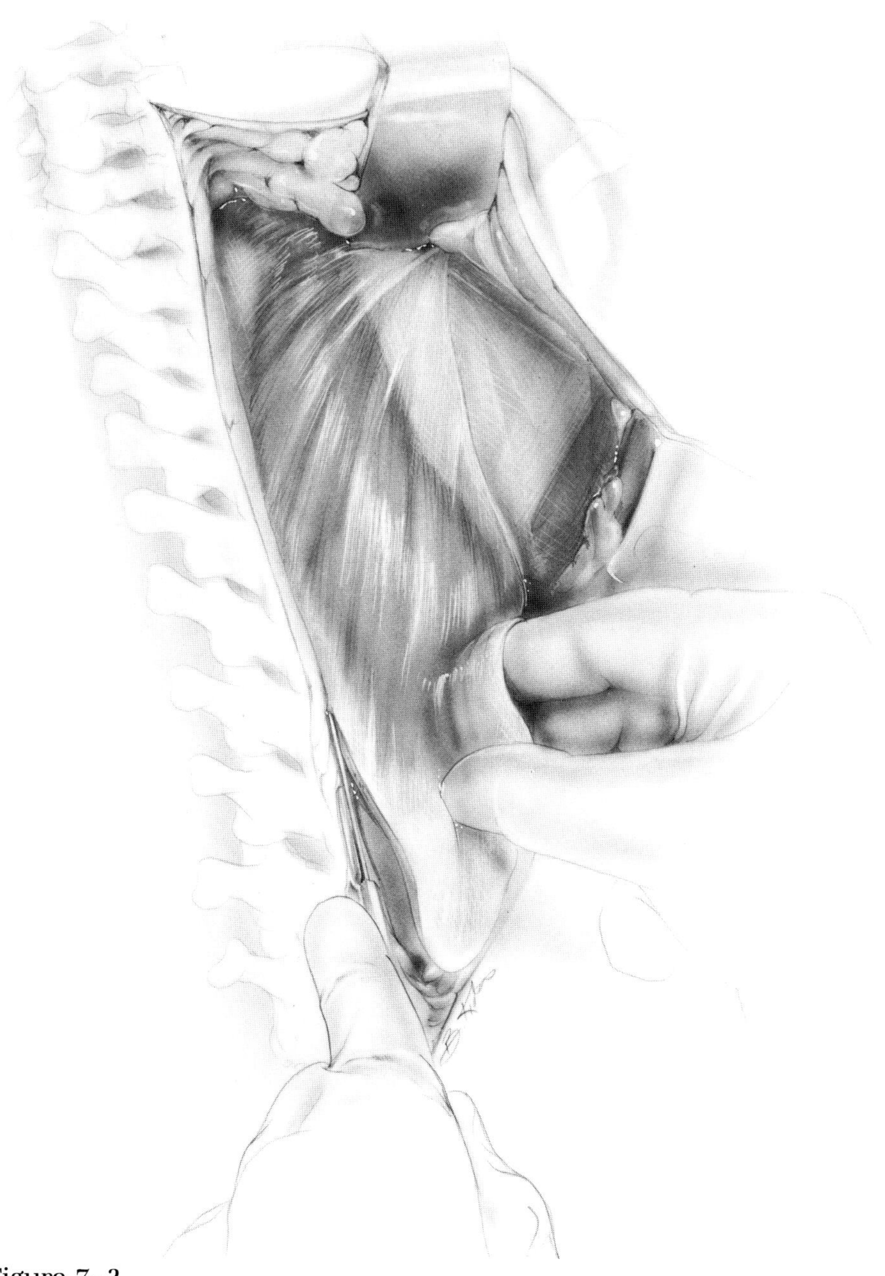

Figure 7–2

Figure 7–3. With the trapezius muscle retracted laterally, the levator scapula muscle can be identified as that structure originating from the superior medial corner of the scapula and running toward the cervical spine (***Figure 7–3A***). Although it lies in the same plane as the rhomboids muscles, it may be difficult to identify as a distinct structure. In about one third of the cases an omovertebral bone (not illustrated here) consisting of actual bone, cartilage, or dense fibrous tissue may take origin from this corner of the scapula, usually lying beneath the levator scapulae muscle. If present, it is rarely connected to the cervical spine by bone and can usually be detached by sharp dissection after the bone has been exposed by extraperiosteal dissection. It is essential to release all structures in this region because they will prevent downward displacement of the scapula. Fibrous bands as well as the levator scapulae muscle are most easily isolated and divided at the superior medial border of the scapula. Notice the transverse cervical artery running deep to the levator scapulae muscle. Care should be taken to avoid cutting it by inserting a finger behind the muscle before dividing it (***Figure 7–3B***).

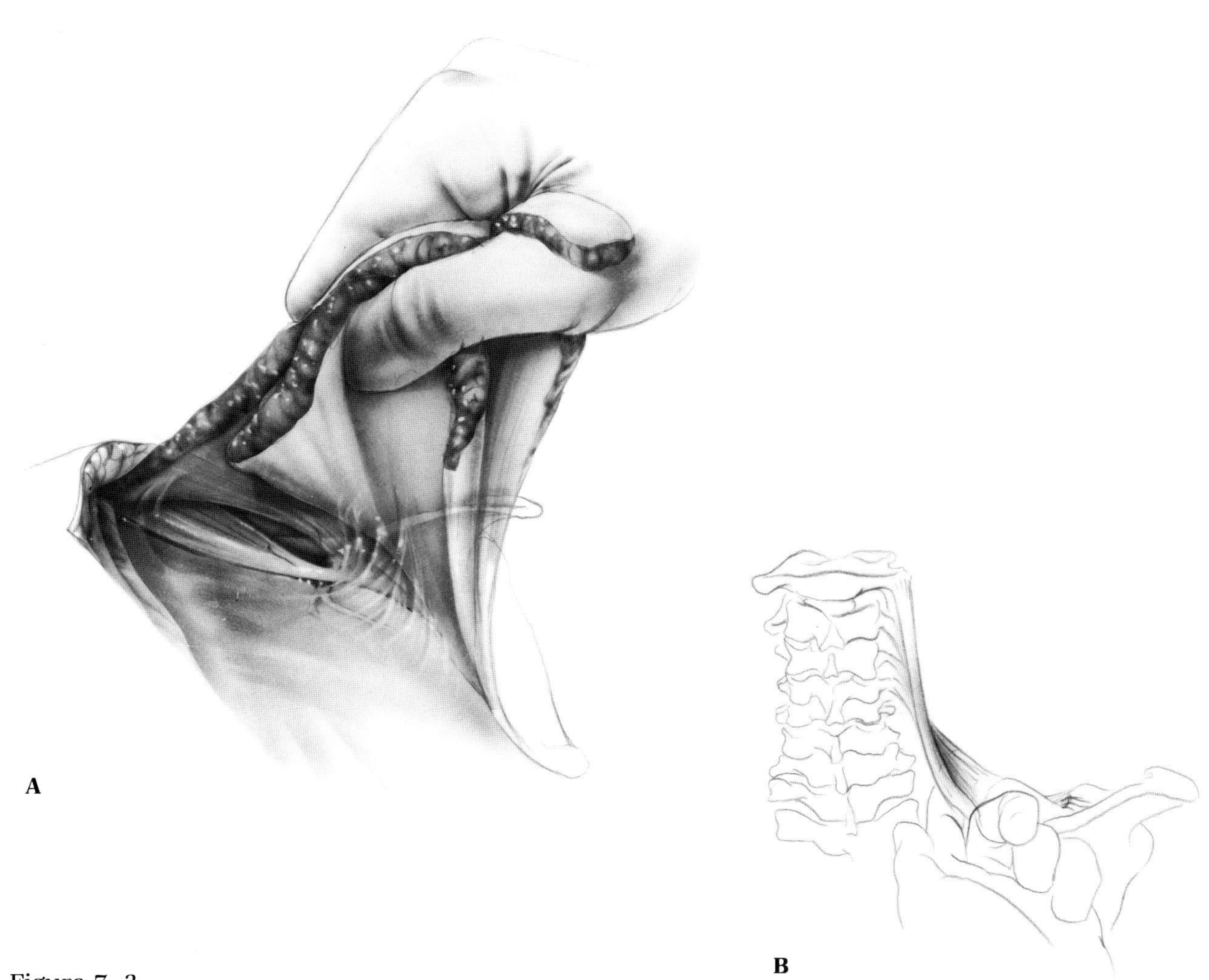

Figure 7–3

Figure 7–4. With the structures originating from the superior medial border of the scapula divided it becomes easier to appreciate the contribution that the large anterior curving medial supraspinous portion of the scapula makes to the deformity. This portion of the scapula should be exposed extraperiosteally and excised with a large bone-cutting forceps. Care should be used to extend no further laterally than the scapular notch to avoid injury to the suprascapular artery or nerve.

With this completed, the scapula can be everted. This will usually reveal multiple fibrous adhesion between the scapula and the chest wall. This is especially true in cases with associated anomalies of the chest wall (*eg*, missing ribs). These adhesions should be divided. The scapula can now be pushed downward and observation made for any other tight structures. In severe cases it may be necessary to divide a portion of the serratus muscle insertion into the scapula.

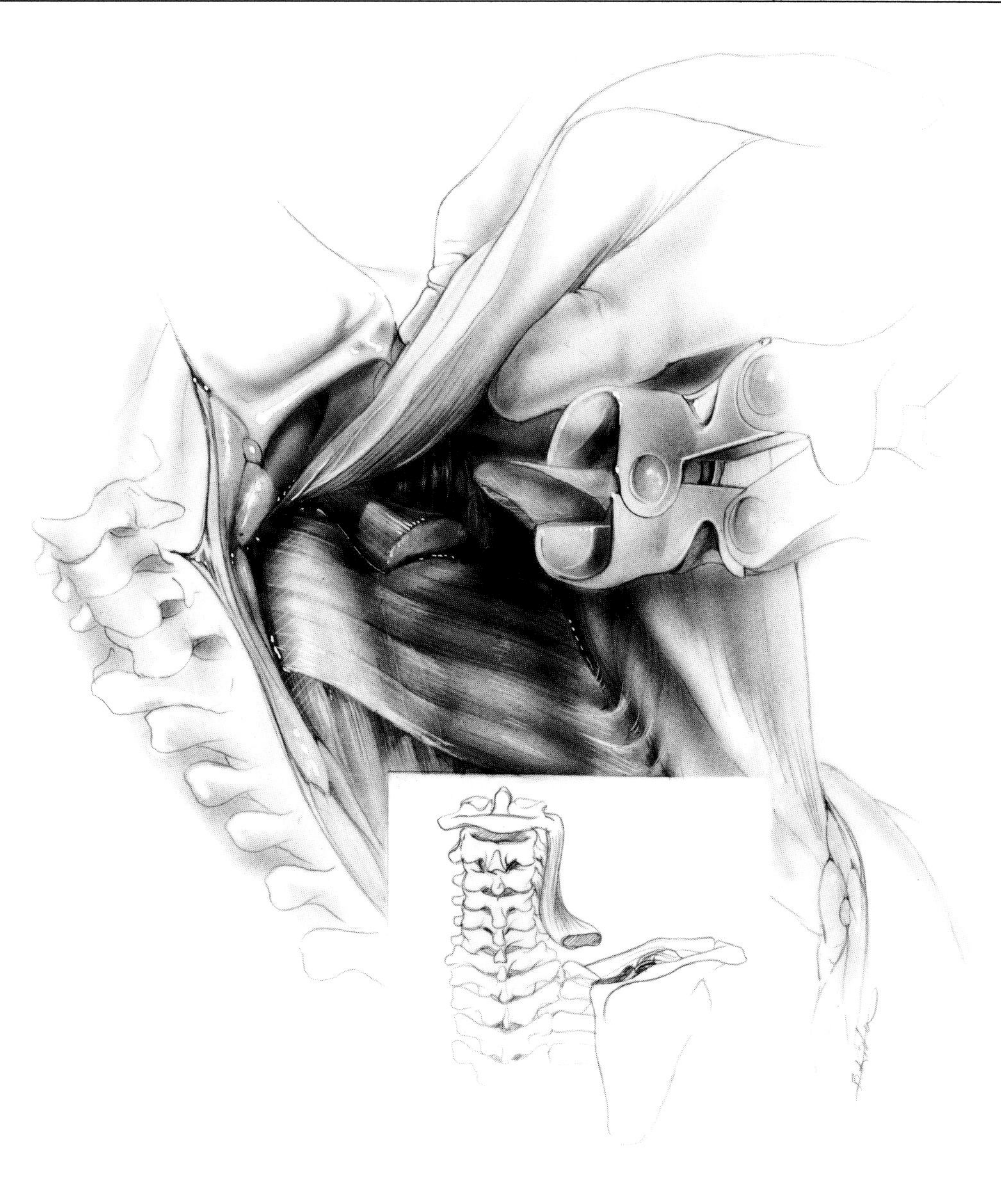

Figure 7–4

Figure 7–5. The latissimus dorsi muscle is elevated to allow the scapula to be displaced beneath it. The rhomboid and trapezius muscles are now pulled downward, displacing the scapula to the desired level. It is important at this point to realize that the affected scapula is smaller than normal. Therefore, displacing it so that its inferior border is level with the inferior border of the opposite normal scapula would result in overdisplacement. Rather, it should be displaced so that the spines of the two scapulae lie on the same level.

The suprascapularis and subscapularis muscles can be repaired by suturing them together over the resected area of the superior medial border of the scapula. If the serratus muscles were detached they can be resutured to the scapula in a more cephalad location. The rhomboid and trapezius muscles are now reattached to their midline origin in a new, more caudad location. Because the most distal origin of the trapezius muscle (extending to T12) was left intact, there will be a redundant segment of muscle and fascia distally. This can be excised. If desired the tip of the scapula can be sutured to an underlying rib by an absorbable suture as a temporary means of fixation. The author finds this useful in maintaining proper rotation of the scapula. Finally, the latissimus dorsi muscle is reattached to the tip of the scapula. The wound is closed over a suction drain.

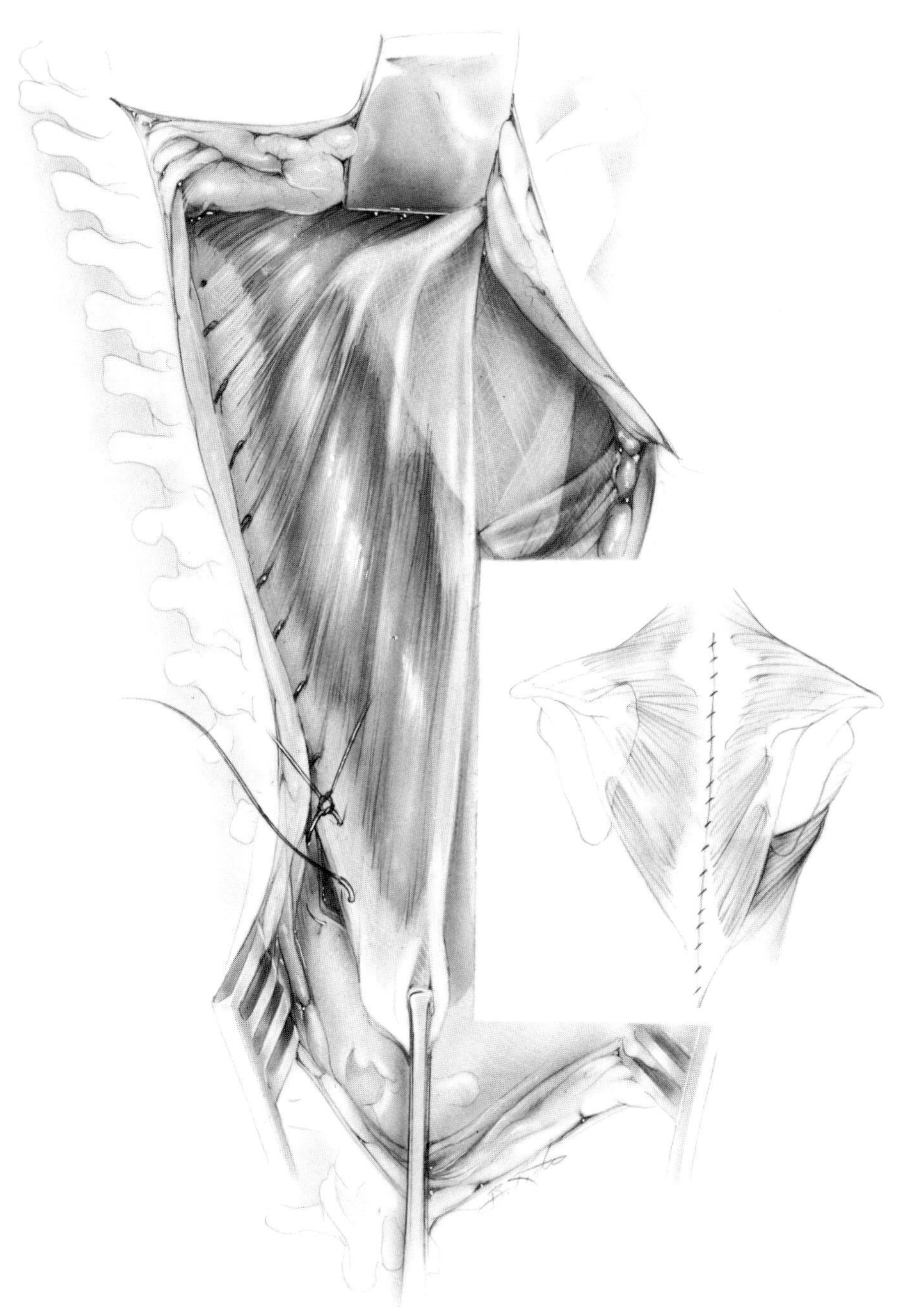

Figure 7–5

Figure 7–6. NH is a 4-year, 8-month-old girl who presented with her parents because of a high left shoulder and restricted motion, which they had recently noted in her shoulder. They had consulted an orthopaedic surgeon 2 years ago and were told that treatment would not be advisable because she would just be trading a slightly high shoulder for a very large scar. They were convinced the deformity was becoming worse, however.

Figure 7–6A is a preoperative radiograph that shows many of the skeletal anomalies seen in association with the congenital elevation of the scapula. The most obvious is that the scapula is high, but it is also smaller than the opposite scapula. There is a defect in the chest wall with missing and deformed ribs, and a mild scoliosis with a vertebral anomaly above are also present.

Postoperatively (***Figure 7–6B***) the spine of the left scapula is on the same level as the normal scapula. The fact that it is smaller is more obvious and demonstrates the point that the affected scapula should not be brought so far inferior that the inferior angle is on the same level as the normal scapula.

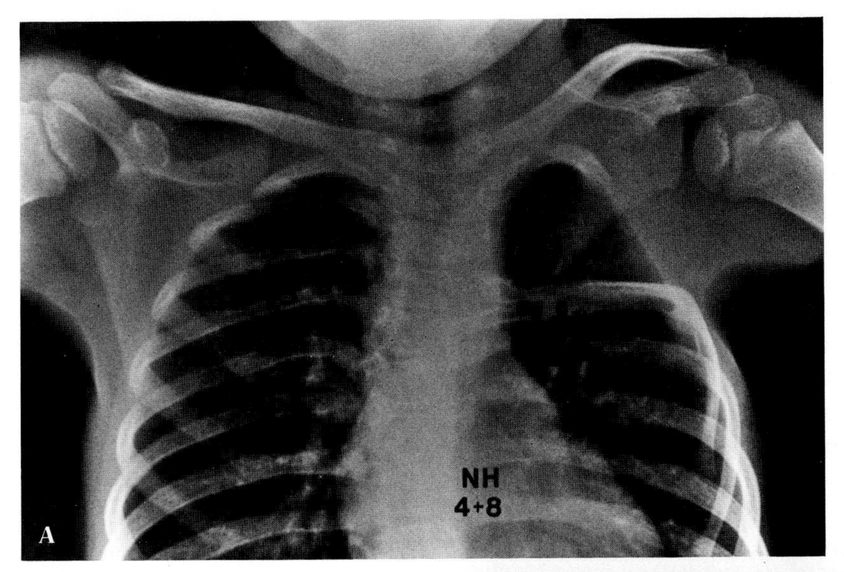

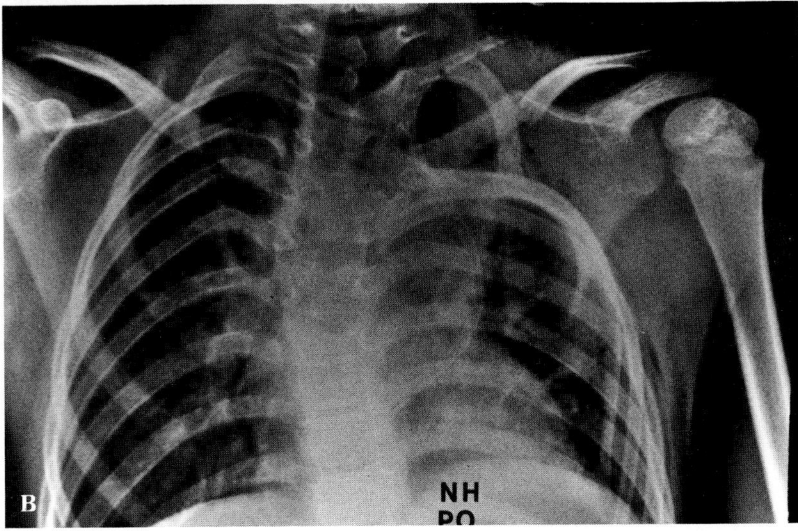

Figure 7–6

POSTOPERATIVE CARE

The patient is placed in a Velpeau-type bandage to immobilize the arm for a period of 4 weeks. The drain can usually be removed on the first or second postoperative day because it is not difficult to secure hemostasis. The patient is allowed to ambulate the day following surgery and is usually ready for discharge on the second or third postoperative day. Following removal of the immobilization at 4 weeks the patient is started on physical therapy that emphasizes glenohumeral range of motion and active strengthening of the shoulder and scapular muscles.

REFERENCES

1. Robinson RA, Braun RM, Mack P, Zadek R. The surgical importance of the clavicular component of Sprengle's deformity. J Bone Joint Surg 1967;49A:1481.
2. Green WT. The surgical correction of congenital elevation of the scapula (Sprengel's deformity). J Bone Joint Surg 1957;39A:1439.
3. Tachdjian MO. Pediatric Orthopedics, 2nd ed. Philadelphia: WB Saunders, 1990:148.
4. Crenshaw AH, ed. Campbell's Operative Orthopaedics, 7th ed. St Louis: CV Mosby, 1987:2764.
5. Woodward JW. Congenital elevation of the scapula: correction by release and transplantation of muscle origins. J Bone Joint Surg 1961;43A:219.
6. Chung SMK, Nissenbaum MM. Congenital and developmental defects of the shoulder. Orthop Clin North Am 1975;6:381.
7. Ross DM, Cruess RL. The surgical correction of congenital elevation of the scapula: a review of seventy-seven cases. Clin Orthop 1977;125:17.
8. Grogan DP, Stanley EA, Bobechko WP. The congenital undescended scapula: surgical correction by the Woodware procedure. J Bone Joint Surg 1983;65B:598.

7.2 Congenital Pseudarthrosis of the Clavicle

Congenital pseudarthrosis of the clavicle is an unusual condition of unknown etiology. Although the name often causes congenital pseudarthrosis of the clavicle to be confused with congenital pseudarthrosis of the tibia in terms of its resistance to repair, this is not the case. The pathology, unlike congenital pseudarthrosis of the tibia, is of two bone ends covered with cartilage and often encapsulated with synovial tissue and fluid. It is clear, however, that resection of the pseudarthrosis, bone graft, and internal fixation are necessary to obtain union.[1–4]

Patients may present at any age with a painless lump in the clavicle. Although usually mild in terms of cosmetic deformity and asymptomatic in younger children, the deformity worsens with age, and discomfort with activities usually will develop in adolescents. For these reasons surgical repair is usually recommended. The ideal time to repair the pseudarthrosis is around 3 to 4 years of age to take advantage of remodeling with growth. Repair can be accomplished with improved cosmesis and elimination of discomfort at any age, however.

Figure 7–7. The patient is placed supine on the operating table with a sand bag under the upper thoracic spine to allow the head and shoulder to fall posterior and improve exposure of the clavicle. The arm, shoulder, and the clavicle are draped free. The anterior iliac crest is also prepared for the bone graft, which will be necessary in the repair. The skin incision is placed along the cephalad edge of the clavicle. Its length will depend on the size of the child, but because the skin in this region is so mobile it need not be excessively long.

Figure 7–8. After dividing the skin, the periosteal surface of the clavicle is exposed below the platysma muscle. The normal clavicle and as much as possible of the bulbous ends of the pseudarthrosis should be exposed subperiosteally. In older children the bulbous ends may be quite large, in which case it is impossible to remain subperiosteally. Great care should be used in the dissection because of the proximity of the subclavian artery and vein as well as the apex of the pleural cavity. The pseudarthrosis is then excised with a rongeur. If the surgeon wishes to preserve the entire pseudarthrosis for histology, a Giggli saw or bone biter may be used provided the circumferential dissection is sufficient.

Figure 7–9. After resection of the pseudarthrosis, a bone graft will be necessary to both secure osteosynthesis and maintain the length of the clavicle. A full-thickness (tricortical) piece of bone can be harvested from the anterior iliac crest just behind the anterosuperior iliac spine. The portion of bone just beneath the apophysis will be thicker than the thin plates of bone that make up most of the iliac wing and thus will provide a better fit with the two ends of the resected pseudarthrosis. A larger piece of bone than is judged necessary should be removed to allow it to be fashioned to the appropriate size and contour.

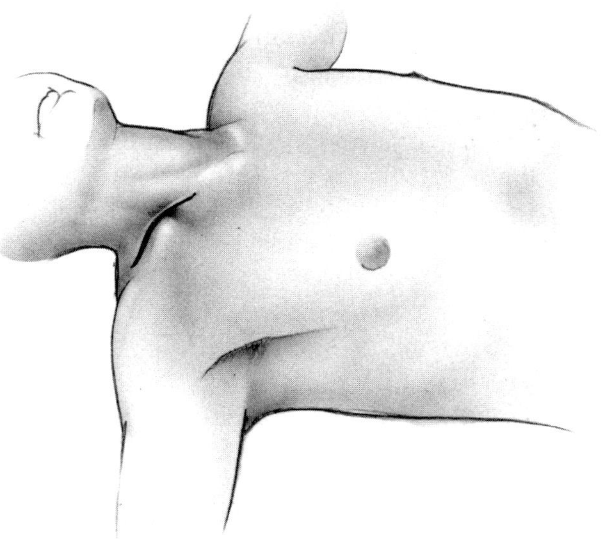
Figure 7–7

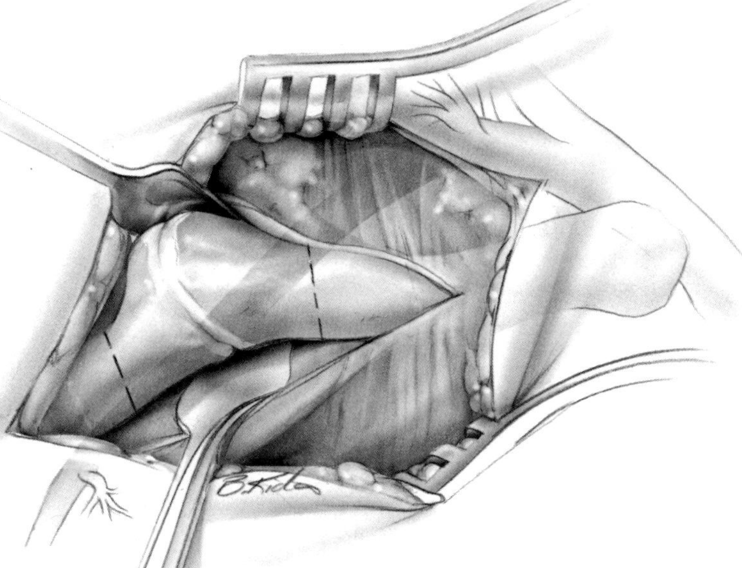
Figure 7–8

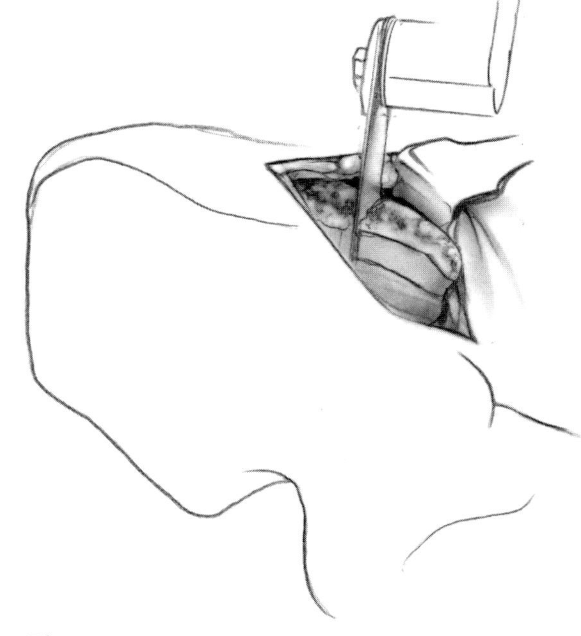
Figure 7–9

Figure 7–10. It has been suggested that the clavicle and graft may be fixed by either an intramedullary Kirschner wire or Steinmann pin or by a plate. Because of the complex shape of the clavicle it is impossible to keep a pin or wire of any strength within the medullary canal of the clavicle. A thin Kirschner wire that can be passed (with difficulty) through the medullary canal of the bone will provide little fixation. The use of a pin or wire also risks migration.

For children the author has found the reconstruction plates to be ideal. They come in two sizes, 2.7 mm and 3.5 mm. Their flexibility makes it possible to contour them exactly to the shape of the clavicle and graft. Because immobilization is required in an active child regardless of the method of fixation, they are sufficiently strong.

With the graft held temporarily in place between the two resected ends of the clavicle by a small Kirschner wire, the appropriate-sized reconstruction plate is contoured using the template provided (***Figure 7–10A, B***).

When the proper shape has been achieved, the plate is attached by screws to both ends of the clavicle and the graft. Each end of the clavicle should be fixed with a minimum of two screws, and at least one screw should hold the graft (***Figure 7–10C***).

The wound is irrigated, a small drain is placed adjacent to the clavicle and brought out through the skin lateral to the incision, and the wound is carefully closed in layers. In small children a Valpeau dressing is applied and reinforced with a roll of plaster if deemed necessary. In older children who may be more cooperative with the postoperative immobilization a commercial sling with a strap that passes around the waist to hold the arm next to the trunk is sufficient.

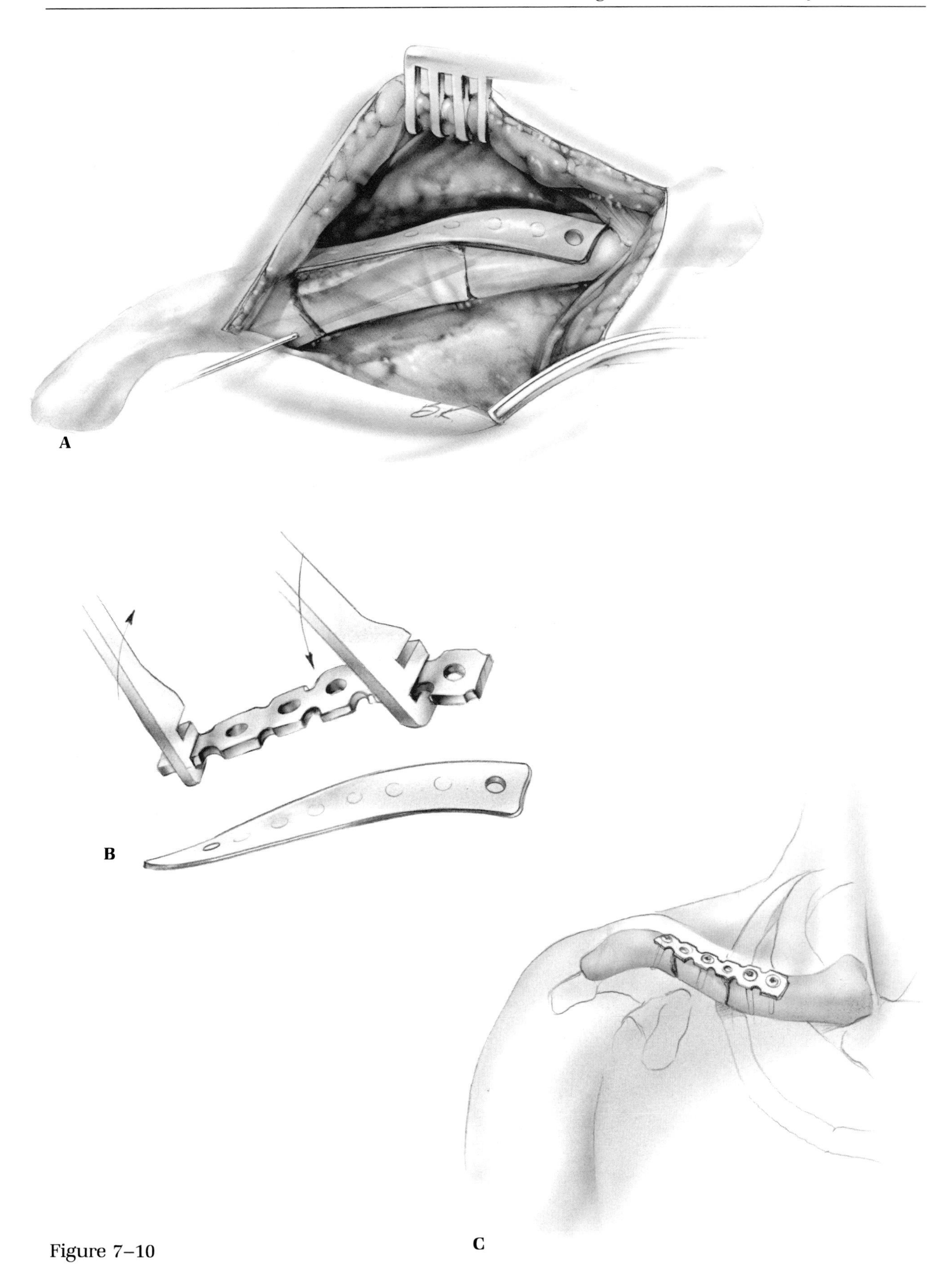

Figure 7–10

Figure 7–11. BC is a 10-year-old boy who noticed a lump on his collar bone and discomfort with throwing activities since an injury 3 years previously. At the time of injury he was told that he had fractured his clavicle and now was referred for a persistent non-union. Radiographs demonstrated a typical congenital pseudarthrosis of the right clavicle (***Figure 7–11A***). The results of excision, grafting, and plating are shown (***Figure 7–11B***). Healing was prompt, and return to all activities without discomfort accomplished in 6 months.

POSTOPERATIVE CARE

The drain can usually be removed the day following surgery. The patient is usually ready for discharge the same day. Immobilization should be continued until radiographic evidence of union is seen. This will usually be sufficient by 6 weeks. The plate can be removed electively 6 to 12 months later as an outpatient.

REFERENCES

1. Jinkins WJ. Congenital pseudarthrosis of the clavicle. Clin Orthop 1969;62:183.
2. Gibson DA, Carroll N. Congenital pseudarthrosis of the clavicle. J Bone Joint Surg 1970;52B:629.
3. Quinlan WR, Brady PG, Regan BF. Congenital pseudarthrosis of the clavicle. Acta Orthop Scand 1980;51:489.
4. Schnall SB, King JD, Marrero G. Congenital pseudarthrosis of the clavicle: A review of the literature and surgical results of six cases. J Pediatr Orthop 1988;8:316.

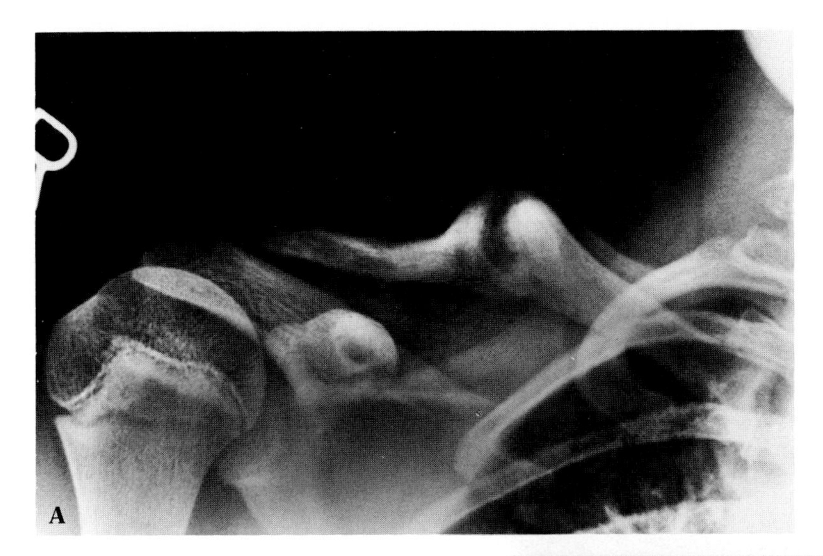

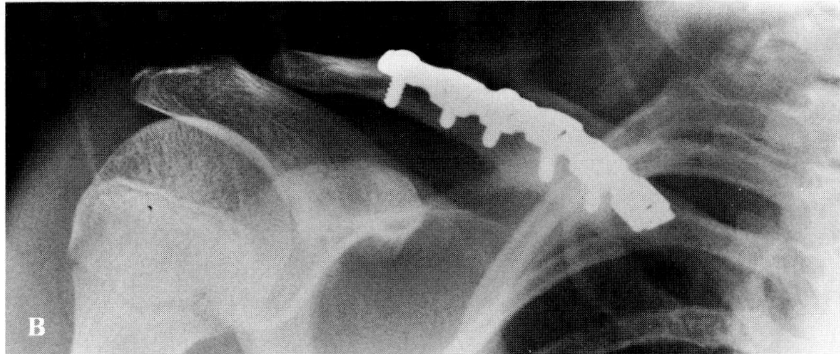

Figure 7–11

7.3 Correction of Cubitus Varus Following Supracondylar Fractures of the Humerus

Of all the complications that are possible following supracondylar fractures of the humerus, none is commoner than cubitus varus. The deformity results from either incomplete reduction or loss of reduction. The mechanism of the deformity explains the components.[1] The distal fragment is internally rotated, allowing the distal fragment to tip into varus and often some hyperextension. The usual 10 degrees of hyperextension with concomitant loss of flexion is seldom noticed by the patient and is not a significant problem. The internal rotation of the distal fragment may result in slight loss of external rotation, but the rotation arch of the shoulder is so great that this also goes unnoticed by the patient. The varus tilt of the distal fragment, however, reverses the usual carrying angle of the elbow from slight valgus to varus. This result, combined with the prominence of the lateral condyle that is also accentuated by the rotation of the distal fragment, produces a very noticeable deformity but rarely any functional loss. Often the cubitus varus deformity will not be apparent for several months leading some to speculate that it is due to a growth disturbance. This is not the case, however. The deformity is not noticed until extension of the elbow joint is restored, and it becomes increasingly obvious as the last degrees of extension are gained.

The importance of understanding the various components of the deformity in relation to the problem the patient experiences is important to the surgical correction. It is rarely necessary to attempt to correct either the rotation or the posterior angulation and to do so greatly increases the difficulty of the osteotomy and leads to a greater complication rate.[2] The patient's problem is the carrying angle of the elbow and the prominence of the lateral condyle. Removal of a simple laterally based wedge of bone from the supracondylar region will correct the cubitus varus. As in correction of ankle valgus by a supramalleolar osteotomy (see Osteotomy of the Distal Tibia; Wiltse Technique) simply closing the wedge without medially displacing the distal fragment will often make the prominence of the lateral condyle greater, however. Attempting to correct rotation will make internal fixation very difficult. Medial displacement of the distal fragment will eliminate the stability of the periosteal hinge that is achieved with a simple closing wedge osteotomy but does not complicate fixation any more than in a fresh supracondylar humeral fracture. The author's preference is to perform a simple closing lateral wedge osteotomy, fix it with a single lateral Kirschner wire, and inspect the arm in full extension. If the prominence of the lateral condyle is objectionable, the wire is removed, the distal fragment medially displaced, and the osteotomy is fixed with both medial and lateral pins.

Figure 7–12. The size of the wedge of bone to be removed is determined by obtaining radiographs of both arms in full extension and supination. A simple method to estimate the wedge is described by Oppenheim et al.[2] A tracing of the normal arm is reversed and superimposed on the abnormal arm. The approximate size of the wedge can now be determined. If the distal limb of the osteotomy is greater than the proximal limb, the prominence of the lateral condyle will be accentuated. Therefore, plan the limbs to be of equal length.

Figure 7–13. The osteotomy may be performed through either a posterior triceps splitting approach or a lateral incision. The author has found the latter to be the easiest and to be associated with the quickest postoperative recovery of motion. The patient is supine with the arm on a narrow translucent hand board. The incision is approximately 4 to 5 cm in length and is placed slightly posterior to the epicondylar ridge to make the scar less noticeable.

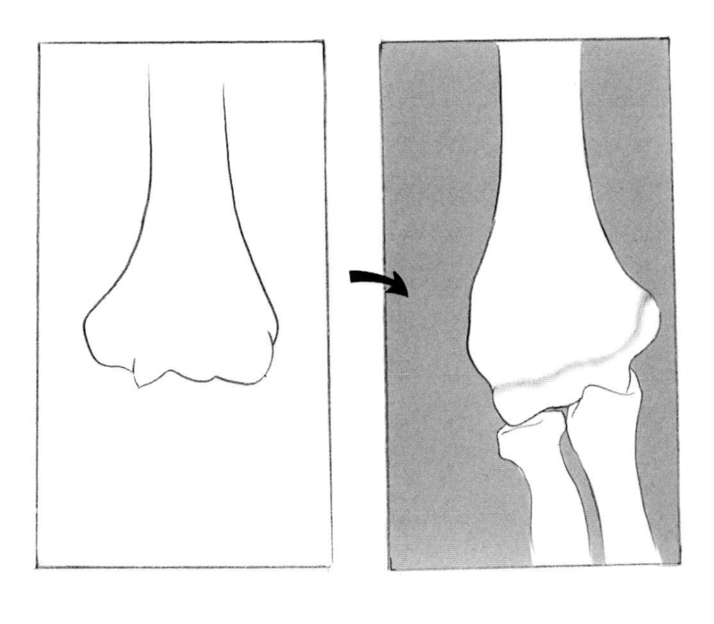

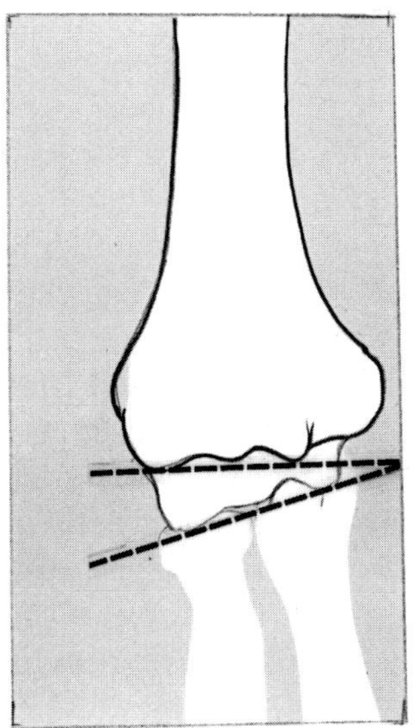

Figure 7–12

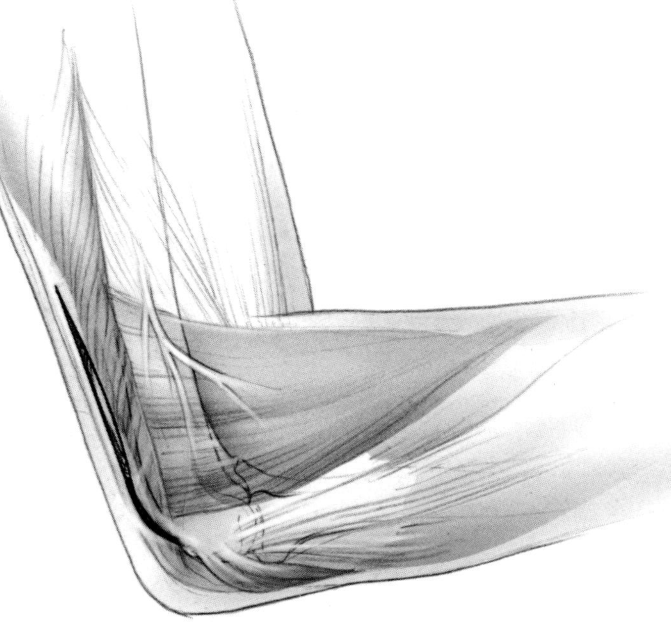

Figure 7–13

Figure 7–14. The incision is carried down to the epicondylar ridge with the triceps muscle posterior and the extensor carpi radialis longus muscle anterior (***Figure 7–14A***). The periosteum is split, and the distal humerus is exposed subperiosteally both anteriorly and posteriorly to the medial side (***Figure 7–14B***). If desired small Kirschner wires can be drilled into the bone along the proposed limbs of the osteotomy, and the location and size of the wedge verified on the image intensifier.

Figure 7–15. A small power saw is used to remove the wedge of bone. If no displacement of the distal fragment is planned, a small portion of the medial cortex is left intact and "green-sticked" to close the wedge. This will greatly enhance the stability and allow fixation with only one lateral Kirschner wire. The surgeon should be certain that the fracture of the medial cortex is complete, however, and there is no tendency for the osteotomy to spring open.

With the osteotomy fixed the arm is extended and inspected for the desired correction. Stability at the osteotomy site is also assessed, and if necessary a Kirschner wire is placed medially. The image intensifier should be used to be certain both of the wires have transfixed both fragments.

The wound is irrigated and closed. A small drain can be used if desired. The Kirschner wires are left protruding through the skin and are bent over. A long arm cast is applied with the elbow at 90 degrees of flexion and the forearm in pronation just as would be done for a medially displaced supracondylar fracture. Several cotton balls placed in the antecubital space next to the skin under the cast padding will permit swelling to occur without restriction from the cast.

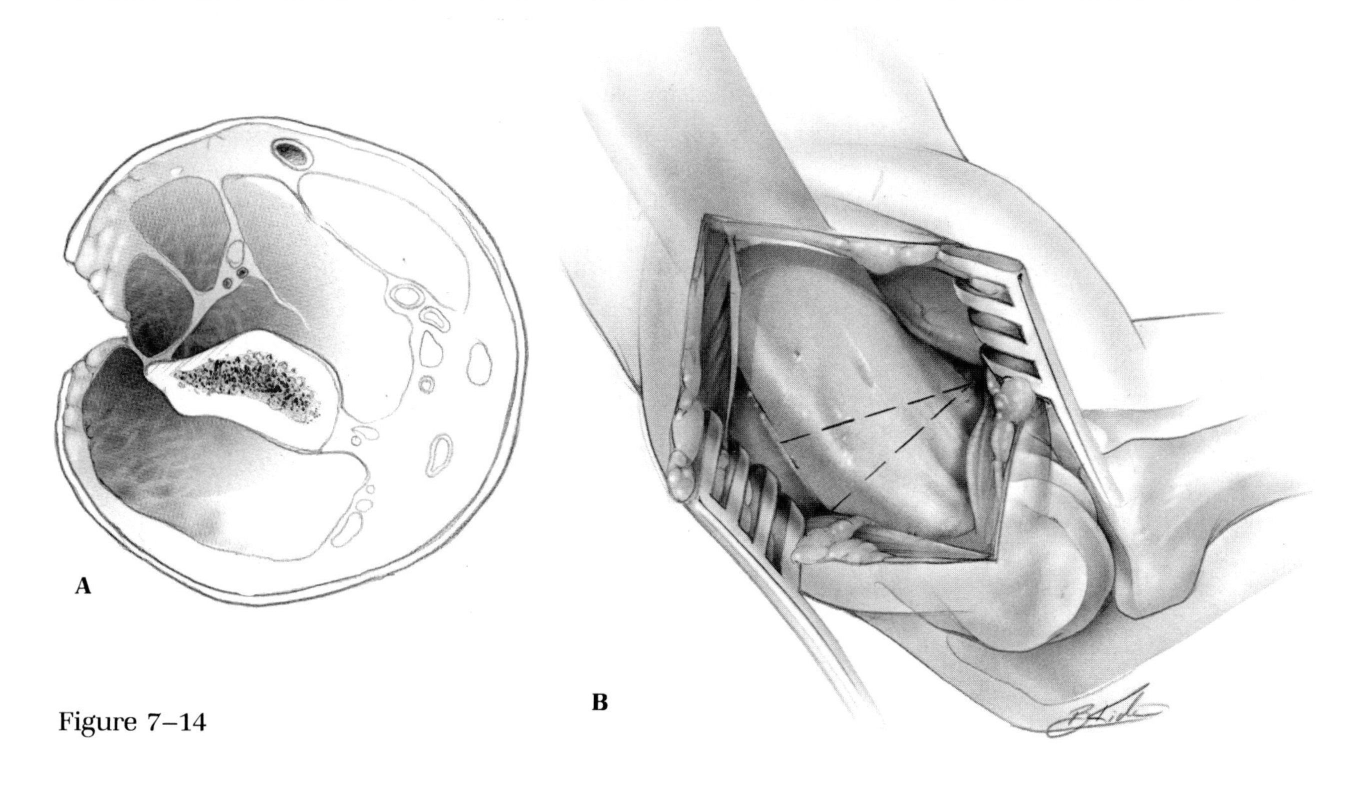

Figure 7–14

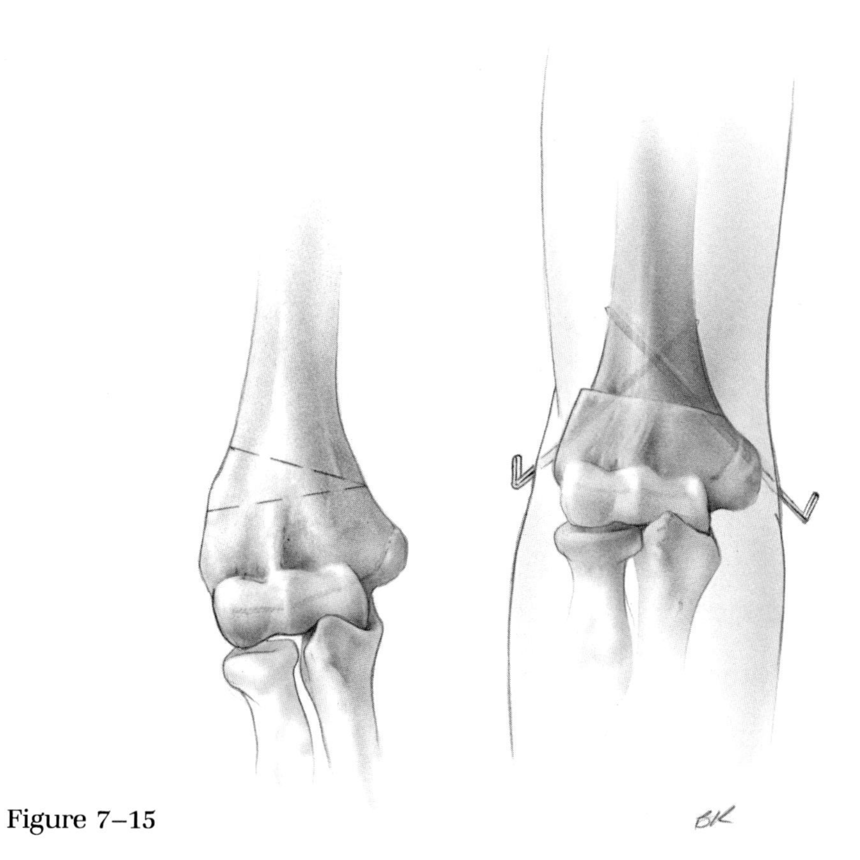

Figure 7–15

Figure 7–16. AW is a 7-year-old girl who presented with a moderate cubitus varus deformity of the arm 1 year after closed reduction of a supracondylar fracture of the humerus (***Figure 7-16A***). The osteotomy was planned to remove a wedge of bone slightly less than 1 cm. Because a large wedge was not required, it was easier to plan the cuts to be of near equal length. With the wedge closed and no medial displacement, the arm showed no lateral prominence (***Figure 7–16B***). Six months later healing is complete and full motion regained (***Figure 7–16C***).

POSTOPERATIVE CARE

The treatment is the same as following supracondylar fracture except the healing may be anticipated to be slightly slower. At approximately 4 weeks there should be sufficient callus to allow the pins to be removed. The patient is left out of a cast or splint, and wears a sling for the next 3 weeks while starting active range-of-motion exercises. When radiographic union is achieved the sling is discontinued, and the patient may resume full activities once full motion is restored.

REFERENCES

1. Wilkins KE. Fractures and dislocations of the elbow region. In: Rockwook CA Jr, Wilkins KE, King RE, eds. Fractures in Children. Philadelphia: JB Lippincott, 1987:426.
2. Oppenheim WL, Clader TJ, Smith C, Bayer M. Supracondylar humeral osteotomy for traumatic childhood cubitus varus deformity. Clin Orthop 1984;188:34.

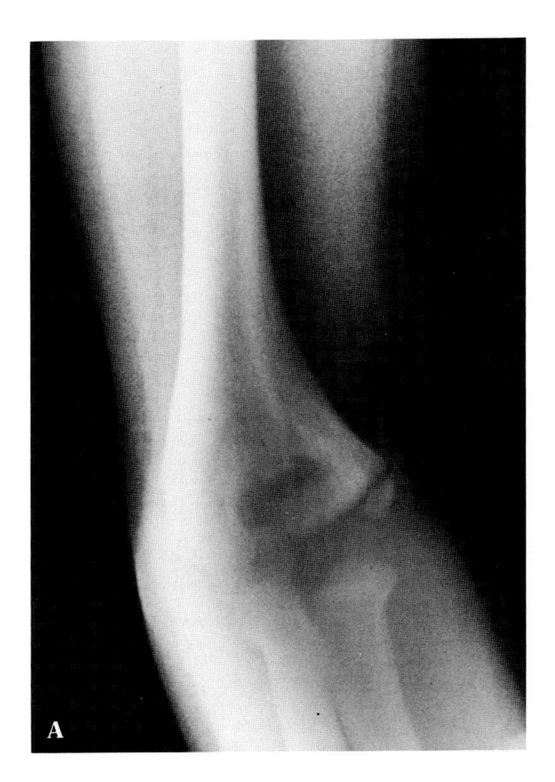

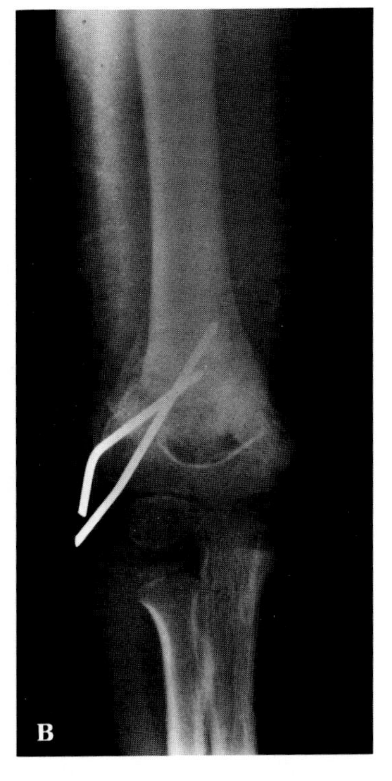

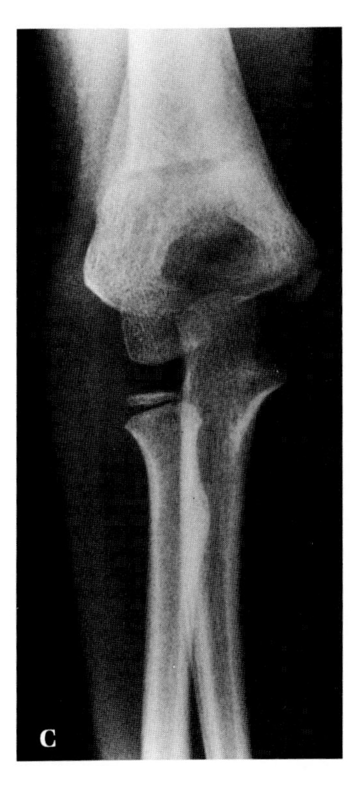

Figure 7–16

7.4
Release of Congenital Constriction Band

Congenital constriction bands may occur in any location on a limb. In addition, they occur with varying degrees of severity ranging from incomplete partial rings that may require no treatment to deep rings that completely encircle the part creating distal edema and cyanosis.

It is important to recognize that this ring of abnormal constriction has breadth as well as depth and consists of abnormal dense scarlike tissue. For this reason the constriction band must be excised rather than merely incised. If it is not excised, the dense scar tissue will merely be rotated into the flaps. In excising the constriction ring, especially in areas such as the fingers or when it appears to go down to the bone, great care must be taken not to divide vital structures that lie beneath. This is especially troublesome in the fingers. It is also important that no more than one half of the circumference of the constriction ring be excised at one time to avoid complete disruption of the lymphatic and vascular drainage from the distal part. An interval of 2 to 3 months is usually adequate.

It is usually never acceptable simply to excise the ring, no matter how minor it appears, and attempt to repair the defect in a linear matter as the resultant scar will contract, creating a cosmetic problem. Thus, the treatment of congenital constriction bands lies in the application of the principles of Z-plasty.

Figure 7–17. The excision of the constriction band can be marked, although it is usually so obvious that this is not necessary. The flaps of the Z-plasty are then planned. They should be as large as feasible. The angle of 60 degrees is thought to provide the optimal balance between the vascular supply to the tip of the flap and the mobility of the base of the flap. Ideally the length of the flap should be no more than two times the width of the base of the flap.

Figure 7–18. Once the constriction band is excised and the flaps mobilized, they are transposed as illustrated. In children it is best to use fine absorbable suture to avoid the arduous task of suture removal.

POSTOPERATIVE CARE

It is wise to provide maximum soft-tissue immobilization during the initial period of healing. This is accomplished with a pressure dressing of fluffed gauze beneath a rigid plaster dressing. Adjacent joints should be immobilized as well. The dressing can usually be removed in 1 week and the second stage performed in 2 to 3 months.

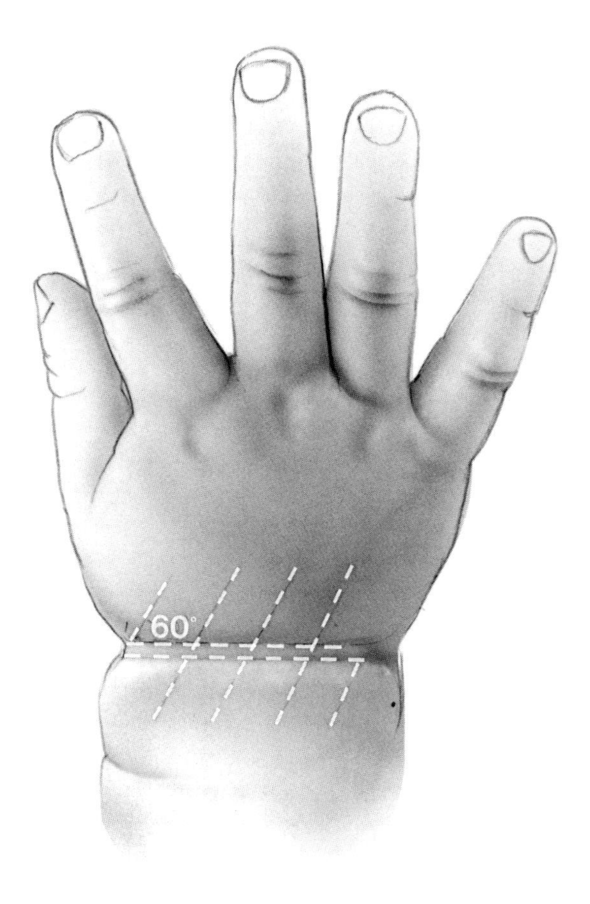

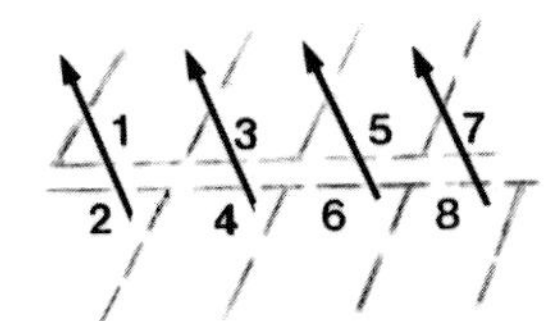

Figure 7–17

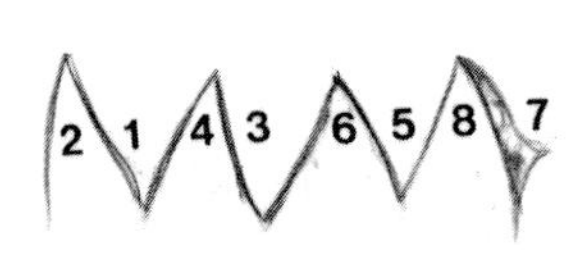

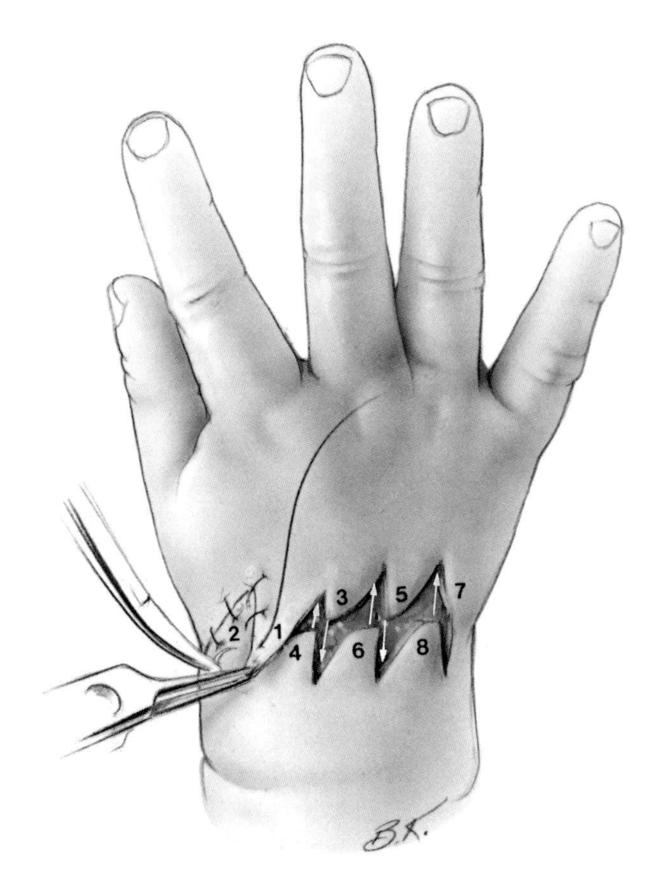

Figure 7–18

7.5 Release of Simple Syndactyly

Syndactyly is the commonest congenital anomaly of the hand following polydactyly. As would be expected, excellent discussions of this topic can be found in standard texts.[1,2] Only separation of a simple syndactyly will be described here.

There is disagreement regarding the age at which each particular syndactyly should be separated as well as which is the best method, but there is no disagreement about several important principles.

1. The surgery should be done in a bloodless field.
2. Loupe magnification is required.
3. The use of angled and zigzag incisions is necessary.
4. Additional skin in the form of either split- or full-thickness graft is required.
5. Local skin flap and not graft should be used to reconstruct the commissure.
6. Rigid and adequate postoperative dressings are needed to ensure healing of the skin.

Figure 7–19. The first part of the operation is to plan the incisions. There are many different incisions that work well, and it is said that a surgeon will prefer the one he or she is taught. The planning begins with the flap that will be used to reconstruct a commissure. The broad dorsal flap first described by Bauer, Tondra, and Trusler[3] has received wide acceptance and will be described. The flap begins at the metacarpophalangeal joint and extends about two thirds of the way to the proximal interphalangeal joint. It will be approximately 1 cm in width and should taper slightly from base to tip (***Figure 7–19A***).

Before the volar incisions are made it is first necessary to determine the location of the commissure on the volar surface. This can be done by examining the hand from the radial side in the clenched fist position. It will be observed that in the normal hand the commissure is approximately midway between the metacarpal head and the distal condyle of the proximal phalanx (***Figure 17–19B***). This point can be marked by passing a small needle from the dorsal to volar surface along this midway mark. At this point a transverse incision can be made to provide the area where the dorsal flap will be sutured.

After this, dorsal and volar zigzag incisions are made out to the distal interphalangeal (DIP) joint in such a manner that the base of the triangle of the volar flap matches the tip of the dorsal flap and vice versa (***Figure 17–19C***). The planning of this interdigitation can be aided by passing a small 27-gauge needle through the dorsal and volar skin to mark the tips of the flaps.

From the DIP joint to the tip of the fingers a straight longitudinal incision is made to complete the separation of the skin. Care should be taken not to damage the nail plate if it is joined by making one clean, sharp, decisive incision through it.

As these flaps are developed it is extremely important that they be defatted. This increases their mobility and decreases the postoperative swelling.

Figure 7–20. There is usually a clear line of separation between the two fingers in a simple syndactyly, with little crossing of fibrous bands or blood vessels (***Figure 7–20A***). In some cases, however, the digital vessels or nerves may divide more distal than usual. It is therefore necessary to isolate the neurovascular bundles. This should start distal, following these structures proximal until their junction is found (***Figure 7–20B***). If the nerve is found to divide more distal than desirable, it can be split. If the vessels divide more distal, the surgeon must choose whether or not to divide one of these to allow the commissure to be moved more proximal to the correct location. Some surgeons do not advocate this, but it is commonly done. If one vessel is divided, it should be carefully recorded in the operative note so that further surgical planning can account for the fact that only one artery supplies the digit. This is especially important if there is a syndactyly on the other side of the affected finger.

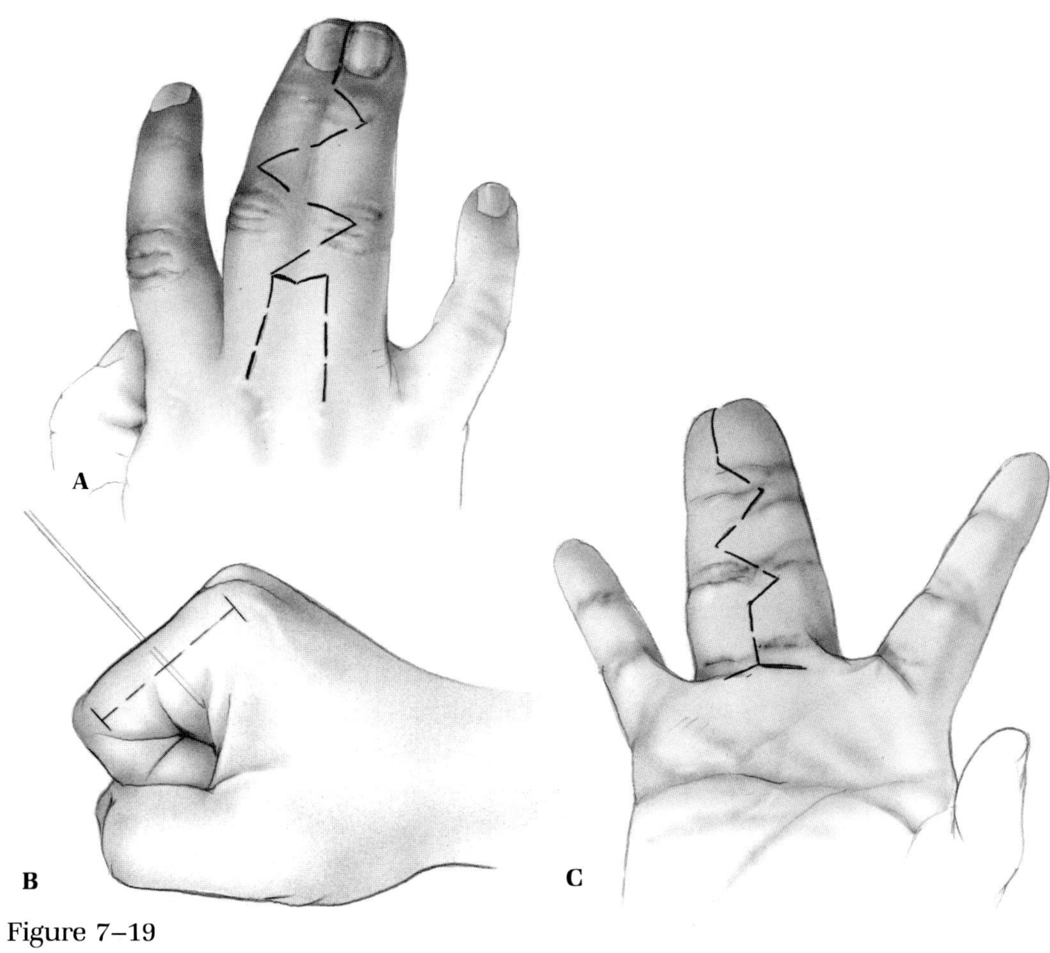

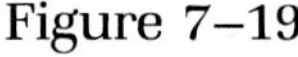
Figure 7–19

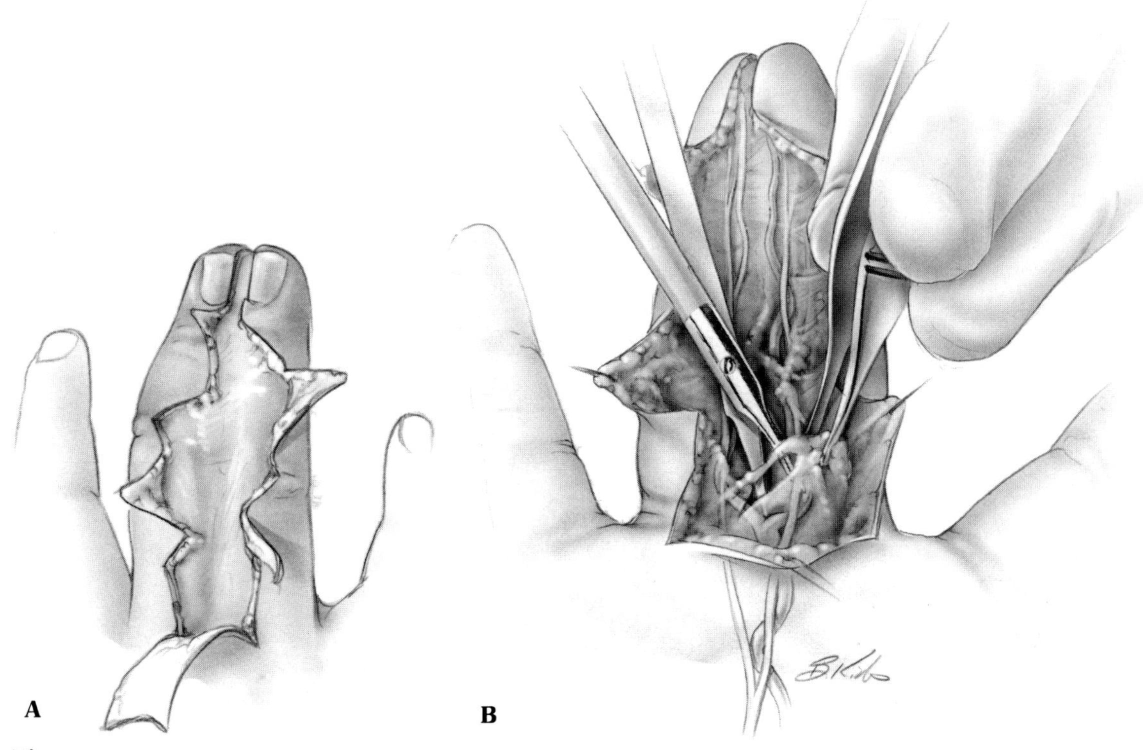

Figure 7–20

Figure 7–21. The flaps are now sutured into place starting with the dorsal flap. Before this is done, it is important to be sure that the flaps are defatted. The flaps should be sutured with a fine, absorbable material so that these sutures will not have to be removed (***Figure 7–21A***).

This will leave two areas on each finger to be grafted, the most distal and most proximal portion of each finger. Thin full-thickness skin should be used for this coverage (***Figure 7–21B***). It can most easily be obtained from the groin crease with care to stay far enough lateral to avoid skin that will later grow hair. This wiil have to be at least lateral to the femoral artery, and preferably more lateral below and just medial to the anterosuperior iliac spine. The defect from which the graft is obtained is closed primarily and the graft sutured into the recipient areas.

A pressure dressing that will apply gentle compression to the flaps and the skin grafts is essential. This should be covered with a rigid plaster that extends above the elbow to immobilize the child's arm.

POSTOPERATIVE CARE

The dressing is usually left in place for 10 to 14 days to allow good healing of the grafts and flaps. If deemed necessary, an additional dressing can be applied for 1 to 2 weeks to allow further stabilization of the grafts. Following this there is usually no need for further immobilization, and the patient is allowed full use of the hand.

REFERENCES

1. Bayne LG, Costas BL. Malformations of the upper limb. In: Morrissy RT, ed. Lovell and Winter's Pediatric Orthopaedics, 3rd ed. Philadelphia: JB Lippincott, 1990:577.
2. Flatt AE. The care of congenital anomalies of the hand. St. Louis: CV Mosby, 1977:170.
3. Bauer TB, Tondra JM, Trusler HM. Technical modification in repair of syndactylism. Plast Reconstr Surg 1956;17:385.

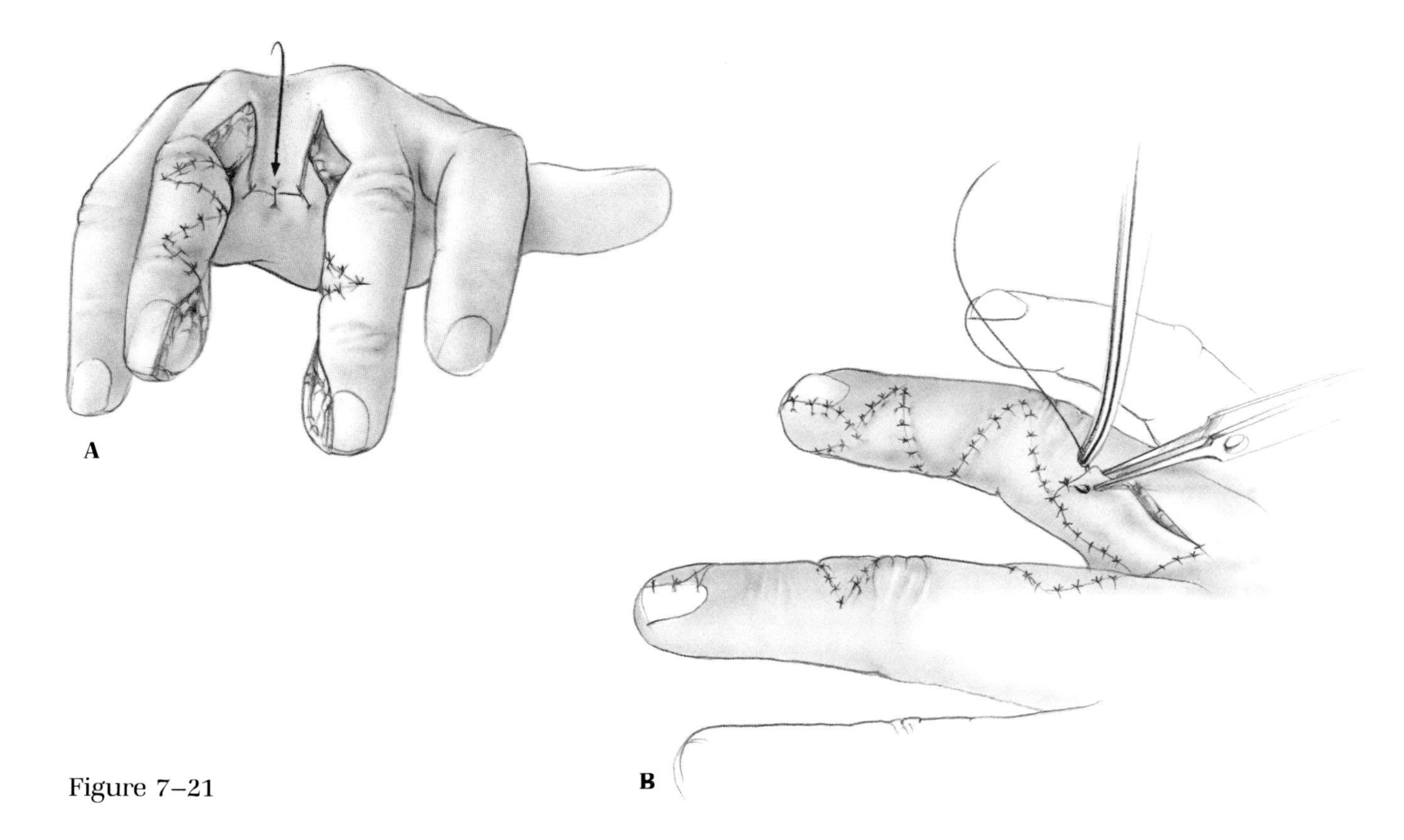

Figure 7–21

7.6 Release of Congenital Trigger Thumb

Congenital trigger thumb is usually noted by the parent sometime after birth. In some cases it may be possible to extend the thumb, in which case a trial of nonoperative treatment is indicated.[1] A course of observation is usually indicated in most circumstances because about 40% of the cases will resolve, and full motion will result after surgery if it is performed in the first 3 years of life.

Figure 7–22. Although this release can be done through a simple transverse incision, an ulnar-based zigzag incision over the flexor crease of the metacarpophalangeal joint will give better exposure. The incision is perhaps the most difficult part of the operation for the radial digital nerve crosses the midline at exactly this point, and because it lies just beneath the skin it can easily be divided while making the skin incision.

Figure 7–23. After the dermis is divided a small, sharp scissors or hemostat is used to disect out the radial digital nerve.

Figure 7–24. Once it is safely retracted out of the way, the A-1 pully is incised. It is usually not necessary to excise a portion of this pully nor to shave the nodule, which will disappear following the release.

Figure 7–25. The thumb is extended fully to be certain that the release is complete. The release should not be extended too far distal so as to avoid bow stringing of the flexor pollicis longus tendon. Only the skin is closed.

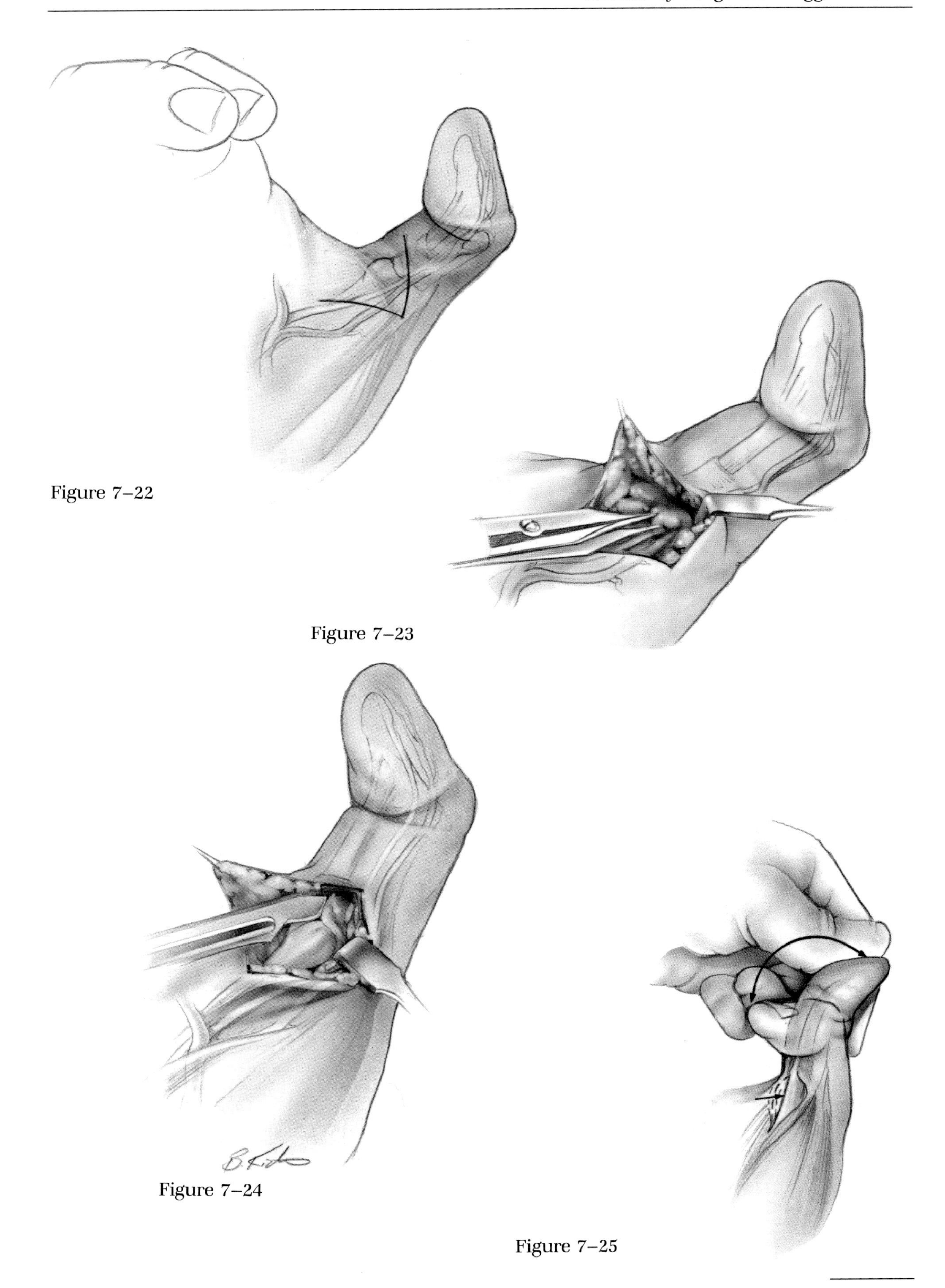

Figure 7–22

Figure 7–23

Figure 7–24

Figure 7–25

POSTOPERATIVE CARE

The thumb is placed in a light (child-proof) dressing for 1 week and then removed to allow return to the usual activities. No further treatment is required.

REFERENCE

1. Bayne LG, Costas BL. Malformations of the upper extremity. In: Morrissy RT, ed. Lovell and Winter's Pediatric Orthopaedics, 3rd ed. Philadelphia: JB Lippincott, 1990:583.

7.7
Excision of Duplicate Thumb

Duplication of the thumb or preaxial polydactyly is not very common. Because polydactyly is the commonest congenital anomaly of the hand, however, most orthopaedic surgeons will encounter this anomaly. The treatment of this condition may hold a trap for the physician who is unaware of the unique anatomy of this condition. Because of the anatomic reasons discussed subsequently, simple excision of the smaller thumb will rarely produce a satisfactory result.[1]

The selection of which digit to remove may be difficult if both are of near the same size and function. Both function and cosmesis should be considered. In general the radial digit will be the smaller and will be removed. This confers the advantage of leaving the ulnar collateral ligament intact for stability during pinch. Despite the fact that both thumbs will have their own flexor and extensor motors, however, the thenar musculature will attach to the radial-most digit. It is therefore necessary that these attachments be preserved and reattached to the remaining digit. If the ulnar digit is removed, it is necessary that a periosteal and ligamentous flap from the radial border of this digit be preserved to reconstruct an ulnar-collateral ligament for the remaining digit.

The wide variety of anomalies encountered under the term *duplicate thumb* makes careful assessment and planning imperative. Wassel[2] has classified these anomalies into seven types, whereas Marks and Bayne[3] have devised a simpler classification based on the level of duplication. These authors and others have discussed the principles involved as well as the results.[4,5]

The surgeon must plan an incision that will not leave a linear scar that will later contract, correct all rotational and angular deformity in the retained digit, carefully plan a reconstruction of the joint that will impart lasting stability, centralize the flexor and extensor tendons, and plan to keep the attachments of the thenar muscles on the retained digit.

These principles are illustrated on the commonest type of thumb duplication: a Wassel type IV, or a Marks and Baynes type I in which there is complete duplication of the proximal phalanx.

Figure 7–26. The incision is planned in such a way as to avoid a straight scar. The incision illustrated has committed the surgeon to removal of the radial thumb. This incision will permit exposure of all of the structures to both thumbs.

If the surgeon is uncertain at the beginning of the case as to which thumb is to be retained, a different incision should be planned. This might occur if both digits were small, or there was a question of the blood supply to the digit that might be retained.

Figure 7–27. After the flaps are developed, the neurovascular bundles are identified and traced to their respective digits. This is to be certain they are protected, and that the digit to be retained is innervated and vascularized. At this point the thenar muscles are detached from the base of the radial digit. These will attach to the radial side of the radial digit by a fairly broad tendon. Sufficient tendon and, if necessary, periosteum should be retained with the muscles to provide strong attachment to the retained digit.

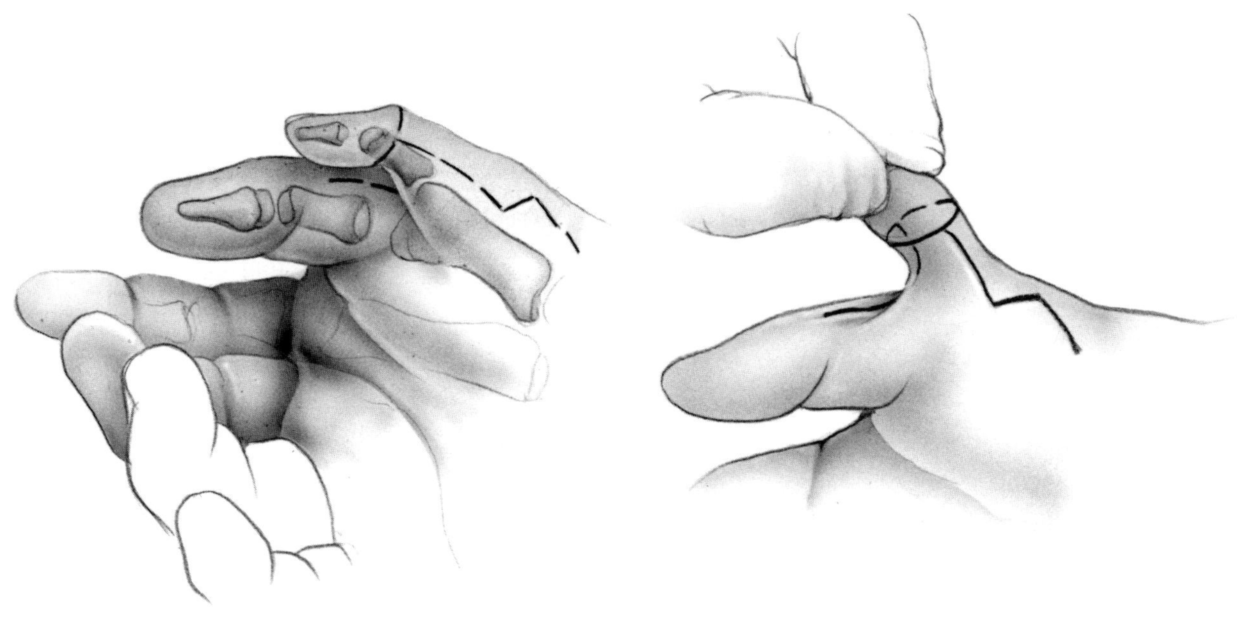

Figure 7–26

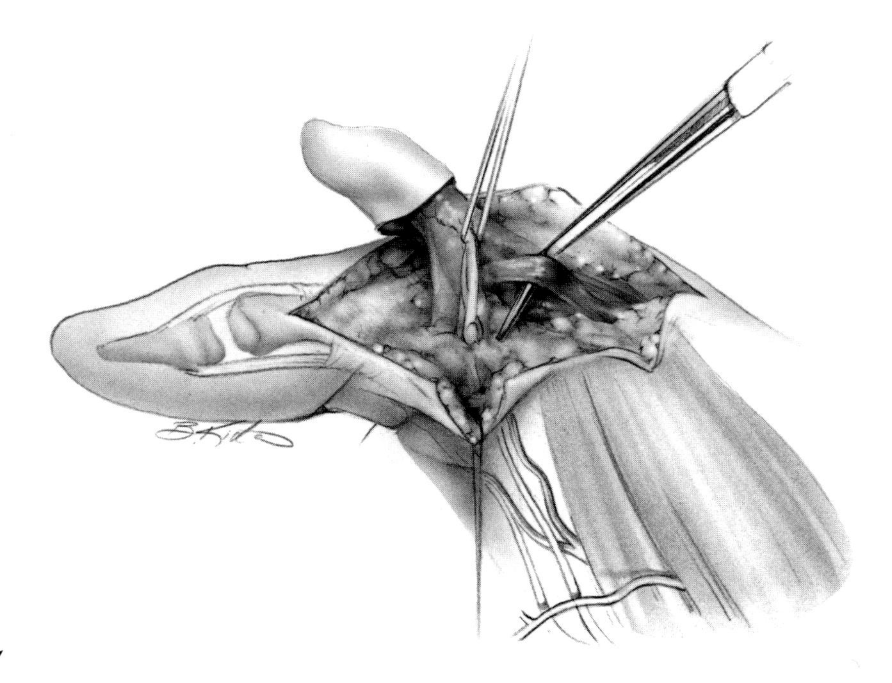

Figure 7–27

Figure 7–28. With the thenar muscles detached and retracted out of the way, a flap of periosteum and ligament from the radial digit is raised. This flap is then dissected proximally off of the metacarpal (***Figure 7–28A***). This will be sutured into the radial side of the retained digit to reconstruct the radial collateral ligament. This is very important because ulnar deviation is one of the commonest complications following this procedure.

The radial digit is now removed, and the remaining ulnar digit subluxated to demonstrate the condyle of the metacarpophalangeal joint (***Figure 7–28***). This condyle is broader than normal and must be narrowed to provide good cosmesis as well as good stability for the retained digit. There is usually a small ridge that will identify that portion of the condyle on which each of the thumbs articulated. In addition there is frequently an ulnar deviation of the metacarpal head. In keeping with the principles outlined, it is necessary to correct this deviation at this time.

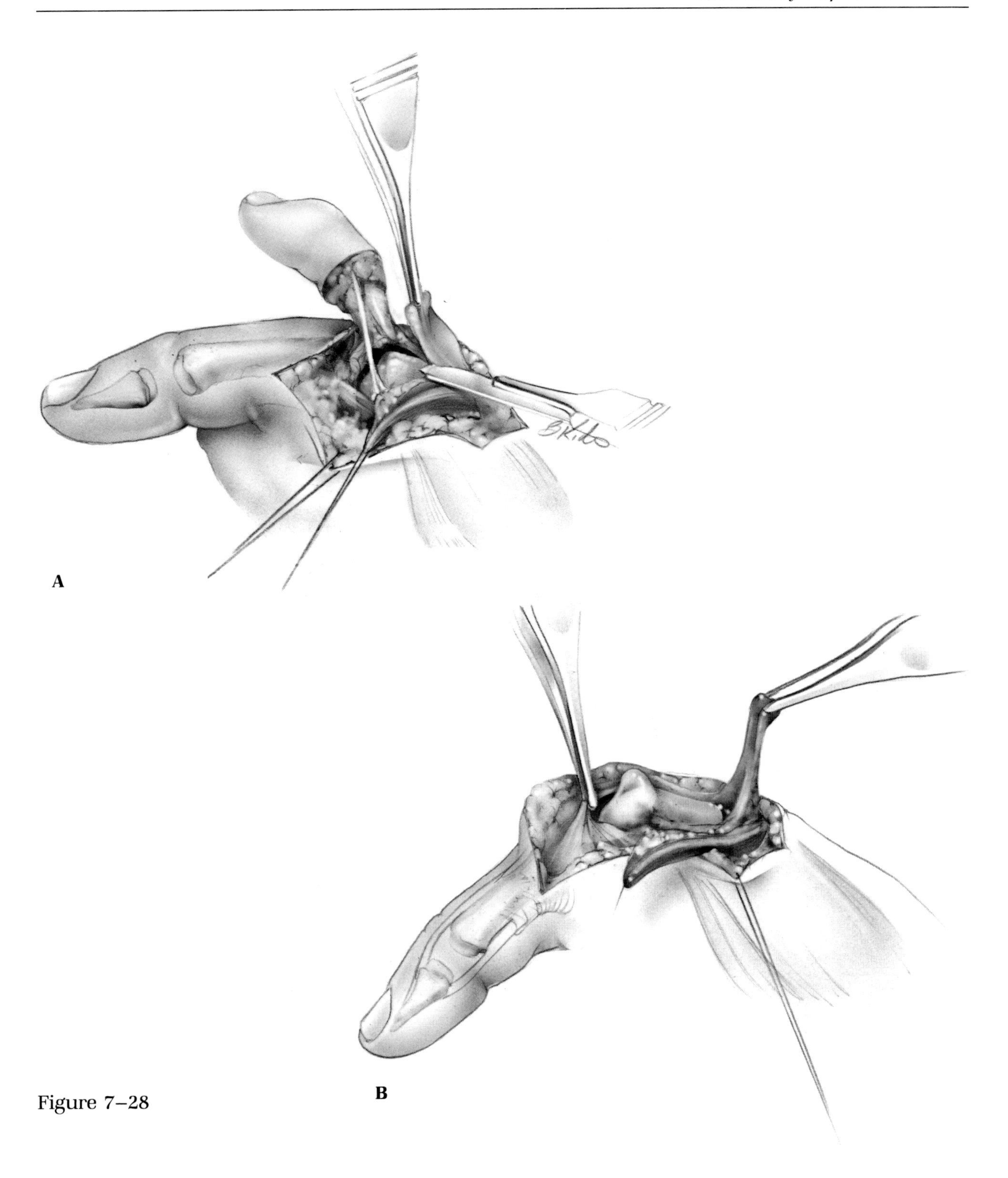

Figure 7–28

Figure 7–29. The excess radial portion of the condyle is removed with a small osteotome. A small closing wedge osteotomy is made just behind the condyle of the metacarpal. This is designed to correct the ulnar deviation. Any rotational malalignment can also be corrected. This osteotomy can usually be fixed with one small Kirschner wire passed from the tip of the distal phalanx.

Figure 7–30. When the osteotomy is fixed, the periosteal and ligamentous flap that was raised from the discarded digit and radial side of the metacarpal is sutured to the radial side of the retained digit. Care should be taken in adjusting the tension of this repair. Subsequently, the thenar muscles are sutured over this to the base of the retained digit.

Figure 7–31. The skin is closed. There is no problem with a shortage of skin but often some excess. This can be trimmed. The resulting suture line should not be linear. A rigid dressing and long arm cast are applied.

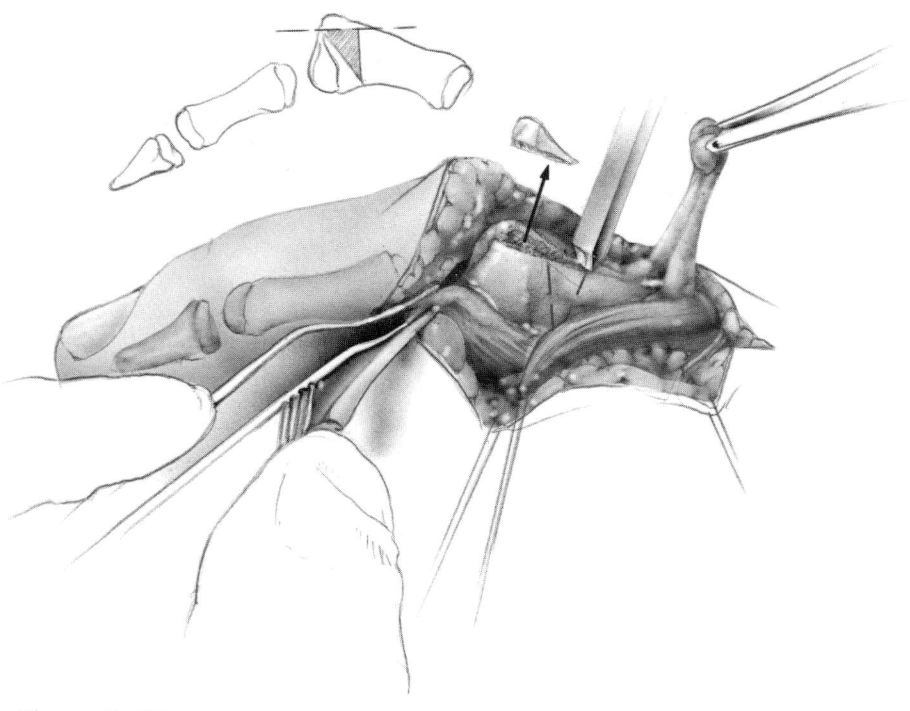

Figure 7–29

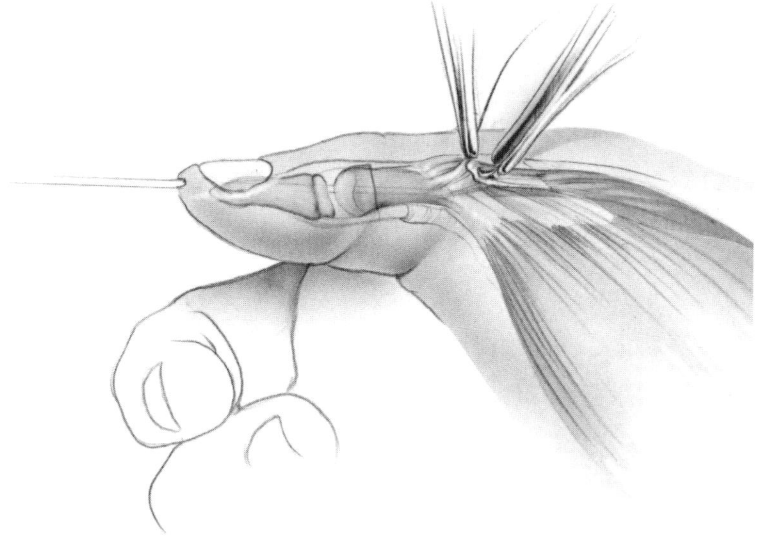

Figure 7–30

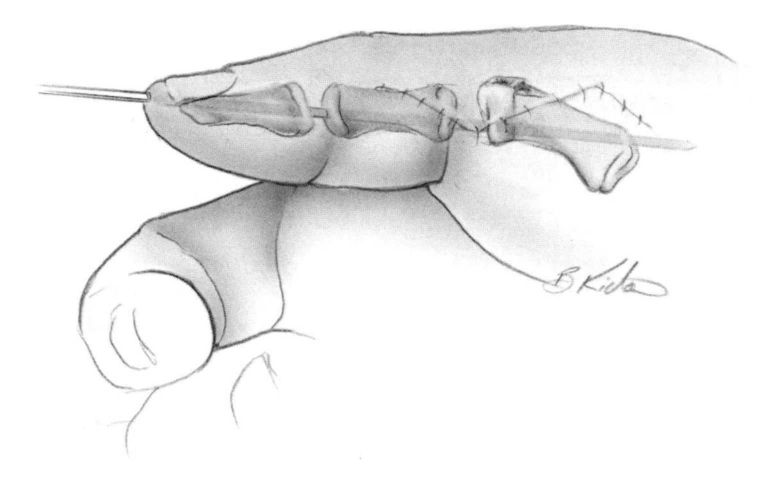

Figure 7–31

POSTOPERATIVE CARE

The cast is removed at 6 weeks, and a splint is fabricated to protect the repair of the radial collateral ligament. The splint is worn full time for the first month while motion is started. Following this the splint is continued at night for 6 months.

REFERENCES

1. Dobyns JH, Lipscomb PR, Cooney WP. Management of thumb duplication. Clin Orthop 1985;195:26.
2. Wassel HD. The results of surgery for polydactyly of the thumb: a review. Clin Orthop 1969;64:175.
3. Marks TW, Bayne LG. Polydactyly of the thumb: abnormal anatomy and treatment. J Hand Surg 1978;3:107.
4. Tada K et al. Duplication of the thumb. J Bone Joint Surg 1983;65A:584.
5. Cheng JCY, Chan KM, Ma GFY, Leung PC. Polydactyly of the thumb: a surgical plan based on ninety-five cases. J Hand Surg 1984;9A:155.

7.8
Transfer of Flexor Carpi Ulnaris for Wrist Flexion Deformity

Wrist flexion deformity is a frequent problem in children with cerebral palsy. There are two aspects to the problem. The first and the one discussed most often in relation to correction of the deformity is function. The wrist is often held in flexion, pronation, and ulnar deviation with inability to dorsiflex the wrist or release a grasp. The second problem is cosmetic. This is rarely considered by most authors on the subject to be a worthwhile goal of surgery. For many patients, especially those with hemiparesis who are attending regular schools, this can be a very important consideration.

The criteria for obtaining a good result with this operation were briefly mentioned in the follow-up article of the original patients.[1] Tachdjian lists eight prerequisites for this procedure. They are mentioned here as factors to be considered, some more strongly than others, rather than as absolute prerequisites.

- The flexor carpi ulnaris should have good motor power.
- There should be good passive dorsiflexion of the wrist, extension of the fingers, and supination of the forearm.
- The patient should be able to extend the fingers actively with the wrist held in neutral.
- The patient should have good voluntary control over placement of the arm.
- There should be adequate sensory function in the hand.
- The patient should have reasonable intellect.
- The patient should be old enough to comply with the postoperative therapy program.
- No movement disorder, eg, athetosis should be present.

Hoffer et al[2] studied spastic patients with dynamic electromyography and noted that the flexor carpi ulnaris co-contracted with the finger extensors. Because release is often more of a problem than grasp, they suggested transferring the flexor carpi ulnaris into the extensor digitorum communis to improve both release of grasp and wrist extension. In a subsequent report Hoffer et al[3] demonstrated the effectiveness of this in carefully selected patients and described the indications. Besides failure to achieve the desired functional goals, the commonest complication of this procedure is a wrist extension contracture. Hoffer et al[3] claim that transferring the flexor carpi ulnaris into the extensor digitorum communis obviates this problem.

Figure 7–32. Although the procedure is usually done with the patient in the supine position, the prone position may facilitate exposure in the occasional patient with an internal rotation contracture of the shoulder coupled with a pronation contracture of the forearm.

The procedure begins by detaching the flexor carpi ulnaris tendon and freeing up the muscle belly from its extensive origin along the ulna. Although initially being described as done through two separate incisions, it makes more sense to make one incision because most of the dissection is done in the distal aspect of the forearm. The incision starts distal at the flexor crease of the wrist and directly over the flexor carpi ulnaris tendon where it inserts into the pisiform bone. It extends about midway up the forearm. A right-angled retractor can be used to elevate the skin at the proximal extent of the wound, allowing dissection as far proximal as the junction of the middle and distal one third of the forearm. The fascia over the tendon and the lateral aspect of the muscle are divided. The ulnar nerve will lie directly under the tendon, so caution must be used in freeing it from the pisiform bone.

Once the tendon is divided, the muscle fibers along the lateral aspect of the muscle originating from the ulna are easily identified. These fibers must be freed by dissecting them off the periosteum of the ulna. The flexor carpi ulnaris receives its nerve supply from the underlying ulnar nerve. As the dissection proceeds proximally, it is important to identify and protect these branches. This dissection will need to extend proximally at least to the upper one third of the forearm—far enough to allow the muscle belly to be directed around the medial border of the ulna in a straight line.

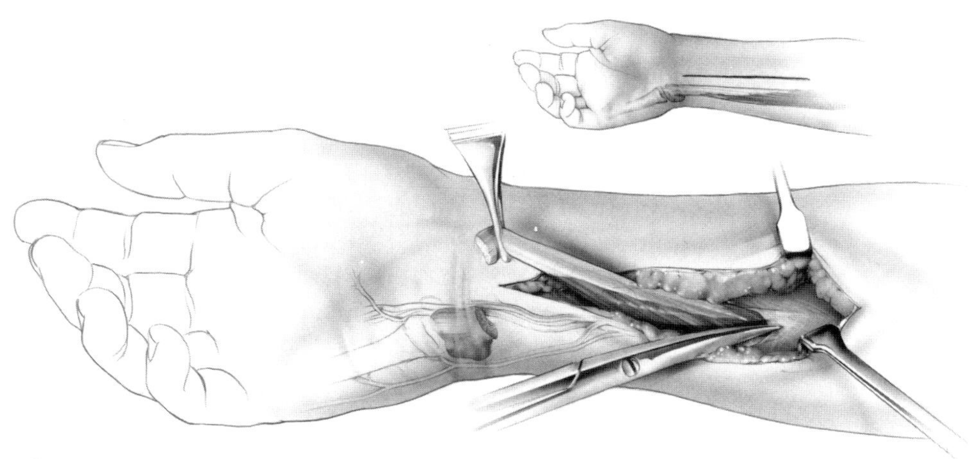

Figure 7–32

Figure 7–33. The second incision is made directly over the extensor carpi radialis and brevis tendons starting at the extensor crease of the wrist and extending proximally for 3 to 4 cm. After incising the fascia the two tendons can be identified: the most radial is the extensor carpi radialis longus, and the more ulnar is the brevis. Inserting the transfer into the extensor carpi radialis longus gives a better supination force and is more effective at overcoming ulnar deviation, whereas inserting the transfer into the brevis will give a more central pull. A subcutaneous tunnel is dissected from the proximal extent of the volar incision around the subcutaneous medial border of the ulna. A tendon forceps is used to bring the flexor carpi ulnaris around the medial aspect of the ulna through the subcutaneous tunnel and into the second incision on the dorsal aspect of the wrist. After the surgeon assures himself or herself that a sufficient portion of the intermuscular septum has been excised and that the tendon is running along a relatively straight path, the first incision is closed.

Figure 7–34. The flexor carpi ulnaris is then sutured into the desired tendon. As this is done the wrist is held in approximately 45 degrees of extension, and the forearm is held in maximum supination. After the tendon anastomosis is complete, the wrist should passively flex at least 15 degrees past neutral with the fingers simultaneously going into extension.

The second wound is closed, and the patient is placed in a long arm cast with the wrist in slightly less than maximum dorsiflexion and the forearm in full supination. Because the underlying pathology is spasticity, the thumb should be incorporated in the cast in a position of abduction, and the metacarpal joints should be flexed about 15 degrees while the interphalangeal joints are in neutral.

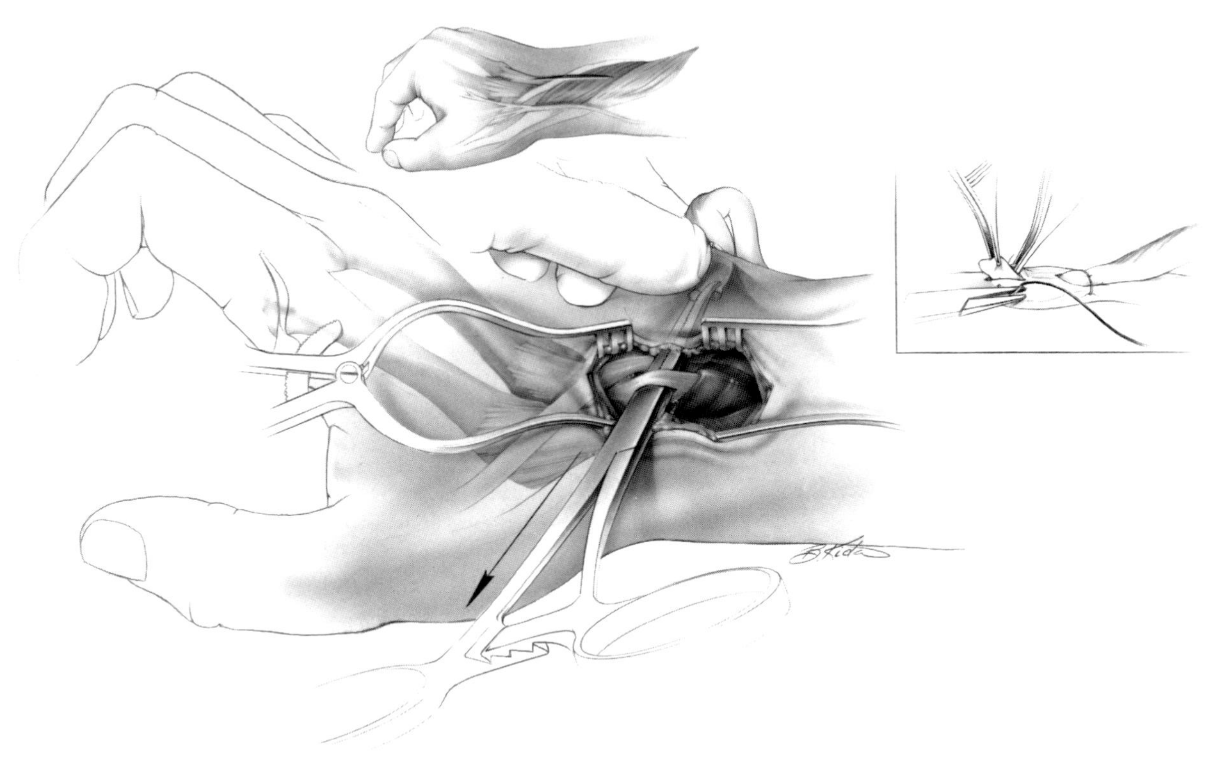

Figure 7–33

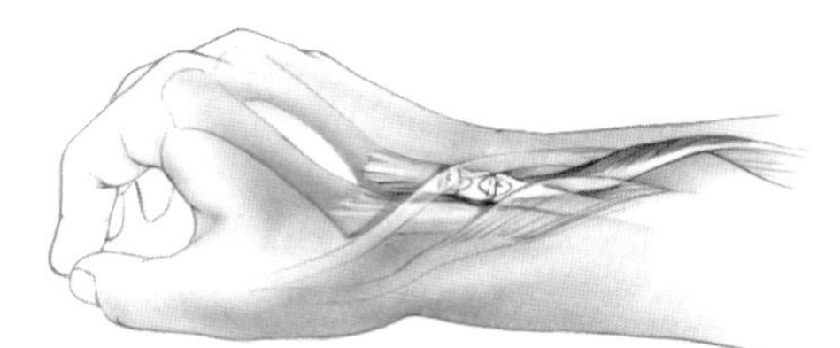

Figure 7–34

POSTOPERATIVE CARE

The cast is removed in 4 weeks. A removable splint is fitted, which allows the wrist to be removed for therapy. Retraining of wrist extension, grasp, and release is begun at this time. Splinting of the wrist in extension is continued for up to 6 months.

REFERENCES

1. Green WT, Banks HH. Flexor carpi ulnaris transplant and its use in cerebral palsy. J Bone Joint Surg 1962;44A:1343.
2. Hoffer MM, Perry J, Melkonian GJ. Dynamic electromyography and decision-making for surgery in the upper extremity of patients with cerebral palsy. J Hand Surg 1979;4:424.
3. Hoffer MM, Lehman M, Mitani M. Long-term follow-up on tendon transfers to the extensors of the wrist and fingers in patients with cerebral palsy. J Hand Surg 1986;11:836.

7.9 Correction of Thumb-in-Palm Deformity in Cerebral Palsy

Children with cerebral palsy frequently have difficulty with hand function, and often most noticeable is the thumb deformity. The indications for correction of such deformities have been discussed in detail by several authors.[1–3] Most authors have stressed the importance of the preoperative evaluation in the outcome with assessment of voluntary control, sensation, cognition, and the ability to cooperate with a postoperative program being the most important factors.

House et al[2] have classified the various deformities by an assessment of the function of the thumb rather than its static position.

Type I: Metacarpal adduction contracture. This is the commonest deformity and is usually associated with a contracture of the first thumb web space. It is caused by spasticity and contracture of the adductor pollicis and first dorsal interosseous muscles.

Type II: Metacarpal adduction contracture and metacarpophalangeal flexion deformity. In this deformity the interphalangeal joint remains mobile while the metacarpophalangeal joint is fixed in flexion by contracture of the flexor pollicis longus.

Type III: Metacarpal adduction contracture combined with a metacarpophalangeal hyperextension deformity or instability. This deformity is caused by spasticity of the extensor pollicis longus in the absence of spasticity in the flexor pollicis longus.

Type IV: Metacarpal adduction contracture combined with metacarpophalangeal and interphalangeal flexion deformities. This is usually caused by spasticity of the flexor pollicis longus and the intrinsic muscles of the thumb, but may be caused by isolated spasticity of the flexor pollicis longus.

The various steps that are taken in the correction of the various deformities may be considered in three categories: release of the skin and muscle contractures, augmentation of the weak muscles, and stabilization of joints.

Figure 7–35. The release of the contracted first thumb web space is achieved by Z-plasty incision through which both the tight dorsal fascia and the muscles causing the contracture in the first place, the adductor pollicis longus and the first dorsal interosseous muscles, can be divided. The incision is a "four-flap Z-plasty." This Z-plasty has been variously described using angles of 120 degrees and 60 degrees, or as illustrated here 90 degrees and 45 degrees. It is important that each limb of the incision be of equal length. The first limb of the incision is made along the line of the maximum contracture. At each end of this incision and at 90 degrees to it another incision is made (***Figure 7–35A***). This limb should be equal in length to one-half of the length of the longitudinal limb. Finally, a third limb is added to each end of the incision, which bisects the right angle made by the first two limbs. This should be equal in length to the second limb. The incision is closed by transposing the flaps (***Figure 7–35B***).

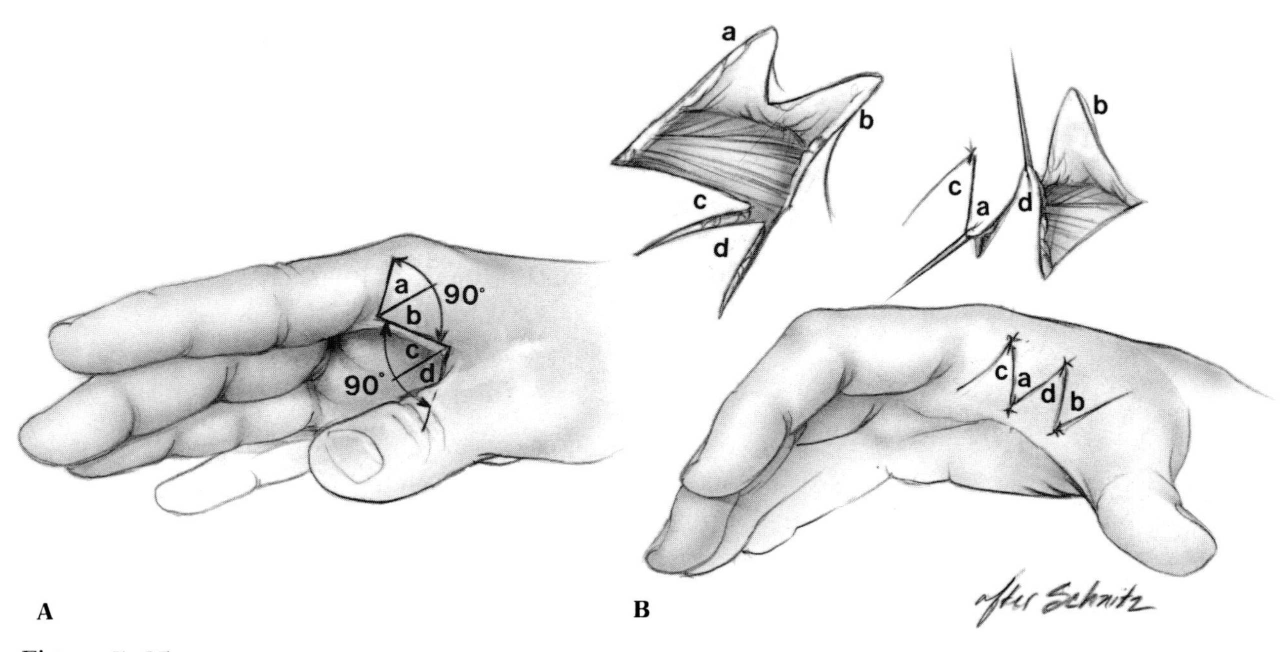

Figure 7–35

Figure 7–36. Once the flaps of the incision are developed and retracted and the dorsal fascia is divided, the tight adductor pollicis and the first dorsal interosseous muscle are easily identified (***Figure 7–36A***). The origin of the first dorsal interosseous muscle that arises from two heads, one on the first metacarpal and one on the second metacarpal, is released first. Care must be taken as the radial artery passes between these two heads to form the deep palmar arch. The portion inserting on the first metacarpal is released first. It will usually be necessary to release at least a portion of the head originating on the second metacarpal also because the two heads join together close to their origin (***Figure 7–36B***).

Following this the adductor pollicis muscle is released by partially dividing it in its intramuscular portion. This muscle can be found running obliquely beneath the first dorsal interosseous muscle. Its division is more easily accomplished, however, from the palmar aspect of the wound (***Figure 7–36C***). If this does not provide sufficient abduction, it will be necessary to release it from its origin on the third metacarpal as described subsequently.

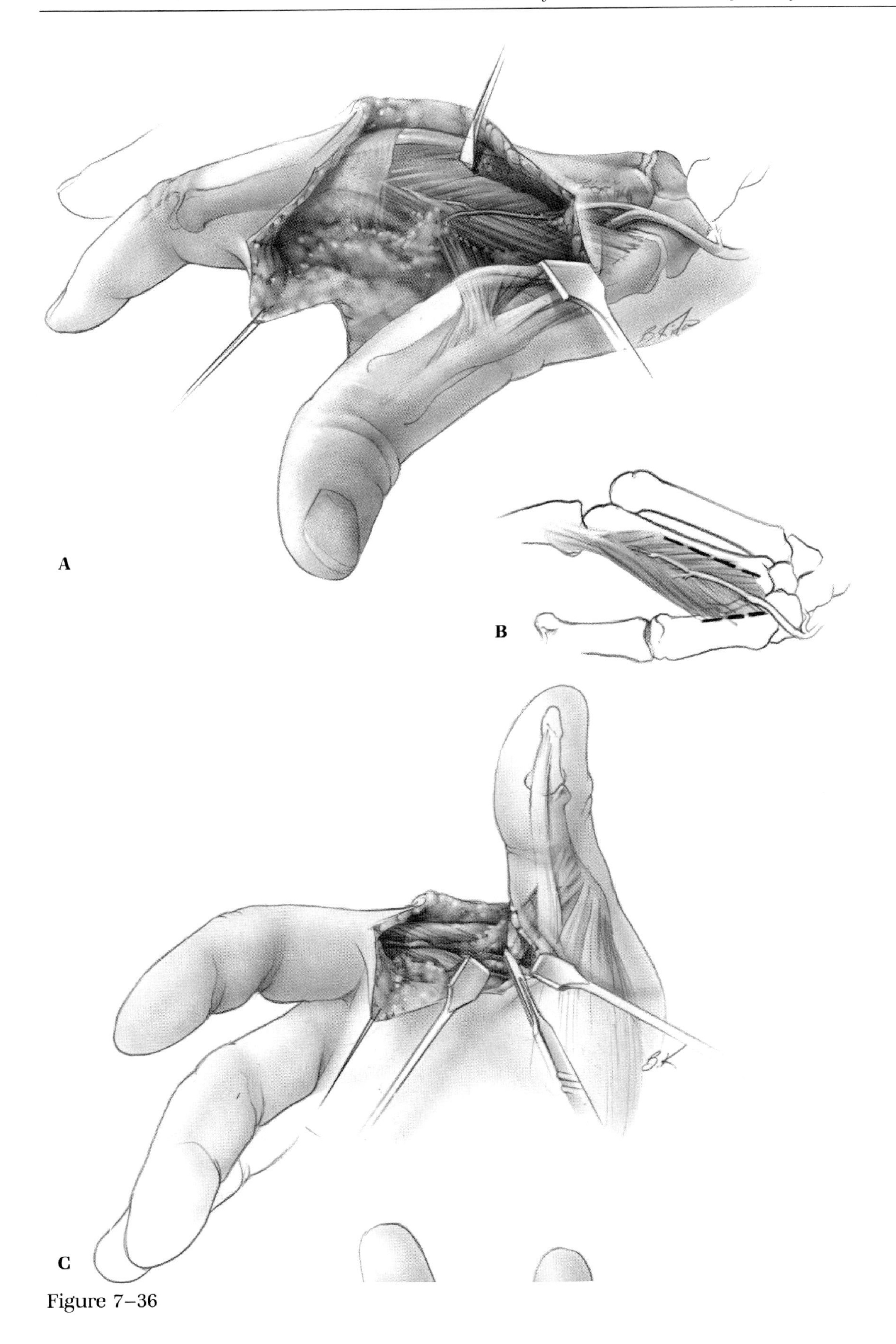

Figure 7–36

Figure 7–37. In the severer type II deformities, it is usually necessary to release the origin of the adductor pollicis muscle from the third metacarpal and the origin of the flexor pollicis brevis from the flexor retinaculum. If necessary, a portion of the abductor pollicis brevis can also be released. This procedure was described by Matev.[4]

A palmar incision following the crease of the thenar eminence is used. The proximal portion of this incision will come to lie over the third metacarpal (***Figure 7–37A***). After the skin and fascia are divided, the flexor tendons of the middle finger are retracted ulnarward, whereas the neurovascular bundle and superficial palmar that arch along with the flexor tendons of the index finger are retracted radialward (***Figure 7–37B***). This will expose (from distal to proximal) the transverse head of the adductor pollicis, the oblique head of the adductor pollicis, the flexor pollicis brevis, and the abductor pollicis brevis overlying the opponens pollicis muscle. The adductor pollicis muscle is stripped off of the third metacarpal while the origin of the flexor pollicis brevis is detached from the flexor retinaculum (transverse carpal ligament) (***Figure 7–37C***).

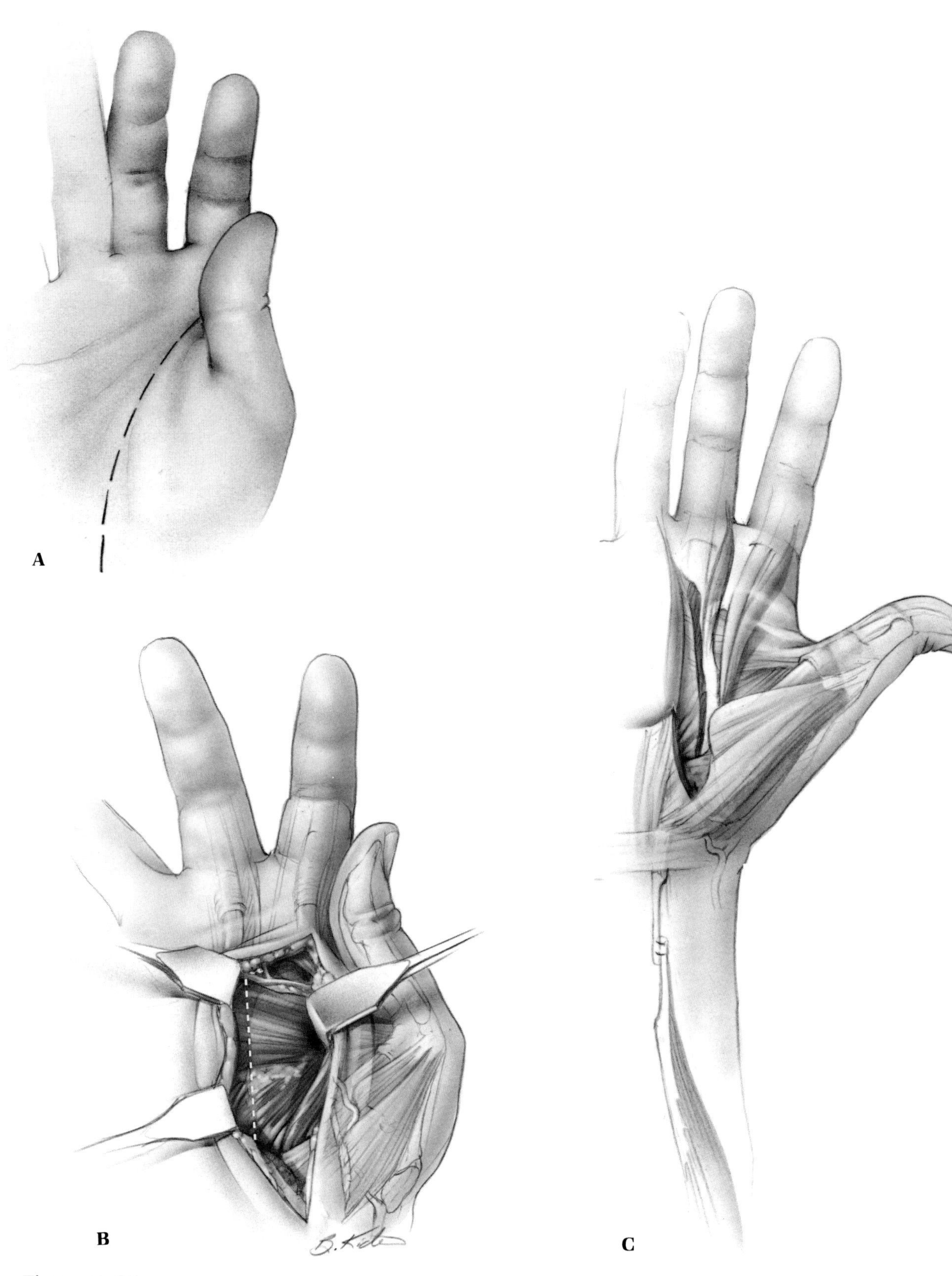

Figure 7–37

Figure 7–38. In type III deformities it may be necessary to stabilize the thumb metacarpophalangeal joint. This may be done by arthrodesis. In the growing child this can be accomplished by denuding the cartilage from the joint surface and fixing the joint with an intramedullary pin. This will spare the growth of the physis.

Another method that preserves more of the function of the thumb, however, is described by Filler, Stark, and Boyes.[5] Through a V-shaped incision over the volar aspect of the metacarpophalangeal joint as described for release of trigger thumb, the sheath of the flexor pollicis longus is partially excised to expose the tendon. As with release of trigger thumb, it is important to identify and retract the neurovascular bundles carefully, particularly the radial digital nerve that lies just beneath the skin and crosses the operative site. This will expose the volar plate or capsule. Its proximal insertion is incised and freed (***Figure 7–38A***). Then both sides are incised just outside of the sesamoid bones so that only the distal attachment remains. The joint is flexed 30 to 35 degrees and transfixed with a small Kirschner wire. The capsule is advanced proximally until it is taut. At this new point of insertion a small groove is cut into the cortical bone, and a small drill hole is made from this groove to the dorsal surface of the metacarpal. A pull-out wire or strong, absorbable suture is passed through this hole and tied over a button on the dorsum of the thumb to secure the insertion of the volar plate into this groove (***Figure 7–38B***).

In the type IV deformity it will be necessary to lengthen the flexor pollicis longus. A Z-lengthening is easily accomplished proximal to the wrist.

There are numerous motors that can be used to augment the abductor pollicis longus, extensor pollicis brevis, or extensor pollicis longus as may be necessary. The palmaris longus, brachioradialis, and flexor carpi radialis muscles are some of the more commonly used.

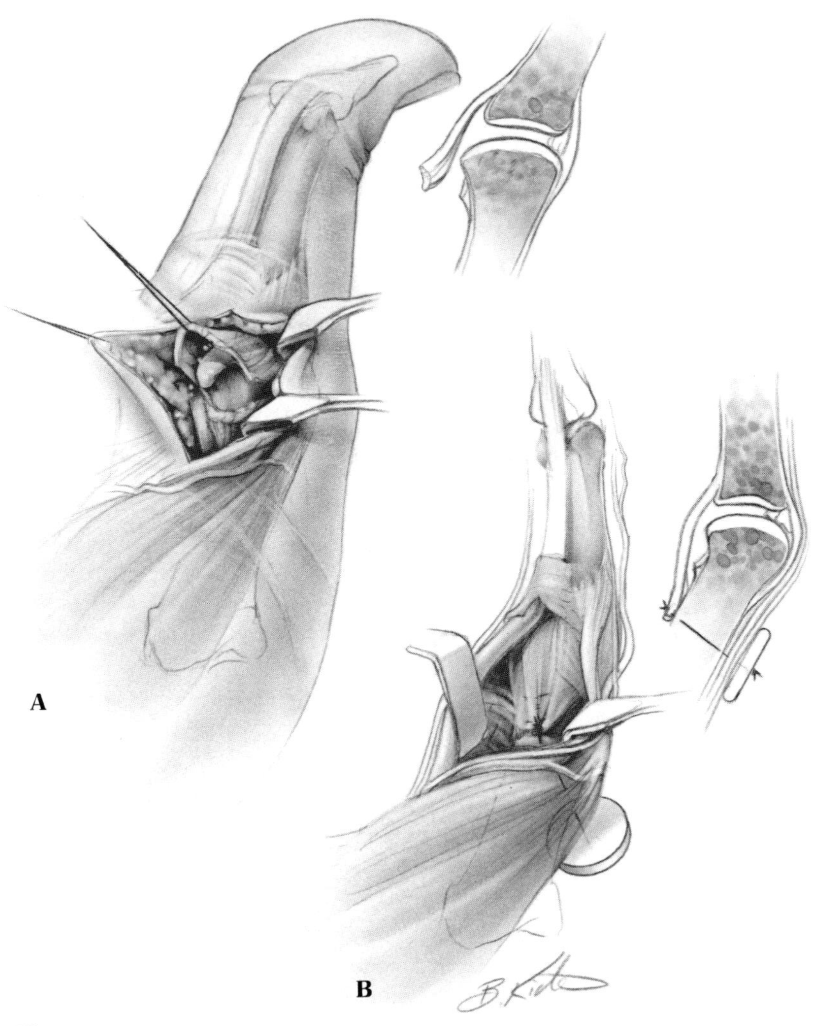

Figure 7–38

POSTOPERATIVE CARE

Patients who have had only release or lengthening of contracted muscles are immobilized in a plaster splint or cast with the thumb in abduction and extension for 4 weeks. If arthrodesis or capsulodesis has been performed, immobilization may need to be continued for as long as 8 weeks. After immobilization is discontinued, the patient is started on a therapy program to mobilize and improve the function of the thumb as well as the fingers and wrist. An abduction splint is used continuously except during therapy for the next 6 to 12 weeks and then at nighttime only until dynamic balance has been achieved.

REFERENCES

1. Goldner JL. Reconstructive surgery of the hand in cerebral palsy and spastic paralysis resulting from injury to the spinal cord. J Bone Joint Surg 1955;37A:1141.
2. House JH, Gwathmey FW, Fidler MO. A dynamic approach to the thumb-in-palm deformity in cerebral palsy: evaluation and results in fifty-six patients. J Bone Joint Surg 1981;63A:216.
3. Rang M. Cerebral palsy. In: Morrissy RT, ed. Lovell and Winter's Pediatric Orthopaedics, 3rd ed. Philadelphia: JB Lippincott, 1990:495.
4. Matev IB. Surgical treatment of flexion-adduction contracture of the thumb in cerebral palsy. Acta Orthop Scand 1970;41:439.
5. Filler BC, Stark HH, Boyes JH. Capsulodesis on the metacarpophalangeal joint of the thumb in children with cerebral palsy. J Bone Joint Surg 1976;58A:667.

Index

Page numbers followed by *f* indicate figures; those followed by *t* indicate tabular material.

H

P

S

ISBN 0-397-50969-3